Functional Nanomaterials in Biomedicine

Functional Nanomaterials in Biomedicine

Editors

Wansong Chen
Jianhua Zhang

MDPI • Basel • Beijing • Wuhan • Barcelona • Belgrade • Manchester • Tokyo • Cluj • Tianjin

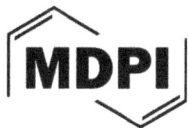

Editors
Wansong Chen
Chemistry and Chemical
Engineering
Central South University
Changsha
China

Jianhua Zhang
Chemical Engineering
Tianjin University
Tianjin
China

Editorial Office
MDPI
St. Alban-Anlage 66
4052 Basel, Switzerland

This is a reprint of articles from the Special Issue published online in the open access journal *Molecules* (ISSN 1420-3049) (available at: www.mdpi.com/journal/molecules/special_issues/nanomater_biomed).

For citation purposes, cite each article independently as indicated on the article page online and as indicated below:

LastName, A.A.; LastName, B.B.; LastName, C.C. Article Title. *Journal Name* **Year**, *Volume Number*, Page Range.

ISBN 978-3-0365-6020-5 (Hbk)
ISBN 978-3-0365-6019-9 (PDF)

© 2022 by the authors. Articles in this book are Open Access and distributed under the Creative Commons Attribution (CC BY) license, which allows users to download, copy and build upon published articles, as long as the author and publisher are properly credited, which ensures maximum dissemination and a wider impact of our publications.

The book as a whole is distributed by MDPI under the terms and conditions of the Creative Commons license CC BY-NC-ND.

Contents

Wansong Chen, Keyin Liu and Jianhua Zhang
Functional Nanomaterials: From Structures to Biomedical Applications
Reprinted from: *Molecules* **2022**, *27*, 7492, doi:10.3390/molecules27217492 1

Ganesh Gollavelli, Anil V. Ghule and Yong-Chien Ling
Multimodal Imaging and Phototherapy of Cancer and Bacterial Infection by Graphene and Related Nanocomposites
Reprinted from: *Molecules* **2022**, *27*, 5588, doi:10.3390/molecules27175588 5

Haojun Li, Meng Xu, Rui Shi, Aiying Zhang and Jiatao Zhang
Advances in Electrostatic Spinning of Polymer Fibers Functionalized with Metal-Based Nanocrystals and Biomedical Applications
Reprinted from: *Molecules* **2022**, *27*, 5548, doi:10.3390/molecules27175548 39

Haihan Song, Mengli Zhang and Weijun Tong
Single-Atom Nanozymes: Fabrication, Characterization, Surface Modification and Applications of ROS Scavenging and Antibacterial
Reprinted from: *Molecules* **2022**, *27*, 5426, doi:10.3390/molecules27175426 57

Bassam Felipe Mogharbel, Marco André Cardoso, Ana Carolina Irioda, Priscila Elias Ferreira Stricker, Robson Camilotti Slompo and Julia Maurer Appel et al.
Biodegradable Nanoparticles Loaded with Levodopa and Curcumin for Treatment of Parkinson's Disease
Reprinted from: *Molecules* **2022**, *27*, 2811, doi:10.3390/molecules27092811 79

Aleksandra Sentkowska and Krystyna Pyrzyńska
The Influence of Synthesis Conditions on the Antioxidant Activity of Selenium Nanoparticles
Reprinted from: *Molecules* **2022**, *27*, 2486, doi:10.3390/molecules27082486 103

Yunxiao Feng, Gang Liu, Ming La and Lin Liu
Colorimetric and Electrochemical Methods for the Detection of SARS-CoV-2 Main Protease by Peptide-Triggered Assembly of Gold Nanoparticles
Reprinted from: *Molecules* **2022**, *27*, 615, doi:10.3390/molecules27030615 117

Peng Zhang, Xinyu Ma, Ruiwei Guo, Zhanpeng Ye, Han Fu and Naikuan Fu et al.
Organic Nanoplatforms for Iodinated Contrast Media in CT Imaging
Reprinted from: *Molecules* **2021**, *26*, 7063, doi:10.3390/molecules26237063 127

Yaliang Huang, Yong Chang, Lin Liu and Jianxiu Wang
Nanomaterials for Modulating the Aggregation of β-Amyloid Peptides
Reprinted from: *Molecules* **2021**, *26*, 4301, doi:10.3390/molecules26144301 159

Yangmun Bae, Yoonyoung Kim and Eun Seong Lee
Endosomal pH-Responsive Fe-Based Hyaluronate Nanoparticles for Doxorubicin Delivery
Reprinted from: *Molecules* **2021**, *26*, 3547, doi:10.3390/molecules26123547 191

Chaojie Zhu, Junkai Ma, Zhiheng Ji, Jie Shen and Qiwen Wang
Recent Advances of Cell Membrane Coated Nanoparticles in Treating Cardiovascular Disorders
Reprinted from: *Molecules* **2021**, *26*, 3428, doi:10.3390/molecules26113428 203

Yanting Sun, Yuling Li, Shuo Shi and Chunyan Dong
Exploiting a New Approach to Destroy the Barrier of Tumor Microenvironment: Nano-Architecture Delivery Systems
Reprinted from: *Molecules* **2021**, *26*, 2703, doi:10.3390/molecules26092703 223

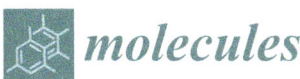

Editorial

Functional Nanomaterials: From Structures to Biomedical Applications

Wansong Chen [1,2,*], Keyin Liu [1] and Jianhua Zhang [3,*]

1. State Key Laboratory of Biobased Material and Green Papermaking, Qilu University of Technology, Shandong Academy of Sciences, Jinan 250316, China
2. College of Chemistry and Chemical Engineering, Central South University, Changsha 410017, China
3. Department of Polymer Science and Engineering, School of Chemical Engineering and Technology, Tianjin University, Tianjin 300072, China
* Correspondence: chenws@csu.edu.cn (W.C.); jhuazhang@tju.edu.cn (J.Z.)

In recent decades, a number of functional nanomaterials have attracted a great amount of attention and exhibited excellent performance for biomedical and pharmaceutical applications. Functional nanomaterials usually display unique physicochemical properties, nano-sized characteristics, controlled shape and versatile modification possibilities as well as well-defined multifunctionalities. A wide variety of nanomaterials, such as liposomes, polymer-based nanoparticles (NPs), carbon-based NPs, silica-based NPs, metal and metal–oxide NPs (e.g., Au, Ag and iron oxides), covalent organic frameworks and metal–organic frameworks NPs, have been developed and employed for the treatment of various diseases. These functional nanomaterials offer unprecedented opportunities for the site-specific and controllable delivery of drugs, genes, proteins and other bioactive agents. Moreover, functional nanomaterials with unique photoelectric properties can be used for photoacoustic, photothermal or photodynamic as well as hyperthermal therapy. In addition, some functional NPs can find applications for a new generation of intelligent biosensing, bioseparation, bioimaging, cell labeling and diagnosis methods as well as for monitoring cells and tissues.

Despite these tremendous advantages and great advances, clinical applications of nanomaterials as therapeutic, imaging and diagnostic agents still remain limited. For example, nanocarriers such as liposomes, micelles, dendrimers and polymeric NPs often suffer from the premature release of drugs under complex physiological conditions and uncontrollable drug release rate in vivo. From the injection site to the targeted sites, nanomedicines will be confronted with sequential drug delivery barriers, the fast clearance of blood circulation, extravasation from the blood vessels, enhanced penetration into the deep part of the nidus, effective internalization and controlled drug release inside the targeted cells. Especially for the treatment of cancer, it is necessary to develop novel and effective nanocarriers with the ability to efficiently overcome the physiological barriers for drug delivery in the body as soon as possible; especially to resolve the poor tumoral accumulation and penetration caused by the dense extracellular matrix and high interstitial fluid pressure in tumor tissues. Moreover, to overcome drug resistance, it is highly desirable to develop multifunctional nanomedicines with the combination of multiple therapeutic modalities, such as chemotherapy, photothermal therapy, photodynamic therapy, chemodynamic therapy, radiotherapy, starving therapy, and immunotherapy. Additionally, the stability and degradability as well as biosafety of most nanomedicines in biofluids should be carefully evaluated before their administration to humans. In light of the above-mentioned issues, it is imperative to develop novel and effective nanomaterials for biomedical and pharmaceutical applications.

In this Special Issue, we present original research and review articles with a focus on functional nanomaterials in biomedicine. In the direction of functional nanocarriers,

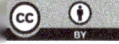

Carvalho et al. reported a type of dual functionalized NPs for the synergistic delivery of levodopa and curcumin. The NPs were derived from the self-assembly of positively charged diblock copolymer NH_2–poly(ethylene oxide)- poly(ε-caprolactone) (NH_2–PEO–PCL) and were then modified by the addition of glutathione on the outer surface. The results indicate that the developed biodegradable NPs with blood compatibility and low cytotoxicity can pass the blood–brain barrier, target the brain tissue, and provide a more sustained release of drugs for potential application in the treatment of Parkinson's disease [1]. Lee et al. reported on pH-responsive metal-based biopolymer NPs for tumor-specific chemotherapy. The aminated hyaluronic acid (aHA) chains were coupled with pH-responsive 2,3-dimethylmaleic anhydride (DMA). Then, the obtained aHA-DMA was electrostatically complexed with ferrous chloride tetrahydrate ($FeCl_2/4H_2O$) and doxorubicin (DOX). The produced DOX-loaded Fe-based hyaluronate nanoparticles (DOX@aHA-DMA/Fe NPs) were found to be able to improve tumor cellular uptake due to HA-mediated endocytosis for tumor cells. The nanoparticles selectively release DOX in the acidic environment of tumor cells due to ionic repulsion, which demonstrates that they can serve as promising tumor-targeting drug carriers [2]. Dong et al. summarized the advances in the tumor microenvironment (TME)-targeted nano-delivery system, which was demonstrated to be able to regulate the distribution of drugs in the body; specifically increase the concentration of drugs in the tumor site; enhance efficacy; and reduce adverse reactions, leading to a significant improvement in the effect of tumor therapy. This comprehensive review exhibited the principles and strategies of the design and utilization of the particular microenvironment of tumors to design functional NPs for the treatment and diagnosis of tumors [3].

In the direction of multimodal imaging and phototherapy of cancer and bacterial infections, Ling et al. summarized the recent progress of the general preparation and functionalization of graphene and related nanocomposites as theranostic materials. The graphene nanocomposites act as outstanding carriers for various therapeutic organic drugs or imaging probes. Moreover, graphene nanocomposites provide a robust platform for self-acting luminescent for confocal laser scanning microscopy, magnetic resonance imaging, computed tomography, positron emission tomography and photoacoustic imaging. Additionally, graphene nanocomposites can be applied in photothermal and photodynamic therapies against different cancers and bacterial infections [4]. Zhang et al. comprehensively summarized the strategies and applications of organic NPs, especially polymer-based NPs, for the delivery of iodinated contrast media in X-ray computed tomography (CT) imaging. They mainly focused on the use of polymeric nanoplatforms to prolong circulation time, reduce toxicity and enhance the targetability of iodinated contrast media. These organic NPs, such as PEGylated liposomes, nanoemulsions, micelles, polymersomes, dendrimers and natural NPs, have exhibited great potential in the development of functionalized contrast media with better biocompatibility, a longer circulation time and more efficient targeting capabilities [5].

In the direction of antibacterial, antimicrobial, antiviral and antioxidant applications of functional NPs, Tong et al. systematically summarized the preparation, characterization and regulation of single-atom nanozymes (SAzymes) through pyrolysis and defect engineering. The strategies of surface modification for SAzymes for their biomedical applications were also discussed. Due to their high atom utilization, the unsaturated coordination of active centers, and geometric structures similar to those of natural enzymes, SAzymes were demonstrated to possess tremendous potential for application in the biomedical field, especially in those of reactive oxygen species (ROS) scavenging and antibacterial therapy [6]. Zhang et al. systematically summarized the principles for the preparation and application of electrostatic spinning, especially of electrospun fibers or membranes functionalized with metal-based nanocrystals. The metal-based nanocrystal-modified nanofibers exhibited high potential in many applications, especially for antimicrobial applications [7]. Liu et al. reported that the label-free peptide substrate was able to induce the aggregation of gold nanoparticles (AuNPs) through electrostatic interactions, leading to the cleavage of the peptide by the severe acute respiratory syndrome coronavirus 2 main protease (Mpro).

As a result, the visual analysis of Mpro activity according to color change of the AuNPs suspension can be achieved. Moreover, the co-assembly of AuNPs and peptides was coated on the peptide-covered electrode surface, thereby facilitating the development of a simple and sensitive electrochemical method for Mpro detection in serum samples, which was valuable for the development of effective antiviral drugs [8]. Pyrzyńska et al. investigated the influence of reaction conditions and clean-up procedure on shape, size and antioxidant activity of selenium nanoparticles (SeNPs). They found that the size and morphology of SeNPs can be controlled by the clean-up step. Moreover, the antioxidant activity often depends on the nanoparticles size and homogeneity of SeNPs [9].

In the direction of the treatment of neurogenic disease, Wang et al. comprehensively summarized the recent progress in nanomaterials-based methodologies for inhibiting amyloid-β peptides aggregation. Some nanomaterials, such as gold NPs, carbon-based NPs, transition oxide two-dimensional (2D) nanomaterials, metal–organic frameworks (MOF) and self-assembled nanomaterials were demonstrated to be able to directly interact with amyloid-β peptides to inhibit their aggregation. In addition, some nanomaterials with photosensitive properties can influence the format of amyloid-β peptides, exhibiting great potential in Alzheimer's disease treatment [10]. In the direction of the treatment of cardiovascular disease, Wang et al. systematically summarized the advances in the preparation and utilization of cell-membrane coated nanoparticles (CMCNPs) for the treatment of cardiovascular disease. Due to their biomimetic properties, such CMCNPs can avoid immune clearance and thus prolong nanocarriers' circulation time. Moreover, the functional proteins on the cloaked cell membranes can impart CMCNPs with additional biological properties, such as selective adherence, inflammatory site targeting and endothelium penetration. All these features significantly enhance the therapeutic efficacies of CMCNPs in treating cardiovascular diseases [11].

We hope this Special Issue provides researchers with information to help them understand the advanced strategies of functional nanoplatforms in biomedical and pharmaceutical applications, inspiring new ideas for future research directions and research activities.

Funding: This work was supported by State Key Laboratory of Biobased Material and Green Papermaking, Qilu University of Technology, Shandong Academy of Sciences (GZKF202108), Hunan Provincial Natural Science Foundation of China (2022JJ20052), Natural Science Foundation of Tianjin City (19JCYBJC17200).

Conflicts of Interest: The authors declare no conflict of interest.

References

1. Mogharbel, B.F.; Cardoso, M.A.; Irioda, A.C.; Stricker, P.E.F.; Slompo, R.C.; Appel, J.M.; de Oliveira, N.B.; Perussolo, M.C.; Saçaki, C.S.; da Rosa, N.N.; et al. Biodegradable Nanoparticles Loaded with Levodopa and Curcumin for Treatment of Parkinson&rsquo's Disease. *Molecules* **2022**, *27*, 2811. [PubMed]
2. Bae, Y.; Kim, Y.; Lee, E.S. Endosomal pH-Responsive Fe-Based Hyaluronate Nanoparticles for Doxorubicin Delivery. *Molecules* **2021**, *26*, 3547. [CrossRef] [PubMed]
3. Sun, Y.; Li, Y.; Shi, S.; Dong, C. Exploiting a New Approach to Destroy the Barrier of Tumor Microenvironment: Nano-Architecture Delivery Systems. *Molecules* **2021**, *26*, 2703. [CrossRef] [PubMed]
4. Gollavelli, G.; Ghule, A.V.; Ling, Y.-C. Multimodal Imaging and Phototherapy of Cancer and Bacterial Infection by Graphene and Related Nanocomposites. *Molecules* **2022**, *27*, 5588. [CrossRef] [PubMed]
5. Zhang, P.; Ma, X.; Guo, R.; Ye, Z.; Fu, H.; Fu, N.; Guo, Z.; Zhang, J.; Zhang, J. Organic Nanoplatforms for Iodinated Contrast Media in CT Imaging. *Molecules* **2021**, *26*, 7063. [CrossRef] [PubMed]
6. Song, H.; Zhang, M.; Tong, W. Single-Atom Nanozymes: Fabrication, Characterization, Surface Modification and Applications of ROS Scavenging and Antibacterial. *Molecules* **2022**, *27*, 5426. [CrossRef] [PubMed]
7. Li, H.; Xu, M.; Shi, R.; Zhang, A.; Zhang, J. Advances in Electrostatic Spinning of Polymer Fibers Functionalized with Metal-Based Nanocrystals and Biomedical Applications. *Molecules* **2022**, *27*, 5548. [PubMed]
8. Feng, Y.; Liu, G.; La, M.; Liu, L. Colorimetric and Electrochemical Methods for the Detection of SARS-CoV-2 Main Protease by Peptide-Triggered Assembly of Gold Nanoparticles. *Molecules* **2022**, *3*, 615. [CrossRef] [PubMed]

9. Sentkowska, A.; Pyrzyńska, K. The Influence of Synthesis Conditions on the Antioxidant Activity of Selenium Nanoparticles. *Molecules* **2022**, *27*, 2486. [CrossRef] [PubMed]
10. Huang, Y.; Chang, Y.; Liu, L.; Wang, J. Nanomaterials for Modulating the Aggregation of β-Amyloid Peptides. *Molecules* **2021**, *26*, 4301. [CrossRef] [PubMed]
11. Zhu, C.; Ma, J.; Ji, Z.; Shen, J.; Wang, Q. Recent Advances of Cell Membrane Coated Nanoparticles in Treating Cardiovascular Disorders. *Molecules* **2021**, *26*, 3428. [CrossRef] [PubMed]

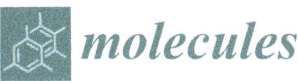

Review

Multimodal Imaging and Phototherapy of Cancer and Bacterial Infection by Graphene and Related Nanocomposites

Ganesh Gollavelli [1], Anil V. Ghule [2] and Yong-Chien Ling [3,*]

[1] Department of Humanities and Basic Sciences, Aditya Engineering College, Surampalem, Jawaharlal Nehru Technological University Kakinada, Kakinada 533437, Andhra Pradesh, India
[2] Department of Chemistry, Shivaji University, Kolhapur 416004, Maharashtra, India
[3] Department of Chemistry, National Tsing Hua University, Hsinchu 30013, Taiwan
* Correspondence: ycling@mx.nthu.edu.tw

Abstract: The advancements in nanotechnology and nanomedicine are projected to solve many glitches in medicine, especially in the fields of cancer and infectious diseases, which are ranked in the top five most dangerous deadly diseases worldwide by the WHO. There is great concern to eradicate these problems with accurate diagnosis and therapies. Among many developed therapeutic models, near infra-red mediated phototherapy is a non-invasive technique used to invade many persistent tumors and bacterial infections with less inflammation compared with traditional therapeutic models such as radiation therapy, chemotherapy, and surgeries. Herein, we firstly summarize the up-to-date research on graphene phototheranostics for a better understanding of this field of research. We discuss the preparation and functionalization of graphene nanomaterials with various biocompatible components, such as metals, metal oxides, polymers, photosensitizers, and drugs, through covalent and noncovalent approaches. The multifunctional nanographene is used to diagnose the disease with confocal laser scanning microscopy, magnetic resonance imaging computed tomography, positron emission tomography, photoacoustic imaging, Raman, and ToF-SMIS to visualize inside the biological system for imaging-guided therapy are discussed. Further, treatment of disease by photothermal and photodynamic therapies against different cancers and bacterial infections are carefully conferred herein along with challenges and future perspectives.

Keywords: graphene; nanocomposites; multimodal imaging; phototherapy; theranostics; cancer; bacterial infection

1. Introduction

Humankind have faced many threats, especially from cancer and infectious diseases, in the past and in the current times. These problems have remained persistent for many decades. Science has provided remedies alongside many religious beliefs, especially during the pandemic times. This scenario increased the need for non-invasive, economic, therapeutic models to fight cancer, Alzheimer's disease, cardiovascular disease, influenza, COVID-19, and other microbial infections, and existing diseases [1–4]. Scientific advancements are required to find solutions to these problems. Innovations in science have provided many therapeutic models, such as chemotherapy and surgeries, after traditional treatment methods such as Chinese medicine and Indian. Innovations in nanotechnology and nanomedicine aim to provide better solutions in medicine [5–8]. Nanotechnology offers small size delivery systems inside cellular and subcellular levels owing to high surface area to carry many therapeutic drugs with biocompatibility and inherent theranostic properties [9].

Theranostics is an emerging field in nanomedicine which may provide simple, economic diagnoses and therapy solutions to many cancers and infectious diseases. Rather than rely on single diagnosis and therapy models, multiple practices are important to provide accurate results of disease confirmation and cure. Nanomaterials with multiple diagnosis and therapeutic characteristics are highly desired in nanomedicine [10,11]. The current diagnosis techniques for cancer and infectious diseases in research are Confocal Laser Scanning Microscopy (CLSM), Magnetic Resonance imaging (MRI), Computed Tomography (CT), Positron Emission Tomography (PET), Raman, and Time-of-Flight Secondary Ion Mass Spectrometry (ToF-SIMS). However, each model has its own advantages and disadvantage [12,13]. Other than multiple imaging guided techniques, multiple therapeutic models are also important, and chemotherapy, immunotherapy, gene therapy, and surgeries which can provide good results [14–17]. However, these treatments may prone to some kind of tissue damage and inevitable side effects [18–21].

In recent years, phototherapy has become emerging research topic in nanomedicine to treat cancer and bacterial infections [22]. Phototherapy is a non-invasive technique due to its usage of low laser powers and short time interactions to the patent [23]. This is due to the utilization of low energy NIR light which has better tissue penetration in biological systems than visible and UV light, which may burn the skin and harm the patient [24]. Any system which can absorb NIR light and create a local heat to burn tumors and bacterial cells would be beneficial to nanomedicine [25]. Many nanomaterials with different size, shape, and biofunctionality have been demonstrated to target cancer and bacterial invasion [26–28]. The most successful photo and chemotherapeutic nanomaterials, such as Au, Ag, Fe, carbon, and polymeric nanomaterials, are well studied [29]. Due to its very good biocompatibility, low toxicity, tunable size, and high surface areas, we selected 2D graphene and reviewed the status quo of this nanomaterial in nanomedicine and theranostics [30].

Graphene is an allotropic form of carbon where the carbons are arranged in a 2D hexagonal chicken-net-like network which can offer high surface area, better electrical and thermal conductivity with optical transparency, and tuneable surface functionality with the olefin carbon network [31,32]. The intriguing properties of size, shape, and toxicity of graphene and graphene-related nanomaterials, such as graphene oxide (GO), reduced graphene oxide (RGO), and functionalized graphene nanocomposites (GNCs), are investigated in this review for multimodal imaging guided targeted phototherapy. Herein, we discuss the preparation of GNCs functionalization with many metals, metal oxides, polymers, photsensitizers, as well as other therapeutic drugs by covalent and non-covalent approaches to treat malignant tumors and antibiotic resistant bacterial infections by NIR triggered photothermal therapy (PTT) and photodynamic therapy (PDT) as well as synergistic effects of other combination therapies (Scheme 1).

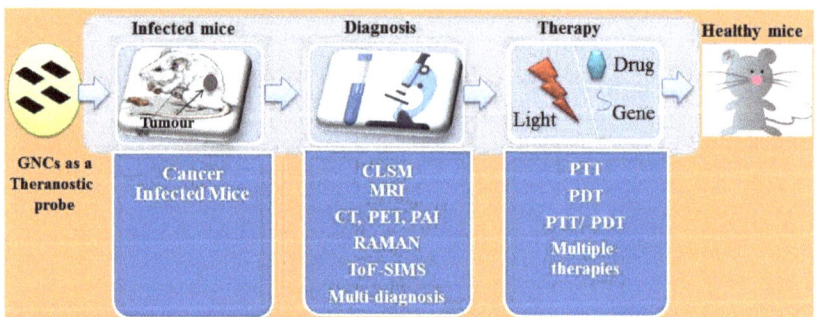

Scheme 1. Graphene nanocomposites for multimodal imaging guided therapy.

2. Preparation of Graphene Nanocomposites
2.1. Graphene Oxide

GO belongs to the graphene family which is a densely packed honeycomb-like structure made from a sheet of sp^2 and sp^3 bonded carbon atoms. Graphene nanomaterials have benefits such as high mechanical strength, Young's modulus, surface area, conductivity, and carrier mobility, making them a perfect nanomaterial for various applications [33]. Graphene and its derivatives are widely used due to their excellent inherent properties and extraordinary composition in drug delivery, cancer treatment, biosensing, and bioimaging. Apart from these advantages of GO, the study has also focused on its toxicity and demonstrates GNCs are less toxic than carbon nanotubes. This outcome supports the use of GNCs for cancer and hyperthermia treatment [34]. Scheme 2 presents the various types of graphene and their composites, preparation, and biological applications. Types, preparation, properties, functionalization, and focused therapeutic applications of graphene nanomaterials are also shown in Scheme 2. Researchers are currently giving particular attention to the preparation of single-layered GO from graphite, by using strong oxidizing agents and concentrated acids, because of its extensive applications in the biomedical field [35]. GO contains epoxy, carboxyl, carbonyl, and hydroxyl functional groups that make it hydrophilic and biocompatible [33].

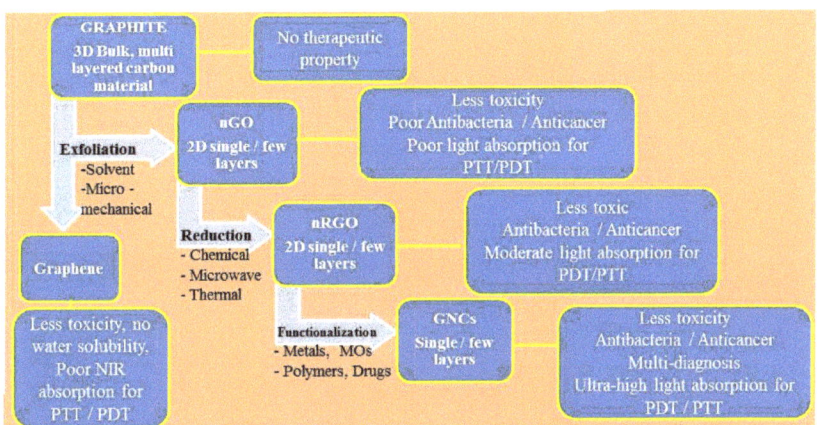

Scheme 2. Exfoliation of graphite into graphene, GO, RGO, and GNCs as well as phototheranostic properties. MOs—metal oxides.

The graphene was synthesized by various methods in which the top–down and bottom–up approaches are generally used. In the top–down method, discrete graphene sheets are synthesized by breaking a stacked layer of graphite. The top–down approach includes micromechanical cleavage, thermal reduction, and electrochemical exfoliation whereas, chemical vapor deposition is included in the bottom–up approach [35]. Among the several preparation methods of graphene, the reduction of GO has gained significant attention because of its low-cost, ease of implementation, as well as variety of reducing agents and synthesis procedures [36]. Moreover, for the preparation of GO the Staudenmaier method, Brodie method, Hummers' method and their modified versions are well known and widely used [37]. However, the Hummers' method showed the degree of oxidation to be more compared with the other methods [38]. In brief, in the Hummers' method the graphite flakes were mixed with H_2SO_4 and $NaNO_3$ solution under an ice bath. Then, $KMnO_4$ was added to the above mixture with constant stirring. Due to the addition of $KMnO_4$, the solution became brown. Next, that solution was diluted with water and then treated with hydrogen peroxide. Lastly, the product was washed with distilled water and 10% HCl solution to remove impurities. An improved form of the Hummers' method for the preparation of GO was reported, by improving the oxidation with the addition of extra $KMnO_4$ without $NaNO_3$ addition, and a reaction was carried out in H_2SO_4/H_3PO_4 with a 9:1 ratio. This improved form of the Hummers' method showed an even carbon network, more oxidized hydrophilic carbon, and no toxic gas production during preparation [39]. The phase purity and functional groups were initially confirmed by X-ray diffraction (XRD) and Fourier transform infrared spectroscopy (FT-IR). The surface morphology and microstructure of GO were confirmed by scanning electron microscopy (SEM) and transmission electron microscopy (TEM). By using Raman spectroscopy various graphene-based nanomaterials were characterized. Moreover, X-ray photoelectron spectroscopy (XPS), thermo-gravimetric analysis (TGA), differential scanning calorimeter (DSG), and atomic force microscopy (AFM) were used to evaluate graphene-based nanomaterials [40].

Graphene and GO have more surface area and strong light absorption properties, hence being considered ideal applicants in cancer therapy. Moreover, graphene has been confirmed to possess better photothermal anticancer efficiency than carbon nanotubes. The authors also concluded easy preparation, low cost, and low toxicity made graphene-based nanomaterials an ideal candidate for cancer treatment [34]. A later work evaluating the cytotoxicity of GO and GO loaded with doxorubicin (DOX) on human multiple myeloma cells suggested low-cytotoxicity GO as a suitable nanocarrier for anticancer drug [41]. Moreover, further work to improve GO biocompatibility was carried out by its initial conjugation with NH$_2$-PEG3500-maleimide. Then, functionalization was performed using peptide (integrin αvβ6-specific HK) through maleimide-thiol coupling, and finally, HPPH was loaded on GO-PEG-HK via π−π stacking (Figure 1A). GO(HPPH)-PEG-HK was capable of killing the tumor cells and lung metastasis [42].

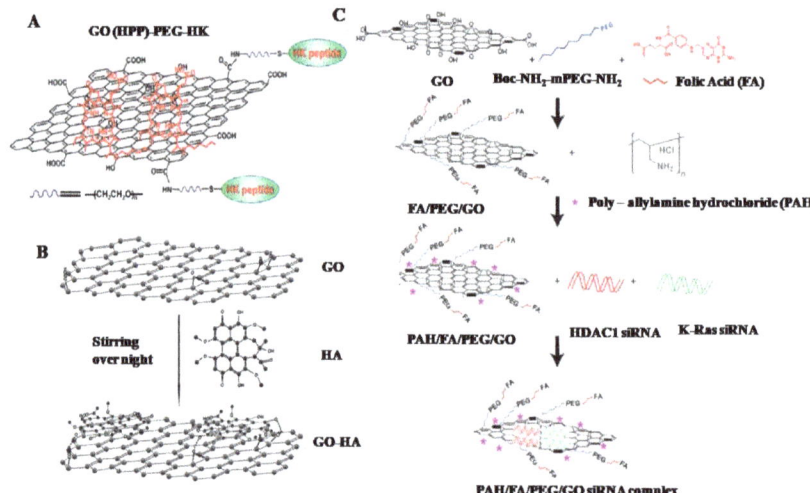

Figure 1. Schematic. (**A**) Structure of GO(HPPH)-PEG-HK [42]. (**B**) Diagram of the synthesis and functionalization to prepare GO-HA hybrid [43]. (**C**) The synthesis and functionalization to prepare PAH/FA/PEG/GO siRNA complex [44]. Reprinted/adapted with permission from Refs. [43,44]. Copy right 2011, copyright Wiley-VCH. Copy right 2017, copyright Ivyspring.

A novel mechanochemical method was developed to synthesize GO-Fe$_3$O$_4$ nanocomposites [45]. An efficient, nontoxic PEGylated GO/epirubicin was designed to destruct tumor cells [46]. In addition, hypocrellin A (HA) was loaded onto GO for anticancer treatment. The carboxyl, hydroxyl, and epoxide groups present on GO were linked with the quinone portion of HA via hydrogen bonding, as shown in Figure 1B [43]. Moreover, a PAH/FA/PEG/GO siRNA complex for gene delivery consistin of a GO monolayer delivering HDAC1 and K-Ras siRNAs to target pancreatic cancer cells was reported. The detailed synthesis procedure for PAH/FA/PEG/GO siRNA is shown in Figure 1C [44]. The combined use of PEG and grafted GO (pGO) enhanced its aqueous stability followed by loading of pGO with chlorin e6 (Ce6) photosensitizer and doxorubicin (DOX). Higher photodynamic anticancer effects as compared with Ce6/pGO or DOX/pGO were found [47]. Additionally, a covalently bonded biocompatible GO-PEG showed toxicity for lung cancer A549 and human breast cancer MCF-7 cells. Further, paclitaxel (PTX) was conjugated with GO-PEG via π-π stacking and hydrophobic interactions, and the results showed high toxicity to A549 and MCF-7 cells [48]. For the cancer cell apoptosis, a multifunctional

FePt-DMSA/GO-PEG-FA (iron platinum-dimercaptosuccinnic acid/PEGylated GO-folic acid) composite was reported [49]. For the breast cancer cells, a PEGylated nGO loaded with PS and two-photon (TP) compound was prepared. The results showed that GO-PEG (TP) has the capability to kill breast cancer cells (4T1) at a 980 nm laser irradiation [50].

For bacterial infection phototherapy, a variety of metals and metal oxides were loaded onto graphene as antibacterial agents. Briefly, the TiO$_2$-Ag/graphene as a ternary nanocomposite was synthesized and its photodynamic effect was carried on *E. coli* bacteria and A375 (melanoma), HaCaT (keratinocyte) cells. The results suggested the ternary composite could be applied for bacterial keratosis or skin tumors [51]. Additionally, different metals such as Zn, Ni, Sn, and steel were coated with GO (Figure 2A). The different metals have different capacities to fight against bacteria: GO-Zn acts as a better antibacterial agent than GO-Ni, followed by GO-Sn and GO-steel [52]. Moreover, a ZnO/GO nanocomposite prepared by loading green-synthesized ZnO NPs to GO nanosheets (Hummers' method) (Figure 2B) has the capacity to kill the bacteria and also serves as an anticancer drug [53].

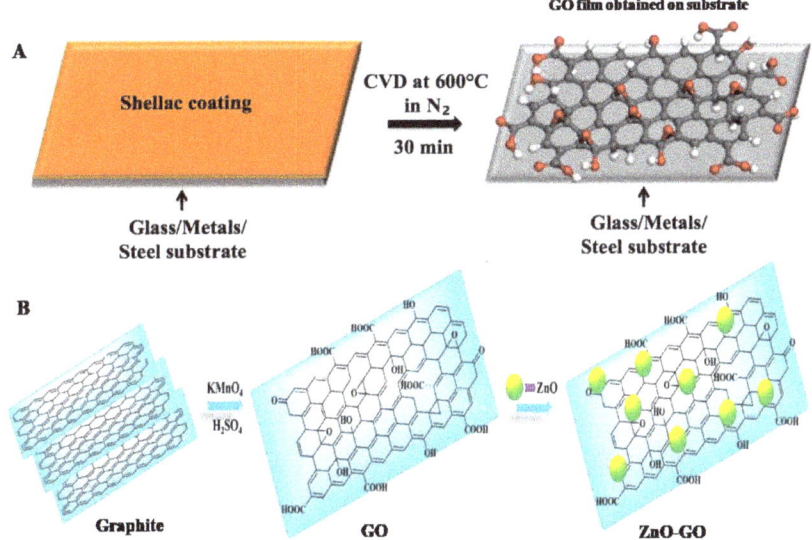

Figure 2. (**A**) Schematic diagram showing synthesis of GO directly on various substrates from natural biopolymer shellac. GO film is shown in ball and stick model; red: oxygen atom, gray: carbon atom, white: hydrogen atom. The shellac-coated substrates were heated at 600 °C under nitrogen atmosphere for 30 min to synthesize GO directly on different substrates [52]. (**B**) The possible mechanism of the transformation of graphite to GO and then to ZnO/GO NC [53]. Reprinted/adapted with permission from Refs. [52,53]. Copy right 2018, copyright Willey-VCH. Copy right 2020, copyright RSC.

Additional advantages of graphene include (1) cross-linked capability with polymers, (2) admirable biocompatibility in in vitro and in vivo, and (3) more surface area, specifically graphene sheets. Hence it makes more contact with the bacteria and leads to more pronounced antibacterial effect. Considering all these advantages, a boronic acid-functionalized graphene and combined with quaternary ammonium salt (B-CG-QAS) acted as a multidrug-resistant to bacterial infection [54]. In addition, GO-PEI-GQDs via layer-by-layer deposition [55] and polyvinyl-N-carbazole-GO (PVK-GO) nanocomposite [56] were also reported. The variation in antibacterial effect due to variation in the combination of the substrate with GO was noticed. The GO fixed titanium with enhanced photoacoustic performance (GO-EPD) showed enhanced antibacterial, activity followed by GO-APS (GO-electrostatic interaction) and GO-D (GO-gravitational effect) [57].

2.2. Reduced Graphene Oxide

The RGO has been used in drug delivery, bioimaging, and anticancer applications due to its high electrical and thermal conductivity. However, GO has less NIR absorption capacity than RGO. Moreover, RGO is superior for high photothermal conversion and optical properties. The hydrophilic nature of RGO is essential in medical applications; hence, several efforts have been researched to enhance its hydrophilicity [58]. Furthermore, RGO was synthesized by chemical or thermal reduction of GO or graphite oxide. The hydrazine, hydrazine hydrate, sodium borohydride, and L-ascorbic acid are used as reducing agents during RGO synthesis [59]. Moreover, the plant extract is also used for the synthesis of RGO due to its non-toxicity, cost-effectiveness, biocompatibility, and environment-friendly nature over chemical and physical approaches (see Scheme 2). As per the report, these biomolecules, such as amino acids, bovine serum albumin, humanin, glucose, melatonin, and ascorbic acid, interact with functional groups present in RGO [60]. Furthermore, humanin has been used for the green synthesis of RGO [61]. Chitosan was used to combine with RGO to reduce and stabilize the GO as well as entrap DOX and IR820 dye. The in vitro and in vivo results confirmed the chit-RGO-DOX-IR820 was applicable for cancer theranostics [62].

Various studies have reported the increased effectiveness of cancer treatment on combination therapies. For instance, GO (from graphene flakes) was partially reduced with NaOH and chloroacetic acid followed by surface modification to form FP-PrGO-Ce6-AuNR by depositing gold nanorods (AuNR) onto FP-PrGO-Ce6. The FP-PrGO-Ce6-AuNR nanocarrier acted as a targeting agent for anticancer theranostics [63]. Moreover, RGO-coated polydopamine doped mesoporous silica was used for anticancer treatment. The RGO/MSN/PDA-loaded DOX helps photothermal activity and shows an antitumor effect [64]. A green approach used an environmentally friendly, non-toxic, natural phenolic resveratrol compound instead of hydrazine and hydrogen sulfide for the formation of RGO [65]. Recently, an HSA/RGO/Cladophora glomerata bio-nano composite was prepared as a PS for study using L929, HeLa cancer cell line, Pseudomonas aeruginosa, and Staphylococcus aureus bacteria. The results showed that the synthesized composite has the capacity to kill bacteria with demonstrated photothermal activity [66].

For bacterial infection problems, silver is a well-known antibacterial agent. Moreover, combination therapies showed increased antibacterial properties. In addition, RGO induces photothermal effect for bacterial treatment. For instance, RGO/Ag composite was prepared as an antibacterial agent [67]. Moreover, the RGO-Cu_2O nanocomposite was synthesized to fight against bacteria [68]. The GO/nitrogen-doped carbon dots/hydroxyapatite/titanium film (GO/NCD/Hap/Ti) showed a PTT/PDT approach to bacterial infection [69].

2.3. Functionalization

The synthesis of stable and functional GNCs is the most crucial aspect of the biomedical field. Though GO and RGO are reported as good PTT agents, its NIR absorption capability has to be improved further for more efficient phototherapy results. Moreover, RGO is hydrophobic, which limits its application during cancer treatment [37]. Hence, to fulfil these drawbacks, surface functionalization is the best option in the medical field to treat cancerous cells. Generally, the surface functionalization was carried out by covalent and non-covalent interactions. Non-covalent bonding includes electrostatic interactions, hydrogen bonding, π-π stacking, and van der Waals interactions. For example, a MFG (magnetic and fluorescent graphene)-$SiNc_4$ (silicon napthalocyanine bis(trihexylsilyloxide) via covalent and non-covalent π-π stacking was prepared. MFG showed flat NIR absorption and was reported to have a remarkable PTT/PDT in HeLa cancer cells [70]. GO quantum dots (GOQDs) using hypocretin A (HA) for loading via π-π interaction were applied to detect cancer cells [71]. In addition, nucleophilic substitution, condensation, and electrophilic addition offer alternative paths for the covalent functionalization of GO.

Alternative approaches, such as GO with polyamidoamine dendrimer (GO-PAMAM) loaded with DOX and MMP-9 shRNA plasmid (Figure 3A), were applied for the treatment of breast cancer cells [72]. Moreover, the NGO-COOH prepared using Hummers' method was functionalized with a Gd-DTPA dendrimer and finally loaded with the anticancer drugs epirubicin (EPI) and Let-7g miRNA (Figure 3B) to treat cancer cells [73]. Moreover, the GO-PLL(poly-L-lysine)/DOX/ZnPc acts as an admirable anticancer carrier to transport DOX and ZnPc to detect cancer cells. The synthesized nanocomplex shows not only anticancer activity but also photodynamic and chemotherapeutic effects against cancer cells [74]. Moreover, the GO firstly composited with carboxymethyl chitosan (CMC) followed by conjugation with hyaluronic acid (HA) and fluorescein isothiocyanate (FI) to prepare GO-CMC-FI-HA/DOX. The results proved that the nanocomplex can be used as an anticancer drug with controlled release [75].

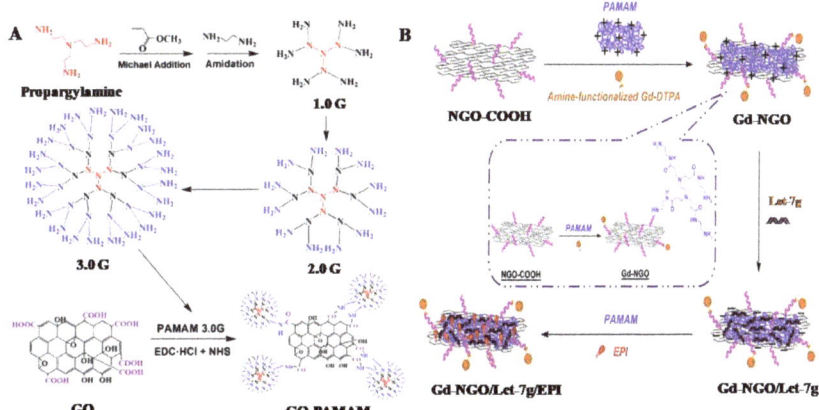

Figure 3. (**A**) Synthetic route of PAMAM 3.0G and GO-PAMAM [72]. (**B**) Schematic of the procedure for preparation of Gd-NGO/Let-7g/EPI [73]. Reprinted/adapted with permission from Refs. [72,73]. Copy right 2017, copyright Elsevier. Copy right 2014, copyright Elsevier.

The increase in bacterial infections is a serious problem for human health. Hence, the synthesis of multifunctional materials would be beneficial for surgical operations. Concerning this situation, GO functionalized (noncovalent) PEGylated phthalocyanines were synthesized for antibacterial phototherapy (ZnPc-TEGMME@GO) (Figure 4A) [76]. Moreover, RGO was functionalized with polycationic poly-L-lysine (PLL) to increase its drug loading capability with colloidal stability, as shown in Figure 4B. Further, RGO-PLL was labelled with anti-HER2 to form a bond with HER2 receptors to detect breast cancer cells [77]. The GO/AuNRs was synthesized and functionalized with polystyrene sulfonate (PSS) which showed tumor-killing capacity [78]. Furthermore, functionalization of RGO with hyaluronic acid increases the stability and cytocompatibility, as well as induce cancer cell ablation [79]. Moreover, the ZnO QDs-GO nanocomposite was prepared as an antibacterial agent. The author has combined chitosan with ZnOQDs@GO to enhance drug delivery capacity, biodegradability, and biocompatibility [80].

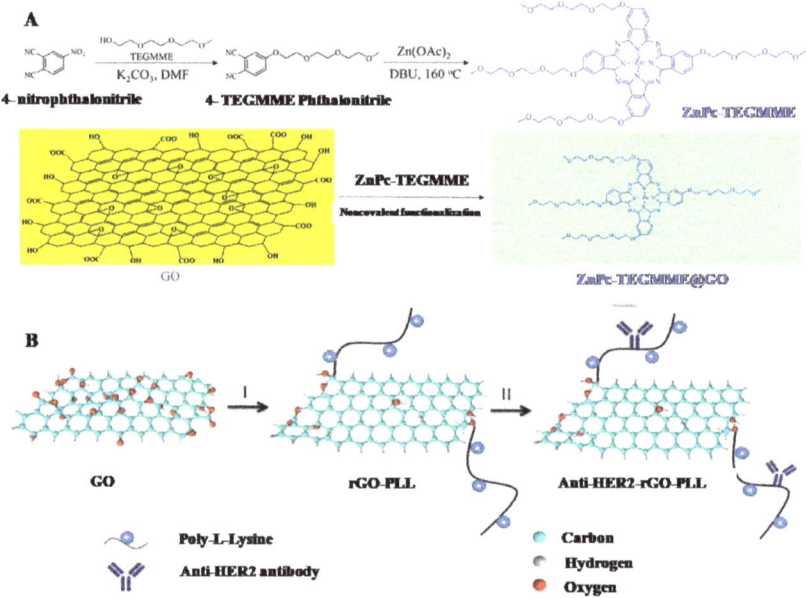

Figure 4. (**A**) Schematic Illustration of the Preparation of ZnPc-TEGMME@GO [76]. (**B**) Synthesis of anti-HER2-rGO-PLL is performed in two steps: (I) GO is functionalized with PLL under alkaline conditions followed by NaBH$_4$ reduction to form rGO-PLL and (II) rGO-PLL is subsequently conjugated with anti-HER2 antibodies via glutaldehyde bifunctional linkers [77]. Reprinted/adapted with permission from Refs. [76,77]. Copy right 2017, copyright ACS. Copy right 2016, copyright Elsevier.

3. Graphene Nanocomposite Theranostics for Multimodal Imaging Guided Phototherapy

Nanomaterials-based theranostics are the future of personalized medicine as a single nanoplatform can provide multiple imaging and therapies in a short time by simplifying the cost and the amount of the drug required for multiple diseases [81]. Multimodal imaging-based diagnosis is the most reliable technique to identify the problems in cancer- and bacteria-infected patients, and it will be helpful to surgeons and clinicians to make better predictions and conclusions about the problem, thus will improve treatment confidence. Several imaging techniques have been adopted in the research, such as CLSM, MRI, CT, PET, PAI, Raman, ToF-SIMS, and other imaging techniques for early diagnosis (Scheme 3) [82–85].

Phototherapy (PT) involves light interaction (Vis-NIR) with nanomaterials to generate heat or reactive oxygen to destruct cancer and bacterial infection. If the therapy process involves generation of heat from nanomaterials which can suppress or burn the tumor/bacteria is called PTT. If the PT involves reactive oxygen species (ROS) and singlet oxygen ($^1O_2$) generation to destruct the cellular components, it is called PDT. If the nanomaterial inherently cannot generate ROS and $^1O_2$, it has to functionalize with PS [70]. The NIR light has high tissue penetration and low absorption by the biological medium. Hence, we usually adopt the NIR lasers for PT. Apart from PT, combination therapies with chemo and gene therapies could also enhance the treatment results [86]. Various PT agents have been explored by researchers including inorganic, organic, and composite nanomaterials [24]. The extensive publication record of functionalized nanographene composites on imaging guide therapy shows they are a focus in this field of theranostics due to their effectiveness in disease eradication. To overcome the individual drawbacks of diagnosis and therapy, integration of independent techniques has become a major challenge in nanomedicine.

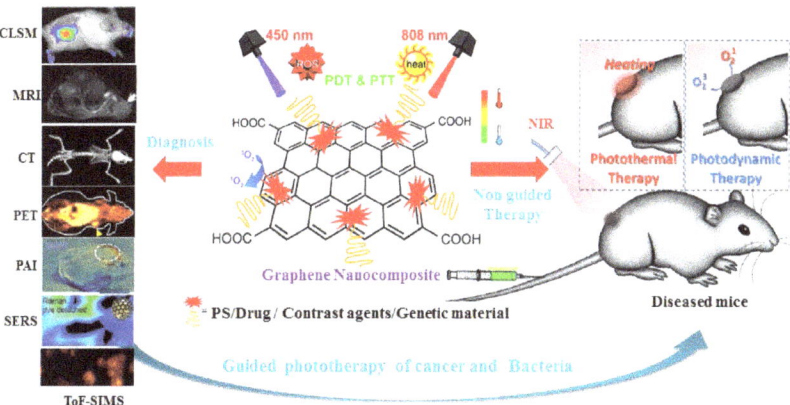

Scheme 3. Multimodal imaging guided phototherapy of bacteria and cancer bearing mice with graphene nanocomposite. Reprinted/adapted with permission from Refs. [85,86]. Copy right 2017, copyright ACS. Copy right 2014, copyright ACS.

3.1. CLSM for Imaging Guided Therapy

Typically, scientists rely on CLSM to identify cell morphology and drug internalizations as they are economic and the most available handy preliminary techniques in the lab. When the nanodrug is added to the cells before going to the CLSM, optical microscopes-based imaging is highly important to check the cell structure and morphology. After that, CLSM is helpful to identify the fluorescent drug molecule's internalization, its location in the cells, and whether it was entered into the cytoplasm and thereby nucleolus or was hindered at the cell wall.

Quantum dots (QDs)-based imaging has drawn the attention of nanomedicine scientists due to its tunable size and variable colors with stable fluorescence emissions [87]. On the other hand, its toxicity issues lead to a focus on alternate materials. In this perspective, Au nanomaterials are said to be a hallmark for imaging guided therapy due to their tunable size and stable emissions with good biocompatibility [88,89]. However, carbon-based nanomaterials, such as graphene and CQDs, are emerging and attractive nanomaterials due to their high surface area and versatile surface chemistry to functionalize inorganic and organic imaging and drug molecules for multimodal imaging-guided therapy for cancer and bacterial infection. They are also reported to be highly biocompatible and antibacterial [90]. In order to be an imaging probe, graphene must be functionalized with luminescent inorganic or organic materials. In pioneering works by Dai et al. on the preparation of nanoGO-based imaging probes for imaging and therapy of cancer, GO was functionalized with PEG- and B-cell-specific Rituxan antibody for targeted cell imaging and cancer therapy [91,92]. Later, GO was functionalized with PEG and fluorescein to make the GO as highly biocompatible and fluorescent to monitor its internalization into the cells. Few more GO-based fluorescence imaging probes have been successfully reported [93,94].

We prepared a multifunctional graphene (MFG) by functionalization with polyacrylic acid, FeNPs, and fluorescein ortho-methacrylate to impart both magnetic and fluorescence properties for CLSM imaging in HeLa cells and in zebrafish whole-body imaging (Figure 5). The MFG showed good biodispersability, biocompatability, and stable green fluorescence emission inside the biological system. These results confirmed that the MFG could be a good candidate for imaging guided PTT of cancer and bacterial infection as it also possessed flat absorption in the entire VU-Vis-NIR region [95,96]. In order to make it a PDT drug, we functionalized a PS (SiNc$_4$) to offer MFG-SiNC$_4$ and the synergistic effects of PTT/PDT and PTT, as shown in Figure 5C,D, with 98% efficacy in light [70]. Very recently, mesoporous silica (MS) coated RGO was synthesized and functionalized with indocyanine green (ICG), PEG (MS-RGO-ICG-PEG), and folic acid (MS-RGO-ICG-PEG-FA) for targeted imaging and phototherapy of cancer. Figure 5G shows the increase in the temperature with laser irradiation at the tumor site of mice injected with MS-RGO-ICG-PEG-FA. Hence, it could be a good candidate for phototherapy, which was evident after the experiments. Figure 5H marks that there is a decrease in the tumor volume of the mice treated with MS-RGO-ICG-PEG-FA compared to MS-RGO-FA alone, without PS ICG. The effectiveness of tumor suppression can be explained by the synergistic effects of PTT from rGO and PDT from ICG. The experiments are performed using an 808 nm laser with 1 W/cm^2 for 10 min [97]. Irrespective of this progress, fluorescence-based techniques are still limited to the laboratory stage presumably due to the limitations of poor resolution, and because the drug molecules should be fluorescent.

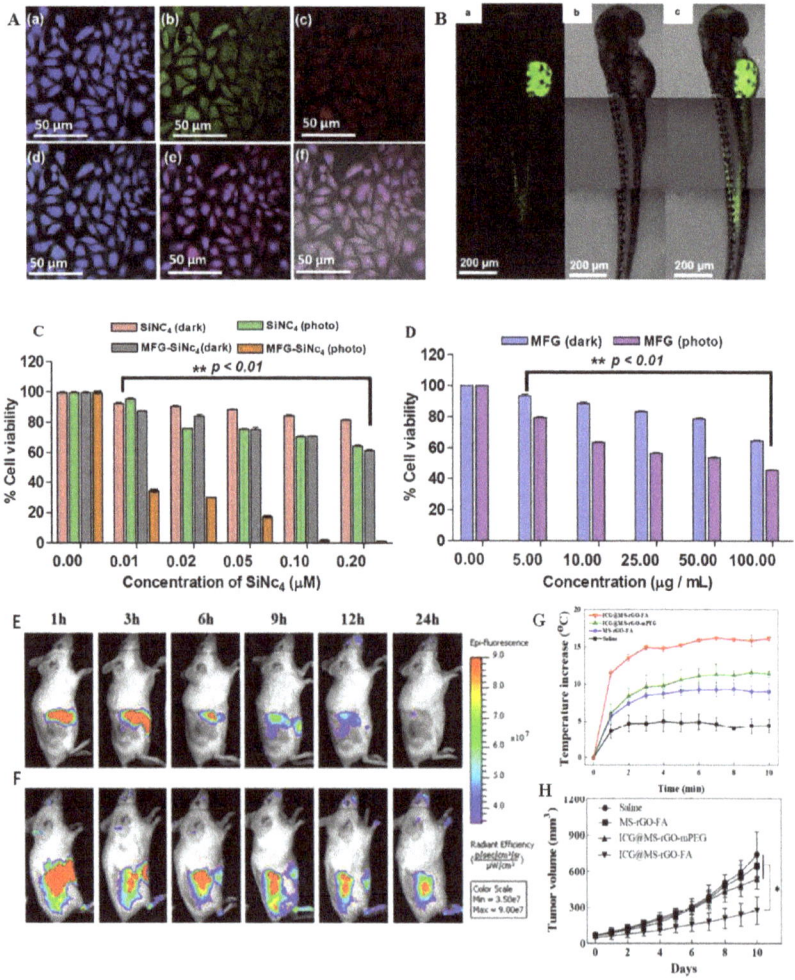

Figure 5. CLSM images of functionalized graphene composites. (**A**) In vitro images of MFG-SiNC$_4$ in HeLa cells where the images reveal very good biodistribution throughout the cell ((a) control stained with DAPI, (b) green, and (c) red emissions from the MFG-SiNC$_4$ and, (d,e) are the combined images of ab andac. (f) The combined images of abc with DIC). (**B**) In vivo whole-body zebrafish images with MFG, where the green fluorescence is observed throughout the body due to its very good bio-distribution [70,95]. (**C,D**) The combined PTT/PDT and PTT of MFG-SiNc$_4$ and MFG [70,95]. (**E,F**) Time dependent in vivo mice non-targeting and targeting images of MS-RGO-ICG-PEG and

MS-RGO-ICG-PEG-FA. The image taken at 24 h reveals that the FA functionalized GO, (**E**) has shown bright luminescence and very good tumor specificity whereas it is not observed in non FA targeted GO (**F**). (**G**) Time vs. temperature at tumor bearing mice. (**H**) Tumor volume after irradiation with laser up to 10 days [97]. Reprinted/adapted with permission from Refs. [70,95]. Copy right 2012 and 2014, copyright Elsevier. Reprinted/adapted with permission from Ref. [97]. Copy right 2022, copyright MDPI.

3.2. MRI for Imaging Guided Therapy

Among all imaging techniques, MRI and CT scans are clinically versatile and best used so far for imaging-based diagnosis purpose. These techniques do not rely on any fictionalization of fluorophores and QDs. MRI works based on the radio waves and magnetic field to identify damaged (cancer) tissue from the healthy tissues based on activating the local proton environment. It has the great advantage of ease of use for X-ray imaging techniques. However, it has the limitations of poor sensitivity and lengthy signal recording times. The proton magnetic moment of tissue is environment-dependent and the T1 and T2 times may not produce a better image, hence some external contrast agents are frequently used. The well-known Gd^{3+} for bright contrast and superparamagnetic iron oxide NPs for dark contrast are used [98].

Graphene-related nanomaterial magnetic composites have a great advantage in helping these imaging guided therapy processes to improve the signals or contrasts to provide enhanced resolution in the final images during disease identification [99]. GO has been a scaffold for many imaging probes and drug loadings, and there are several works that have discussed magnetic nanoparticles-loaded GO, creating a better contrast agent due to its high loading capacity [100]. Recently, the oxidation of ball-milled graphite producing a nanoGO was reported. The extent of oxidation along with the presence of Mn^{2+} ions from $KMnO_4$ are responsible for better proton relaxivity and displayed very good T1- and T2-weighted MRI contrast images [101]. Moreover, the RGO and created structural defects and oxygen functionalities are reported too. The destruction of symmetry in RGOs sublattices created a paramagnetic property, and it was demonstrated to be a good MRI contrast agent. The authors have suggested that the amount of the defects and the oxygen functionality determines the paramagnetism [102]. A nonmagnetic particles-based GO by the fuctionalization of GO with fluorine for MRI with NIR absorption capability for photo therapy of cancer was reported [103]. Apart from this, metal-free, magnetic graphene QDs doped with boron provided very good MR imaging results in both in vitro and in vivo [104]. Moreover, a GO-DTP-Gd magnetic complex for T1 MRI was prepared and demonstrated to be a better contrast agent than commercially used Magnevist. The complex has further functionalized with doxorubicin through physorption and shows very good toxicity towards cancer [105]. In addition, graphene encapsulated cupper probes were prepared and used as neural electrodes to image neural-cell activities in the brain [106]. Further, $^{99m}Tc^{I}$ and Gd-based pegylated ultrasmall nano GO ($^{99m}Tc^{-}$ and Gd-usNGO-PEG) were prepared for the multimodal MRI and SPECT/CT imaging of lymph nodes. The preparation approach is claimed to be chelator free, and the final product has been utilized for multimodal purposes [107].

In brief, many authors have reported that GO- and RGO-based iron oxide nanocomposites are excellent for MR imaging and guided therapy of cancer [100]. As discussed earlier, we also prepared an MFG-SiNC4 with excellent superperamagnetic properties, fluorescence, biocompatibility, and water dispersability for in vitro MRI to serve as a good contrast agent, as shown in Figure 6A,B. Later, we demonstrated this material for guided PT of cancer (Figure 5C,D) [70,95]. Further, polyethylene glycol and super paramagnetic iron oxide nanoparticles functionalized rGO (rGO-IONPs-PEG) was prepared for multimodal imaging, such as the MRI-, CLSM-, and PAI-guided PTT of breast cancer in both in vitro and in vivo. The prepared GNC had excellent magnetic properties for MRI imaging, with good fluorescence and PAI imaging capabilities and good drug loading capability. Figure 6C,D show the PT efficiency of RGO-IONPs-PEG-Laser and greater tumor reduction was observed after the laser ablation compared to controls. Figure 6E shows the guided MRI images of mice before and after injection, and during therapy, with and without lasers. The day 7 laser-treated MRI reveals the complete tumor absence compared to untreated mice at the same duration of time. The study [108] is among the papers which have demonstrated imaging-guided therapy with reliable MR imaging in a systematic manner for theranostics, as shown in Figure 6.

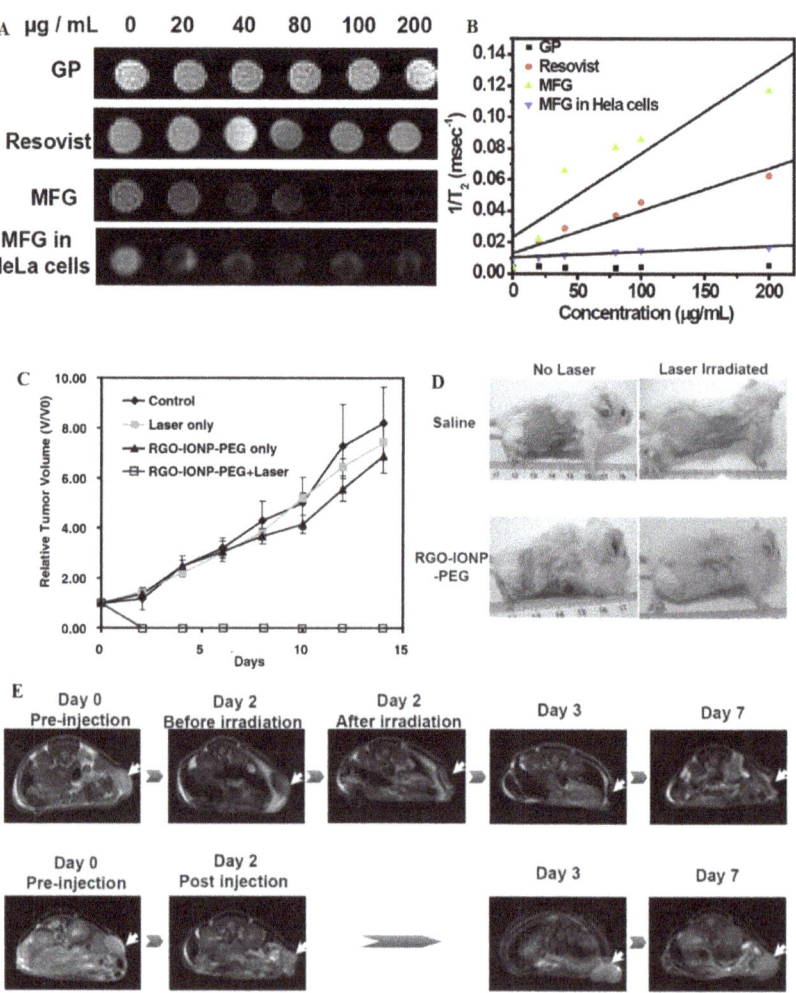

Figure 6. MR images of GNCs in vitro and in vivo imaging guided phototherapy. (**A**) In vitro MRI of MFG and in HeLa cells. The contrast of the images increases with the concentration of MFG and MFG-SiNc$_4$ than clinically accepted resovist. (**B**) The corresponding 1/T2 intensities with concentration [70]. (**C**) Relative tumor volume with respective to the graphene photodrug and duration of therapy up to 14 days. (**D**) The pictorial representation of mice bearing tumor before and after PT, where the tumor has vanished within a few days of therapy than compared to the control experiments with out RGO-IONPs-PEG and laser. (**E**). Upper row is the MR images of tumor (indicates with white arrow) before and after PT and its suppression monitoring with time (0–7 days). The lower row is for without laser irradiation after injection of RGO-IONPs-PEG [108]. Reprinted/adapted with permission from Ref. [70]. Copy right 2014, copyright Elsevier. Reprinted/adapted with permission from Ref. [108]. Copy right 2012, copyright Wiley-VCH.

Apart from these, many researchers have synthesized GO/RGO based magnetic nanocomposite for MR imaging [109–111]. In addition to GO and rGO based IONPs, Gd doped graphene QDs also has been prepared and demonstrated for MR imaging [112,113], which could also offer good loading of imaging and drugs molecules and less toxicity to serve as a theranostic material. According to the literature the contrast agents improve the image quality and here the IONPs produce better contrast than Gd or other magnetic nanomateial composites.

3.3. CT for Imaging Guided Therapy

CT scan is an alternative 3D imaging technique whch works based on the X-ray attenuation of molecular tissues to identify tumors at lower cost than an MRI. It can also provide good spatial–temporal resolution of cancer tissues, and the image recording time is shorter than MRI. Usually, barium sulphate and iodine-based contrast agents are used when CT lacks the necessary sensitivity to image some soft, low-density tissues. The literature on various nanomaterials for CT scan is available. Carbon-based nanomaterials have a unique role due to their biocompatibility and high contrast agent's immobilization capability. Among the few nanomaterials reported for CT scanning, Bi nanomaterial is exclusively studied, though CuS and some of its composites are also explored for CT and MR imaging together [98].

However, the available literature is limited regarding GNCs for CT scanning along with MR imaging. GNCs are synthesized from the oxidation of graphite with $KMnO_4$ and reduced with HCl before being further functionalized with iodine, and have shown good CT and MR imaging contrast [114]. It has been reported that Bi NPs functionalized graphene QDs was prepared with good dispersibility and low toxicity for improved CT imaging followed by PT of cancer [115]. GO functionalized with FePt NPs composite was made and successfully demonstrated for both MR and CT imaging followed by in situ pH responsive targeted cancer inactivation [116]. A nanocomposite of $BaHoF_5$ decorated GO-PEG was prepared with good biocompatibility, and was well demonstrated as a CT and MR imaging agent followed by PTT therapy [117]. GO decorated with ultra-small $ZnFe_2O_4$ and upconversion luminescence nanoparticles (UCNPs) have been well demonstrated for CT scanning along with MRI, PAI, and fluorescence imaging guided photothearpy as a unique multi diagnosis platform [118].

Recently, GO decorated with AuNPs, SPIONPs, along with DOX-loaded 1-tetradecanol (TD) was prepared (called smart nanocomposite, NC) and successfully demonstrated for CT- and MRI-guided controlled chemo-phototherapy of cancer in vitro and in vivo. The advantage of this material is that the Au NPs on GO can act as a CT contrast agent and provide better emission of X-rays due to its high atomic number (Figure 7A) with good house-filed values (Figure 7B). The FeNPs can act as dual CT and MRI contrast agents (Figure 7C,D). Hence, the combination of these two materials on top of GO has provided a great advantage of dual modal imaging and revealed increased contrast in concentration, after 24 h, at the post-intratumoral site (i.t) compared to the post intraperitonial site in the images of Figure 7C,D. Figure 7E shows a reduction in tumor volume within a few days after PT with DOX-NCs+NIR. Figure 7F shows the corresponding morphology of tumor and total mice view from pre injection to 90 days of PT [119].

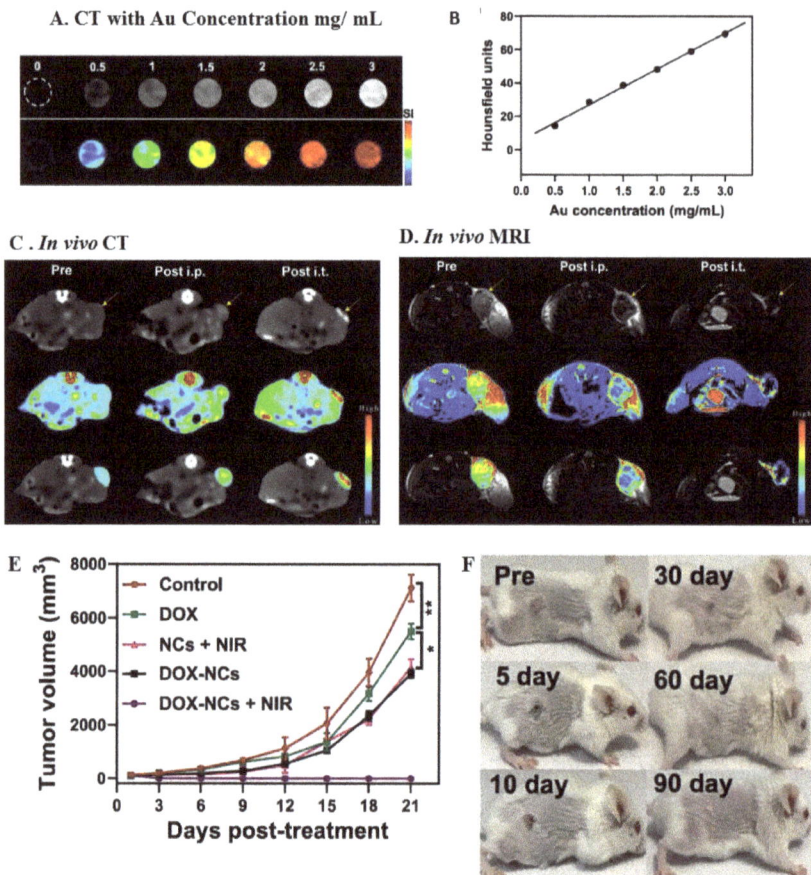

Figure 7. In vivo CT and MR imaging of NCs containing AuNPs and SPIOs. (**A**) CT images of CNs with increasing concentration of AuNPs from 0–3 mg/mL. (**B**) The corresponding graph of Hounsfield values with AuNPs concentration. In vivo (**C**) CT scan and (**D**) MR images of CT26 tumor bearing mice, pre and post injections at post i.p and post i.t. The upper, middle, and lower images are for original, intensity mapping, and merged images of all. (**E**) Corresponding results after PT where the graph shows reduction in tumor volume within few days of time with DOX-NCs+NIR. (**F**) The morphology of tumor and total mice view from pre injection to 90 days of therapy. The stars (*) represents the statistical significance of the data (* for 0.05, ** for 0.01). Reprinted/adapted with permission from Ref. [119]. Copy right 2022, copyright Ivyspring.

Apart from these three (CLSM, MRI, and CT) well used techniques PET, PAI, and ToF-SIMS, and combined MRI/CT, CT/PEI, MRI/CT/PL/PAI, and MRI/CT/EPR, could also be important tools to the earlier diagnosis. These are currently of great interest to nanomedicine researchers.

3.4. PET for Imaging Guided Therapy

Radio labelling techniques such as PET and CT have great sensitivity due to the low background, requirement of low signal amplification, and good penetration depth in vivo. As said earlier, nanographene-based scaffolds have a greater importance in radio imaging technology with the functionalization of radioactive elements such as ^{198,199}Au, ^{64}Cu, ^{66}Ga, ^{111}In, and ^{121}I. In this regard of PET imaging, for the first time GO-based targeting and non-targeting imaging agents such as ^{64}Cu-NOTA functionalized GO-PEG (^{64}Cu-NOTA-GO) and ^{64}Cu-NOTA-GO conjugated with TRC105 (^{64}Cu-NOTA-GO-TRC105) for targeting a CD105 (endogline) has been synthesized. ^{64}Cu was linked with GO-PEG via 1,4,7-triazacyclo nonane-1,4,7 triacetic acid (NOTA, a chelating agent of ^{64}Cu). As shown in Figure 8A–D, the ^{64}Cu-NOTA-GO-TRC105 has very good biodistribution and targeting ability towards 4T1 tumor-bearing mice compared to non-targeting ^{64}Cu-NOTA-GO, pre injected TRC105 blocking dosed mice, and CD105-negative MCF7 human breast cancer cells. The combined CT and PET images also can be seen in the images [120].

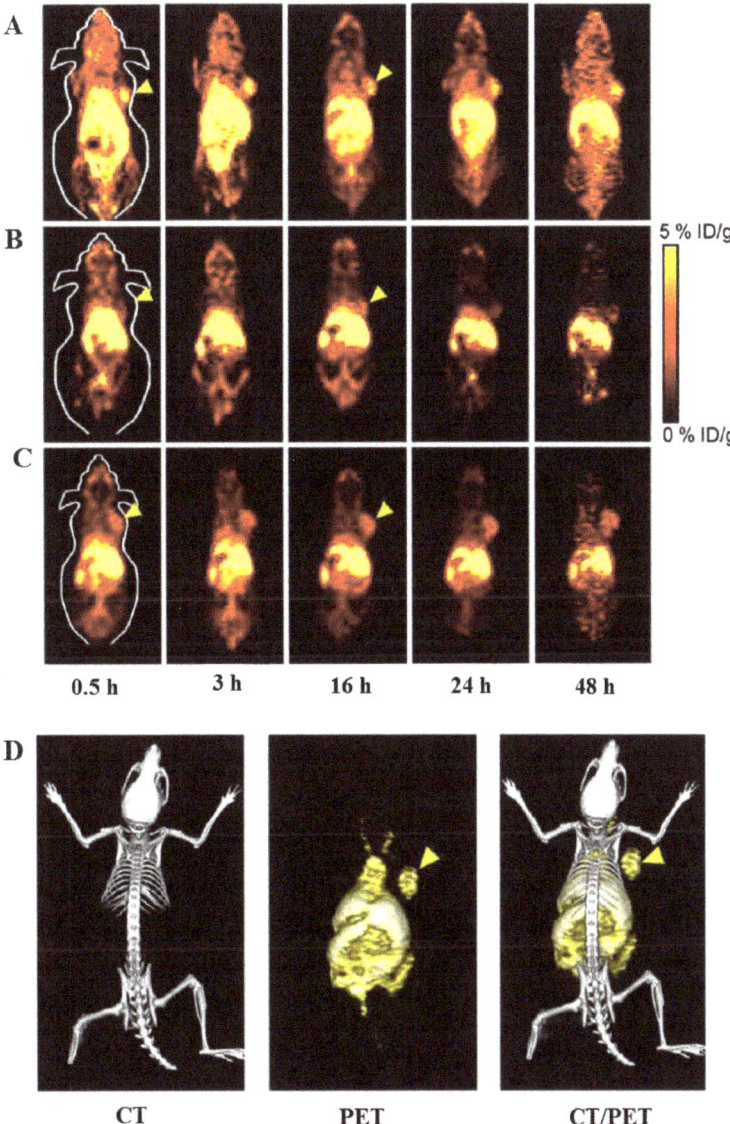

Figure 8. PET and CT in vivo 4T1 tumor containing mice images of GO labelled with ^{64}Cu isotope and tumor targeting TRC105 bioconjugate. (**A**) The post injected ^{64}Cu-NOTA-GO-TRC105 PET images with different time intervals from 0.5 h to 48 h. The arrows at the right corners of the images

indicate the tumor. (**B**) ^{64}Cu-NOTA-GO alone TRC105, and (**C**) Preinjected blocking dose of TRC105. The tumor specificity is very apparent in case of GO functionalized with TRC105 than not functionalized GO. (**D**) The CT, PET, and combined CT/PET images of ^{64}Cu-NOTA-GO-TRC105. Reprinted/adapted with permission from Ref. [120]. Copy right 2012, copyright ACS.

After that ^{66}Ga was functionalized to GO and obtained the same result with similar strategy of PET imaging of 4T1 cells in vitro, in vivo and ex vivo with good distribution in the body without toxicity [121]. Later, the same researchers labelled the ^{64}Cu to the rGO with the same synthetic adaption to prepare ^{64}Cu-NOTA-rGO-TRC105 for targeting 4T1 murine breast cancer cells and obtained successful results than with non-targeting rGO nanodrug [122]. Very recently, radioactive iodine (^{124}I)-labelled GO nanocomposite has been reported for PET imaging and boron delivery inside mice. The images reveal that time-dependent biodistribution in the liver, spleen, stomach, and heart for long-time circulation inside the body, up to 48 h. The in vitro studies of *C. elegans* confirmed that the ^{124}I-GO does not show any significant toxicity. Hence ^{124}I-GO could be a better candidate for boron neutron capture therapy of cancer [123].

3.5. PAI for Imaging Guided Therapy

PAI is another non-invasive imaging model to monitor the tumor environment with greater resolution and high tissue penetration depth. The PA signal production involves the following process. The light energy absorbed by the material converts into heat and increases the temperature, followed by thermoelastic expansion which causes the generation of acoustic waves (AWs). The AW generates an image contrast respective to the concentration of the absorbing material. In this regard, light absorbing nanomaterials have an advantage of converting photo energy into thermal energy and generation of AWs for better PAI imaging [124,125]. Among carbon nanomaterials, graphene-based 2D nanomaterials and their composites draw great interest in the study of PAI imaging due to their unique light absorption from UV, VIS, to NIR-I and NIR-II regions. Based on the belief of the light absorption of graphene, RGO are highly advantageous than GO as the later has a poor absorption of light in the visible and NIR regions [126]. Graphene-based nanoplatelets and nanoribbons (GNRs) are tested for PAI and thermal acoustic imaging (TAI) imaging. The oxidized GNRs were found to reveal dual modal PAI and TAI imaging [127]. Similar results of NIR absorption of microwaves reducing RGO-based PAI has been reported, and it is believed that the imaging intensities are wavelength-independent [128]. In the same year, dye-enhanced NIR absorption of GO was reported to overcome the limitations of GO absorption in NIR region to produce PA images for phototherapy of cancer. It was observed that the GO-ICG-FA (indocynine green an NIR absorbing dye and folic acid, a tumor targeting agent) showed better contrast, and no contrast was observed with GO-ICG or GO-FA alone [129]. Graphene microbubbles as an enhanced NIR PAI contrast agent was also reported with good biocompatibility and spatial resolution [130]. Another work describes that GO functionalized with chitosan–FA (GO-CS-FA) has good success as a PA and fluorescence tumor vascular imaging guided therapy for cancer in vivo [131].

A dual modal PAI and photothermal imaging probe rGADA nanocomposite was fabricated by the rGO functionalized with AuNS (gold nanostars), bilayered lipids, FA (rGADA), and K-Ras gene plasmid (KrasI) rGADA-KrasI, for targeted imaging guided photothermal and gene therapy of pancreatic cancer. The Figure 9A shows that there is a good PAI contrast with increasing concentrations of rGADA. The Figure 9B reveals in vivo tumor PAI imaging at different times from 0–48 h showing that a distinct rGADA at tumor has been apparent with time. Figure 9C,D are photothermal curves for the temperature rise of the nanocomposite and photothermal images at 808 nm. From the information obtained from the above experiments it is evident that the rGADA has successfully internalized and distributed at the tumor site for PTT and gene transfection of cancer in vivo. In vivo PTT experiments showed 76.1% tumor suppression under laser with rGADA+L, whereas the gene therapy results in 55.2% with rGADA-KrasI. The combined PTT and gene therapies ofrGADA-KrasI + L with laser resulted in very good tumor suppression of 98.5% compared individual therapy and therapy without a laser. The measured comparative weights are shown in Figure 9E of the tumors for controls and rGADA-KrasI after laser irradiation. They demonstrate that a negligible and completely vanished tumor was evidenced [132]. Similarly, rGO–AuNPs also reported to PAI for NIR–II phototherapy [133]. Hence, graphene-based targeted multiple imaging guided combination therapies could be a very good idea in the implementation of non-invasive theranostic probes.

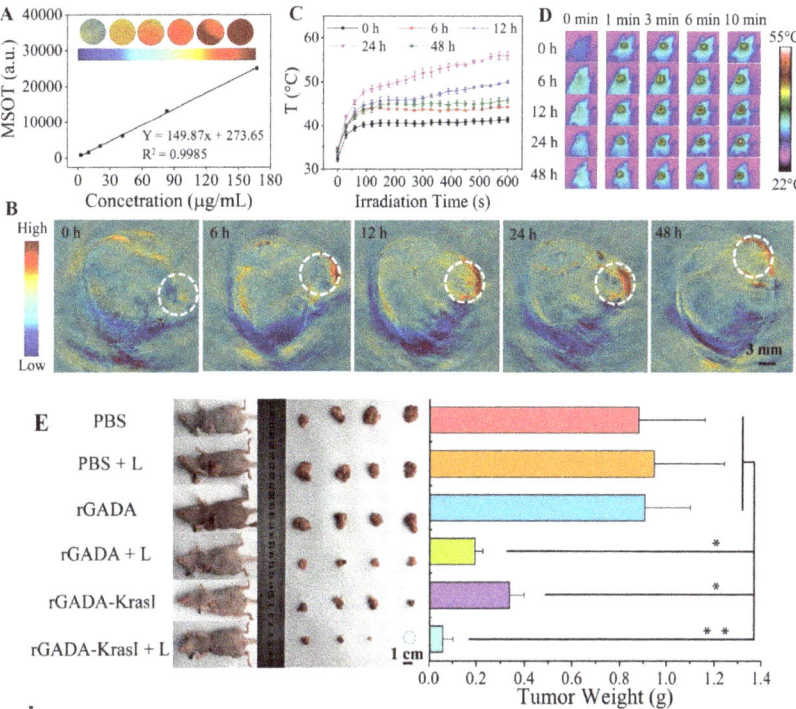

Figure 9. PAI and PT images of rGADA with different concentration and, at different time after intravenous injection to mice containing Capan-1 tumor and, PT and gene therapies with RGADA-KrasI. (**A,B**) are for PAI images of samples and in mice. The white circles represent the tumor region. (**C,D**) are temperature curves of tumor with different irradiation times (0–48 h) and thermographic images from in vivo tumor site at the irradiation time of 10 min with 808 nm laser with 1.2 W/cm^2 power densities. (**E**) Tumor bearing mice and its weights before and after laser treatment with PBS-L, rGADA + L, and rGADA-KrasI + L. The stars (*) represents the statistical significance of the data (* for 0.05, ** for 0.01). Reprinted/adapted with permission from Ref. [132]. Copy right 2020, copyright Wiley-VCH.

3.6. Raman for Imaging Guided Therapy

Raman is a spectroscopic technique named by its inventor Sir. C. V. Raman in 1928 who proposed the Raman Effect. The phenomenon is based on the inelastic and elastic scattering of light from the vibrations of objects such as nanomaterials, drugs, and other biological molecules. When this technique is coupled with microscopy it is called Raman microscopy, and can be used to visualize in vitro and in vivo biological components, internalized nanomaterials, and drugs with high specificity and sensitivity at workable spatial resolutions. However, high sample concentration is required for better resolution and fast image acquisition due to the weak scattering signals. To overcome this hurdle, Resonance Raman (RR), Surface-Enhanced Raman Spectroscopy (SERS), and Coherent Raman spectroscopy (CRS) were developed. Scientists have mostly adopted SERS in nanomedicine due to its signal enhancement in the presence of rough surface nanomaterials such as Au, Ag, and Cu in the sample system [134].

A GO@Au and fluorescent tag functionalized dual modal luminescent and Raman imaging has been reported [135]. Moreover, the GO-Ag nanocomposite for a SERS-based imaging cellular probe and FA for targeting the tumor to impart was prepared. The GO-Ag-FA treated cells have shown excellent uptake and cellular internalization and evidenced by SERS images taken after 2 h of incubation time [136]. In addition, a AuNR@GO nanocomposite functionalized with DOX to obtain DOX@GO@AuNRs for chemo and PT of HeLa cancer cells was reported. The GO and AuNRs showed strong SERS signals, but the DOX signals decreased within the cells due to the phagocytosis and the acidic environment inside the cells. The prepared nanomaterial showed good SERS signals and temperature changes upon laser irradiation. Hence it demonstrated good chemo-PTT results under light and was titled as a two-step Raman guided therapy [137]. After GO, an RGO-based, SERS-guided, low laser-powered, targeted PT was reported by preparing anti-EGFR-PEG-rGO@CPSS-Au-R6G. The RGO was functionalized with PEG, CPSS (carbon porous silica nanosheets), Au nanosheets, R6G, (Rhodamine 6G a Raman reporter), and anti-EGFR (epidermal growth factor receptor for targeting tumor) for sensitive low-powered laser-efficient NIR PT therapy against A549 and MRC-5 cells [138].

Recently, a SERS-guided multi modal chemo, gene, and PT of cancer with Au@GO-NP-NACs was reported, where the NP stands for nanoparticles and NACs for nucleic acid components ex. BCL2 mRNA. Figure 10A shows the schematic image of the guided SERS imaging and therapy in vivo. There is a tumor microenvironment which depicts the heterogeneity of the tumor, and the laser illumination of the tumor and normal tissue projects the effectiveness of the tumor eradication with Au@GO-NP-NACs. Figure 10B is for schematic representation of SERS signals at non-tumor and tumor site and the SERS intensity mapping, where the intensity of Cy5 is high at non-tumor tissues and less at the tumor. Figure 10C shows the corresponding Raman spectrum intensities at 1120 cm of Raman dye in different tissues. From the observation of the mapping and the spectral intensity, the SERS was varied, and we observed very weak signal at tumor in vivo due to the over expression of BCL2 in mice after the injection of the graphene drug. This kind of analysis is indispensable to evaluate drug distribution and its circulation in healthy and unhealthy tissues for specific and effective eradication of cancer. After the therapy process, the tumor from tissue has removed and observed its volume compared with untreated tumors. It was found that there is a great reduction in its volume in (Au@GO-NP-NACs) NP-NIR-treated mice, as shown in Figure 10D. The comparative tumor volume and time of therapy with control, NIR, and non-NIR treated NPs (Au@GO-NP-NACs) was plotted and it was apparent that the therapy was highly effective with NIR laser and NPs after 3 weeks (Figure 10E). The same material was functionalized with DOX and other types of genetic materials to evaluate the combined chemo-gene–PT of cancer to provide a better outlook of the therapy results in a single and minimal dosage of a drug, within a short time, with non-invasive NIR lasers. Such efforts for evaluating the potential of single material theranostic ability are highly warranted in nanomedicine to clear the hurdles of clinical trials [139].

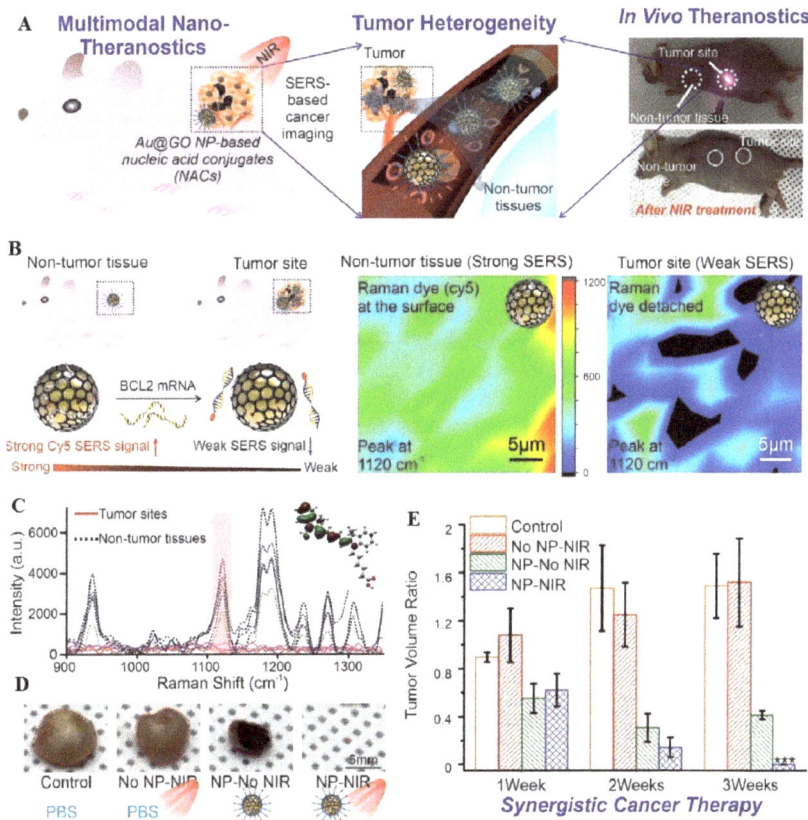

Figure 10. In vivo Raman (SERS) imaging and multimodal therapy of cancer. (**A**) Au@GO NP-NACs injected mice, tumor heterogeneity and PT. (**B**) Schematic diagram for non-tumor and tumor tissue and corresponding SERS mappings. (**C**) Raman shifts and SERS intensities at tumor sites and non-tumor tissues. (**D**) Extracted tumor from mice after 3 days of PT, the images are for control, without NP and NIR laser, with NP and without NIR laser, with NP and with NIR laser treated tumor and its volume. The NP-NIR treated tumor has shown a complete shrinkage of tumor. (**E**) The tumor volume ratio with synergistic cancer therapies of control, no NP-NIR, NP-No NIR, and NP-NIR. After 3 weeks of the therapy, the NP-NIR gave a remarkable therapy result of close to zero tumor volume ratio. Reprinted/adapted with permission from Ref. [139]. Copy right 2020, copyright Wiley-VCH.

3.7. ToF-SIMS for Cellular Imaging and Guided Cancer Therapy

ToF-SIMS imaging is one of the most surface-sensitive techniques to analyze chemical compositions of materials and biological systems containing chemical components. It has great capability to map low molecular weight components (<500 KD) and submicron resolution. ToF-SIMS involves sputtering the primary ion beam (Bi_3^+, Ar_n^+, and C_{60}^+) with the sample surface, and the secondary ions generated from the sample will be collected according to their flight times and its mass/charge. The chemical compositions can be predicted based on their respective masses in comparison with the reference library. This technique is unique in imaging single cells, human tissues, and skin and cancer cells, and could be an important label-free tool to diagnosis the cancer cells from healthy normal cells. It is helpful in studying the toxicity of nanomaterials, drug internalization into the cells, apoptosis, and to predict other cellular killing mechanisms by collecting and imaging the cellular components' mass/time values [140,141]. The information obtained also has great importance in predicting the drug and cellular interactions, hence also in drug development and pharmacology studies [142]. However, it has a limitation of low sensitivity in analyzing the very low molecular weight components in wet samples, as the large molecules' excessive fragmentation obtained with a high energy ion beam is not very accurate. As a result, any material which could enhance the signal sensitivity has priority, as every single fragment is indispensable in predicting the disease information. GO and graphene have been used as a matrix material for enhancing surface sensitivity and signal intensity in analyzing small lipid molecules [143].

The potential toxicity by ZnO NPs in sun cream is of increasing concern. We have developed ToF-SIMS and CLSM imaging methods using human skin equivalent HaCaT cells as a model system for rapid and sensitive ZnO NPs cytotoxicity study (Figure 11A). The CLSM images (Figure 11B) revealed the absorption and localization of ZnO NPs in the cytoplasm and nuclei. The TOF-SIMS images demonstrated elevated levels of intracellular ZnO concentration and associated Zn concentration-dependent 40Ca/39K ratio, presumably caused by the dissolution behavior of ZnO NPs (Figure 11C). The imaging results demonstrated spatially-resolved cytotoxicity relationship between intracellular ZnO NPs, ^{40}Ca/^{39}K ratio, phosphocholine fragments, and glutathione fragments [144].

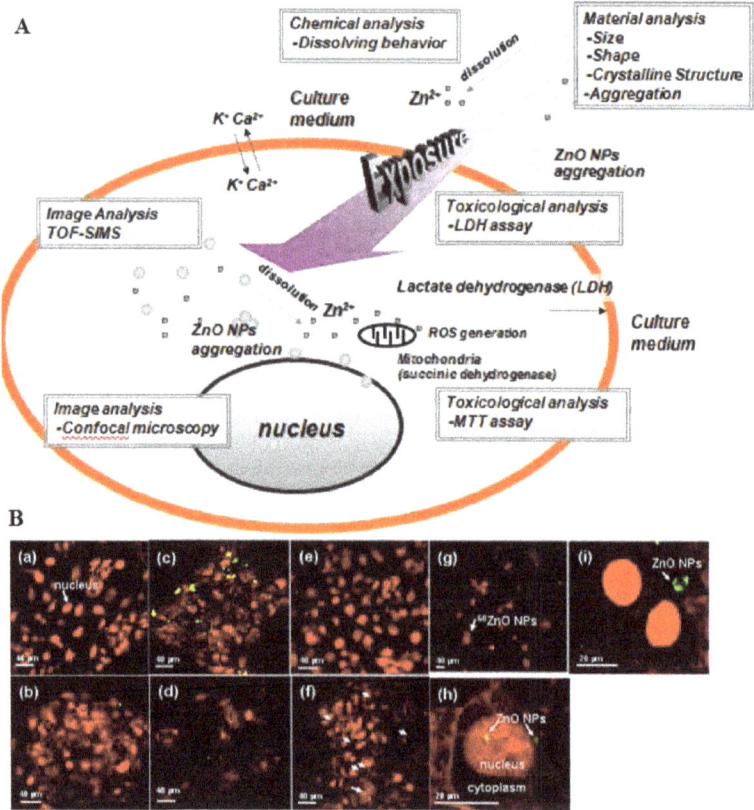

Figure 11. Cont.

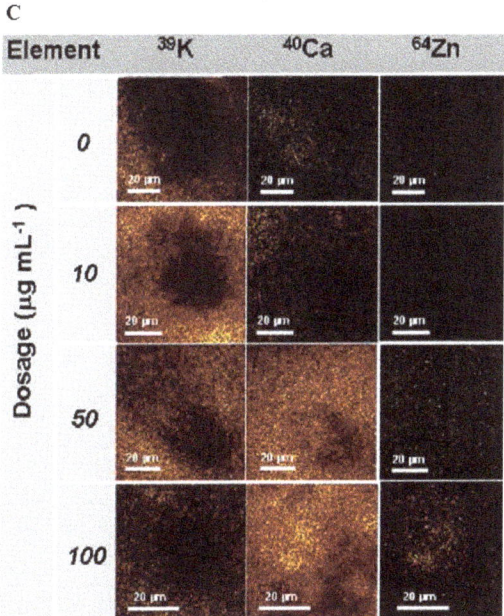

Figure 11. (**A**) Schematic illustration of integrating CLSM and Tof-SIMS image analyses for cytotoxicity study of ZnO NPs in HaCaT cells. (**B**) The confocal images of HaCaT cells treated with different ZnO NPs concentration (**a**) 0, (**b**) 10, (**c**) 50, and (**d**) 100 µg/mL; ^{68}ZnO NPs (**e**) 10, (**f**) 50, and (**g**) 100; (**h**,**i**) enlarged images of individual cells treated with 50 and 100 µg/mL ZnO NPs. Green fluorescence and red color, respectively, represent the ZnO (^{68}ZnO) NPs and nuclei of HaCaT cells (highlighted by arrow mark in (**f**): ^{68}ZnO NPs). (**C**) The TOF-SIMS ion images of ^{39}K$^+$, ^{40}Ca$^+$, and ^{64}Zn$^+$ of HaCaT cells treated with 0, 10, 50, and 100 µg/mL ZnO NPs. Scale bar is 20 µm [144]. Reprinted/adapted with permission from Ref. [144]. Copy right 2014, copyright Elsevier.

In a recent study, the ToF-SIMS signal enhancement of the single layer graphene covered wet cells with Bi$_3^+$ as a primary ion source was reported. The secondary ion imaging of cholesterol at *m/z* 369.25, phosphoethanolamine at *m/z* 142.05, palmitic acid at *m/z* 255.25, and oleic acid at *m/z* 281.26 are mapped [145]. An earlier study on the signal enhancement of ToF-SIMS by amine functionalized graphene quantum dots (GQDs) also show a better signal enhancement compared to hydroxyl GQDs in a comparative study [146]. From the above discussion it was evident that, GO, GQDs, and graphene have a remarkable effect on the quality of ToF-SIMS spectra and imaging and can overcome the hurdles of wet cell imaging's complex matrix effects. Non-invasive multimodal imaging by a single nanoprobe could offer a greater advantage of gathering the diagnosis information from each technique by providing its advantage where an individual imaging technique cannot. It will improve diagnosis accuracy and efficiency. Moreover, the multiple nanoprobe-based nanotheranostic material offers minimal toxicity and provides body–blood clearance easily by avoiding multiple drug dosages. In brief, each technique has its advantages and disadvantages. However, highly sensitive, non-invasive techniques could take a greater importance than other techniques in nanomedicine in the future.

3.8. Guided Phototherapy of Bacteria

Bacterial infections have led to millions of patients dying every year all over the world. Generally, antibiotic treatment has been used for bacterial infections. However, inappropriate and overuse of antibiotics has led to an increase in the drug-fighting capacity of bacteria [146]. Notably, antibiotic resistance is related to structure transformation, gene mutation, and bacterial biofilm formation. Additionally, biofilm is a multicellular bacterial group surrounded by its own synthesized extracellular polymeric material composed of proteins, polysaccharides, lipids, and extracellular DNA [147]. The extracellular polymeric material provides an appropriate microenvironment for bacterial growth, and protection against antibiotics, and hence, bacterial infection control becomes an obstinate challenge. Thus, there is an urgent need to find new strategies to combat bacterial infections [148]. PTT gained increasing demand in the medical field over conventional antibiotic therapy because it destructs bacteria and their biofilm. Specifically, PTT combined with NIR light has various benefits, including deep tissue penetration, spatiotemporal controllability, and little light absorption in tissue. Nevertheless, the disadvantage of PTT is that a nonselective thermal effect may arise due to the weak affinity between pathogenic bacteria and a photothermal agent that may damage healthy cells during irradiation [149].

Increasing bacterial infections are a serious problem for human health. Hence, the synthesis of multifunctional antibacterial materials is needed for surgical operations. Concerning this situation, we prepared non-targeted and targeted magnetic graphene and carbon nanotubes against *S. aureus* and *E. coli* for PTT. Excellent bacterial capturing efficiency (Figure 12A,B) was observed with MRGOGA (magnetic RGO functionalized with glutaraldehyde). This was also evident from the SEM images shown in Figure 12C. The batch-mode- and continuous-mode PTT showed 99% killing efficiency under NIR laser irradiation at 808 nm, shown in Figure 12B. The plate count method, shown in Figure 12D, demonstrated that both the strains had completely vanished after laser treatment with MRGOGA [150,151].

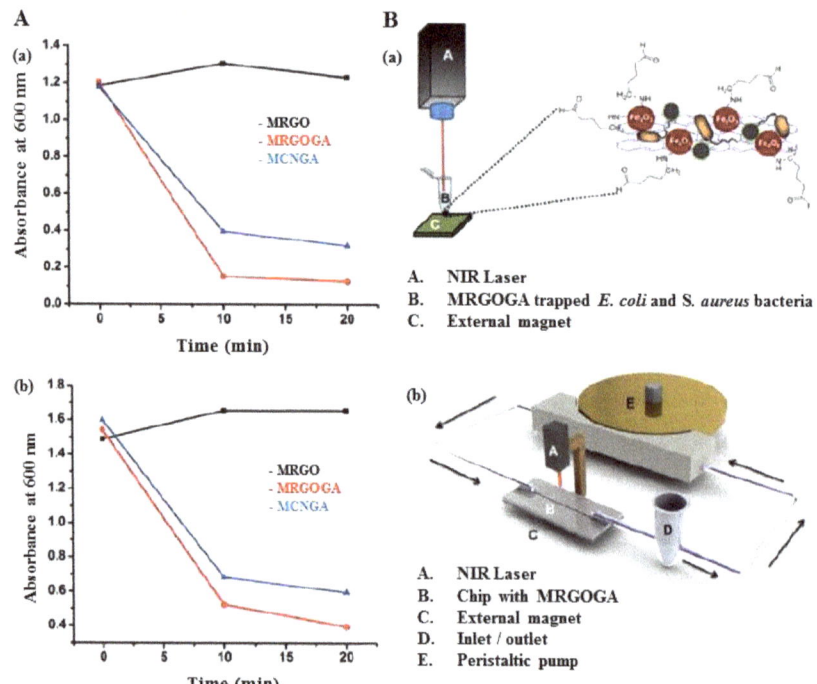

Figure 12. *Cont.*

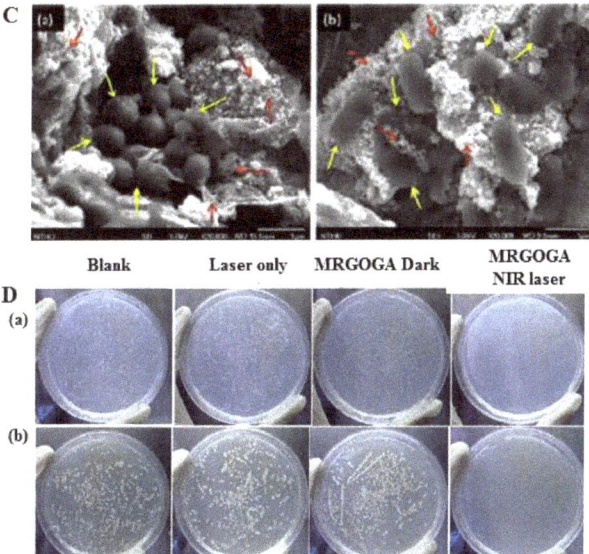

Figure 12. Efficient capture and targeted PTT of bacteria by MRGO, MRGOGA, and MCNGA. (**A**) The capturing capability of *S. aureus* (**a**) and *E. coli* (**b**). (**B**) The batch mode and dynamic mode (lab on chip) PTT with laser irradiated at 808 nm. (**C**) SEM of *E. coli* (**a**) and *S. aureus* (**b**) after capturing by MRGOGA. (**D**) Bacterial plates for both *S. aureus* (**a**) and *E. coli* (**b**), blank, laser only, MRGOGA dark, and MRGOGA with NIR laser. Reprinted/adapted with permission from Ref. [150]. Copy right 2013, copyright ACS 2013.

We have started working on phototherapy of bacterial infection with progressive achievements firstly using ZnO NPs [152] followed by using modified carbon nanotubes [153] and lastly extends to biomimetic applications using graphene nanomaterials [154–157]. The trend of using graphene nanomaterials is just at the beginning. For instance, the preparation of GO-functionalized (noncovalent) PEGylated phthalocyanines was used for antibacterial phototherapy (ZnPc-TEGMME@GO). The antibacterial activity against *E. coli* and *S. aureus* bacteria at different illumination was shown in Figure 13A,B. As reported, the synthesized nanocomposite showed PTT/PDT capacity with antibacterial activity. The authors further recorded SEM images before and after the treatment of nanocomposites against bacteria. The formation of holes on the bacterial surface confirmed the damage to the cell membrane. Further, the material was demonstrated in vivo by considering mice as a model animal. From the thermographic images it was confirmed that the material was internalized and can create local heating around the wound. Hence, it favors the in vivo PT/PDT, and the results after irradiation with 450 nm (PTT) and 680 nm (PDT) confirmed complete wound healing after 12 days of treatment. Whereas the control mice has the persistent wound even after laser irradiation without photodrug (Figure 13C–E) [76]. In addition, the concept of targeted nanoparticles in cancer therapy with in vivo biocompatibility of graphene-based nanomaterials is summarized. The detailed chemistry and properties of GO as well as the review of functionalized GO and GO-metal nanoparticle composites in nanomedicine for anticancer drug delivery and cancer treatment is reviewed [158]. Moreover, the concept of targeted nanoparticles in cancer therapy with in vivo biocompatibility of graphene-based nanomaterials is summarized. The detailed chemistry and properties of GO as well as the functionalized GO and GO-metal nanoparticle composites in nanomedicine for anticancer drug delivery and cancer treatment is reviewed [159].

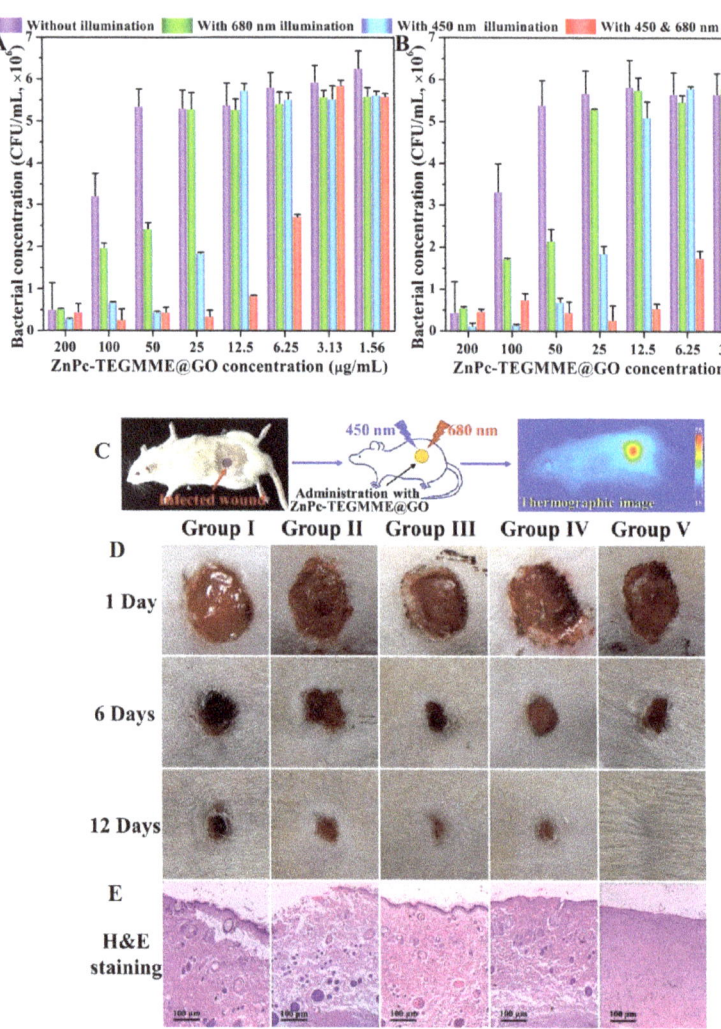

Figure 13. (**A**,**B**) for *S. aureus* and *E. coli* antibacterial activity with ZnPc-TEGMME@GO at different lasers (450 nm and 680 nm) triggered combined PTT/PDT. (**C**) In vivo antibacterial activity to infected mice treated with ZnPc-TEGMME@GO and its thermographic images. (**D**) Infected wound area before and after PT from Day 1 to day 12 represented in five groups. Group I with saline water and dark. Group II is ZnPc-TEGMME@GO and dark. Group III is ZnPc-TEGMME@GO 680 nm laser. Group IV is for ZnPc-TEGMME@GO and 450 nm lasers and finally Group V is for ZnPc-TEGMME@GO with 680 nm and 450 nm laser. (**E**) H&E (Hematoxylin and Eosin) Staining [76]. Reprinted/adapted with permission from Ref. [76]. Copy right 2021, copyright ACS 2021.

In another study, the RGO was functionalized with polycationic poly-L-lysine (PLL) because of more drug loading capability with colloidal stability. Further, rGO-PLL is labeled with anti-HER2 to form a bond with HER2 receptors to detect breast cancer cells [159].

3.9. Comparison among GNCs

According to the above research discussion, every author made their contribution towards this field. Dai et al., for the first time, introduced the GO and RGO to the theranostic applications, thereby extensively contributing to this important research. Later, other researchers gave their insights to fuel the graphene nanomedicine. For instance, we have prepared MFG to impart long-range absorption of graphene in both biological window I and II, along with demonstrating the CLSM/MRI and both single light induced PTT/PDT [70,95,96]. Choi et al., Yang et al., Mirrahimi et al., Hong et al., Jia et al., Yang et al., Belu et al., and Lim et al. demonstrated multimodal imaging (CLSM, MRI, CT, PET, PAI, RAMAN and ToF-SIMS) and multimodal therapies including chemo, gene, and PTs. Most of these researchers have also given tremendous efforts to improve the therapeutic capabilities by minimizing GNCs concentration, laser wavelengths from the first biological windows to the second biological window, and less laser powers and irradiation times [84,97,107,108,119,120,132,139,145,146]. Keshav et al., provided excellent pharmacokinetic data to take the material towards preclinical trials. Table 1 represents some of the interesting works discussed. Based on the comparison of the tabulated literature, 808 nm laser with irradiation time of 5–15 min with ~1 W/cm^2 and ~100 µg/mL were the most suitable parameters for phototheranostics. In the case of bacteria, the same parameters are good for photodisinfection. However, according to us and to Liang et al., experiments with very low powers and GNCs dosage have also shown great therapeutic effects [96,150,158]. As each datum is indispensable, we appreciate the existing literature greatly. Apart from GNCs, there are several nanomaterials which have been reported for nanomedicine. Among the reported carbon, Au, Fe, Si, dendrimer, and polymer nanomaterials are highly suitable as novel theranostic agents [160–164]. Graphene has a great advantage over other nanomaterials due its tunable size, dimensionality, tunable surface, covalent and non-covalent chemistry, atomic sensitivity and <nm thickness, easy synthesis, and its economic availability for both cancer therapy and antibacterial activity [165–167].

Table 1. Self-comparison of GNCs phototheranostic ability for cancer and bacterial infection.

No	GNCs	Imaging	Cell/Animal Model	Light and Power
	Time (min)	Therapy	Dose	Ref. No
1	MFG-SiNC$_4$	CLSM and MRI	HeLa cells/Zebrafish	Tungsten halogen lamp, 1 W/cm^2, 775 nm
	20	PTT/PDT	100 µg/mL	[70,95]
2	MS-RGO-ICG-PEG-FA	CLSM and IVIS	CT-26 cells/mice	808 nm laser, 2.0 W/cm^2
	10	PTT/PDT	100 µg/mL	[97]
3	GO (^{99m}Tc$^-$ and Gd-usNGO-PEG)	MRI and SPECT/CT	Lymph nodes	
	-	-	-	[107]
4	RGO-IONP-PEG	CLSM, MRI and PAT	4T1 tumor cells/mice	808 nm laser, 0.5 W cm^2
	5	PTT/PDT	2 mg/mL	[108]
5	ZnFe$_2$O$_4$/UCNPs	UCL, CT, MRI, PAT.	U14 cells/mice	980 nm laser, 0.8 W/cm^2
	15	PTT/PDT	250 µg/mL	[118]
6	DOX-NCs	CT and MRI	CT26 cells/mice	808 nm laser, 0.7 W/cm^2
	15	Chemo and PTT	20 µg/mL	[119]
7	^{64}Cu-NOTA-GO-TRC105	CT/PET	4T1 tumor cells/mice	
	-	-	-	[120]

Table 1. *Cont.*

No	GNCs	Imaging	Cell/Animal Model	Light and Power
	Time (min)	Therapy	Dose	Ref. No
8	rGADA-KrasI	PAI/PT	Pancreatic cancer cells/mice	808 nm laser, 1.2 W/cm^2
	10	PTT and gene therapy	0.6 mg/mL	[132]
9	anti-EGFR-PEG-rGO@CPSS-Au-R6G	Optical microscope/CLSM/SERS	A549 cells	808 nm laser, 0.5 W/cm^2
	5	PTT	100 µg/mL	[138]
10	Single layer graphene	ToF-SIMS	A549 cells	-
	-	-	-	[84]
11	GQDs	ToF-SIMS	MCF-7 cell	-
	-	-	-	[146]
12	MRGOGA	SEM and CLSM	*S. aureus* and *E. coli*	808 nm laser, 1.2 W/cm^2
	10	PTT	80 µg/mL	[150]
13	ZnPc-TEGMME@GO	SEM/Thermographic imaging	*S. aureus* and *E. coli*	450 nm and 680 nm lasers, 0.0142 W/cm^2
	10	PTT/PDT	50 µg/mL	[76]
14	RGO-PAA	CLSM	HeLa cells/*S. aureus* and *E. coli*	808 nm/1064 nm laser, 0.4 mW/cm^2
	10	PTT	3 mg/mL	[96]
15	Chitosan with ZnOQDs@GO	SEM/Thermographic imaging	*S. aureus* and *E. coli*	808 nm laser, 2 W/cm^2
	6	PTT	500 µg/mL	[158]

4. Conclusions and Future Perspectives

We summarized the recent progress of the general preparation and functionalization of GO, RGO, and GNCs as theranostic materials to provide simple and advanced imaging-guided therapeutic drugs to invade malignant tumors and bacterial infections. The water solubility, low toxicity, and high surface area of GO made a very good nanoplatform to carry many therapeutic organic drugs and to load different imaging probes. However, its low NIR absorption is unlikely, and not very favorable to the phototherapy of cancer and bacteria. Hence, RGO or functionalized nanocomposites of graphene-related materials provide a better solution to overcome the difficulties where GO cannot. The multi-modal imaging and PS functionalized nanographene composite provide a very accurate diagnostic confidence to proceed with the therapy of combined PTT/PDT, which may require in less time and smaller drug concentrations. Among the nanotherapies reported, phototherapy has good results, with less intensive time and energy, and without any side effects and damage to healthy tissues.

Graphene/GO/GQDs can offer diversified chemistry for self-acting luminescent for CLSM, magnetic for MRI, surface plasmonic state for SERS and ToF-SIMS signal enhancement, PAI imaging, and inherent PTT, PDT agent. It has great potential to carry many chemical drugs and genes for chemo- and gene therapies with very good biocompatibility. However, much research is required to move GNCs towards clinical implementation, as their size, shape, no of carbons, layers, number of oxygen functional groups, accurate mass, and photo yield to generate ROS and heat have to be optimized precisely. In perspective of PT, the biological windows must be explored in NIR-I and NIR-II. Overall, nanotechnology scientists could use flexible GNCs in whatever they want to fabricate.

Author Contributions: All authors conceptualized the outline and agreed on the content of the manuscript. G.G. and A.V.G. prepared the manuscript. Y.-C.L. revised the manuscript. All authors have read and agreed to the published version of the manuscript.

Funding: This research received no external funding.

Institutional Review Board Statement: Not applicable.

Informed Consent Statement: Not applicable.

Data Availability Statement: Not applicable.

Conflicts of Interest: The authors declare no conflict of interest.

References

1. Editorial: Reflecting on 20 years of progress. *Nat. Rev. Cancer* **2021**, *21*, 605. [CrossRef] [PubMed]
2. Knopman, D.S.; Amieva, H.; Petersen, R.C.; Chételat, G.; Holtzman, D.M.; Hyman, B.T.; Nixon, R.A.; Jones, D.T. Alzheimer disease. *Nat. Rev. Dis. Primers* **2021**, *7*, 33. [CrossRef]
3. Flora, G.D.; Nayak, M.K. A Brief Review of Cardiovascular Diseases. Associated Risk Factors and Current Treatment Regimes. *Curr. Pharm. Des.* **2019**, *25*, 4063–4084. [CrossRef] [PubMed]
4. Baker, R.E.; Mahmud, A.S.; Miller, I.F.; Rajeev, M.; Rasambainarivo, F.; Rice, B.L.; Takahashi, S.; Tatem, A.J.; Wagner, C.E.; Wang, L.F.; et al. Infectious disease in an era of global change. *Nat. Rev. Microbiol.* **2022**, *20*, 193–205. [CrossRef] [PubMed]
5. Salata, O.V. Applications of nanoparticles in biology and medicine. *J. Nanobiotechnol.* **2004**, *2*, 3. [CrossRef] [PubMed]
6. Gu, L.; Mooney, D.J. Biomaterials and emerging anticancer therapeutics: Engineering the microenvironment. *Nat. Rev. Cancer* **2016**, *16*, 56–66. [CrossRef]
7. Shi, J.; Kantoff, P.W.; Wooster, R.; Farokhzad, O.C. Cancer nanomedicine: Progress, challenges and opportunities. *Nat. Rev. Cancer* **2017**, *17*, 20–37. [CrossRef] [PubMed]
8. Chen, G.; Roy, I.; Yang, C.; Prasad, P.N. Nanochemistry and Nanomedicine for Nanoparticle-based Diagnostics and Therapy. *Chem. Rev.* **2016**, *116*, 2826–2885. [CrossRef]
9. Soares, S.; Sousa, J.; Pais, A.; Vitorino, C. Nanomedicine: Principles, Properties, and Regulatory Issues. *Front. Chem.* **2018**, *6*, 360. [CrossRef]
10. Rakhshandehroo, T.; Smith, B.R.; Glockner, H.J.; Rashidian, M.; Pandit-Taskar, N. Molecular Immune Targeted Imaging of Tumour Microenvironment. *Nanotheranostics* **2022**, *6*, 286. [CrossRef]
11. Chen, H.; Zhang, W.; Zhu, G.; Xie, J.; Chen, X. Rethinking cancer nanotheranostics. *Nat. Rev. Mater.* **2017**, *2*, 17024. [CrossRef]
12. Robson, A.L.; Dastoor, P.C.; Flynn, J.; Palmer, W.; Martin, A.; Smith, D.W.; Woldu, A.; Hua, S. Advantages and Limitations of Current Imaging Techniques for Characterizing Liposome Morphology. *Front. Pharmacol.* **2018**, *9*, 80. [CrossRef]
13. Man, F.; Lammers, T.; de Rosales, R.T.M. Imaging Nanomedicine-Based Drug Delivery: A Review of Clinical Studies. *Mol. Imaging Biol.* **2018**, *20*, 683–695. [CrossRef]
14. Adeel, M.; Duzagac, F.; Canzonieri, V.; Rizzolio, F. Self-therapeutic nanomaterials for cancer therapy: A review. *ACS Appl. Nano Mater.* **2020**, *3*, 4962–4971. [CrossRef]
15. Chabner, B.A., Jr.; Roberts, T.G. Chemotherapy and the war on cancer. *Nat. Rev. Cancer* **2005**, *5*, 65–72. [CrossRef]
16. Akkın, S.; Varan, G.; Bilensoy, E. A review on cancer immunotherapy and applications of nanotechnology to chemoimmunotherapy of different cancers. *Molecules* **2021**, *11*, 3382. [CrossRef]
17. Waldman, A.D.; Fritz, J.M.; Lenardo, M.J. A guide to cancer immunotherapy: From T cell basic science to clinical practice. *Nat. Rev. Immunol.* **2020**, *20*, 651–668. [CrossRef]
18. Bulaklak, K.; Gersbach, C.A. The once and future gene therapy. *Nat. Commun.* **2020**, *11*, 5820. [CrossRef]
19. Altun, İ.; Sonkaya, A. The most common side effects experienced by patients were receiving first cycle of chemotherapy. *Iran. J. Public Health* **2018**, *47*, 1218–1219.
20. Nurgali, K.; Jagoe, R.T.; Abalo, R. Editorial: Adverse effects of cancer chemotherapy: Anything new to improve tolerance and reduce sequelae? *Front. Pharmacol.* **2018**, *9*, 245. [CrossRef]
21. Schirrmacher, V. From chemotherapy to biological therapy: A review of novel concepts to reduce the side effects of systemic cancer treatment (Review). *Int. J. Oncol.* **2019**, *54*, 407–419.
22. Amjad, M.T.; Chidharla, A.; Kasi, A. *Cancer Chemotherapy*; StatPearls Publishing: Treasure Island, CA, USA, 2022.
23. Shi, H.; Sadler, P.J. How promising is phototherapy for cancer? *Br. J. Cancer* **2020**, *123*, 871–873. [CrossRef]
24. Chitgupi, U.; Qin, Y.; Lovell, J.F. Targeted nanomaterials for phototherapy. *Nanotheranostics* **2017**, *1*, 38–58. [CrossRef]
25. Ma, Y.; Zhang, Y.; Li, X.; Zhao, Y.; Li, M.; Jiang, W.; Tang, X.; Dou, J.; Lu, L.; Wang, F.; et al. Near-Infrared II phototherapy induces deep tissue immunogenic cell death and potentiates cancer immunotherapy. *ACS Nano* **2019**, *13*, 11967–11980. [CrossRef]
26. Zhang, X.; Wang, S.; Cheng, G.; Yu, P.; Chang, J. Light-responsive nanomaterials for cancer therapy. *Engineering* **2022**, *13*, 18–30. [CrossRef]
27. Albanese, A.; Tang, P.S.; Chan, W.C.W. The effect of nanoparticle size, shape, and surface chemistry on biological systems. *Annu. Rev. Biomed. Eng.* **2012**, *14*, 1–16. [CrossRef]

28. Renero-Lecuna, C.; Iturrioz-Rodríguez, N.; González-Lavado, E.; Padín-González, E.; Navarro-Palomares, E.; Valdivia-Fernández, L.; García-Hevia, L.; Fanarraga, M.L. Effect of size, shape, and composition on the interaction of different nanomaterials with Hela cells. *Hindawi J. Nanomater.* **2019**, *11*, 7518482. [CrossRef]
29. Raza, M.A.; Kanwal, Z.; Rauf, A.; Sabri, A.N.; Riaz, S.; Naseem, S. Size- and shape-dependent antibacterial studies of silver nanoparticles synthesized by wet chemical routes. *Nanomaterials* **2016**, *6*, 74. [CrossRef]
30. Garg, B.; Sung, C.H.; Ling, Y.C. Graphene-based nanomaterials as molecular imaging agents. *Wiley Interdiscip. Rev. Nanomed. Nanobiotechnol.* **2015**, *7*, 737–758. [CrossRef]
31. Mao, H.Y.; Laurent, S.; Chen, W.; Akhavan, O.; Imani, M.; Ashkarran, A.A.; Mahmoudi, M. Graphene: Promises, facts, opportunities, and challenges in nanomedicine. *Chem. Rev.* **2013**, *113*, 3407–3424. [CrossRef]
32. Gollavelli, G.; Ling, Y.C. Chapter 21 Ultrathin graphene structure, fabrication and characterization for clinical diagnosis applications. In *Smart Nanodevices for Point-of-Care Applications*; SuvardhanKanchi, S., Chokkareddy, R., Rezakazemi, M., Eds.; CRC Press: Boca Raton, FL, USA, 2022; pp. 263–280.
33. Yin, P.T.; Shah, S.; Chhowalla, M.; Lee, K.B. Design, synthesis, and characterization of graphene-nanoparticle hybrid materials for bioapplications. *Chem. Rev.* **2015**, *115*, 2483–2531. [CrossRef]
34. Markovic, Z.M.; Harhaji-Trajkovic, L.M.; Todorovic-Markovic, B.M.; Kepić, D.P.; Arsikin, K.M.; Jovanović, S.P.; Pantovic, A.C.; Dramićanin, M.D.; Trajkovic, V.S. In vitro comparison of the photothermal anticancer activity of graphene nanoparticles and carbon nanotubes. *Biomaterials* **2011**, *32*, 1121–1129. [CrossRef]
35. Edwards, R.S.; Coleman, K.S. Graphene synthesis: Relationship to applications. *Nanoscale* **2013**, *5*, 38–51. [CrossRef]
36. Tang, L.; Li, X.; Ji, R.; Teng, K.S.; Tai, G.; Ye, J.; Wei, C.; Lau, S.P. Bottom-up synthesis of large-scale graphene oxide nanosheets. *J. Mater. Chem.* **2012**, *22*, 5676–5683. [CrossRef]
37. Eskiizmir, G.; Baskın, Y.; Yapıcı, K. Chapter 9 Graphene-based nanomaterials in cancer treatment and diagnosis. In *Fullerens, Graphenes and Nanotubes: A Pharmaceutical Approach*; Grumezescu, A.M., Ed.; Elsevier: Amsterdam, The Netherlands, 2018; pp. 331–374.
38. Shamaila, S.; Sajjad, A.K.L.; Iqbal, A. Modifications in development of graphene oxide synthetic routes. *Chem. Eng. J.* **2016**, *294*, 458–477. [CrossRef]
39. Marcano, D.C.; Kosynkin, D.V.; Berlin, J.M.; Sinitskii, A.; Sun, Z.; Slesarev, A.; Alemany, L.; Lu, W.; Tour, M.M. Improved synthesis of graphene oxide. *ACS Nano* **2010**, *4*, 4806–4814. [CrossRef]
40. Naeem, H.; Ajmal, M.; Muntha, S.; Ambreen, J.; Siddiq, M. Synthesis and characterization of graphene oxide sheets integrated with gold nanoparticles and their applications to adsorptive removal and catalytic reduction of water contaminants. *RSC Adv.* **2018**, *8*, 3599–3610. [CrossRef]
41. Wu, S.; Zhao, X.; Cui, Z. Cytotoxicity of graphene oxide and graphene oxide loaded with doxorubicin on human multiple myeloma cells. *Int. J. Nanomed.* **2014**, *9*, 1413–1421.
42. Yu, X.; Gao, D.; Gao, L.; Lai, J.; Zhang, C.; Zhao, Y.; Zhong, L.; Jia, B.; Wang, F.; Chen, X.; et al. Inhibiting Metastasis and Preventing Tumor Relapse by Triggering Host Immunity with Tumor-Targeted Photodynamic Therapy Using Photosensitizer-Loaded Functional Nanographenes. *ACS Nano* **2017**, *11*, 10147–10158. [CrossRef]
43. Zhou, L.; Wang, W.; Tang, J.; Zhou, J.H.; Jiang, H.J.; Shen, J. Graphene oxide noncovalent photosensitizer and its anticancer activity in vitro. *Chem. Eur. J.* **2011**, *17*, 12084–12091. [CrossRef]
44. Yin, F.; Hu, K.; Chen, Y. SiRNA Delivery with PEGylated Graphene Oxide Nanosheets for Combined Photothermal and Genetherapy for Pancreatic Cancer. *Theranostics* **2017**, *7*, 1133–1148. [CrossRef] [PubMed]
45. Narayanaswamy, V.; Obaidat, I.M.; Kamzin, A.S.; Latiyan, S.; Jain, S.; Kumar, H.; Srivastava, C.; Alaabed, S.; Issa, B. Synthesis of Graphene Oxide-Fe$_3$O$_4$ Based Nanocomposites Using the Mechanochemical Method and In Vitro Magnetic Hyperthermia. *Int. J. Mol. Sci.* **2019**, *20*, 3368. [CrossRef] [PubMed]
46. Yang, H.W.; Lu, Y.J.; Lin, K.J.; Hsu, S.C.; Huang, C.Y.; She, S.H.; Liu, H.L.; Lin, C.W.; Xiao, M.C.; Wey, S.P.; et al. Biomaterials EGRF conjugated PEGylated nanographene oxide for targeted chemotherapy and photothermal therapy. *Biomaterials* **2013**, *34*, 7204–7214. [CrossRef]
47. Miao, W.; Shim, G.; Lee, S.; Lee, S.; Choe, Y.S.; Oh, Y.K. Safety and tumor tissue accumulation of pegylated graphene oxide nanosheets for co-delivery of anticancer drug and photosensitizer. *Biomaterials* **2013**, *34*, 3402–3410. [CrossRef]
48. Xu, Z.; Wang, S.; Li, Y.; Wang, M.; Shi, P.; Huang, X. Covalent functionalization of graphene oxide with biocompatible poly(ethylene glycol) for delivery of paclitaxel. *ACS Appl. Mater. Interfaces* **2014**, *6*, 17268–17276. [CrossRef]
49. Yue, L.; Wang, J.; Dai, Z.; Hu, Z.; Chen, X.; Qi, Y.; Zheng, X.; Yu, D. pH-Responsive, Self-Sacrificial Nanotheranostic Agent for Potential n Vivo and in Vitro Dual Modal MRI/CT Imaging, Real-Time, and in Situ Monitoring of Cancer Therapy. *Bioconjug. Chem.* **2017**, *28*, 400–409. [CrossRef]
50. Liu, J.; Yuan, X.; Deng, L.; Yin, Z.; Tian, X.; Bhattacharyya, S. Graphene oxide activated by 980 nm laser for cascading two-photon photodynamic therapy and photothermal therapy against breast cancer. *Appl. Mater. Today* **2020**, *20*, 100665. [CrossRef]
51. Suciu, M.; Porav, S.; Radu, T. Photodynamic effect of light emitting diodes on *E. coli* and human skin cells induced by a graphene-based ternary composite. *J. Photochem. Photobiol. B Biol.* **2021**, *223*, 12298. [CrossRef]
52. Panda, S.; Rout, T.K.; Prusty, A.D.; Ajayan, P.M.; Nayak, S. Electron transfer directed antibacterial properties of graphene oxide on metals. *Adv. Mater.* **2018**, *30*, 1702149. [CrossRef]

53. Nagaraj, E.; Shanmugam, P.; Karuppannan, K.; Chinnasamy, T.; Venugopal, S. The biosynthesis of a graphene oxide-based zinc oxide nanocomposite using Dalbergia latifolia leaf extract and its biological applications. *New J. Chem.* **2020**, *44*, 2166–2179. [CrossRef]
54. Wang, H.; Zhao, B.; Dong, W.; Zhong, Y.; Zhang, X.; Gong, Y.; Zhan, R.; Xing, M.; Zhang, J.; Luo, G.; et al. A dual-targeted platform based on graphene for synergistic chemo-photothermal therapy against multidrug-resistant Gram-negative bacteria and their biofilms. *Chem. Eng. J.* **2020**, *393*, 124595. [CrossRef]
55. Kumar, M.; Thakur, M.; Bahadur, R.; Kaku, T. Preparation of graphene oxide-graphene quantum dots hybrid and its application in cancer theranostics. *Mater. Sci. Eng. C* **2019**, *103*, 109774.
56. Mej, I.E.; Santos, C.M.; Rodrigues, D.F. Toxicity of a polymer-graphene oxide composite against bacterial planktonic. *Nanoscale* **2012**, *4*, 4746–4756.
57. Qiu, J.; Liu, L.; Zhu, H.; Liu, X. Bioactive Materials Combination types between graphene oxide and substrate affect the antibacterial activity. *Bioact. Mater.* **2018**, *3*, 341–346. [CrossRef]
58. Liu, T.; Tong, L.; Lv, N.; Ge, X.; Fu, Q.; Gao, S.; Ma, Q.; Song, J. Two-Stage Size Decrease and Enhanced Photoacoustic Performance of Stimuli-Responsive Polymer-Gold Nanorod Assembly for Increased Tumour Penetration. *Adv. Funct. Mater.* **2019**, *29*, 1806429. [CrossRef]
59. Pei, S.; Cheng, H.M. The reduction of graphene oxide. *Carbon* **2012**, *50*, 3210–3228. [CrossRef]
60. Mathew, T.; Sree, R.A.; Aishwarya, S.; Kounaina, K.; Patil, A.G.; Satapathy, P.; Hudeda, S.P.; More, S.S.; Muthucheliyan, K.; Kumar, T.N.; et al. Graphene-based functional nanomaterials for biomedical and bioanalysis applications. *FlatChem* **2020**, *23*, 00184. [CrossRef]
61. Gurunathan, S.; Han, J.; Kim, J.H. A novel functional molecule for the green synthesis of graphene. *Colloids Surf. B Biointerfaces* **2013**, *111*, 376–383. [CrossRef] [PubMed]
62. Zaharie-butucel, D.; Potara, M.; Suarasan, S.; Licarete, E.; Astilean, S. Efficient combined near-infrared-triggered therapy: Phototherapy over chemotherapy in chitosan-reduced graphene oxide-IR820 dye-doxorubicin nanoplatforms. *J. Colloid Interface Sci.* **2019**, *552*, 218–229. [CrossRef]
63. Lee, S.; Kim, S.Y. Gold Nanorod/Reduced Graphene Oxide Composite Nanocarriers for Near-Infrared-Induced Cancer Therapy and Photoacoustic Imaging. *ACS Appl. Nano Mater.* **2021**, *4*, 11849–11860. [CrossRef]
64. Liu, R.; Zhang, H.; Zhang, F.; Wang, X.; Liu, X.; Zhang, Y. Polydopamine doped reduced graphene oxide/mesoporous silica nanosheets for chemo-photothermal and enhanced photothermal therapy. *Mater. Sci. Eng. C* **2019**, *96*, 138–145. [CrossRef] [PubMed]
65. Gurunathan, S.; Han, J.W.; Kim, E.S.; Park, J.H.; Kim, J.H. Reduction of graphene oxide by resveratrol: A novel and simple biological method for the synthesis of an effective anticancer nanotherapeutic molecule. *Int. J. Nanomed.* **2015**, *2015*, 2951–2969. [CrossRef] [PubMed]
66. Amina, M.; Al Musayeib, N.M.; Alarfaj, N.A.; El-tohamy, M.F.; Al-hamoud, G.A. Facile multifunctional-mode of fabricated biocompatible human serum albumin/reduced graphene oxide/Cladophora glomerata nanoparticles for bacteriostatic photothrapy, bacterial tracking and antioxidant potential. *Nanotechnology* **2021**, *32*, 315301. [CrossRef] [PubMed]
67. Tan, S.; Wu, X.; Xing, Y.; Lilak, S.; Wu, M.; Zhao, J.X. Enhanced synergetic antibacterial activity by a reduce graphene oxide/Ag nanocomposite through the photothermal effect. *J. Colloids Surf. B Biointerfaces* **2020**, *185*, 110616. [CrossRef]
68. Yang, Z.; Hao, X.; Chen, S.; Ma, Z.; Wang, W.; Wang, C.; Yue, L.; Sun, H.; Shao, Q.; Murugadoss, V.; et al. Long-term antibacterial stable reduced graphene oxide nanocomposites loaded with cuprous oxide nanoparticles. *J. Colloid Interface Sci.* **2019**, *533*, 13–23. [CrossRef]
69. Li, Y.; Xu, X.; Liu, X.; Zheng, Y.; Chen, D.F.; Yeung, K.W.K.; Chiu, Z.; Li, Z.; Liang, Y.; Zhu, S.; et al. Photoelectrons Mediating Angiogenesis and Immunotherapy through Heterojunction Film for Noninvasive Disinfection. *Adv. Sci.* **2020**, *7*, 2000023. [CrossRef]
70. Gollavelli, G.; Ling, Y.C. Magnetic and fluorescent graphene for dual modal imaging and single light induced photothermal and photodynamic therapy of cancer cells. *Biomaterials* **2014**, *35*, 4499–4507. [CrossRef]
71. Choi, S.Y.; Baek, S.H.; Chang, S.J.; Song, Y.; Rafique, R.; Lee, K.T.; Park, T.J. Synthesis of upconversion nanoparticles conjugated with graphene oxide quantum dots and their use against cancer cell imaging and photodynamic therapy. *Biosens. Bioelectron.* **2017**, *93*, 267–273. [CrossRef]
72. Gu, Y.; Guo, Y.; Wang, C.; Xu, J.; Wu, J.; Kirk, T.B.; Ma, D.; Xue, W. A polyamidoamne dendrimer functionalized graphene oxide for DOX and MMP-9 shRNA plasmid co-delivery. *Mater. Sci. Eng. C* **2017**, *70*, 572–585. [CrossRef]
73. Yang, H.W.; Huang, C.Y.; Lin, C.W. Gadolinium-functionalized nanographene oxide for combined drug and microRNA delivery and magnetic resonance imaging. *Biomaterials* **2014**, *35*, 6534–6542. [CrossRef]
74. Wu, C.; He, Q.; Zhu, A.; Li, D.; Xu, M.; Yang, H.; Liu, Y. Synergistic anticancer activity of photo- and chemoresponsive nanoformulation based on polylysine-functionalized graphene. *ACS Appl. Mater Interfaces* **2014**, *6*, 21615–21623. [CrossRef]
75. Yang, H.; Bremner, D.H.; Tao, L.; Li, H.; Hu, J.; Zhu, L. Carboxymethyl chitosan-mediated synthesis of hyaluronic acid-targeted graphene oxide for cancer drug delivery. *Carbohydr. Polym.* **2016**, *135*, 72–78. [CrossRef]
76. Mei, L.; Shi, Y.; Cao, F.; Liu, X.; Li, X.M.; Xu, Z.; Miao, Z. PEGylated phthalocyanine-functionalized graphene oxide with ultrahigh-efficient photothermal performance for triple-mode antibacterial therapy. *ACS Biomater. Sci. Eng.* **2021**, *7*, 2638–2648. [CrossRef]

77. Zheng, X.T.; Ma, X.Q.; Li, C.M. Highly efficient nuclear delivery of anti-cancer drugs using a bio-functionalized reduced graphene oxide. *J. Colloid Interface Sci.* **2016**, *467*, 35–42. [CrossRef]
78. Sun, B.; Wu, J.; Cui, S.; Zhu, H.; An, W.; Fu, Q.; Shao, C.; Yao, A.; Chen, B.; Shi, D. In situ synthesis of graphene oxide/gold nanorods theranostic hybrids for efficient tumor computed tomography imaging and photothermal therapy. *Nano Res.* **2017**, *10*, 37–48. [CrossRef]
79. Lima-Sousa, R.; de Melo-Diogo, D.; Alves, C.G.; Costa, E.C.; Ferreira, P.; Louro, R.O.; Correia, I.J. Hyaluronic acid functionalized green reduced graphene oxide for targeted cancer photothermal therapy. *Carbohydr. Polym.* **2018**, *200*, 93–99. [CrossRef]
80. Liang, Y.; Wang, M.; Zhang, Z.; Ren, G.; Liu, Y.; Wu, S.; Shen, J. Facile synthesis of ZnO QDs@GO-CS hydrogel for synergetic antibacterial applications and enhanced wound healing. *Chem. Eng. J.* **2019**, *378*, 122043. [CrossRef]
81. Siddique, S.; Chow, J.C.L. Application of Nanomaterials in Biomedical Imaging and Cancer Therapy. *Nanomaterials* **2020**, *10*, 1700. [CrossRef]
82. Kunjachan, S.; Ehling, J.; Storm, G.; Kiessling, F.; Lammers, T. Noninvasive imaging of nanomedicines and nanotheranostics: Principles, progress, and prospects. *Chem. Rev.* **2015**, *14*, 10907–10937. [CrossRef]
83. Lim, H.; Lee, S.Y.; Moon, D.W.; Kim, J.Y. Preparation of cellular samples using graphene cover and air-plasma treatment for time-of-flight secondary ion mass spectrometry imaging. *RSC Adv.* **2019**, *9*, 28432–28438. [CrossRef]
84. Lim, H.; Lee, S.Y.; Park, Y.; Jin, H.; Seo, D.; Jang, Y.H.; Moon, D.W. Mass spectrometry imaging of untreated wet cell membranes in solution using single-layer Graphene. *Nat. Methods* **2021**, *18*, 316–320. [CrossRef] [PubMed]
85. Zhang, D.Y.; Zheng, Y.; Tan, C.P.; Sun, J.H.; Zhang, W.; Ji, L.N.; Mao, Z.W. Graphene oxide decorated with Ru(II)-polyethylene glycol complex for lysosome-targeted imaging and photodynamic/photothermal therapy. *ACS Appl. Mater. Interfaces* **2017**, *9*, 6761–6771. [CrossRef] [PubMed]
86. Cheng, L.; Wang, C.; Feng, L.; Kai, Y.; Liu, Z. Functional Nanomaterials for Phototherapies of Cancer. *Chem. Rev.* **2014**, *114*, 10869–10939. [CrossRef] [PubMed]
87. Xu, Q.; Gao, J.; Wang, S.; Wang, Y.; Liu, D.; Wang, J. Quantum dots in cell imaging and their safety issues. *J. Mater. Chem. B* **2021**, *9*, 5765–5779. [CrossRef]
88. Boisselier, E.; Astruc, D. Gold nanoparticles in nanomedicine: Preparations, imaging, diagnostics, therapies and toxicity. *Chem. Soc. Rev.* **2009**, *38*, 1759–1782. [CrossRef]
89. Si, P.; Razmi, N.; Nur, O.; Solanki, S.; Pandey, C.M.; Gupta, R.K.; Malhotra, B.D.; Willander, M.; Zerda, A. Gold nanomaterials for optical biosensing and bioimaging. *Nanoscale Adv.* **2021**, *3*, 2679–2698. [CrossRef]
90. Alavi, M.; Jabari, E.; Jabbari, E. Functionalized carbon-based nanomaterials and quantum dots with antibacterial activity: A review. *Expert Rev. Anti Infect. Ther.* **2021**, *19*, 35–44. [CrossRef]
91. Liu, Z.; Robinson, J.T.; Sun, X.M.; Dai, H. PEGylated nanographene oxide for delivery of water-insoluble cancer drugs. *J. Am. Chem. Soc.* **2008**, *130*, 10876–10877. [CrossRef]
92. Sun, X.; Liu, Z.; Welsher, K.; Welsher, K.; Robinson, J.T.; Goodwin, A.; Zaric, S.; Dai, H. Nano-graphene oxide for cellular imaging and drug delivery. *Nano Res.* **2008**, *1*, 203–212. [CrossRef]
93. Peng, C.; Hu, W.; Zhou, Y.; Fan, C.; Huang, Q. Intracellular imaging with a graphene-based fluorescent probe. *Small* **2010**, *2*, 1686–1692. [CrossRef]
94. Li, J.L.; Tang, B.; Yuan, B.; Sun, L.; Wang, X.G. A review of optical imaging and therapy using nanosized graphene and graphene oxide. *Biomaterials* **2013**, *34*, 9519–9534. [CrossRef]
95. Gollavelli, G.; Ling, Y.C. Multi-functional graphene as an in vitro and in vivo imaging probe. *Biomaterials* **2012**, *33*, 2532–2545. [CrossRef]
96. Sinha, M.; Gollavelli, G.; Ling, Y.C. Exploring the photothermal hot spots of graphene in the first and second biological window to inactivate cancer cells and pathogens. *RSC Adv.* **2016**, *6*, 63859–63866. [CrossRef]
97. Choi, H.W.; Lim, J.H.; Kim, C.W.; Lee, E.; Kim, J.M.; Chang, K.; Chung, B.G. Near-Infrared Light-triggered generation of reactive oxygen species and induction of local hyperthermia from indocyanine green encapsulated mesoporous silica-coated graphene oxide for colorectal cancer therapy. *Antioxidants* **2022**, *11*, 174. [CrossRef]
98. Molkenova, A.; Atabaev, T.S.; Hong, S.W.; Mao, C.; Han, D.W.; Kim, K.S. Designing inorganic nanoparticles into computed tomography and magnetic resonance (CT/MR) imaging-guidable photomedicines. *Mater. Today Nano* **2022**, *18*, 100187. [CrossRef]
99. Younis, M.R.; He, G.; Lin, J.; Huang, P. Recent Advances on Graphene Quantum Dots for Bioimaging Applications. *Front. Chem.* **2020**, *8*, 424. [CrossRef]
100. Gulati, S.; Mansi; Vijayan, S.; Kumar, S.; Agarwal, V.; Harikumar, B.; Varma, R.S. Magnetic nanocarriers adorned on graphene: Promising contrast-enhancing agents with state-of-the-art performance in magnetic resonance imaging (MRI) and theranostics. *Mater. Adv.* **2022**, *3*, 2971–2989. [CrossRef]
101. Mohanta, Z.; Gaonkar, S.K.; Kumar, M.; Saini, J.; Tiwari, V.; Srivastava, C.; Atreya, H.S. Influence of oxidation degree of graphene oxide on its nuclear relaxivity and contrast in MRI. *ACS Omega* **2020**, *5*, 22131–22139. [CrossRef]
102. Enayati, M.; Nemati, A.; Zarrabi, A.; Shokrgozar, M.A. Reduced graphene oxide: An alternative for magnetic resonance imaging contrast agent. *Mater. Lett.* **2018**, *233*, 363–366. [CrossRef]
103. Hu, Y.H. The first magnetic-nanoparticle-free carbon-based contrast agent of magnetic-resonance imaging fluorinated graphene oxide. *Small* **2014**, *10*, 1451–1452. [CrossRef]

104. Wang, H.; Revia, R.; Wang, K.; Kant, R.J.; Mu, Q.; Gai, Z.; Hong, K.; Zhang, M. Paramagnetic properties of metal-free boron-doped graphene quantum dots and their application for safe magnetic resonance imaging. *Adv. Mater.* **2017**, *29*, 1605416. [CrossRef] [PubMed]
105. Zhang, M.; Cao, Y.; Chong, Y.; Ma, Y.; Zhang, H.; Deng, Z.; Hu, C.; Zhang, Z. Graphene oxide based theranostic platform for t1-weighted magnetic resonance imaging and drug delivery. *ACS Appl. Mater. Interfaces* **2013**, *5*, 13325–13332. [CrossRef] [PubMed]
106. Zhao, S.; Liu, X.; Xu, Z.; Ren, H.; Deng, B.; Tang, M.; Lu, L.; Fu, X.; Peng, H.; Liu, Z.; et al. Graphene encapsulated copper microwires as highly MRI compatible neural electrodes. *Nano Lett.* **2016**, *16*, 7731–7738. [CrossRef] [PubMed]
107. Cao, T.; Zhou, X.; Zheng, Y.; Sun, Y.; Zhang, J.; Chen, W.; Zhang, J.; Zhou, Z.; Yang, S. Chelator-free conjugation of ^{99m}Tc and Gd^{3+} to PEGylated nanographene oxide for 3 dual-modality SPECT/MR imaging of lymph nodes. *ACS Appl. Mater. Interfaces* **2017**, *9*, 42612–42621. [CrossRef] [PubMed]
108. Yang, K.; Hu, L.; Ma, X.; Ye, S.; Cheng, L.; Shi, X.; Li, C.; Li, Y.; Liu, Z. Multimodal imaging guided photothermal therapy using functionalized graphene nanosheets anchored with magnetic nanoparticles. *Adv. Mater.* **2012**, *24*, 11868–11872. [CrossRef]
109. Lin, C.H.; Chen, Y.C.; Huang, P.I. Preparation of multifunctional dopamine-coated zerovalent iron/reduced graphene oxide for targeted phototheragnosis in breast cancer. *Nanomaterials* **2020**, *10*, 1957. [CrossRef]
110. Sadighian, S.; Bayat, N.; Najaflou, S.; Kermanian, M.; Hamidi, M. Preparation of graphene oxide/Fe_3O_4 nanocomposite as a potential magnetic nanocarrier and MRI contrast agent. *Chem. Sel.* **2021**, *6*, 2862–2868.
111. Peng, E.; Choo, E.S.G.; Chandrasekharan, P.; Yang, C.T.; Ding, J.; Chuang, K.H.; Xue, J.M. Synthesis of manganese ferrite/graphene oxide nanocomposites for biomedical applications. *Small* **2012**, *8*, 3620–3630. [CrossRef]
112. Yang, Y.; Chen, S.; Li, H.; Yuan, Y.; Zhang, Z.; Xie, J.; Hwang, D.W.; Zhang, A.; Liu, M.; Zhou, X. Engineered paramagnetic graphene quantum dots with enhanced relaxivity for tumour imaging. *Nano Lett.* **2019**, *9*, 441–448. [CrossRef]
113. Ding, H.; Wang, D.; Sadat, A.; Li, Z.; Hu, X.; Xu, M.; Morais, P.C.; Ge, B.; Sun, S.; Ge, J.; et al. Single-atom gadolinium anchored on graphene quantum dots as a magnetic resonance signal amplifier. *ACS Appl. Bio Mater.* **2021**, *4*, 2798–2809. [CrossRef]
114. Lalwani, G.; Sundararaj, J.L.; Schaefer, K.; Button, T.; Sitharaman, B. Synthesis, characterization, In vitro phantom imaging, and cytotoxicity of a novel graphene-based multimodal magnetic resonance imaging-x-ray computed tomography contrast agent. *J. Mater. Chem. B* **2014**, *2*, 3519–3530. [CrossRef]
115. Badrigilan, S.; Shaabani, B.; Aghaji, N.G.; Mesbahi, A. Graphene quantum dots-coated bismuth nanoparticles for improved CT imaging and photothermal performance. *Int. J. Nanosci.* **2020**, *19*, 1850043.
116. Li, W.M.; Wei, D.M.; Wushouer, A.; Cao, S.D.; Zhao, T.T.; Yu, D.X.; Lei, D.P. Discovery and Validation of a CT-Based Radiomic Signature for Preoperative Prediction of Early Recurrence in Hypopharyngeal Carcinoma. *BioMed Res. Int.* **2020**, *2020*, 4340521. [CrossRef]
117. Chang, X.; Zhang, M.; Wang, C.; Zhang, J.; Wu, H.; Yang, S. Graphene oxide/$BaHoF_5$/PEG nanocomposite for dual-modal imaging and heat shock protein inhibitor-sensitized tumour photothermal therapy. *Carbon* **2020**, *158*, 372–385. [CrossRef]
118. Bi, H.; He, F.; Dai, Y.; Xu, J.; Dong, Y.; Yang, D.; Gai, S.; Li, L.; Li, C.; Yang, P. Quad-model imaging-guided high-efficiency phototherapy based on upconversion nanoparticles and $ZnFe_2O_4$ integrated graphene oxide. *Inorg. Chem.* **2018**, *57*, 9988–9998. [CrossRef]
119. Mirrahimi, M.; Alamzadeh, Z.; Beik, J.; Sarikhani, A.; Mousavi, M.; Irajirad, R.; Khani, T.; Davani, E.S.; Farashahi, A.; Ardakani, T.S.; et al. A 2D nanotheranostic platform based on graphene oxide and phase-change materials for bimodal CT/MR imaging, NIR-activated drug release, and synergistic thermo-chemotherapy. *Nanotheranostics* **2022**, *6*, 350–364. [CrossRef]
120. Hong, H.; Yang, K.; Zhang, Y.; Engle, J.W.; Feng, L.; Yang, Y.; Tapas, R.; Goel, N.S.; Bean, J.; Theuer, C.P.; et al. In vivo targeting and imaging of tumour vasculature with radiolabeled, antibody-conjugated nanographene. *ACS Nano* **2012**, *6*, 2361–2370. [CrossRef]
121. Hong, H.; Zhang, Y.; Engle, J.W.; Nayak, T.R.; Theuer, C.P.; Nickles, R.J.; Barnhart, T.E.; Cai, W. In vivo targeting and positron emission tomography imaging of tumour vasculature with ^{66}Ga-labeled nano-graphene. *Biomaterials* **2012**, *33*, 4147–4156. [CrossRef]
122. Shi, S.; Yang, K.; Hong, H.; Valdovinos, H.F.; Nayak, T.R.; Zhang, Y.; Theuer, C.P.; Barnhart, T.E.; Liu, Z.; Cai, W. Tumour vasculature targeting and imaging in living mice with reduced graphene oxide. *Biomaterials* **2013**, *34*, 3002–3009. [CrossRef]
123. Ugalde, A.F.; Sandoval, S.; Pulagam, K.R.; Juan, A.M.; Laromaine, A.; Llop, J.; Tobias, G.; Núñez, R. Radiolabeled obaltabis (dicarbollide) anion-graphene oxide nanocomposites for in vivo bioimaging and boron delivery. *ACS Appl. Nano Mater.* **2021**, *4*, 1613–1625. [CrossRef]
124. Binte, A.; Balasundaram, G.; Moothanchery, M.; Dinish, U.S.; Renzhe, B.; Ntziachristos, V.; Olivo, M. A review of clinical photoacoustic imaging: Current and future trends. *Photoacoustics* **2019**, *16*, 100–144.
125. Han, S.H. Review of photoacoustic imaging for imaging-guided spinal surgery. *Neurospine* **2018**, *15*, 306–322. [CrossRef] [PubMed]
126. Huang, K.; Zhang, Y.; Lin, J.; Huang, P. Nanomaterials for photoacoustic imaging in the second near-infrared window. *Biomater. Sci.* **2019**, *7*, 472–479. [CrossRef] [PubMed]
127. Lalwani, G.; Cai, X.; Nie, L.; Wang, L.V. Balaji Sitharaman. Graphene-based contrast agents for photoacoustic and thermoacoustic tomography. *Photoacoustics* **2013**, *1*, 62–67. [CrossRef]
128. Patel, M.A.; Yang, H.; Chiu, P.L.; Mastrogiovanni, D.D.T.; Flach, C.R.; Savaram, K.; Gomez, L.; Hemnarine, A.; Mendelsohn, R.; Garfunkel, E.; et al. Direct Production of graphene nanosheets for near infrared photoacoustic imaging. *ACS Nano* **2013**, *7*, 8147–8157. [CrossRef]

129. Wang, Y.W.; Fu, Y.Y.; Peng, Q.; Guo, S.S.; Liu, G.; Li, J.; Yang, H.H.; Chen, G.N. Dye-enhanced graphene oxide for photothermal therapy and photoacoustic imaging. *J. Mater. Chem. B* **2013**, *1*, 5762–5767. [CrossRef]
130. Toumia, Y.; Domenici, F.; Orlanducci, S.; Mura, F.; Grishenkov, D.; Trochet, P.; Lacerenza, S.; Bordi, F.; Paradossi, G. Graphene meets microbubbles: A superior contrast agent for photoacoustic imaging. *ACS Appl. Mater. Interfaces* **2016**, *8*, 16465–16475. [CrossRef]
131. Jun, S.W.; Manivasagan, P.; Kwon, J.; Nguyen, V.T.; Mondal, S.; Ly, C.D.; Lee, J.; Kang, J.H.; Kim, C.S.; Oh, J. Folic acid-conjugated chitosan-functionalized graphene oxide for highly efficient photoacoustic imaging-guided tumour-targeted photothermal therapy. *Int. J. Biol. Macromol.* **2020**, *155*, 961–971. [CrossRef]
132. Jia, X.; Xu, W.; Ye, Z.; Wang, Y.; Dong, Q.; Wang, E.; Li, D.; Wang, J. Functionalized graphene@goldnanostar/lipid for pancreatic cancer gene and photothermal synergistic therapy under photoacoustic/photothermal imaging dual-modal guidance. *Small* **2020**, *16*, e2003707. [CrossRef]
133. Wang, Z.; Sun, X.; Huang, T.; Song, J.; Wang, Y. A Sandwich nanostructure of gold nanoparticle coated reduced graphene oxide for photoacoustic imaging-guided photothermal therapy in the second NIR window. *Front. Bioeng. Biotechnol.* **2020**, *8*, 655. [CrossRef]
134. El-Mashtoly, S.F.; Gerwert, K. Diagnostics and Therapy Assessment Using Label-Free Raman Imaging. *Anal. Chem.* **2022**, *94*, 120–142. [CrossRef] [PubMed]
135. Zhang, Z.; Liu, Q.; Gao, D.; Luo, D.; Niu, Y.; Yang, J.; Li, Y. Graphene oxide as a multifunctional platform for Raman and fluorescence imaging of cells. *Small* **2015**, *11*, 3000–3005. [CrossRef]
136. Liu, Z.; Guo, Z.; Zhong, H.; Qin, X.; Wan, M.; Yang, B. Graphene oxide based surface-enhanced Raman scattering probes for cancer cell imaging. *Phys. Chem. Chem. Phys.* **2013**, *15*, 2961–2966. [CrossRef]
137. Deng, L.; Li, Q.; Yang, Y.; Omar, H.; Tang, N.; Zhang, J.; Nie, Z.; Khashab, N.M. "Two-step" Raman imaging technique to guide chemo-photothermal cancer therapy. *Chem. Eur. J.* **2015**, *21*, 17274–17281. [CrossRef]
138. Chen, Y.W.; Liu, T.Y.; Chen, P.J.; Chang, P.H.; Chen, S.Y. A high-sensitivity and low-power theranostic nanosystem for cell SERS imaging and selectively photothermal therapy using anti-egfr-conjugated reduced graphene oxide/mesoporous Silica/AuNPs nanosheets. *Small* **2016**, *12*, 1458–1468. [CrossRef]
139. Yang, L.; Kim, T.H.; Cho, H.Y.; Luo, J.; Lee, J.M.; Chueng, S.T.D.; Hou, Y.; Yin, P.T.T.; Han, J.; Kim, J.H.; et al. Hybrid graphene-gold nanoparticle-based nucleic acid conjugates for cancer-specific multimodal imaging and combined therapeutics. *Adv. Funct. Mater.* **2020**, *31*, 2006918. [CrossRef]
140. Cai, L.; Sheng, L.; Xia, M.; Li, Z.; Zhang, S.; Zhang, X.; Chen, H. Graphene oxide as a novel evenly continuous phase matrix for TOF-SIMS. *J. Am. Soc. Mass Spectrom.* **2016**, *28*, 399–408. [CrossRef]
141. Colliver, T.L.; Brummel, C.L.; Pacholski, M.L.; Swanek, F.D.; Ewing, A.G.; Winograd, N. Atomic and molecular imaging at the single-cell level with TOF-SIMS. *Anal. Chem.* **1997**, *69*, 2225–2231. [CrossRef]
142. Lee, T.G.; Park, J.W.; Shon, H.K.; Moon, D.W.; Choi, W.W.; Li, K.; Chung, J.H. Biochemical imaging of tissues by SIMS for biomedical applications. *Appl. Surf. Sci.* **2008**, *255*, 1241–1248. [CrossRef]
143. Belu, A.M.; Davies, M.C.; Newton, J.M.; Patel, N. TOF-SIMS characterization and imaging of controlled-release drug delivery systems. *Anal. Chem.* **2000**, *72*, 5625–5638. [CrossRef]
144. Lee, P.L.; Chen, B.C.; Gollavelli, G.; Shen, S.Y.; Yin, Y.S.; Lei, S.L.; Jhang, C.L.; Lee, W.R.; Ling, Y.C. Development and validation of TOF-SIMS and CLSM imaging method for cytotoxicity study of ZnO nanoparticles in HaCaT cells. *J. Hazard. Mater.* **2014**, *277*, 3012. [CrossRef] [PubMed]
145. Kim, J.Y.; Lim, H.; Moon, D.W. Mass spectrometry imaging of small molecules from live cells and tissues using nanomaterials. *Surf. Interface Anal.* **2022**, *54*, 381–388. [CrossRef]
146. Li, H.W.; Hua1, X.; Long, Y.T. Graphene quantum dots enhanced ToF-SIMS for single-cell imaging. *Anal. Bioanal. Chem.* **2019**, *411*, 4025–4030. [CrossRef] [PubMed]
147. Roope, L.S.J.; Smith, R.D.; Pouwels, K.B.; Buchanan, J.; Abel, L.; Eibich, P.; Butler, C.C.; Tan, P.S.; Walker, A.S.; Robotham, J.V.; et al. The challenge of antimicrobial resistance: What economics can contribute. *Science* **2019**, *364*, eaau4679. [CrossRef] [PubMed]
148. Costerton, J.W.; Stewart, P.S.; Greenberg, E.P. Bacterial Biofilms: A Common Cause of Persistent Infections. *Science* **1999**, *284*, 1318–1322. [CrossRef]
149. Qian, W.; Yan, C.; He, D.; Yu, X.; Yuan, L.; Liu, M.; Luo, G.; Deng, J. pH-triggered charge-reversible of glycol chitosan conjugated carboxyl graphene for enhancing photothermal ablation of focal infection. *Acta Biomater.* **2018**, *69*, 256–264. [CrossRef]
150. Wu, M.C.; Deokar, A.R.; Liao, J.H.; Shih, P.Y.; Ling, Y.C. Graphene-based photothermal agent for rapid and effective killing of bacteria. *ACS Nano* **2013**, *7*, 1281–1290. [CrossRef]
151. Gollavelli, G.; Chang, C.C.; Ling, Y.C. Facile synthesis of smart magnetic graphene for safe drinking water: Heavy metal removal and disinfection control. *ACS Sustain. Chem. Eng.* **2013**, *1*, 462–472. [CrossRef]
152. Ghule, K.; Ghule, A.V.; Chen, B.J.; Ling, Y.C. Preparation and characterization of ZnO nanoparticles coated paper and its antibacterial activity study. *Green Chem.* **2006**, *8*, 1034–1041. [CrossRef]
153. Deokar, A.R.; Lin, L.Y.; Chang, C.C.; Ling, Y.C. Single-walled carbon nanotube coated antibacterial paper: Preparation and mechanistic study. *J. Mater. Chem. B* **2013**, *20*, 2639–2646. [CrossRef]

154. Deokar, A.R.; Madhulika, S.; Ganesh, G.; Ling, Y.C. Chapter 3 Antimicrobial Perspectives for Graphene-Based Nanomaterial. In *Graphene Science Handbook*; Applications and Industrialization; Aliofkhazraei, M., Ali, N., Milne, W.I., Ozkan, G.S., Mitura, S., Gervasoni, J.L., Eds.; CRC Press: Boca Raton, FL, USA, 2016; Volume 6, pp. 27–40.
155. Bhaskar, G.; Ling, Y.C. Chapter 10 Richness of Graphene-Based Materials in Biomimetic Applications. In *Graphene Science Handbook*; Applications and Industrialization; Aliofkhazraei, M., Ali, N., Milne, W.I., Ozkan, G.S., Mitura, S., Gervasoni, J.L., Eds.; CRC Press: Boca Raton, FL, USA, 2016; Volume 6, pp. 125–142.
156. Bhaskar, G.; Ling, Y.C. Chapter 14 Carbon-based nanomaterials as nanozymes. In *Carbon Nanomaterials Sourcebook: Nanoparticles, Nanocapsules, Nanofibers, Nanoporous Structures, and Nanocomposites*; Sattler, B.K., Ed.; CRC Press: Boca Raton, FL, USA, 2016; Volume 2, pp. 309–333.
157. Wen, Y.J.; Yan, L.Y.; Ling, Y.C. The designing strategies of graphene-based peroxidase mimetic materials. *Sci. China Chem.* **2018**, *61*, 266–275. [CrossRef]
158. Feng, W.J.; Wang, Z.K. Biomedical applications of chitosan-graphene oxide nanocomposites. *iScience* **2022**, *25*, 103629. [CrossRef]
159. Sharma, H.; Mondal, S. Functionalized Graphene Oxide for Chemotherapeutic Drug Delivery and Cancer Treatment: A Promising Material in Nanomedicine. *Int. J. Mol. Sci.* **2020**, *21*, 6280. [CrossRef]
160. Manzano, M.; Vallet-Regí, M. Mesoporous Silica Nanoparticles for Drug Delivery. *Adv. Funct. Mater.* **2020**, *30*, 1902634. [CrossRef]
161. Zhang, Y.; Li, S.; Xu, Y.; Shi, X.; Zhang, M.; Huang, Y.; Liang, Y.; Chen, Y.; Ji, W.; Kim, J.R.; et al. Engineering of hollow polymeric nanosphere-supported imidazolium-based ionic liquids with enhanced antimicrobial activities. *Nano Res.* **2022**, *15*, 5556–5568. [CrossRef]
162. Zhang, Y.; Song, W.; Lu, Y.; Xu, Y.; Wang, C.; Yu, D.G.; Kim, I. Recent Advances in Poly (α-L-glutamic acid)-Based Nanomaterials for Drug Delivery. *Biomolecules* **2022**, *12*, 636. [CrossRef]
163. Tang, Y.; Varyambath, A.; Ding, Y.; Chen, B.; Huang, X.; Zhang, Y.; Yu, D.G.; Kim, I.; Song, W. Porous organic polymers for drug delivery: Hierarchical pore structures, variable morphologies, and biological properties. *Biomater. Sci.* **2022**; *advance article*.
164. Zhang, Y.; Kim, I.; Lu, Y.; Xu, Y.; Yu, D.G.; Song, W. Intelligent poly (l-histidine)-based nanovehicles for controlled drug delivery. *J. Control. Release* **2022**, *10*, 963–982. [CrossRef]
165. Chen, H.; Chen, Z.; Yang, H.; Wen, L.; Yi, Z.; Zhou, Z.; Dai, B.; Zhang, J.; Wue, X.; Wu, P. Multi-mode surface plasmon resonance absorber based on dart-type single-layer graphene. *RSC Adv.* **2022**, *12*, 7821. [CrossRef]
166. Cai, L.; Zhang, Z.; Xiao, H.; Chena, S.; Fua, J. An eco-friendly imprinted polymer based on graphene quantum dots for fluorescent detection of *p*-nitroaniline. *RSC Adv.* **2019**, *9*, 41383. [CrossRef]
167. Tang, N.; Li, Y.; Chen, F.; Han, Z. In situ fabrication of a direct Z-scheme photocatalyst by immobilizing CdS quantum dots in the channels of graphene-hybridized and supported mesoporous titanium nanocrystals for high photocatalytic performance under visible light. *RSC Adv.* **2018**, *8*, 42233. [CrossRef]

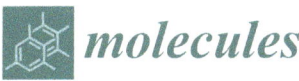

Review

Advances in Electrostatic Spinning of Polymer Fibers Functionalized with Metal-Based Nanocrystals and Biomedical Applications

Haojun Li [1], Meng Xu [1], Rui Shi [2], Aiying Zhang [1] and Jiatao Zhang [1,3,*]

[1] Institute of Medical-Industrial Integration, Beijing Key Laboratory of Structurally Controllable Advanced Functional Materials and Green Applications, School of Materials Science and Engineering, Beijing Institute of Technology, Beijing 100081, China
[2] Jishuitan Hospital, Beijing 100035, China
[3] Key Laboratory of Medical Molecule Science and Pharmaceutics Engineering, Ministry of Industry and Information Technology, School of Chemistry and Chemical Engineering, Beijing Institute of Technology, Beijing 100081, China
* Correspondence: zhangjt@bit.edu.cn

Abstract: Considering the metal-based nanocrystal (NC) hierarchical structure requirements in many real applications, starting from basic synthesis principles of electrostatic spinning technology, the formation of functionalized fibrous materials with inorganic metallic and semiconductor nanocrystalline materials by electrostatic spinning synthesis technology in recent years was reviewed. Several typical electrostatic spinning synthesis methods for nanocrystalline materials in polymers are presented. Finally, the specific applications and perspectives of such electrostatic spun nanofibers in the biomedical field are reviewed in terms of antimicrobial fibers, biosensing and so on.

Keywords: electrostatic spinning; inorganic nanocrystals; polymer fibers; antimicrobial; biomedical

1. Introduction

In recent decades, electrostatic spinning has received more and more attention as an important technology for the preparation of micro/nanomaterials due to the rapid demand for fiber-based applications. Electrostatic spinning is a process in which a polymer solution is stretched into nanofibers by applying a high-voltage electric field. The concept of electrostatic spinning was conceived as early as 1600 by Gilbert, who observed in a study that polymer solutions could form conical droplets under an electric field [1]. In 1882, Taylor published a series of seminal papers stating that as the electric field strength increased to a critical level, the spherical droplet would gradually evolve into a cone [2] (now commonly referred to as a "Taylor cone") and emit a liquid jet. The application of the electrojet process to the preparation of fibers eventually evolved into electrostatic spinning technology. After 1990, Reneker's group and Rutledge's group conducted more in-depth research on electrostatic spinning technology and applications [3,4]. Recently, more and more attention has been paid to electrostatic spinning by using new materials to fabricate composite materials and ceramic nanofibers, due to the fact that new applications in electrostatic spinning fibers are used in in soft electronic devices [5–7], biomedicine [8,9], energy harvesting, conversion and storage [10,11]. The number of publications on electrospinning keeps increasing, as shown in Figure 1A, which also indicates the new opportunities in the development of electrostatic spinning.

The ability to encapsulate hydrophobic and hydrophilic compounds and functional nanomaterials directly into fibers is a major advantage in electrostatic spinning technology [12–14]. This is because electrostatic spinning can be performed under relatively mild environmental conditions, which could retain the activity of the loaded substances during the forming process, making them more suitable for encapsulating active nanomaterials that are sensitive to heat than other conventional processing strategies. As for bio-applications, it has been demonstrated that cells could also be processed by electrostatic spinning without loss of their activities [15–17]. In addition, electrospun fibers, with tunable diameters from submicron to nanometer level and high specific surface area, can also facilitate the dispersion of their loaded compounds into the surrounding medium, thereby controlling the release of active substances (e.g., drugs) [18–21]. In addition, electrospun fibers can mimic the microstructure of the human extracellular matrix, thus, greatly improving the biocompatibility of the material and making it more stable for the loaded bio-nanomaterials and drugs [22].

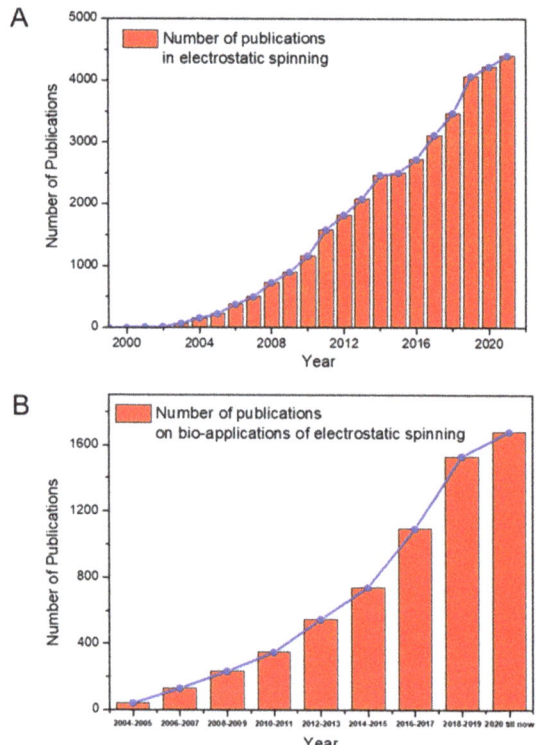

Figure 1. Number of publications on (**A**) electrostatic spinning and (**B**) bio-applications of electrostatic spinning indexed by Web of Science.

Due to the aforementioned properties, electrospun fibers have promising applications in the field of biomedical materials, especially in the controlled release of compounds in drug delivery [23,24], scaffolds in tissue engineering [25,26] and wound dressings [27,28]. The number of publications on the bio-application of electrospinning technology also keeps increasing in the most recent 20 years, as shown in Figure 1B. In this work, we summarize the principles of electrostatic spinning, with emphasis on the two main methods of loading inorganic NCs onto electrospun membranes and their advantages and limitations. Then, we review the applications of electrospun fiber membranes loaded with inorganic NCs in the field of antibacterial and biosensing directions, especially publications reported in the last 10 years. Finally, we discuss the challenges and opportunities of electrostatic spinning, especially for nanosynthesis.

2. The Principle of Electrostatic Spinning Technology

2.1. Principle of Electrostatic Spinning

A schematic diagram of the electrostatic spinning for preparing nanofibers is shown in Figure 2, including strategies, such as directly mixing, in situ growth and assembly of inorganic NCs. The equipment of electrostatic spinning generally consists of three parts: the spinneret, the high-voltage power supply and the receiving device [29]. In general, the electrostatic spinning process can be divided into the following four steps: (i) the polymer solution forms a Taylor cone under an electric field; (ii) the charged jet extends along a straight line under the electric field; (iii) the jet becomes finer under the electric field and the electric bending instability (also called agitation instability) increases; and (iv) the jet condenses into solid fibers and is collected on a grounded collector [30]. Among them, the formation of the Taylor cone is the most critical step in this process, which determines the quality of the fibers. In the electrospinning process, the metal whiskers are easily formed. The static polarization of the wire in the electric field brings about an energy gain, resulting in a metal whisker that appears as a hair-like protrusion on the surface of some metal [31]. In spite of the potential weakness caused by metal whiskers in the electronic industry, the mechanisms in the formation of metal whiskers still need further investigation.

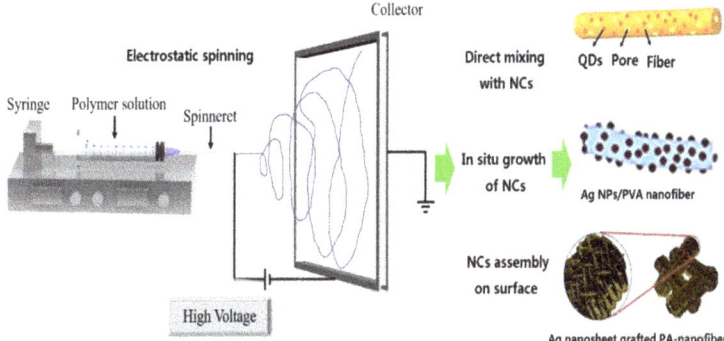

Figure 2. Schematic diagram of nanofibers electrostatic spinning and their direct mixing, in situ growth and assembly of inorganic NCs.

2.2. Main Factors Influencing the Formation of Electrostatic Spinning Nanofibers

The formation of electrospun fibers and the control of their diameters depend largely on the processing parameters, including the polymer solution concentration, applied voltage, liquid flow rates, distance between the spinneret tip and the collector, etc.

2.2.1. Polymer Solution Concentration

As the concentration of the polymer solution increases, the viscosity and surface tension of the solution also increase, resulting in a less stretchable solution, and the jets formed in the electric field become less likely to split and become finer, resulting in a larger diameter for the collected fibers. Thus, under the same conditions, the diameter of nanofibers increases with an increase in polymer concentration. When the concentration of the solution is too low, the viscosity of the solution is also low, which could be easy electrostatic atomization, resulting in the presence of a large number of string beads in the fiber [32]. Therefore, in order to obtain the ideal electrospun fibers, it is necessary to find the most suitable polymer concentration for electrospinning.

2.2.2. Liquid Flow Rate and Receiving Distance

The injection rate also affects the structures of fibers by influencing the formation of Taylor cones. In general, as the injection rates increase, the fiber diameter also increases.

Typically, the jet needs a long enough distance to extend and coagulate before forming solid fibers. Normally, the fibers become finer as the receiving distance increases. After a certain distance, the fibers will no longer become finer due to the solidification of the jet [30].

2.2.3. Electric Field Voltage

A static high-voltage direct current is usually applied to the spinneret to generate an electric field. The magnitude of the voltage determines the amount of charge carried by the jet and the strength of the electric field. Applying a high voltage usually tends to form thinner fibers [33], while it might also cause more liquid to be injected, resulting in larger fiber diameters [34].

3. Noble Metal, Semiconductor Nanocrystalline Materials and Their Electrostatic Spinning into Polymers

3.1. Noble Metal, Semiconductor Nanocrystalline Materials

With the rapid development of nanotechnology and science, colloidal inorganic NCs with different morphologies, sizes and functions (Figure 3) have been investigated, including noble metal nanoparticles (NPs) [35–37], semiconducting metal oxides [38,39], single-atom catalysts [40–43], hybrid NCs [44–46], noble metal nanoclusters [47] and semiconductor quantum dots (QDs) [48–52], etc. These kinds of nanomaterials are widely used in the fields of energy [53,54], catalysis [55,56], sensing [57], electronic information [58], optoelectronic devices [59], biomedicine and imaging [60–62] because of their unique optical, electronic, magnetic, thermal and mechanical properties. Dispersing nanomaterials into a bulk matrix, such as large-scale polymer fibers, with low concentrations but well-maintained intrinsic nano effect and properties, has been regarded as a promising strategy to further explore their potential applications in our daily life.

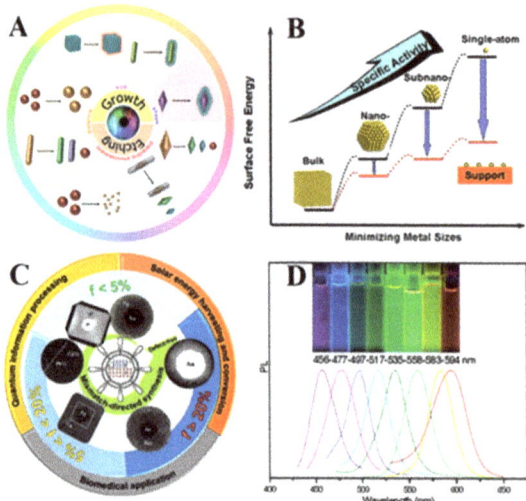

Figure 3. Various nanocrystalline materials. (**A**) Various shapes of noble metal NCs [40]. Copyright 2019 American Chemical Society. (**B**) Subnano- to single-atom catalysts [48]. Copyright 2013 American Chemical Society. (**C**) Hybrid NCs [49]. Copyright 2020 American Chemical Society. (**D**) QDs [57]. Copyright 2008 American Chemical Society.

3.2. Preparation of Nanocrystalline Functionalized Electrospun Composite Fibers

There are many strategies to assemble NCs into electrospun fibers and direct mixing and in situ growth are two most representative strategies. By combining inorganic NCs with electrospun nanofibers, the stability of many kinds of such NCs can be effectively improved. Moreover, their intrinsic properties could be well maintained. In addition, the advantages and disadvantages of each of these two methods are listed in Table 1.

Table 1. Advantages and disadvantages of direct mixing method and in situ growth method.

Methods	Advantages	Disadvantages
Direct mixing method	(i) Faster and simpler than other compared methods; (ii) Particle sizes and categories depending on pre-synthesized NCs.	(i) Easy to aggregation; (ii) Post-treatment process needed (purification, extractions, etc.); (iii) Lacking size homogeneity in dense matrices; (iv) Restrained connection between NCs and fibers.
In situ growth method	(i) Easy to perform; (ii) Not necessarily extra time in polymeric solution preparation; (iii) No additional solvents required; (iv) Adjustable particle size determined by precursors.	(i) Multi-step reaction; (ii) Additional post-processing time; (iii) Not applicable to all NCs.

3.2.1. Direct Mixing with NCs in Polymer Precursors

Due to the properties of small size effect and high surface energy, NCs could be aggregated in long-term practical applications. However, when mixing these inorganic NCs with the solutions of electrospinning polymers, NCs would be coordinated and stabilized by the surficial ligands of electrospun polymers, which could inhibit the aggregations of NCs. At present, many kinds of inorganic NCs, such as noble metal, metal oxygen/sulfide and semiconductor NCs, have been directly mixed and blended in electrospun nanofibers [63–66]. For example, El-Hefnawy et al. reported the synthesis of Ag NC dispersed polymer fibers [67]. The fabricated Ag NCs were made into a monodisperse form with a diameter of no more than 6 nm. Prior to the electrospinning process, they added different volumes of Ag NCs dropwise into the polymer mixture solution to obtain nanofiber sheets containing different concentrations of Ag NCs. They found that the fibers containing Ag NCs were uniform and the diameter of the fibers could be tunable by increasing the concentration of Ag NCs.

Similarly, Manjumeena et al. reported the synthesis of Au NCs deposited on polyvinyl alcohol (PVA) nanofibers enabled by the dispersion of PVA and Au NCs in distilled water by controlling the corresponding electrospun conditions [68]. Electrospun nanofibers loaded with Au NCs were obtained and the scanning electron microscope (SEM) and high-resolution transmission electron microscope (HRTEM) results indicated that Au NCs were located on the surface of the electrospun fiber. They concluded that the PVA could become more hydrophilic after being loaded with a small amount of Au NPs. Another study, by Li et al., reported the synthesis of Fe_3O_4-modified electrospun fibers [69]. They found that at high voltages, Fe_3O_4 could improve the arrangement of fibers compared to pristine electrospun fibers. Two-dimensional NCs could also be deposited on nanofibers, as reported by Somia et al. (Figure 4) [70]. Cellulose nanocrystalline-ZnO (CNC-ZnO) hybrids were obtained using the hydrothermal method followed by dispersion in chloroform/DMF mixed solvent with additionally dissolved pl (PHBV). PHBV/CNC-ZnO composite nanofibers were successfully obtained through the electrospinning strategy. It was found that after the combination of sheet-like CNC-ZnO and PHBV, the nucleation density, overall crystallinity and crystallinity in PHBV composite nanofibers were significantly improved and their thermal degradation temperature also increased.

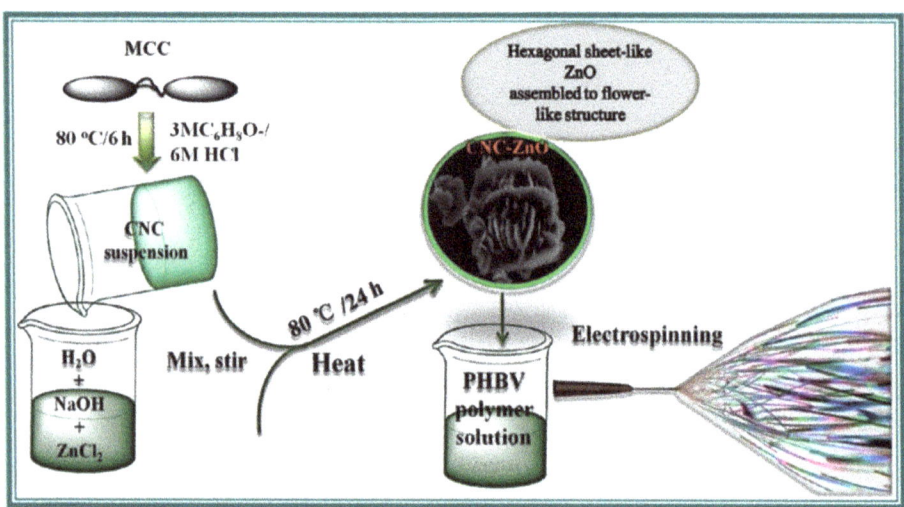

Figure 4. Schematic illustration of possible experimental preparation procedure of sheet-like CNC-ZnO nanohybrids and their electrospinning process [69]. Copyright 2018 American Chemical Society.

3.2.2. In Situ Growth of NCs on Electrospun Fibers

In situ growth of NCs on electrospun fibers is another efficient strategy to achieve NC-modified nanofibers. Generally, the precursor solution of the metal salt is dissolved in the electrospinning solution followed by using light, electricity, heat, chemical reduction and other methods to trigger the reduction in and oxidation of metal ions in the electrospun solution or electrospinning fiber. As shown in Figure 5, Song Lin et al. reported two in situ growth methods to obtain Ag NC-loaded PVA nanofiber pads. The first method was to reflux the $AgNO_3$-soluble PVA solution at 105 °C for 1 h, resulting in Ag NCs being generated in this process, and then the nanofibers were obtained by the electrospinning process. The second method was to dissolve PVA in deionized water to obtain a viscous solution and then add $AgNO_3$ as an electrospinning solution. After the end of electrospinning, Ag NCs could be formed inside the nanofibers under full ultraviolet (UV) lamp illumination. Among them, the size and yield of doped Ag NCs can be adjusted by controlling preheating treatment or UV irradiation [71]. Soon et al. prepared polyacrylonitrile (PAN) electrospun fiber membranes supporting Pt NTHFPs (NPs) by in situ calcination [72]. The PAN electrospun fibers were prepared first followed by immersion in $Pt(acac)_2$ acetone solution to load Pt. After heat treatment in an inert atmosphere, the nanofibers loaded with Pt NPs were carbonized at high temperatures. In another representative study by Dakota et al., Ag NP-modified polycaprolactone (PCL) nanofibers were fabricated by in situ plasma treatment [73]. First, the PCL and $AgNO_3$ were dissolved in acetone followed by electrospinning under appropriate conditions. The electrospun fibers were then treated with air plasma, which could be a simple and effective method to generate Ag NPs on fiber membranes.

Similarly, Wang et al. dissolved polylactic acid (PLA)/PCL and Cu_2S NPs in a N-N dimethylformamide/tetrahydrofuran (DMF/THF) solvent mixture forming Cu_2S NC-mixed polymer fibers, as shown in Figure 6A [74]. It was shown that these fiber films exhibited excellent and controllable photothermal properties under NP (NIR) irradiation, showing great promise in tumor-induced wound healing applications. Compared to single-component-modified nanofibers, Yu's group reported the fabrication of assembled binary component NC-modified nanofibers by embedding Au nanorods (NRs) and silver nanowire (Ag NW) assemblies into PVA electrospun nanofibers to improve the stability of Au NRs/Ag NWs, as shown in Figure 6B [75]. When using a woven-structured copper mesh as the receiver device, the Au NRs/Ag NW assemblies were mostly distributed in a directional manner within the electrospun fibers. Furthermore, because of the polarization effect of the Ag NP-polymer solution under the high-voltage power supply, they distributed the dimer and small aggregates of Ag NPs directionally inside the PVA fiber and the composite fiber finally produced a more desirable surface-enhanced Raman scattering (SERS) effect [76].

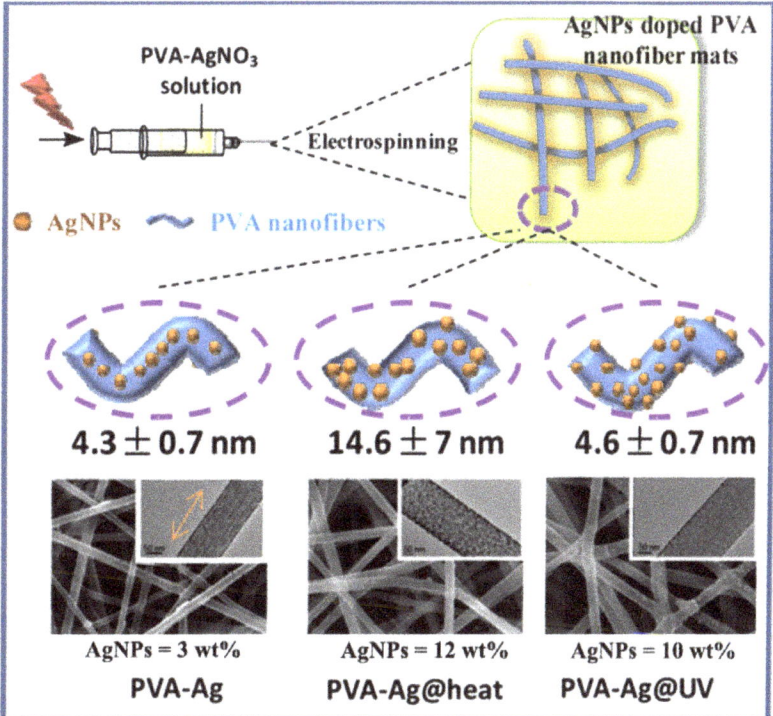

Figure 5. Overview of electrospinning process of Ag NP-doped PVA nanofiber mats under different prepared conditions [70]. Copyright 2022 Dove Press Ltd.

As for the synthesis of semiconductor NC-modified nanofibers, as shown in Figure 7A, Kampara et al. used an in situ calcination strategy to obtain a PVA electrospun fiber membrane loaded with CdO semiconductor NCs [77]. The precursor to synthesize CdO NCs was cadmium acetate dihydrate. After the initial electrospinning, the original nanofiber membranes were transferred to the muffle furnace and calcined at high temperature to obtain the product. As shown in Figure 7B, Kamal et al. prepared PLA/titanium dioxide hybrid nanofibers using the in situ hydrothermal method. The coated fibers were obtained by combining electrospinning and electrospraying techniques. The electrospinning solution was prepared by dissolving PLA in a mixed solvent of dichloromethane/methanol. A mixture of tetraisopropoxide Ti(O-iPr)$_4$ (TIP), ethanol and hydrochloric acid was used for electrospraying, as a precursor to Ti. The obtained coating fibers were sufficiently dried under vacuum and then transferred to an autoclave for hydrothermal treatment and the Ti precursors were finally converted into TiO$_2$ NPs [78].

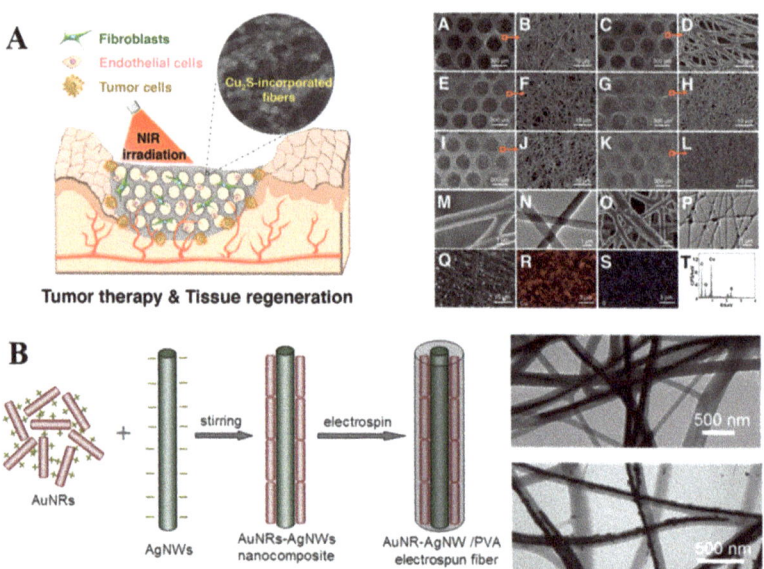

Figure 6. Preparation of nanocrystalline/electrospun composite fibers by direct mixing method. (**A**) Cu2S-incorporated PLA/PCL fiber membrane [74]; Copyright 2017 American Chemical Society. (**B**) Au NR-Ag NWs/PVA electrospun fibers [75]. Copyright 2012 The Royal Society of Chemistry.

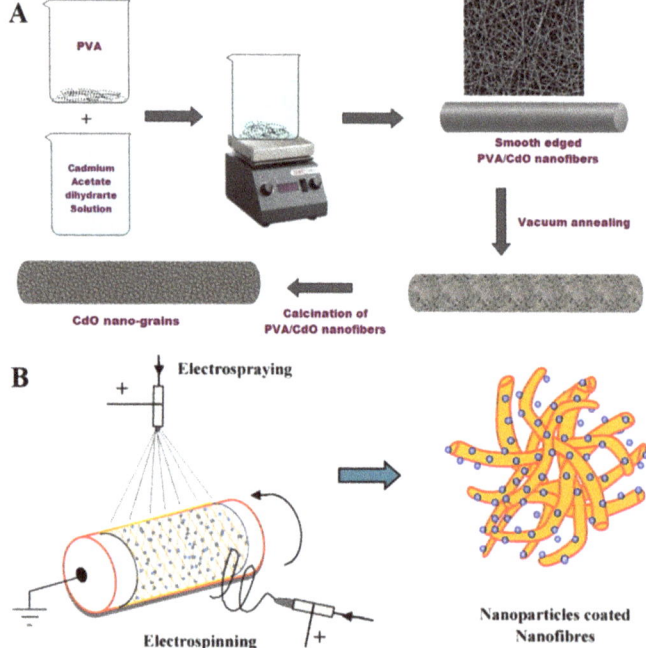

Figure 7. (**A**) Experimental procedure for electrospinning of CdO nanograins [77]. Copyright 2020 Elsevier Ltd. (**B**) Schematic diagram nanoparticle coating on nanofibers using electrospinning and electrospraying [78]. Copyright 2012 Elsevier B.V.

4. Functionalized Electrostatic Spinning Composite Fibers for Biomedical Applications

By virtue of the aforementioned advantages of electrospun nanofibers, such as nanoscale size, high porosity and large specific surface area, their potential applications have been widely studied in many fields [5–11]. Specifically, nontoxic electrospun nanofibers were regarded as promising candidates for biomedicines [23–28], with adjustable properties, such as drug release, wound dressing, tissue engineering and trauma repair.

4.1. Electrostatic Spun Nano-Antimicrobial Fibers

Many kinds of noble metals and oxides of some metals can exhibit certain antimicrobial properties [79–81]. Ag NPs are some of the most typical antibacterial NCs by virtue of the advantages of adjustable size, excellent antibacterial effect, continuous antibacterial effect, etc., which exhibits a wide range of applications in the field of antibacterial biology. As shown in Figure 8A, Yan et al. prepared PVA nanofibers loaded with Ag NPs using an in situ hydrothermal assay [82]. They assessed the bactericidal properties of pure PVA and Ag NPs/PVA through turbidity and absorption methods for E. coli and S. aureus. Their results indicated that the latter exhibited more excellent antibacterial properties. The amount of fiber-loaded Ag NPs was also controlled by adjusting the concentration of $AgNO_3$, which indicated that samples with a concentration of $AgNO_3$ at 0.066 mol/L had the highest antimicrobial rates against E. coli and S. aureus, at 98% and 99%, respectively. By direct mixing, Erick et al. incorporated Ag NPs into PCL electrospun nanofibers to study their antimicrobial properties. They demonstrated the antibacterial activity of fiber scaffolds by agar diffusion and the results indicated that the antibacterial activity of fiber scaffolds on S. aureus, E. coli, K. pneumoniae and P. aeruginosa was directly proportional to the concentration of Ag NPs. Compared with Gram-negative bacteria (E. coli, P. aeruginosa and K. pneumoniae), Gram-positive strains (S. Aureus, S. mutans, B. subtilis) were more sensitive to PLA-Ag NPs nanofibers [83]. Reza et al. studied the wound healing effects of compound nanofibers embedded with Ag NPs. The antibacterial activity of the product against E. coli, P. aeruginosa and S. aureus was studied in vitro and the results indicated that the higher the silver content, the better the antibacterial effect. The product was tested for cytotoxicity in vitro using the MTT assay and the results showed that the fiber scaffold was nontoxic and had good biocompatibility. They used nanofiber pads on wounds caused by resection of white rabbits in New Zealand to study their effects as wound dressings. Silver-containing nanofiber membranes showed good healing properties compared to Ag-free polyvinylalcohol/polyvinylpyrrolidone/pectin/mafenide acetate (PVA/PVP/PEC/MF) nanofibers and obtained the best wound healing effect when the composition ratio of Ag NPs/PVA/PVP/PEC/MF was 0.7:91.8:2.5:2.5 wt% [84]. As shown in Figure 8B, Qian et al. developed a novel Ag-modified/collagen-coated electrospun p/polycaprolactone (PLGA/PCL) scaffold (PP-pDA-Ag-COL) with improved antimicrobial and osteogenic properties [85]. The scaffold was generated by electrospinning a basic PLGA/PCL matrix, followed by Ag NPs impregnation via in situ reduction, polydopamine coating and then coating by collagen I. The three intermediate materials involved in the fabrication of the scaffolds, namely, PLGA/PCL (PP), PLGA/PCL-polydopamine (PP-pDA) and PLGA/PCL-polydopamine-Ag (PP-pDA-Ag), were used as control scaffolds. There was a wider antibacterial zone associated in PP-pDA-Ag-COL and PP-pDA-Ag scaffolds versus control scaffolds ($p < 0.05$) and bacterial fluorescence was reduced on the Ag-modified scaffolds after 24 h inoculation against Staphylococcus aureus and Streptococcus mutans. In a mouse periodontal disease model, the PP-pDA-Ag-COL scaffold enhanced alveolar bone regeneration (31.8%) and was effective for periodontitis treatment. These results demonstrate that this novel PP-pDA-Ag-COL scaffold enhanced biocompatibility and osteogenic and antibacterial properties.

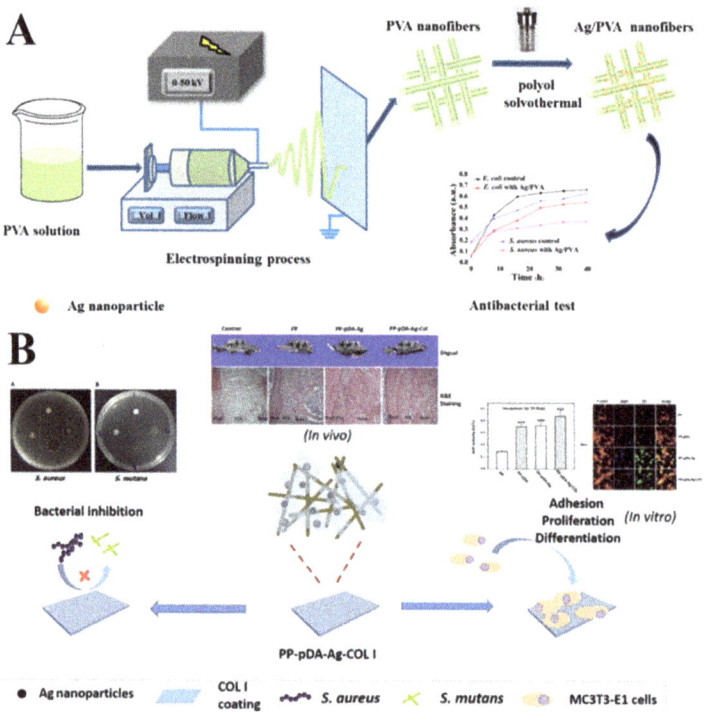

Figure 8. (**A**) Schematic illustration of fabrication and antibacterial test for Ag/PVA composite nanofibers through the electrospinning and solvothermal methods [82]. Copyright 2020 by the authors. (**B**) Triple PLGA/PCL scaffold modification including silver impregnation, collagen coating and electrospinning significantly improve biocompatibility, antimicrobial and osteogenic properties for orofacial tissue regeneration [85]. Copyright 2019 American Chemical Society.

TiO_2 NCs, as an inorganic antibacterial agent, especially under light irradiation, have also gradually received attention as a promising nano-antibacterial material by virtue of their advantages of high stability, nontoxicity and easily manipulated properties. Pant et al. prepared TiO_2-containing nylon-6 nanofibers using electrospinning technology and experimentally demonstrated that the nanofibers had good antibacterial properties [86]. Toniatto et al. reported the synthesis of TiO_2-modified PLA by direct mixing [87]. The prepared composite nanofibers were tested using thiazole blue colorimetry (MTT method) and the results showed that the composite nanofibers had no significant cytotoxicity. Through the evaluation of antibacterial experiments, the composite nanofibers with a content of 5 wt% show strong bactericidal properties.

In addition to the above materials being widely used in the field of antibacterial biology, nanomaterials, such as Au NPs [88], Se NPs [89] and ZnO NCs [90], also exhibit excellent performance in this field.

4.2. Biosensing Applications

Biosensing is an important branch of chemical sensing, which has been applied for the detection of small biological molecules, enzymes, nucleic acids, disease markers, cells, bacteria, etc. As for different biological reactions, designing and constructing suitable NC/electrospun composite fiber membranes are important for biosensing applications.

In a recent study reported by Beak et al., Cu nanoflower-modified Au NP-graphene oxide (GO) nanofibers were synthesized as electrochemical biosensors for glucose detection using a novel electrospinning method [91]. Electrochemical experiments showed that Cu-nanoflower@AuNPs-GO nanofibers have the advantages of high sensitivity, low detection limit and good reproducibility and selectivity in detecting glucose. In addition to the special catalytic properties, metal oxides could also facilitate electron transfer, which could provide a more friendly electroactive surface, thus, enabling the direct transfer of electrons to the electrode. For example, Li et al. prepared uniformly dispersed Pd NPs anchored on CuO nanofibers through the electrostatic spinning method, which were used to construct enzyme-free glucose sensors, with the advantages of fast response, high sensitivity and low detection limit [92]. Liu et al. also used ZnO nanostructures as an immobilized substrate for an enzyme glucose sensor and immobilized glucose oxidase on it, thus, enabling it to directly undergo electron transfer with the electrode and exhibit high catalytic activity, with a wide linear range and high sensitivity [93]. Perovskite NCs with high optoelectronic properties were also applied for biosensing applications. For example, Wang et al. prepared monolithic superhydrophobic polystyrene fiber membranes encapsulated with $CsPbBr_3$ quantums (CPBQD) by one-step electrospinning [94]. The fiber membrane composite coupled CPBQD with a polystyrene (PS) matrix and showed high quantum yield (~91%), narrow half-peak width (~16 nm) and ~100% fluorescence retention after 10 days of exposure to water. Thanks to the excellent optical properties of CPBQD, an ultra-low detection limit of 0.01 ppm was obtained for Rhodamine 6G (R6G) detection and the HRTEM (FRET) efficiency was calculated as 18.80% at 1 ppm R6G in aqueous solution.

Hybrid materials composed of polymer nanofibers and plasmonic noble metal NCs have also developed significantly in recent years for biosensing. For example, as shown in Figure 9, Yang et al. designed a plasma-independent substrate consisting of Ag NPs supported on PAN electrospun nanofiber membranes as a bacterial-detection sensor [95]. The substrate exhibited highly sensitive SERS performance for bacterial identification in the absence of specific bacterial-aptamer coupling. The substrate exhibited good homogeneity of SERS response to bacterial organelles. The antimicrobial properties were also evaluated, which indicated that Ag@PAN nanofiber mats have good antimicrobial properties against both Escherichia coli and Staphylococcus aureus. Anitha et al. synthesized a composite nanofiber membrane loaded with Au NPs by a simple direct mixing method for the detection of H_2O_2 [96]. By virtue of the uniform distribution and large surface area of the Au NPs in the nanofibers, the Au NP-composite electrodes enabled greatly improved electrochemical properties, compared to Au NP-free composite electrodes. When they were employed as reservoirs for immobilizing horseradish peroxidase, reliable and sensitive electrochemical detection by the enzyme reaction was achieved. Their experimental results demonstrated that the detection sensitivity to H_2O_2 could be an order of magnitude higher than other previously reported electrochemical sensors.

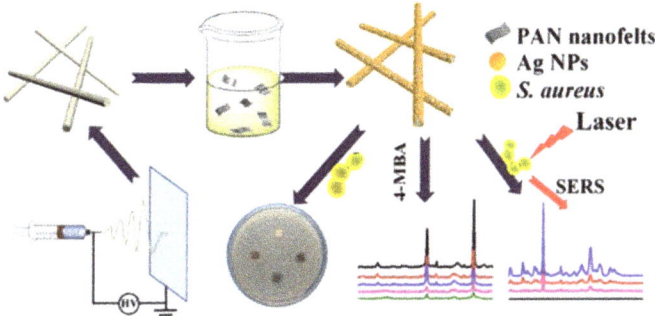

Figure 9. A simple electrostatic spinning technique to prepare Ag@PAN nanofiber membranes for bacterial detection [95]. Copyright 2020 American Chemical Society.

4.3. Other Applications

In addition to antimicrobial applications and biosensing, NC-loaded electrospun fiber membranes were also applied in other biomedical fields. For example, Ming et al. synthesized an electrospun fiber membrane loaded with Au NRs for photothermal treatment of cancer [97]. This strategy not only utilizes the excellent photothermal properties of Au NRs to selectively kill cancer cells, but also utilizes widely used biodegradable electrospinning membranes as Au NRs carriers and surgical recovery materials. Polyethylene glycol (PEG)-modified Au NRs are embedded in an electrospun fiber membrane consisting of PLGA and PLA-b-PEG. After incubation with the cells in the cell culture medium, the PEG-Au NRs were released from the membrane and taken up by cancer cells, allowing the generation of heat upon NIR irradiation to induce cancer cell death (as shown in Figure 10). For another example, biomaterial-based scaffolds fabricated using the electrospinning technique are promising platforms for bone tissue engineering. In the study of Huang et al., citrate-stabilized Au NPs were encapsulated into polyvinylpyrrolidone/ethylcellulose (P/E) scaffolds fabricated by the coaxial electrospinning technique [98]. The results showed that Au NPs were successfully wrapped in electrospinning brackets and the addition hardly affected fiber morphology, but improved porosity and mechanical properties. In vitro studies revealed that Au NP-incorporated electrospun scaffolds showed excellent biocompatibility and osteogenic bioactivities, wherein the alkaline phosphatase activity, mineralized nodule formation and the osteogenic-related genes expression were enhanced in Ag NP-incorporated electrospun scaffolds compared to the neat P/E electrospun nanofibers. Then, the Ag NP-incorporated electrospun scaffolds were surgically implanted into the defect area of the rat skull bone to test their in vivo bone repairing effect. It was observed that Ag NP-incorporated scaffolds rapidly accelerated bone regeneration in vivo.

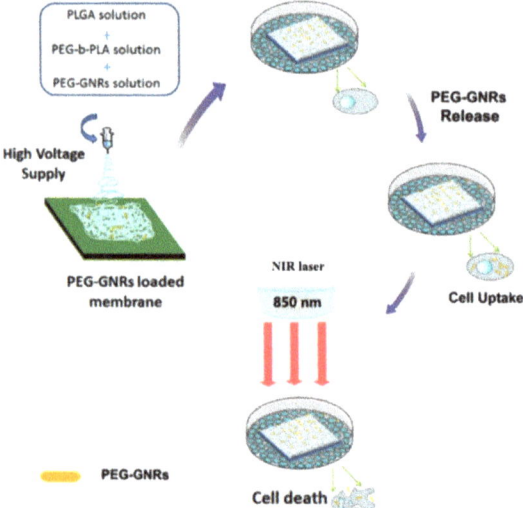

Figure 10. Schematic illustration depicting the strategy of using PEG-GNRs membrane for the photothermal therapy of cancer cells in vitro [97]. Copyright 2014 American Chemical Society.

5. Conclusions

Considering the huge requirements in applications of flexible electronic devices, biomedicine and energy harvesting and conversion, etc., the organization of inorganic NCs as building blocks coordinated into hierarchical cross-dimensional and cross-size micro/nano matrix with maintained high performances would be attractive. In this review, taking advantage of electrostatic spinning technologies induced polymer fibers, the research progress of inorganic NCs/polymer fibers synthesis and biomedical applications were reviewed. As mentioned above, electrostatic spinning, as a kind of simple but effective fiber production technology, has been widely used in medical releasing, biosensing and other fields. However, inorganic NC/polymer fiber composites still have many challenges to explore, even in biomedical fields, as illustrated in Figure 11.

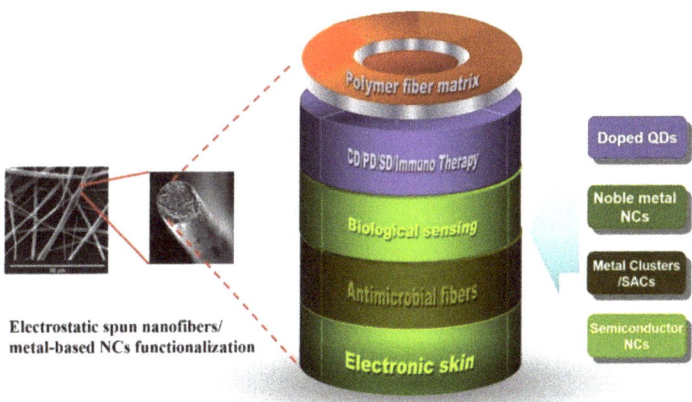

Figure 11. The outlook of metal-based NC functionalization in electrostatic spun nanofibers for extended applications.

(1) Though NC-modified nanofibers have exhibited high potential in many applications, how to modulate the depositing position of NCs is still challenging. Based on the reported strategies, a portion of NCs could be located inside the nanofibers, which could restrain their access to reactive molecules for efficient catalysis or biomedical applications. Hence, efficient strategies to precisely modulate the depositing sites of NCs on nanofibers could be helpful to further explore their applications [99,100].

(2) Compared to single-component modified nanofibers, composites consisting of an electrospun fiber membrane with multicomponent NCs could be developed for more biomedical applications, such as wound dressing applications [101]. Though there are several related papers, the mechanism of synergistic and potential coupling effects between the different introduced NCs within the electrospun fibers on the catalytic, optical and biocompatible properties should be further investigated, which could play an important role in designing reasonable multi-functional NCs/electrospun composite fiber membranes.

(3) Functional NC-modified electrospun fibers, incorporated with sensing and therapeutic capabilities, could be a potential approach in the development of personalized healthcare [102]. For example, "Electronic skin" has become a hotspot in the field of flexible and wearable electronics. Functional NC-modified electrospun composite fibers could be candidates to realize electronic devices and systems with skin-like properties and functions [103,104].

(4) Hybrid NCs, such as Au/semiconductors hetero-NCs with plasmon enhancement, could also exhibit unique biomedical applications when coupled with nanofibers, such as multi-level enhanced chemodynamic, sonodynamic and therapy applications, based on their sonosensitizers and photodynamic functionalities [49–52,105–109]. It is believed that with the further development of multi-functional inorganic NC/polymer fibers, electrostatic spinning technology will become one of the most widely used technologies in the medical field.

Author Contributions: J.Z. supervised the project, H.L. wrote and edited the manuscript, J.Z. revised the manuscript and provided financial support. H.L., M.X., R.S., A.Z. and J.Z. participated in the discussion and approved for publication of this work. All authors have read and agreed to the published version of the manuscript.

Funding: This work was supported by the National Natural Science Foundation of China (Grant No. 51872030, 52072035, 22005027, 51631001, 52173232, 22105116, 51902023).

Institutional Review Board Statement: Not applicable.

Informed Consent Statement: Not applicable.

Data Availability Statement: Not applicable.

Conflicts of Interest: The authors declare no conflict of interest.

Abbreviations

DMF	N-N dimethylformamide
FRET	Fluorescence resonance energy transfer
HRTEM	High-resolution transmission electron microscope
MF	Mafenide acetate
NCs	Nanocrystals
NIR	Near infrared
NPs	Nanoparticles
NRs	Nanorods
PAN	Polyacrylonitrile
PCL	Polycaprolactone
PEC	Pectin
PEG	Polyethylene glycol
PHBV	Poly(3-hydroxybutyrate-3-hydroxyvalerate)
PLA	Polylactic acid
PLGA	Poly-lactic-co-glycolic acid
PS	Polystyrene
PVA	Polyvinyl alcohol
PVP	Polyvinylpyrrolidone
QD	Quantum
R6G	Rhodamine 6G
SEM	Scanning electron microscope
SERS	Surface-enhanced Raman scattering
THF	Tetrahydrofuran
TIP	Ti(O-iPr)$_4$
UV	Ultraviolet

References

1. Gilbert, W. *De Magnete*; Courier: New York, NY, USA, 1958.
2. Taylor, G. Disintegration of water drops in an electric field. *Proc. R. Soc. Lond. A* **1964**, *280*, 383.
3. Reneker, D.H.; Chun, I. Nanometre diameter fibres of polymer, produced by electrospinning. *Nanotechnology* **1996**, *7*, 216. [CrossRef]
4. Shin, Y.M.; Hohman, M.M.; Brenner, M.P.; Rutledge, G.C. Electrospinning: A whipping fluid jet generates submicron polymer fibers. *Appl. Phys. Lett.* **2001**, *78*, 1149. [CrossRef]
5. Ding, X.T.; Zhao, Y.; Hu, C.G.; Hu, Y.; Dong, Z.L.; Chen, N.; Zhang, Z.P.; Qu, L.T. Spinning fabrication of graphene/polypyrrole composite fibers for all-solid-state, flexible fibriform supercapacitors. *J. Mater. Chem. A* **2014**, *2*, 12355. [CrossRef]
6. Someya, T.; Amagai, M. Toward a new generation of smart skins. *Nat. Biotechnol.* **2019**, *37*, 382. [CrossRef]
7. Wang, Y.; Yokota, T.; Someya, T. Electrospun nanofiber-based soft electronics. *NPG Asia Mater.* **2021**, *13*, 22. [CrossRef]
8. Bianka, G.; Kalaoglu-Altan, O.I.; Sanyal, R.; Sanyal, A. Hydrophilic cross-linked polymeric nanofibers using electrospinning: Imparting aqueous stability to enable biomedical applications. *ACS Appl. Polym. Mater.* **2022**, *4*, 1.
9. Eom, S.; Sang, M.P.; Hong, H.; Kwon, J.; Dong, S.K. Hydrogel-assisted electrospinning for fabrication of a 3D complex tailored nanofiber macrostructure. *ACS Appl. Mater. Interfaces* **2020**, *12*, 51212. [CrossRef]
10. Sang, H.J.; Lee, W.; Ji, S.Y. All-in-one piezo-triboelectric energy harvester module based on piezoceramic nanofibers for wearable devices. *ACS Appl. Mater. Interfaces* **2020**, *12*, 18609.

11. Parangusan, H.; Bhadra, J.; Al-Thani, N. Flexible piezoelectric nanogenerator based on [P(VDF-HFP)]/PANI-ZnS electrospun nanofibers for electrical energy harvesting. *J. Mater. Sci. Mater. Electron.* **2021**, *32*, 6358. [CrossRef]
12. Baskapan, B.; Callanan, A. Electrospinning fabrication methods to incorporate laminin in polycaprolactone for kidney tissue engineering. *Tissue Eng. Regen. Med.* **2022**, *19*, 73. [CrossRef] [PubMed]
13. Frizzell, H.; Ohlsen, T.J.; Woodrow, K.A. Protein-loaded emulsion electrospun fibers optimized for bioactivity retention and pH-controlled release for peroral delivery of biologic therapeutics. *Int. J. Pharm.* **2017**, *533*, 99. [CrossRef] [PubMed]
14. Wang, J.; Windbergs, M. Controlled dual drug release by coaxial electrospun fibers-Impact of the core fluid on drug encapsulation and release. *Int. J. Pharm.* **2019**, *556*, 363. [CrossRef]
15. Ehler, E.; Jayasinghe, S.N. Cell electrospinning cardiac patches for tissue engineering the heart. *Analyst* **2014**, *139*, 4449. [CrossRef] [PubMed]
16. Sampson, S.; Saraiva, L.; Gustafsson, K.; Jayasinghe, S.; Robertson, B. Cell electrospinning: An in vitro and in vivo study. *Small* **2014**, *10*, 78. [CrossRef] [PubMed]
17. Jayasinghe, S.N. Cell electrospinning: A novel tool for functionalising fibres, scaffolds and membranes with living cells and other advanced materials for regenerative biology and medicine. *Analyst* **2013**, *138*, 2215. [CrossRef] [PubMed]
18. Illangakoon, U.E.; Gill, H.; Shearman, G.C.; Parhizkar, M.; Mahalingam, S.; Chatterton, N.P.; Williams, G.R. Fast dissolving paracetamol/caffeine nanofibers prepared by electrospinning. *Int. J. Pharm.* **2014**, *477*, 369. [CrossRef]
19. Alshaya, H.A.; Alfahad, A.J.; Alsulaihem, F.M.; Aodah, A.H.; Alshehri, A.A.; Almughem, F.A.; Alfassam, H.A.; Aldossary, A.M.; Halwani, A.A.; Bukhary, H.A.; et al. Fast-dissolving nifedipine and atorvastatin calcium electrospun nanofibers as a potential buccal delivery system. *Pharmaceutics* **2022**, *14*, 358. [CrossRef]
20. Hu, J.; Li, H.Y.; Williams, G.R.; Yang, H.H.; Tao, L.; Zhu, L.M. Electrospun poly(N-isopropylacrylamide)/ethyl cellulose nanofibers as thermoresponsive drug delivery systems. *J. Pharm. Sci.* **2016**, *105*, 1104. [CrossRef]
21. Li, H.; Sang, Q.; Wu, J.; Williams, G.R.; Wang, H.; Niu, S.; Wu, J.; Zhu, L.M. Dual-responsive drug delivery systems prepared by blend electrospinning. *Int. J. Pharm.* **2018**, *543*, 1. [CrossRef]
22. Dziemidowicz, K.; Sang, Q.; Wu, J.; Zhang, Z.; Zhou, F.; Lagaron, J.M.; Mo, X.; Parker, G.J.M.; Yu, D.G.; Zhu, L.M.; et al. Electrospinning for healthcare: Recent advancements. *J. Mater. Chem. B* **2021**, *9*, 939. [CrossRef] [PubMed]
23. Jia, D.; Gao, Y.; Williams, G.R. Core/shell poly(ethylene oxide)/Eudragit fibers for site-specific release. *Int. J. Pharm.* **2017**, *523*, 376. [CrossRef] [PubMed]
24. Pant, B.; Park, M.; Park, S.J. Drug delivery applications of core-sheath nanofibers prepared by coaxial electrospinning: A review. *Pharmaceutics* **2019**, *11*, 305. [CrossRef] [PubMed]
25. Hu, J.J.; Liu, C.C.; Lin, C.H.; Tuan-Mu, H.-Y. Synthesis, characterization, and electrospinning of a functionalizable, polycaprolactone-based polyurethane for soft tissue engineering. *Polymers* **2021**, *13*, 1527. [CrossRef]
26. Fang, J.; Zhang, J.; Du, J.; Pan, Y.; Shi, J.; Peng, Y.; Chen, W.; Yuan, L.; Ye, S.H.; Wagner, W.R.; et al. Orthogonally functionalizable polyurethane with subsequent modification with heparin and endothelium-inducing peptide aiming for vascular reconstruction. *ACS Appl. Mater. Interfaces* **2016**, *8*, 14442. [CrossRef]
27. Yu, B.; He, C.; Wang, W.; Ren, Y.; Yang, J.; Guo, S.; Zheng, Y.; Shi, X. Asymmetric wettable composite wound dressing prepared by electrospinning with bioinspired micropatterning enhances diabetic wound healing. *ACS Appl. Bio Mater.* **2020**, *3*, 5383. [CrossRef] [PubMed]
28. Huang, Y.P.; Dan, N.H.; Dan, W.H.; Zhao, W.F.; Bai, Z.X.; Chen, Y.N.; Yang, C.K. Bilayered antimicrobial nanofiber membranes for wound dressings via in situ cross-linking polymerization and electrospinning. *Ind. Eng. Chem. Res.* **2018**, *57*, 17048. [CrossRef]
29. Bhardwaj, N.; Kundu, S.C. Electrospinning: A fascinating fiber fabrication technique. *Biotechnol. Adv.* **2010**, *28*, 325. [CrossRef]
30. Xue, J.; Wu, T.; Dai, Y.; Xia, Y. Electrospinning and electrospun nanofibers: Methods, materials, and applications. *Chem. Rev.* **2019**, *119*, 5298. [CrossRef]
31. Karpov, V.G. Electrostatic theory of metal whiskers. *Phys. Rev. Appl.* **2014**, *1*, 044001. [CrossRef]
32. Zubir, A.A.M.; Khairunnisa, M.P.; Atiqah Surib, N.; NorRuwaida, J.; Ali, A.H.M.; Rashid, M. Electrospinning of PLA with DMF: Effect of polymer concentration on the bead diameter of the electrospun fibre. *IOP Conf. Ser. Mater. Sci. Eng.* **2020**, *778*, 012087. [CrossRef]
33. Hu, J.; Wang, X.; Ding, B.; Lin, J.; Yu, J.; Sun, G. One-step electrospinning/netting technique for controllably preparing polyurethane nano-fiber/net. *Macromol. Rapid Commun.* **2011**, *32*, 1729–1734. [CrossRef]
34. Demir, M.M.; Yilgor, I.; Yilgor, E.; Erman, B. Electrospinning of polyurethane fibers. *Polymer* **2002**, *43*, 3303. [CrossRef]
35. Ma, X.; He, S.; Qiu, B.; Luo, F.; Guo, L.; Lin, Z. Noble metal nanoparticle-based multicolor immunoassays: An approach toward visual quantification of the analytes with the naked eye. *ACS Sens.* **2019**, *4*, 782. [CrossRef] [PubMed]
36. Wang, H.; Zhou, S.; Gilroy, K.D.; Cai, Z.; Xi, Y. Icosahedral nanocrystals of noble metals: Synthesis and applications. *Nano Today* **2017**, *15*, 121. [CrossRef]
37. Sun, Y.; Xia, Y. Shape-controlled synthesis of gold and silver nanoparticles. *Science* **2002**, *298*, 2176. [CrossRef] [PubMed]
38. Ji, L.; Hsu, H.Y.; Li, X.; Huang, K.; Zhang, Y.; Lee, J.C.; Bard, A.J.; Yu, E.T. Localized dielectric breakdown and antireflection coating in metal–oxide–semiconductor photoelectrodes. *Nat. Mater.* **2017**, *16*, 127. [CrossRef] [PubMed]
39. Shao, M.; Liu, J.J.; Ding, W.J.; Wang, J.Y.; Dong, F.; Zhang, J.T. Oxygen vacancy engineering of self-doped SnO_{2-x} nanocrystals for ultrasensitive NO_2 detection. *J. Mater. Chem. C* **2020**, *8*, 487. [CrossRef]

40. Li, X.Y.; Rong, H.P.; Zhang, J.T.; Wang, D.S.; Li, Y.D. Modulating the local coordination environment of single-atom catalysts for enhanced catalytic performance. *Nano Res.* **2020**, *13*, 1842. [CrossRef]
41. Zhang, E.; Wang, T.; Yu, K.; Liu, J.; Chen, W.; Li, A.; Rong, H.; Lin, R.; Ji, S.; Zheng, X.; et al. Bismuth single atoms resulting from transformation of metal−organic frameworks and their use as electrocatalysts for CO_2 reduction. *J. Am. Chem. Soc.* **2019**, *141*, 16569. [CrossRef]
42. Jiang, Z.; Sun, W.; Shang, H.; Chen, W.; Sun, T.; Li, H.; Dong, J.; Zhou, J.; Li, Z.; Wang, Y.; et al. Atomic interface effect of a single atom copper catalyst for enhanced oxygen reduction reactions. *Energy Environ. Sci.* **2019**, *12*, 3508. [CrossRef]
43. Yang, X.; Wang, A.; Qiao, B.; Li, J.; Liu, J.; Zhang, T. Single-atom catalysts: A new frontier in heterogeneous catalysis. *Acc. Chem. Res.* **2013**, *46*, 1740. [CrossRef] [PubMed]
44. Liu, J.; Zhang, J.T. Nanointerface chemistry: Lattice-mismatch-directed synthesis and application of hybrid nanocrystals. *Chem. Rev.* **2020**, *120*, 2123. [CrossRef] [PubMed]
45. Pan, R.; Liu, J.; Li, Y.; Zhang, E.; Di, Q.; Su, M.; Zhang, J. Electronic doping-enabled transition from n- to ptype conductivity over Au@CdS core–shell nanocrystals toward unassisted photoelectrochemical water splitting. *J. Mater. Chem. A* **2019**, *7*, 23038. [CrossRef]
46. Wang, D.; Wang, H.; Ji, L.; Xu, M.; Bai, B.; Wan, X.; Hou, D.; Qiao, Z.; Wang, H.; Zhang, J. Hybrid plasmonic nanodumbbells engineering for multi-intensified second near-infrared light induced photodynamic therapy. *ACS Nano* **2021**, *15*, 8694. [CrossRef]
47. Anwer, S.; Ji, M.; Qian, H.; Liu, J.; Xu, M.; Zhang, J. Noble metal nanoclusters and their in situ calcination to nanocrystals: Precise control of their size and interface with TiO_2 nanosheets and their versatile catalysis applications. *Nano Res.* **2016**, *9*, 1763.
48. Li, Y.; Liu, J.; Wan, X.; Pan, R.; Bai, B.; Wang, H.; Cao, X.; Zhang, J. Surface passivation enabled-structural engineering of I-III-VI_2 nanocrystal photocatalysts. *J. Mater. Chem. A* **2020**, *8*, 9951. [CrossRef]
49. Di, Q.; Zhu, X.; Liu, J.; Zhang, X.; Shang, H.; Chen, W.; Liu, J.; Rong, H.; Xu, M.; Zhang, J. High-performance quantum dots with synergistic doping and oxide shell protection synthesized by cation exchange conversion of ternary-composition nanoparticles. *J. Phys. Chem. Lett.* **2019**, *10*, 2606. [CrossRef]
50. Chang, Y.; Xu, M.; Huang, L.; Pan, R.; Liu, J.; Liu, J.; Rong, H.; Chen, W.; Zhang, J. Micro-scale 2D quasi-nanosheets formed by 0D nanocrystals: From single to multicomponent building blocks. *Sci. China Mater.* **2020**, *63*, 1265. [CrossRef]
51. Yoshida, K.; Chang, J.F.; Chueh, C.C.; Higashihara, T. Hybridization of an n-type semiconducting polymer with PbS quantum dots and their photovoltaic investigation. *Polym. J.* **2022**, *54*, 323. [CrossRef]
52. Liu, J.; Fan, J.; Gu, Z.; Cui, J.; Xu, X.; Liang, Z.; Luo, S.; Zhu, M. Green chemistry for large-scale synthesis of semiconductor quantum dots. *Langmuir* **2008**, *24*, 5241. [CrossRef] [PubMed]
53. Wu, P.; Xu, Y.; Zhan, J.; Li, Y.; Xue, H.; Pang, H. The research development of quantum dots in electrochemical energy storage. *Small* **2018**, *14*, e1801479. [CrossRef] [PubMed]
54. Maity, P.; Gayathri, T.; Singh, S.P.; Ghosh, H.N. Impact of FRET between molecular aggregates and quantum dots. *Chem. Asian J.* **2019**, *14*, 597. [CrossRef] [PubMed]
55. Yu, S.; Fan, X.B.; Wang, X.; Li, J.; Zhang, Q.; Xia, A.; Wei, S.; Wu, L.Z.; Zhou, Y.; Patzke, G.R. Efficient photocatalytic hydrogen evolution with ligand engineered all-inorganic InP and InP/ZnS colloidal quantum dots. *Nat. Commun.* **2018**, *9*, 4009. [CrossRef]
56. Xiang, H.; Feng, W.; Chen, Y. Single-atom catalysts in catalytic biomedicine. *Adv. Mater.* **2020**, *32*, e1905994. [CrossRef]
57. Chern, M.; Kays, J.C.; Bhuckory, S.; Dennis, A.M. Sensing with photoluminescent semiconductor quantum dots. *Methods Appl. Fluoresc.* **2019**, *7*, 012005. [CrossRef]
58. Kim, S.W.; Kwon, J.; Lee, J.S.; Kang, B.H.; Lee, S.W.; Jung, D.G.; Lee, J.Y.; Han, M.; Kim, O.G.; Saianand, G.; et al. An organic/inorganic nanomaterial and nanocrystal quantum dots-based multi-level resistive memory device. *Nanomaterials* **2021**, *11*, 3004. [CrossRef]
59. Li, R.; Tang, L.; Zhao, Q.; Ly, T.H.; Teng, K.S.; Li, Y.; Hu, Y.; Shu, C.; Lau, S.P. In_2S_3 quantum dots: Preparation, properties and optoelectronic application. *Nanoscale Res. Lett.* **2019**, *14*, 161. [CrossRef]
60. Hashemkhani, M.; Loizidou, M.; MacRobert, A.J.; Yagci Acar, H. One-step aqueous synthesis of anionic and cationic $AgInS_2$ quantum dots and their utility in improving the efficacy of ALA-based photodynamic therapy. *Inorg. Chem.* **2022**, *61*, 2846. [CrossRef]
61. Zhang, M.; Zang, S.; Ge, G.; Jin, L.; Xin, Y.; Li, H.; Liu, P.; Hou, X.; Hao, D.; Chen, L.; et al. Detection of CD22 expression in living cancer cells by semiconductor quantum dots. *J. Biomed. Nanotechnol.* **2019**, *15*, 2149. [CrossRef]
62. Gongalsky, M.B.; Osminkina, L.A.; Pereira, A.; Manankov, A.A.; Fedorenko, A.A.; Vasiliev, A.N.; Solovyev, V.V.; Kudryavtsev, A.A.; Sentis, M.; Kabashin, A.V.; et al. Laser-synthesized oxide-passivated bright Si quantum dots for bioimaging. *Sci. Rep.* **2016**, *6*, 24732. [CrossRef] [PubMed]
63. Duan, Z.; Huang, Y.; Zhang, D.; Chen, S. Electrospinning fabricating Au/TiO_2 network-like nanofibers as visible light activated photocatalyst. *Sci. Rep.* **2019**, *9*, 8008. [CrossRef] [PubMed]
64. Xu, X.; Yang, Q.; Bai, J.; Lu, T.; Li, Y.; Jing, X. Fabrication of biodegradable electrospun poly(L-lactide-co-glycolide) fibers with antimicrobial nanosilver particles. *J. Nanosci. Nanotechnol.* **2008**, *8*, 5066. [CrossRef] [PubMed]
65. Renu, S.; Shivashangari, K.S.; Ravikumar, V. Incorporated plant extract fabricated silver/poly-D,l-lactide-co-glycolide nanocomposites for antimicrobial based wound healing. *Spectrochim. Acta A Mol. Biomol. Spectrosc.* **2020**, *228*, 117673. [CrossRef] [PubMed]

66. Li, P.; Ruan, L.; Wang, R.; Liu, T.; Song, G.; Gao, X.; Jiang, G.; Liu, X. Electrospun scaffold of collagen and polycaprolactone containing ZnO quantum dots for skin wound regeneration. *J. Bionic. Eng.* **2021**, *18*, 1378. [CrossRef] [PubMed]
67. El-Hefnawy, M.E.; Alhayyani, S.; El-Sherbiny, M.M.; Sakran, M.I.; El-Newehy, M.H. Fabrication of nanofibers based on hydroxypropyl starch/polyurethane loaded with the biosynthesized silver nanoparticles for the treatment of pathogenic microbes in wounds. *Polymers* **2022**, *14*, 318. [CrossRef] [PubMed]
68. Manjumeena, R.; Elakkiya, T.; Duraibabu, D.; Feroze Ahamed, A.; Kalaichelvan, P.T.; Venkatesan, R. 'Green' biocompatible organic-inorganic hybrid electrospun nanofibers for potential biomedical applications. *J. Biomater. Appl.* **2015**, *29*, 1039. [CrossRef]
69. Li, P.; Liu, C.G.; Song, Y.H.; Niu, X.F.; Liu, H.F.; Fan, Y.B. Influence of Fe_3O_4 nanoparticles on the preparation of aligned PLGA electrospun fibers induced by magnetic field. *J. Nanomater.* **2013**, *2013*, 483569. [CrossRef]
70. Abdalkarim, S.; Yu, H.Y.; Wang, C.; Yang, L.; Guan, Y.; Huang, L.; Yao, J. Sheet-like cellulose nanocrystal-ZnO nanohybrids as multifunctional reinforcing agents in biopolyester composite nanofibers with ultrahigh UV-shielding and antibacterial performances. *ACS Appl. Bio. Mater.* **2018**, *1*, 714. [CrossRef]
71. Lin, S.; Wang, R.Z.; Yi, Y.; Wang, Z.; Hao, L.M.; Wu, J.H.; Hu, G.H.; He, H. Facile and green fabrication of electrospun poly(vinyl alcohol) nanofibrous mats doped with narrowly dispersed silver nanoparticles. *Int. J. Nanomed.* **2014**, *9*, 3937. [CrossRef]
72. Kwon, S.Y.; Ra, E.; Jung, D.G.; Kong, S.H. Immobilization of Pt nanoparticles on hydrolyzed polyacrylonitrile-based nanofiber paper. *Sci. Rep.* **2021**, *11*, 11501. [CrossRef] [PubMed]
73. Binkley, D.M.; Lee, B.; Saem, S.; Moran-Mirabal, J.; Grandfield, K. Fabrication of polycaprolactone electrospun nanofibers doped with silver nanoparticles formed by air plasma treatment. *Nanotechnology* **2019**, *30*, 215101. [CrossRef] [PubMed]
74. Wang, X.C.; Lv, F.; Li, T.; Han, Y.; Yi, Z.; Liu, M.; Chang, J.; Wu, C. Electrospun micropatterned nanocomposites incorporated with Cu_2S nanoflowers for skin tumor therapy and wound healing. *ACS Nano* **2017**, *11*, 11337. [CrossRef]
75. Zhang, C.-L.; Lv, K.-P.; Huang, H.-T.; Cong, H.-P.; Yu, S.-H. Co-assembly of Au nanorods with Ag nanowires within polymer nanofiber matrix for enhanced SERS property by electrospinning. *Nanoscale* **2012**, *4*, 5348. [CrossRef]
76. He, D.; Hu, B.; Yao, Q.-F.; Wang, K.; Yu, S.-H. Large-scale synthesis of flexible free-standing SERS substrates with high sensitivity: Electrospun PVA nanofibers embedded with controlled alignment of silver nanoparticles. *ACS Nano* **2009**, *3*, 3993. [CrossRef] [PubMed]
77. Kamal, K.G.; Pradeep, K.M.; Pradeep, S.; Mayank, G.; Gopal, N.; Pralay, M. Hydrothermal in situ preparation of TiO_2 particles onto poly(lactic acid) electrospun nanofibers. *Appl. Surf. Sci.* **2013**, *264*, 375.
78. Kishore, K.R.; Balamurugan, D.; Jeyaprakash, B.G. Electrospinning based CdO nanograins for formaldehyde vapour detection by chemiresistive method. *Mater. Sci. Semicond. Processing* **2021**, *121*, 105296. [CrossRef]
79. Lee, S.; Bai, H.; Liu, Z.; Sun, D. Optimization and an insightful properties-activity study of electrospun TiO_2/CuO composite nanofibers for efficient photocatalytic H_2 generation. *Appl. Catal. B-Environ.* **2013**, *140*, 68. [CrossRef]
80. Srisitthiratkul, C.; Yaipimai, W.; Intasanta, V. Environmental remediation and superhydrophilicity of ultrafine antibacterial tungsten oxide-based nanofibers under visible light source. *Appl. Surf. Sci.* **2012**, *259*, 349. [CrossRef]
81. Srisitthiratkul, C.; Pongsorrarith, V.; Intasanta, N. The potential use of nanosilver-decorated titanium dioxide nanofibers for toxin decomposition with antimicrobial and self-cleaning properties. *Appl. Surf. Sci.* **2011**, *257*, 8850. [CrossRef]
82. Yang, Y.; Zhang, Z.; Wan, M.; Wang, Z.; Zou, X.; Zhao, Y.; Sun, L. A facile method for the fabrication of silver nanoparticles surface decorated polyvinyl alcohol electrospun nanofibers and controllable antibacterial activities. *Polymers* **2020**, *12*, 2486. [CrossRef] [PubMed]
83. Pazos, O.E.; Hafid, R.R.J.; Amador, H.M.E.; Lopez, E.J.; Donohue, C.A.; Carlos, C.G.J.; Espinosa-Cristóbal, L.F.; Reyes-López, S.Y. Dose-dependent antimicrobial activity of silver nanoparticles on polycaprolactone fibers against gram-positive and gram-negative bacteria. *J. Nanomater.* **2017**, *2017*, 4752314.
84. Alipour, R.; Khorshidi, A.; Shojaei, A.F.; Mashayekhi, F.; Moghaddam, M.J.M. Skin wound healing acceleration by Ag nanoparticles embedded in PVA/PVP/Pectin/Mafenide acetate composite nanofibers. *Polym. Test.* **2019**, *79*, 106022. [CrossRef]
85. Qian, Y.; Zhou, X.; Zhang, F.; Diekwisch, T.G.H.; Luan, X.; Yang, J. Triple PLGA/PCL scaffold modification including silver impregnation, collagen coating, and electrospinning significantly improve biocompatibility, antimicrobial, and osteogenic properties for orofacial tissue regeneration. *ACS Appl. Mater. Interfaces* **2019**, *11*, 37381. [CrossRef] [PubMed]
86. Pant, H.R.; Bajgai, M.P.; Nam, K.T.; Seo, Y.A.; Pandeya, D.R.; Hong, S.T.; Kim, H.Y. Electrospun nylon-6 spider-net like nanofiber mat containing TiO_2 nanoparticles: A multifunctional nanocomposite textile material. *J. Hazard. Mater.* **2011**, *185*, 124. [CrossRef]
87. Toniatto, T.V.; Rodrigues, B.V.M.; Marsi, T.C.O.; Ricci, R.; Marciano, F.R.; Webster, T.J.; Lobo, A.O. Nanostructured poly (lactic acid) electrospun fiber with high loadings of TiO_2 nanoparticles: Insights into bactericidal activity and cell viability. *Mater. Sci. Eng. C* **2017**, *71*, 381. [CrossRef]
88. Al-Mogbel, M.S.; Elabbasy, M.T.; Menazea, A.A.; Sadek, A.W.; Ahmed, M.K.; Abd El-Kader, M. Conditions adjustment of polycaprolactone nanofibers scaffolds encapsulated with core shells of Au@Se via laser ablation for wound healing applications. *Spectrochim. Acta Part A Mol. Biomol. Spectrosc.* **2021**, *259*, 119899. [CrossRef]
89. Ahmed, M.K.; Moydeen, A.M.; Ismail, A.M.; El Naggar, M.E.; Menazea, A.A.; El Newehy, M.H. Wound dressing properties of functionalized environmentally biopolymer loaded with selenium nanoparticles. *J. Mol. Struct.* **2021**, *1225*, 129138. [CrossRef]
90. Ghiyasi, Y.; Salahi, E.; Esfahani, H. Synergy effect of Urtica dioica and ZnO NPs on microstructure, antibacterial activity and cytotoxicity of electrospun PCL scaffold for wound dressing application. *Mater. Today Commun.* **2021**, *26*, 102163. [CrossRef]

91. Baek, S.H.; Roh, J.; Park, C.Y.; Kim, M.W.; Shi, R.; Kailasa, S.K.; Park, T.J. Cu-nanoflower decorated gold nanoparticles-graphene oxide nanofiber as electrochemical biosensor for glucose detection. *Mater. Sci. Eng. C Mater. Biol. Appl.* **2020**, *107*, 11027. [CrossRef]
92. Sberveglieri, G.; Baratto, C.; Comini, E.; Faglia, G.; Ferroni, M.; Ponzoniet, A.; Vomieroal, A. Synthesis and characterization of semiconducting nanowires for gas sensing. *Sens. Actuators B Chem.* **2007**, *121*, 208. [CrossRef]
93. Liu, X.; Hu, Q.; Wu, Q.; Zhang, W.; Fang, Z.; Xie, Q. Aligned ZnO nanorods: A useful film to fabricate amperometric glucose biosensor. *Colloids Surf. B Biointerfaces* **2009**, *74*, 154. [CrossRef] [PubMed]
94. Wang, Y.; Zhu, Y.; Huang, J.; Cai, J.; Zhu, J.; Yang, X.; Shen, J.; Jiang, H.; Li, C. $CsPbBr_3$ perovskite quantum dots-based monolithic electrospun fiber membrane as an ultrastable and ultrasensitive fluorescent sensor in aqueous medium. *Phys. Chem. Lett.* **2016**, *7*, 4253. [CrossRef]
95. Yang, Y.; Zhang, Z.; Wan, M.; Wang, Z.; Zhao, Y.; Sun, L. Highly sensitive surface-enhanced raman spectroscopy substrates of Ag@PAN electrospinning nanofibrous membranes for direct detection of bacteria. *ACS Omega* **2020**, *5*, 19834. [CrossRef]
96. Anitha, D.; Hyungkyu, H.; Taeseup, S.; Young-Pil, K.; Ungyu, P. Gold nanoparticle-composite nanofibers for enzymatic electrochemical sensing of hydrogen peroxide. *Analyst* **2013**, *138*, 5025.
97. Cheng, M.; Wang, H.; Zhang, Z.; Li, N.; Fang, X.; Xu, S. Gold nanorod-embedded electrospun fibrous membrane as a photothermal therapy platform. *ACS Appl. Mater. Interfaces* **2014**, *6*, 1569. [CrossRef]
98. Huang, C.; Dong, J.; Zhang, Y.; Chai, S.; Wang, X.; Kan, S.; Yu, D.; Wang, P.; Jiang, Q. Gold nanoparticles-loaded polyvinylpyrrolidone/ethylcellulose coaxial electrospun nanofibers with enhanced osteogenic capability for bone tissue regeneration. *Mater. Des.* **2021**, *212*, 110240. [CrossRef]
99. Zhu, H.; Du, M.; Zhang, M.; Wang, P.; Bao, S.; Zou, M.; Fu, Y.; Yao, J. Self-assembly of various Au nanocrystals on functionalized water-stable PVA/PEI nanofibers: A highly efficient surface-enhanced raman scattering substrates with high density of "hot" spots. *Biosens. Bioelectron.* **2014**, *54*, 91. [CrossRef]
100. Qian, Y.; Meng, G.; Huang, Q.; Zhu, C.; Huang, Z.; Sun, K.; Chen, B. Flexible membranes of Ag-nanosheet-grafted polyamide-nanofibers as effective 3D SERS substrates. *Nanoscale* **2014**, *6*, 4781. [CrossRef]
101. Libanori, A.; Chen, G.; Zhao, X.; Zhou, Y.H.; Chen, J. Smart textiles for personalized healthcare. *Nat. Electron.* **2022**, *5*, 142–156. [CrossRef]
102. Wang, D.Y.; Wang, L.L.; Shen, G.Z. Nanofiber/nanowires-based flexible and stretchable sensors. *J. Semicond.* **2020**, *41*, 041605. [CrossRef]
103. Ma, Z.; Kong, D.S.; Pan, L.J.; Bao, Z.N. Skin-inspired electronics: Emerging semiconductor devices and systems. *J. Semicond.* **2020**, *41*, 041601. [CrossRef]
104. Wen, X.; Xiong, J.; Lei, S.; Wang, L.; Qin, X. Diameter refinement of electrospun nanofibers: From mechanism, strategies to applications. *Adv. Fiber Mater.* **2021**, *4*, 145–161. [CrossRef]
105. Fan, Y.; Liu, S.; Yi, Y.; Rong, H.P.; Zhang, J.T. Catalytic nanomaterials toward atomic levels for biomedical applications: From metal clusters to single-atom catalysts. *ACS Nano* **2021**, *15*, 2005. [CrossRef]
106. Wang, D.; Zhu, Y.; Wan, X.; Zhang, X.; Zhang, J.T. Colloidal semiconductor nanocrystals for biological photodynamic therapy applications: Recent progress and perspectives. *Prog. Nat. Sci. Mater. Int.* **2020**, *30*, 443. [CrossRef]
107. Jiang, Q.; Wang, K.; Zhang, X.; Ouyang, B.; Liu, H.; Pang, Z.; Yang, W. Platelet membrane-camouflaged magnetic NPs for ferroptosis-enhanced cancer immunotherapy. *Small* **2020**, *16*, e2001704. [CrossRef]
108. Zhang, F.; Ma, Z.Z.; Shi, Z.F.; Chen, X.; Wu, D.; Li, X.J.; Shan, C.X. Recent advances and opportunities of lead-free perovskite nanocrystal for optoelectronic application. *Energy Mater. Adv.* **2021**, *2021*, 5198145. [CrossRef]
109. Liu, Y.; Molokeev, M.S.; Xia, J. Lattice doping of lanthanide ions in $Cs_2AgInCl_6$ nanocrystals enabling tunable photoluminescence. *Energy Mater. Adv.* **2021**, *2021*, 2585274. [CrossRef]

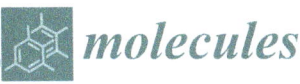

Review

Single-Atom Nanozymes: Fabrication, Characterization, Surface Modification and Applications of ROS Scavenging and Antibacterial

Haihan Song, Mengli Zhang and Weijun Tong *

MOE Key Laboratory of Macromolecular Synthesis and Functionalization, Department of Polymer Science and Engineering, Zhejiang University, Hangzhou 310027, China
* Correspondence: tongwj@zju.edu.cn

Abstract: Nanozymes are nanomaterials with intrinsic natural enzyme-like catalytic properties. They have received extensive attention and have the potential to be an alternative to natural enzymes. Increasing the atom utilization rate of active centers in nanozymes has gradually become a concern of scientists. As the limit of designing nanozymes at the atomic level, single-atom nanozymes (SAzymes) have become the research frontier of the biomedical field recently because of their high atom utilization, well-defined active centers, and good natural enzyme mimicry. In this review, we first introduce the preparation of SAzymes through pyrolysis and defect engineering with regulated activity, then the characterization and surface modification methods of SAzymes are introduced. The possible influences of surface modification on the activity of SAzymes are discussed. Furthermore, we summarize the applications of SAzymes in the biomedical fields, especially in those of reactive oxygen species (ROS) scavenging and antibacterial. Finally, the challenges and opportunities of SAzymes are summarized and prospected.

Keywords: nanozyme; single-atom nanozyme; surface modification; ROS scavenging; antibacterial

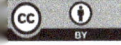

1. Introduction

Enzymes play a very important role in thousands of biochemical reactions carried out in our body from moment to moment. Most enzymes are proteins, and a few are RNA [1], which can specifically catalyze the reaction under mild conditions, and have the characteristics of high catalytic efficiency and good specificity [2]. However, natural enzymes are easily inactivated under harsh conditions, together with complicated preparation process and high cost, which greatly limit their applications [3]. Therefore, people continually develop artificial enzymes as the substitutes of natural enzymes.

In 2007, Yan's group [4] first discovered that Fe_3O_4 nanoparticles (NPs) had peroxidase (POD)-like activity, and their pH and temperature stability were much higher than those of natural horseradish peroxidase (HRP). Since then, the term "nanozyme" has entered the field of vision of scientists. Nanozymes are a class of nanomaterials with catalytic activity similar to natural enzymes, which have the advantages of high stability, low cost, and simple preparation [5]. Scientists have successfully developed a series of carbon-based nanozymes, metal-based nanozymes, metal oxide-based nanozymes, and so on [6], which are widely used in biosensing [7,8], antibacterial [9–11], anti-inflammatory [12–15], cancer treatment [16–19], and other biomedical fields.

Although nanozymes have a wide range of applications in the biomedical field, their catalytic activity, specificity, and affinity for substrates still need to be improved compared with natural enzymes [6,20]. The diversity of protein composition in natural enzymes and the complexity of the folding process endow them with fairly fine structures. Such kind of fine structures are normally absent in nanozymes; thus, their performance in catalytic reactions is far inferior to that of natural enzymes [21]. Furthermore, the internal crystal structure of nanozymes is not uniform and the elemental composition is complex, which makes it difficult to study their active sites, catalytic reaction unit, and catalytic mechanisms [22,23].

In 2011, Zhang's group [24] proposed the concept of single-atom catalysts (SACs). They prepared a new type of catalyst with single Pt atoms atomically dispersed on the surface of iron oxide (FeOx) (denoted as Pt/FeOx). Pt/FeOx exhibited extremely high reactivity in CO oxidation and preferential oxidation. After years of development, SACs are defined as a novel catalyst in which catalytically active isolated metal atoms are immobilized on supports [25]. They combine the advantages of homogeneous catalysis and heterogeneous catalysis [26], and SACs possess the maximized atom utilization, unsaturated coordination of active sites, and adjustable electronic properties, which make them a hot research direction in the field of catalysis [27–29]. Meanwhile, the high atom utilization rate can also reduce the production cost of SACs [30] and the potential toxic and side effects of metal ions [31,32]. More importantly, the isolated and dispersed atoms in SACs are stabilized by surrounding ligands, which is very similar to the geometric structure in some natural enzymes centered on metal atoms [30]; thus, SACs also have been proposed for use as biomimetic single-atom nanozymes (SAzymes). In SAzymes there are well-defined and precisely controlled active sites, so it is easy to determine the catalytic reaction unit, which is particularly important for revealing the structure–activity relationship and studying the catalytic reaction mechanism [22,28].

In this review, we first systematically describe the preparation of SAzymes through pyrolysis and defect engineering and the regulation of their enzyme-like activities, followed by their characterization. In the following part, the strategies of surface modification for SAzymes are further introduced, which is critical for their biomedical applications. Then, the applications of SAzymes in the fields of reactive oxygen species (ROS) scavenging and antibacterial are discussed. Finally, the challenges and opportunities of SAzymes are summarized and prospected.

2. Preparation of SAzymes

Although SAzymes have broad applications in the biomedical fields, the preparation is not easy because of the high surface energy of isolated metal atoms which tend to aggregate into nanoclusters during the preparation process [28,33]. Therefore, preventing the aggregation of metal atoms during the preparation has become the top priority in the development of preparation strategies. Scientists have developed a variety of synthesis strategies, including pyrolysis, defect engineering, atomic layer deposition, photochemical reduction, and so on [28,30], and the advantages and disadvantages of these methods are listed in Table 1. In this review, we mainly focus on the widely used pyrolysis strategy and the defect engineering strategy based on wet chemistry.

Table 1. Advantages and disadvantages of preparation methods of SAzymes.

Methods	Advantages	Disadvantages	Ref.
Pyrolysis	Widely used, high active centers loading, well-defined structure, large-scale manufacture potential.	High energy consuming, uncontrollable particle size, poor biocompatibility.	[20,30]
Defect engineering	Better biocompatibility, controllable particle size, low cost, low energy consuming.	Less application system, more activity modulation methods need to be developed.	[27]
Atomic layer deposition	Precise control of active center deposition, convenient to study the relationship between catalyst structure and performance.	Difficult to achieve mass production, high cost.	[34]
Photochemical reduction	Easy to operate, no professional equipment required.	Relatively low active center loading, difficult to achieve mass production.	[35,36]

2.1. Pyrolysis

As a widely used preparation method for carbon-supported SAzymes [37], pyrolysis is usually a method to prepare SAzymes by thermally pyrolyzing the carrier loaded with the active species precursor in a specified gas atmosphere, which can realize the precise control of structure and high loading of atomically dispersed metal atoms [30]. Classical pyrolysis usually includes three steps. Firstly, the active center precursor is loaded on/into the carrier, and then it is pyrolyzed in a gas atmosphere. During the cracking process, the carbon support is converted into N-doped carbon material and the active centers coordinate with N or C atoms to form an M–N/C structure (M represents a transition metal) [38], and finally the template or unreacted raw materials are removed.

For example, Zhu et al. [39] used aniline, ammonium persulfate, and SiO_2 to synthesize a support, and then added the active center precursor $Pd(CH_3CN)_2Cl_2$ on it. After pyrolysis in Ar, the template was washed away with NaOH, and Pd–C SAzyme with atomically dispersed Pd atoms as active centers was obtained. Pd–C SAzyme showed strong POD-like activity under acidic conditions and excellent photothermal properties. Cheng et al. [40] mixed oxidized carbon nanotubes with pyrrole, added ammonium persulfate to induce the polymerization of pyrrole into polypyrrole, and then added $Fe(NO_3)_3$ and NaCl which would promote the attachment of Fe species on the surface of carbon nanotubes. Afterwards, it was pyrolyzed at 900 °C in N_2, and annealed in NH_3 after removing NaCl and unreacted Fe species with H_2SO_4. Finally, the SAzyme with Fe as the active centers and carbon nanotubes as the carrier (denoted as CNT/FeNC) was obtained (Figure 1A). CNT/FeNC exhibited excellent POD-like activity, enabling sensitive detection of H_2O_2, glucose, and ascorbic acid (AsA).

In addition, metal–organic frameworks (MOFs) are also important support materials which are widely used in the preparation of SAzymes through pyrolysis. Composed of metal nodes and organic ligands, MOFs are a kind of porous crystalline material, and have high specific surface area, well-defined structures, and can be flexibly designed [27]. More importantly, the dispersed metal nodes in MOFs are well defined, which can be directly transformed into isolated metal sites on the carriers due to the carbonization of organic ligands during the pyrolysis process [20]. Therefore, MOFs are excellent carriers for the preparation of SAzymes [28]. The precursor containing the active center also can be easily immobilized in the MOF by ion exchange, etc., and then the metal atom of the active center is coordinated with N or C during the pyrolysis process and transformed into N-doped carbon materials (M–N/C) [30,41].

ZIF-8, with Zn as the metal node and 2-methylimidazole as the organic ligand, has a large specific surface area, numerous pores, and abundant N atoms, which is the preferred MOF for the preparation of SAzyme through pyrolysis [42]. Niu et al. [42] added Fe^{3+} during the synthesis process to obtain Fe-doped ZIF-8, which was subsequently pyrolyzed in N_2 and NH_3 at 900 °C to obtain the SAzyme with atomically distributed Fe as the active center and N-doped carbon material as the carrier (denoted as Fe–N–C SAN) (Figure 1B). Fe–N–C SAN showed good POD-like activity, its activity was comparable to that of HRP, and it was more stable, which could realize the highly sensitive detection of butyrylcholinesterase, a typical biomarker of organophosphorus pesticide exposure [43].

Porphyrin and its derivatives can generate cytotoxic singlet oxygen ($^1O_2$) under irradiation of appropriate light, and are commonly used as photosensitizers in cancer photodynamic therapy [44]. Liu's group used mesoporous silica (m-SiO_2) to coat ZIF-8 and then pyrolyzed to prepare monodisperse mesoporous carbon nanospheres containing porphyrin-like zinc centers (denoted as PMCS) (Figure 1C), in which Zn atoms were atomically dispersed. As a protective layer, m-SiO_2, which could be removed by NaOH etching, will effectively prevent active centers of metal atoms from aggregating during the pyrolysis and ensure the successful synthesis of SAzymes [45]. The PMCS have strong absorption in the near-infrared region and can generate $^1O_2$ under the irradiation of 808 nm laser. Using a similar strategy, Cao et al. [46] fabricated bimetallic MOFs by encapsulating Co species in ZIF-8, followed by pyrolysis in N_2 to obtain PMCS with atomically dispersed

Co as active centers (denoted as Co/PMCS) (Figure 1D). Co/PMCS could mimic superoxide dismutase (SOD), catalase (CAT), and glutathione peroxidase (GPx) to rapidly scavenge reactive oxygen and nitrogen species for the treatment of bacterial-induced sepsis.

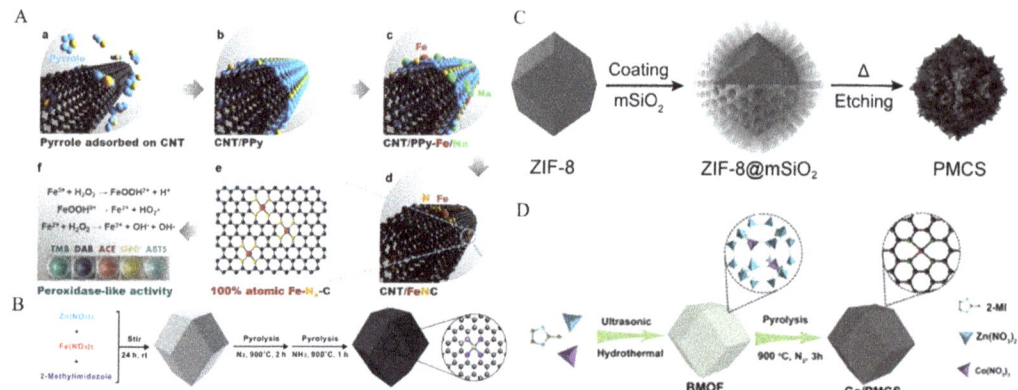

Figure 1. Preparation of SAzymes by pyrolysis. (**A**) CNT/FeNC. (a) Pyrrole adsorbed on CNT. (b) Polypyrrole coated on CNT to form CNT/PPy. (c) Metal cations adsorbed on CNT/PPy. (d) Pyrolysis to form CNT/FeNC. (e) Structure of Fe-Nx-C. (f) POD-like activity of CNT/FeNC. [40]. Copyright 2019, Wiley-VCH. (**B**) Fe–NC SAN [42]. Copyright 2019, Elsevier. (**C**) PMCS [45]. Copyright 2016, Wiley-VCH. (**D**) Co/PMCS [46]. Copyright 2020, Wiley-VCH.

The activity of SAzymes can be adjusted by control of the temperature and gas atmosphere in pyrolysis. Xu et al. [47] prepared PMCS with atomically dispersed Zn as active sites by pyrolysis of ZIF-8, and adjusted the pyrolysis temperature from 600 °C to 1000 °C to obtain a series of SAzymes (denoted as c-ZIF-600, c-ZIF-700, PMCS, c-ZIF-900, and c-ZIF-1000). It was found that c-ZIF-600 and c-ZIF-700 had almost no POD-like activity, c-ZIF-900 and c-ZIF-1000 had weak POD-like activity, and only PMCS exhibited higher POD-like activity. This is due to the increase of the structural defects in pyrolyzed ZIF-8 when the temperature rises. The defects can accelerate the diffusion of substrates to the active sites, thereby improving the catalytic activity. However, the increase of pyrolysis temperature also results in the decrease of Zn, which is the active center. On the whole, the POD-like activity of PMCS obtained by pyrolysis at 800 °C is the highest. The gas atmosphere of pyrolysis also can greatly influence the activity of SAzymes. For example, Wang et al. [48] used TiO_2 as carrier to prepare Co/TiO_2 SAzymes protected by SiO_2 through pyrolysis. By changing the atmosphere of pyrolysis, they obtained two kinds of Co/TiO_2 SAzymes denoted as Co/A–TiO_2 (pyrolysis in air) and Co/N–TiO_2 (pyrolysis in N_2). The oxidase-like (OXD-like) activity of Co/A–TiO_2 was significantly higher than that of Co/N–TiO_2, and Co(II)/Co(III) in Co/A–TiO_2 was higher than that of Co/N–TiO_2, which was also the fundamental reason why the enzyme-like activity of Co/A–TiO_2 was higher than that of Co/N–TiO_2. The different pyrolysis atmospheres can change the coordination environment of the active center, thereby affecting the activity of SAzymes.

Cytocrome P450 and HRP are involved in a variety of biochemical reactions in the body, and their active center is a heme group containing Fe, in which Fe is coordinated by four N atoms in the plane, while it is also coordinated axially with a S or N atom [49]. Therefore, the scientists prepared FeN_5 SAzymes by imitating the structure of cytocrome P450 and introducing axial N coordination into Fe SAzymes. Compared with the common Fe–N_4 SAzymes, the enzyme-like activity of FeN_5 SAzymes was greatly improved [50]. In this study, iron phthalocyanine (FePc) was encapsulated into Zn–MOF to form the host–guest structure of Fe@Zn–MOF, followed by pyrolysis in N_2 to obtain a five-coordinated Fe SAzyme (denoted as FeN_5 SA/CNF) (Figure 2). Its fine structure was characterized by X-ray absorption near-edge spectroscopy (XANES) and extended X-ray absorption fine structure (EXAFS) spectroscopy. The results confirmed the formation of the Fe–N$_5$ structure. The OXD-like activity of FeN$_5$ SA/CNF and the initial reaction rate were much higher than those of FeN$_4$ SA/CNF and its counterparts with different metal ions, indicating that the axial N-coordination structure and the type of metal active center were equally important to its activity. Similarly, Xu et al. [51] prepared FeN$_5$ SAzyme using a melamine-mediated two-step pyrolysis method, in which melamine played a role in providing the axial direction N coordination. The FeN$_5$ SAzyme had much higher POD-like activity than that of the FeN$_4$ SAzyme, indicating that the introduction of axial N significantly enhanced the activity of SAzyme.

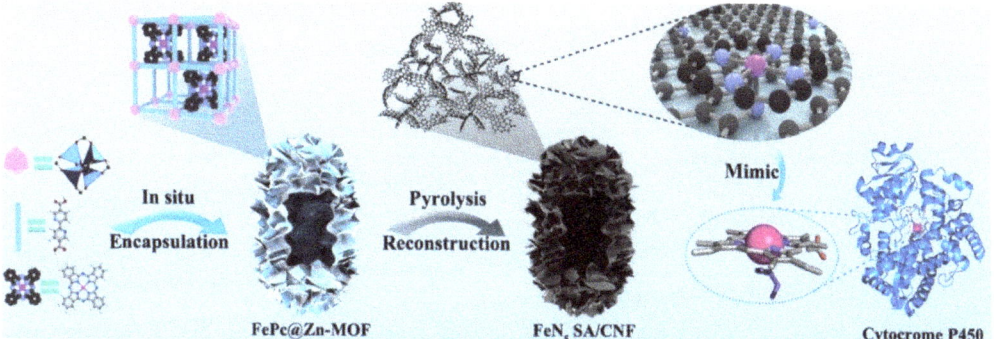

Figure 2. Schematic formation process of carbon nanoframe–confined atomically dispersed Fe sites with axial five-N coordination for mimicking the active center of cytocrome P450 [50]. Copyright 2019, American Association for the Advancement of Science.

The doping of specific elements during the pyrolysis can effectively change the coordination environment of active metal centers in SAzymes and, thus, greatly influence their activities. For example, Jiao et al. [52] used FeCl$_2$ as the Fe source, dicyandiamide as the N source, and boric acid as the B source to prepare B-doped Fe SAzyme (denoted as FeBNC) through pyrolysis. The incorporation of B triggered charge transfer to change the coordination environment of Fe, and thus greatly enhanced the POD-like activity of FeBNC, which provided a new idea for regulating the activity of SAzyme. Feng et al. [53] also prepared a B-doped Zn SAzyme (denoted as ZnBNC) by a similar method. The incorporation of B enhanced the N and O content, water dispersibility, and POD-like activity of ZnBNC, and it was also found that the incorporation of B could tune the catalytic activity by increasing defects.

To sum up, the strategies of changing the temperature and atmosphere of pyrolysis introducing axial coordination or doping during pyrolysis are essentially changing the coordination environment of the active center. Therefore, as long as it is a strategy that can change the coordination environment of the active centers of SAzymes, their activity can be regulated in principle, which lays the foundation for the development of more SAzymes activity regulation strategies.

Pyrolysis has been proved as an effective way to fabricate SAzymes, and their activity also can be facially regulated by tuning the temperature and atmosphere, introducing axial coordination as well as doping of specific elements. Thus, this strategy is widely used for the preparation of SAzymes for diverse applications. However, SAzymes prepared through this method are generally hydrophobic, so further surface modification is necessary for potential biomedical applications [20], and the particles may sinter together under the high temperature of pyrolysis. Thus, how to control the size of obtained SAzymes for a particular application is also a big challenge. Moreover, the pyrolysis process also consumes a lot of energy.

2.2. Defect Engineering

Baerlocher et al. [54] found that the presence of ordered Si vacancies significantly enhanced the catalytic activity of SSZ-74, and the formation of nanoscale ferroelectric domains in relaxor ferroelectrics was also associated with some form of structural disorder in the material induced by defects [55]. Therefore, controlling the generation of defects in materials may maximize the beneficial defects to improve their properties, that is, "defect engineering". Wan et al. [56] synthesized a single-atom gold catalyst based on TiO_2 nanosheets (denoted as Au–SA/Def–TiO_2) (Figure 3A), which had abundant oxygen vacancy defects on its surface detected by electron paramagnetic resonance (EPR) measurement (Figure 3B). Au was effectively stabilized by the formation of Ti–Au–Ti, and the complete conversion temperature of Au–SA/Def–TiO_2 catalyzed CO oxidation was lower than that of single-atom gold catalyst synthesized using perfect TiO_2 without defects, indicating the higher catalytic activity brought by defects.

As a porous crystal, MOFs have inherent defects and complex structure [57], so they also have potential for SAzyme preparations by defect engineering. However, the introduction of defects may inevitably lead to structural instability of MOFs. Jasmina et al. [58] discovered zirconium-based MOFs (Zr-MOFs) UiO66, UiO67, and UiO68 in 2008. Due to the high strength of carboxylate–Zr bonds and the high connectivity of metal clusters [59], Zr-MOFs have excellent thermal [60], solvent [61], and high-pressure stabilities compared with other MOFs [62]. Therefore, Zr-MOFs have become the preferred material for the preparation of SAzymes by defect engineering. There are two main types of defects in MOFs (Figure 3C): the missing-linker defects and the missing-cluster defects [63,64]. Defects are introduced in a variety of ways, which can be divided into two broad categories: "de novo" synthesis and post-synthetic treatment [65–67]. "De novo" synthesis directly synthesizes MOFs with defects by changing the reaction conditions. Among them, the most widely used is the addition of modulators [66], including water [29], HCl [68], Hac [69], trifluoroacetate (TFA) [70], etc. The coordination ability of these modulators to clusters is much greater than that of organic ligands, so they will compete with organic ligands for coordination, resulting in defects. The content of defects in MOFs can be further tuned by changing the amount or type of modulators [68,71]. Post-synthesis treatments include post-synthesis exchange (PSE), the use of etchants, and so on. PSE, also known as solvent-assisted exchange, refers to the exchange of metal ions [72] or linkers [73] in MOFs. The etching method uses some acids, bases, and salts as etchants to introduce defects and even mesoporous or macroporous structures into MOFs, which can significantly adjust the performance of MOFs [74,75].

In the defects engineering strategy, defects are first introduced in MOFs by "de novo" synthesis or post-synthesis treatment, and then active ions or atoms are embedded in the defects. The distance between the metal nodes increases the distance between the defects; thus, the embedded ions or atoms are not easy to aggregate, ensuring the generation of atomically distributed active centers. Li et al. [68] used HCl and HAc as modulators to prepare defective NH_2–UiO66 NPs (denoted as HCl–NH_2–UiO66 NPs and Ac–NH_2–UiO66 NPs, respectively), and then embedded Fe^{3+} in the defects to prepare the SAzymes with atomically dispersed Fe as the active center (denoted as Fe–HCl–NH_2–UiO66 NPs and Fe–Ac–NH_2–UiO66 NPs, respectively) (Figure 3D). The thermogravimetric curve (TGA) (Figure 3E) indicated that there were missing-linker defects in both Fe–HCl–NH_2–UiO66 NPs and Fe–Ac–NH_2–UiO66 NPs and more defects in Fe–HCl–NH_2–UiO66 NPs. Fe–HCl–NH_2–UiO66 NPs showed higher POD-like activity than Fe–Ac–NH_2–UiO66 NPs and could be used for monitoring of trace H_2O_2 in cancer cells.

The amount of modulators used can affect the content of defects and thus the properties of the catalyst. Ma et al. [76] prepared a series of defective NH_2–UiO66 (denoted as UiO66–NH_2–X, where X represented the molar ratio of HAc to linker) by adding different amounts of HAc during the synthesis. The content of defects increased with the increase amount of HAc. In the presence of the cocatalyst Pt (denoted as Pt@UiO66–NH_2–X), the photocatalytic H_2 production first increased and then decreased with the increase of structural defects, and Pt@UiO66–NH$_2$–X exhibited the best catalytic activity and high stability when X was 100. Although Pt@UiO66–NH$_2$–X is not an SAzyme, it shows that the content of defects can be changed by adjusting the amount of the modulator, thereby adjusting the activity of the catalyst, which contributes to a new and important idea for the activity regulation of SAzymes prepared by defect engineering.

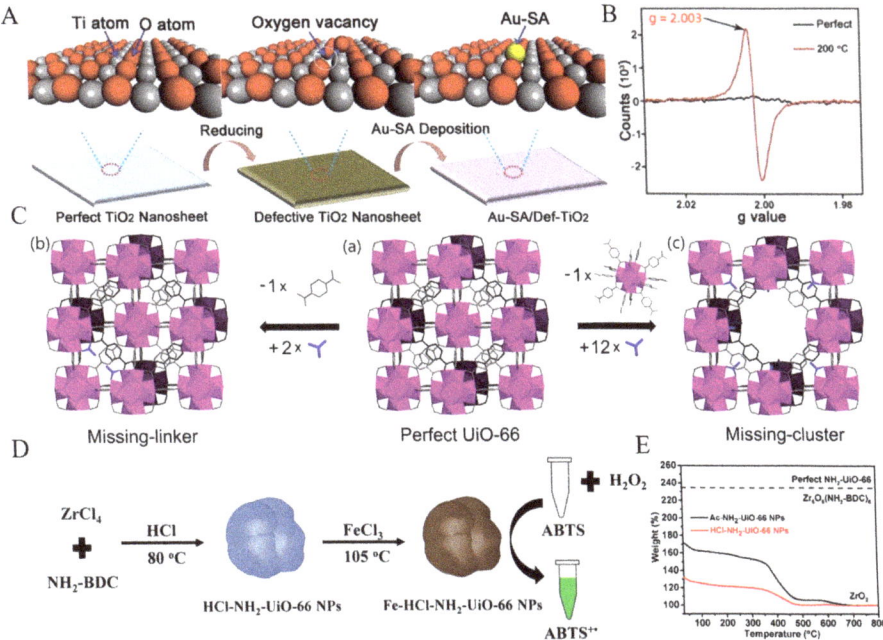

Figure 3. Defect engineering to prepare SAzymes. (**A**) Preparation of Au-SA/Def-TiO$_2$ [56]. Copyright 2018, Wiley-VCH. (**B**) EPR of Per-TiO$_2$ and Def-TiO$_2$ [56]. Copyright 2018, Wiley-VCH. (**C**) Two kinds of defect formation in MOFs. (a) Perfect UiO-66. (b) Replacement of one linker with two monocarboxylic groups, generating one missing-linker defect per unit cell. (c) Replacement of one cluster with twelve monocarboxylic groups, generating one missing-cluster defect per unit cell. [59]. Copyright 2017, Elsevier. (**D**) Preparation of Fe–HCl-NH$_2$-UiO66 NPs [68]. Copyright 2021, Elsevier. (**E**) TGA of Fe-HCl–NH$_2$-UiO66 NPs and Fe-Ac-NH$_2$-UiO66 NPs [68]. Copyright 2021, Elsevier.

Compared with the pyrolysis method, the defect engineering method can be conducted in a wet chemistry way; thus, the obtained SAzymes can be easily dispersed in aqueous solution and their original size can be largely preserved. This feature is quite important for the biomedical applications of SAzymes. However, the strategies to tune the activity of SAzymes fabricated through the defect engineering method are still greatly needed; now, SAzymes prepared by this way in the literature are mainly concentrated in industrial applications [56,77,78], and there are few reports on their biomedical applications. Nonetheless, it provides a new approach of low cost and low energy consumption to prepare SAzymes.

3. Characterizations of SAzymes

With the deepening of SAzymes research and the increasingly mature characterization techniques, more and more characterization techniques for SAzymes have emerged, including integrated electron microscopy, X-ray spectroscopy, infrared spectroscopy, nuclear magnetic resonance spectroscopy, etc. [33,41]. Herein, we focus on three characterization techniques that are most widely used in the field of SAzymes: high-angle annular dark-field scanning transmission electron microscopy (HAADF-STEM), XANES, and EXAFS.

If a characterization method can be used to directly see the uniformly distributed atomic-level active centers on the surface of the carrier, it will greatly promote the research of SAzymes. The electrons emitted inside the HAADF-STEM are partially scattered beyond the angle of convergence, and these high-energy electrons can be collected to image the isolated metal atoms [79]. Both XANES and EXAFS belong to X-ray absorption fine structure (XAFS) spectroscopy. XAFS establishes the relationship between X-ray absorption coefficient $\mu(E)$ and incident X-ray photon energy. The electrons of element atoms are liberated from lower-energy bound states, resulting in an increase in $\mu(E)$, and these energies are called the X-ray absorption edge of the element [80]. XANES is characterized by a signal of 30–50 eV above the X-ray absorption edge of a certain element atom, which reflects the valence of the atom and other information. EXAFS is characterized by the signals of 30–50 eV and 1000 eV above the absorption edges, providing information on the bonding structure around atoms. Structural information, the average atomic coordination number, interatomic distance, and other information can be obtained through Fourier transform-EXAFS (FT-EXAFS) and its fitting image, and wavelet transform-EXAFS (WT-EXAFS) can provide more structural information [27,81]. Examples of SAzymes characterization are shown in Table 2, and we choose two typical ones for detailed introduction.

Table 2. Summary of characterizations of SAzymes.

SAzymes	Characterization	Results	Ref.
Fe–N–C SACs	HAADF-STEM XANES EXAFS	Atomically dispersed Fe Valence state of Fe was between 0 and +3 Only Fe–N existed	[82]
Co/PMCS	HAADF-STEM XANES EXAFS	Atomically dispersed Co Co was positive charged CoN_4 existed	[46]
FeN_5 SA/CNF	HAADF-STEM XANES EXAFS	Atomically dispersed Fe Contained FeN_4 structure FeN_5 existed	[50]
ZnBNC	HAADF-STEM XANES EXAFS	Atomically dispersed Zn Valence state of Zn was between 0 and +2 ZnN_4 existed	[53]
Au-SA/Def–TiO_2	HAADF-STEM XANES EXAFS	Atomically dispersed Au Valence state of Au was +3 Au–O and Au–Ti existed	[56]
Fe–HCl–NH_2–UiO66 NPs	HAADF-STEM XANES EXAFS	Atomically dispersed Fe Valence state of Fe was between +3 Fe–O–Zr existed	[68]
SAFe–NMCNs	HAADF-STEM XANES EXAFS	Atomically dispersed Fe Valence state of Fe was between 0 and +3 FeN_4 existed	[83]

For example, Su et al. [83] used Pluronic F127 as template, $(NH_4)_2Fe(SO_4)_2$ as Fe source, and dopamine as nitrogen source and carbon source to prepare N-doped mesoporous carbon nanospheres with atomically dispersed Fe as active center (denoted as SAFe–NMCNs) through pyrolysis. Atomically dispersed Fe (marked by red circles) could be directly observed in SAFe–NMCNs under the HAADF-STEM (Figure 4A). The coordination environment of Fe in SAFe–NMCNs was characterized by XANES and EXAFS. XANES (Figure 4B) results showed that the K-edge absorption of Fe in SAFe–NMCNs was between that of Fe foil and Fe_2O_3, indicating that it was positively charged and had a valence state between 0 and +3. EXAFS (Figure 4C) results indicated that Fe–N scattering paths (1.55 Å) and no Fe–Fe scattering paths (2.2 Å) existed in SAFe–NMCNs. At the same time, the results of WT-EXAFS (Figure 4D) also showed that there was only Fe–N but no Fe–Fe in SAFe–NMCNs, which further indicated that Fe was atomically dispersed. After fitting, the coordination number of Fe is 4.23, indicating that the Fe–N_4 structure was formed, which meant that Fe in SAFe–NMCNs was coordinated by four N atoms.

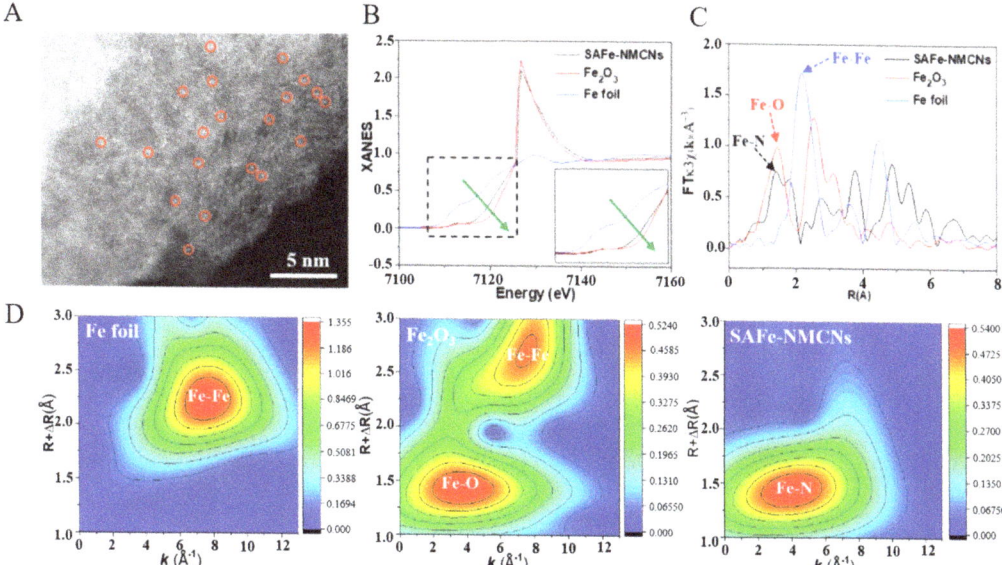

Figure 4. Structure characterization of SAFe-NMCNs (**A**) HAADF-STEM. (**B**) XANES. (**C**) FT-EXAFS. (**D**) WT-EXAFS [83]. Copyright 2022, Elsevier.

Li et al. [68] prepared Fe–HCl–NH_2–UiO66 NPs using defect engineering. No formation of Fe nanoparticles was observed in the HAADF-STEM image, and the element mapping image also confirmed the uniform distribution of Fe in Fe–HCl–NH_2–UiO66 NPs. Moreover, the X-ray photoelectron spectroscopy of Fe 2p showed that Fe(III) characteristic peaks existed in Fe–HCl–NH_2–UiO66 NPs, indicating that Fe had +3 valence. Then, using XAFS for further analysis, the results showed that Fe–HCl–NH_2–UiO66 NPs had similar absorption to Fe_2O_3, which further indicated that Fe had a +3 valence. The coordination environment of Fe was analyzed by FT-EXAFS and the fitting results, which showed coexistence of Fe–O and Fe–Cl and no existence of Fe–Fe, indicating that Fe in Fe–HCl–NH_2–UiO66 NPs was connected to Zr_6 clusters through Fe–O–Zr.

4. Surface Modifications of SAzymes

The catalytic process of nanozymes is different to that of natural enzymes. The catalyzed process of a natural enzyme is (a) substrate binding, (b) catalytic reaction, (c) product release, while that of a nanozyme is similar to heterogeneous catalytic reaction: (a) substrate adsorption, (b) surface reaction, (c) product dissociation and surface active site regeneration [23,84]. Thus, the catalytic process of nanozymes is closely related to their surface [85]. At the same time, since nanozymes are mostly inorganic nanoparticles or carbon materials containing metal elements, their colloidal stability, biocompatibility, and targeting properties need to be improved for biomedical applications [20]. For this purpose, the best choice is the surface modification [30].

For example, polyethylene glycol (PEG) is often used to improve hydrophilicity and biocompatibility of materials. Huo et al. [86] immobilized Fe^{III} acetylacetone in ZIF-8 by hydrothermal method, followed by pyrolysis in Ar to obtain Fe SAzymes with N-doping carbon material as the carrier (denoted as SAF NCs) (Figure 5A) for tumor treatment. To enhance their hydrophilicity and biocompatibility, DSPE–PEG–NH$_2$ was modified on the surface of SAF NCs through hydrophobic–hydrophobic interactions to obtain PEG-modified Fe SAzymes (denoted as PSAF NCs) (Figure 5B). After modification, the distribution of particle size was reduced, the surface potential was more negative, and the dispersion in normal saline was better (Figure 5C). Besides PEG, polyvinyl pyrrolidone is also often used as a surface modifier to improve the dispersity and biocompatibility of SAzymes [87].

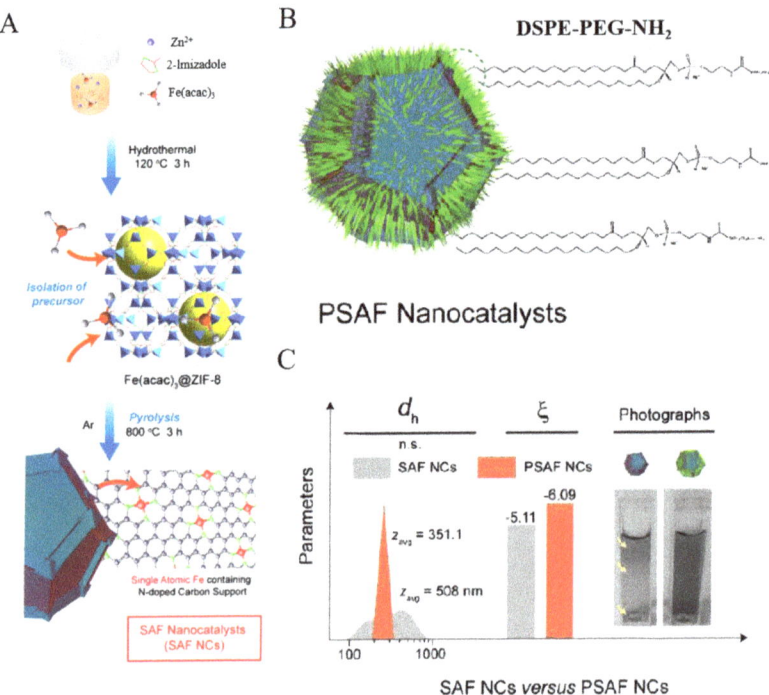

Figure 5. (**A**) Preparation of SAF NCs. (**B**) Structure of PSAF NCs. (**C**) Particle size distribution, zeta potential, and dispersibility in normal saline [86]. Copyright 2019, American Chemical Society.

In addition to enhancing the dispersity and biocompatibility of SAzymes, surface modification also helps to improve targeting. Gong et al. [88] synthesized carbon dots with citric acid and polyene polyamines, which were subsequently loaded with HAuCl$_4$ and reduced with NaBH$_4$ to obtain SAzyme with an active center of Au (denoted as CAT-g). Triphenyl phosphorus (TPP) and cinnamaldehyde (CA) were then modified on its surface, and the modified CAT-g was denoted as MitoCAT-g. TPP could target mitochondria, Au depleted glutathione (GSH) in mitochondria, and CA produced ROS. MitoCAT-g destroyed the redox balance of tumor cells, amplified the effect of ROS to destroy mitochondria, and led to apoptosis, so as to achieve the purpose of tumor treatment. The modification of TPP resulted in the distribution of more particles in mitochondria; thus, they could kill cancer cells more effectively.

The method of cell membrane modification is also widely used in the field of SAzyme. Liu et al. [89] prepared Fe SAzymes (denoted as SAF NPs) by pyrolyzing ZIF-8 loaded with Fe species (Figure 6A). After loaded doxorubicin (DOX) within their porous structure, SAF NPs were modified by human non-small-cell lung cancer cell membrane (A549 CM), denoted as SAF NPs@DOX@CM (Figure 6B). There were specific proteins on the surface of cancer cell membrane (CM), and the influence of homology enabled CM-modified NPs to escape the phagocytosis and immune rejection of macrophages, thereby greatly prolonging their blood circulation time and enhancing tumor targeting. After incubated with human normal hepatocytes and A549 cells for 24 h, respectively, both SAF NPs@CM and SAF NPs@DOX@CM caused extensive apoptosis of A549 cells and the DOX-loaded group caused more (Figure 6C), which was related to the targeting ability of NPs after CM modification and the difference in pH of tumor cells from normal cells. The in vivo experiment also proved that CM modification endowed NPs with the ability to target tumors (Figure 6D).

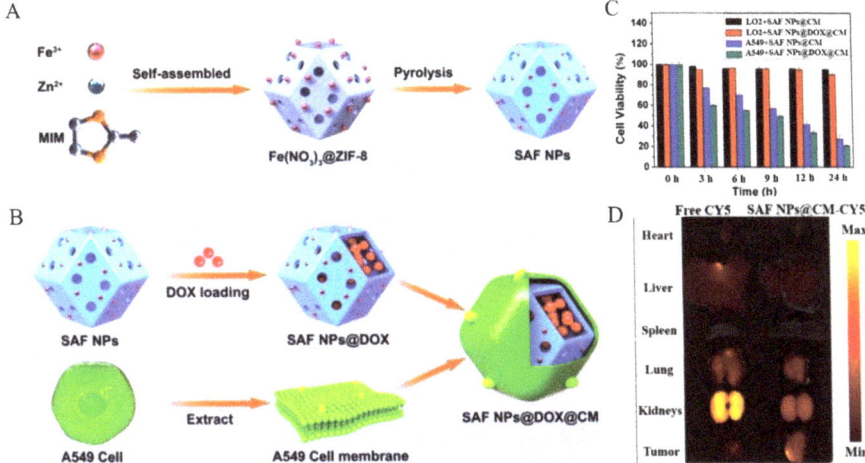

Figure 6. Preparation of SAF NPs (**A**) and SAF NPs@DOX@CM (**B**). (**C**) Viability of cells treated with SAF NPs@CM and SAF NPs@DOX@CM. (**D**) Fluorescence intensities of major organs and tumors after 24 h intravenous injection of free CY5 and SAF NPs@CM-CY5 [89]. Copyright 2021, Wiley-VCH.

Similarly, Qi et al. [90] used platelet membrane (PM) to encapsulate a pyrolyzed mesoporous Fe SAzyme (denoted as PMS). The more negative potential of PMS indicated the successful modification of PM. PMS showed good POD-like activity and photothermal effect, which was expected to realize the combination of chemodynamic therapy and photothermal therapy. More importantly, there is an important protein in PM: P-selectin, which can target tumor cells, thus PMS was selectively endocytosed by 4T1 cells. Meanwhile, PMS was not phagocytosed by Raw264.7 cells, indicating that the homology of PM enabled Fe SAzyme to escape from macrophage phagocytosis.

At present, the surface modification strategies for SAzymes are mostly learned from those already built in the fields of nanomedicine and show great success. However, one should pay special attention to the influence of surface modification on the activity of nanozymes, because the following applications greatly depend on their activity. For example, Sanjay et al. [91] found that CAT-like activity of cerium oxide nanoparticles (CeNPs) increased after they were modified with PO_4^{3-}, but when the concentration of PO_4^{3-} exceeded 100 µM, the SOD-like activity of CeNPs would be significantly inhibited. It was speculated that the inhibition of SOD-like activity might be caused by the reaction of PO_4^{3-} with CeNPs to produce products similar to cerium phosphate. Therefore, the selection of modifiers during surface modification needs careful consideration. More recently, Wang et al. [92] demonstrated that membrane cholesterol depletion could enhance enzymatic activity of cell-membrane-coated MOF NPs. The mechanism behind this phenomenon is that the reducing cholesterol level effectively enhances membrane permeability, thus the substrates are more accessible to the encapsulated enzymes. These findings can provide facile and practical ways for the modulation of the activity of SAzymes through surface modification.

5. Applications of Single-Atom Nanozymes in Biomedicine

Due to its high atom utilization, unsaturated coordination of active centers, and geometric structures similar to those of nature enzymes, SAzymes are widely used in biosensing [40,42,43,82,93,94], cancer treatment [48,51,83,95,96], and so on. In previous review articles, these two types of applications have been comprehensively discussed; thus, this review will not repeat them. Herein, we mainly focus on the applications of SAzymes in ROS scavenging and antibacterial, and the specific mechanism is shown in Figure 7. For ROS scavenging, normally the CAT and SOD-like SAzymes are used, because they can eliminate the excess ROS and alleviate oxidative stress. However, for the antibacterial applications, ROS are produced by SAzymes to damage the membranes or biomacromolecules of bacteria, resulting in the death of them, finally.

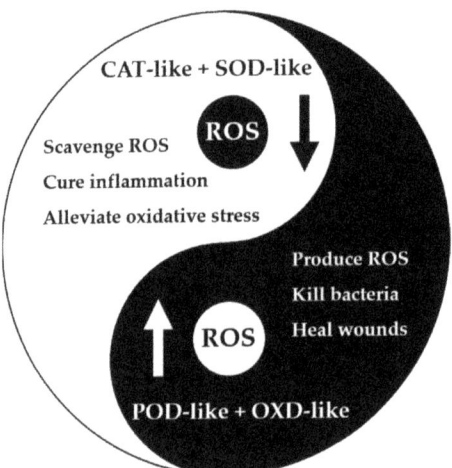

Figure 7. Mechanism of SAzymes for scavenging ROS and antibacterial.

5.1. SAzymes for ROS Scavenging

O_2 participates in thousands of reactions in the human body. Under the catalysis of enzymes in mitochondria, it is reduced to water by transferring four electrons and generates adenosine triphosphate for energy [97], but sometimes a single-electron or double-electron transfer reaction occurs to generate ROS, mainly including $\bullet O_2^-$, H_2O_2, and $\bullet OH$ [98]. ROS is a double-edged sword. Low doses of ROS are essential for the regulation of life, such as cell division [99], signal transmission [100], and so on. However, when the level of ROS exceeds the normal level, it will cause oxidative damage to cells, resulting in hair loss [101], inflammation [46], stroke [14], Parkinson's [12], and other diseases. The level of ROS in the human body is always at a relatively stable level, which depends on the interaction of four enzymes: OXD, POD, CAT, and SOD [102]. OXD and POD can increase ROS, while CAT and SOD can reduce ROS. Therefore, SAzymes with CAT-like and SOD-like activities are expected to scavenge excess ROS and alleviate cellular oxidative damage.

Ma et al. [103] used ZIF-8 to encapsulate FePc followed by pyrolysis to obtain SAzymes with atomically dispersed Fe as the active center (denoted as Fe–SAs/NC) and reported their CAT-like and SOD-like activities. Fe–SAs/NC was modified with DSPE–PEG$_{2000}$ to improve their biocompatibility. The cell experiments proved that Fe–SAs/NC could scavenge ROS and alleviate cellular oxidative damage. Similarly, Lu et al. [104] utilized the pyrolysis of Fe-TPP ⊂ rho-ZIF (Fe-TPP = tetraphenylporphyrin iron; rho-ZIF = zeolitic imidazolate skeleton with rho topology) to obtain atomically dispersed Fe SAzymes (denoted as Fe–N/C SACs). Fe–N/C SACs had multi-enzyme-like activities, including OXD-like, POD-like, CAT-like, and GPx-like activities, which could alleviate cellular oxidative damage.

Yan et al. [105] used CeO_2 as the carrier to load atomically dispersed Pt and obtained Pt@CeO_2 SAzyme. Then, they compounded the SAzyme with polyacrylonitrile fiber and medical polyethylene tape to prepare a Pt@CeO_2 SAzyme-based bandage (Figure 8A) to scavenge excessive ROS and reactive nitrogen species around the traumatic brain injury (TBI) wound in order to alleviate neuroinflammation. Pt@CeO_2 SAzyme had POD-like, CAT-like, SOD-like, and GPx-like activities; thus, they had excellent ability of scavenging ROS inside cells (Figure 8B). At the same time, Pt@CeO_2 was less cytotoxic and could alleviate the oxidative damage of cells caused by H_2O_2 and lipopolysaccharide (LPS) (Figure 8C). Animal experiments showed that the TBI wound healing effect of the Pt@CeO_2 treatment group was significantly better than that of the other groups, indicating the correctness and feasibility of the bandage treatment principle. Similarly, the Co/PMCS also showed SOD-like, CAT-like, and GPx-like activities [46]. It could effectively reduce the content of ROS caused by various stimuli to alleviate oxidative damage of cells, and the animal experiments showed that whether LPS or *Escherichia coli* (*E. coli*) were used to induce sepsis in mice, Co/PMCS had a good therapeutic effect, and the levels of tumor necrosis factor-α and interleukin-6 were significantly decreased.

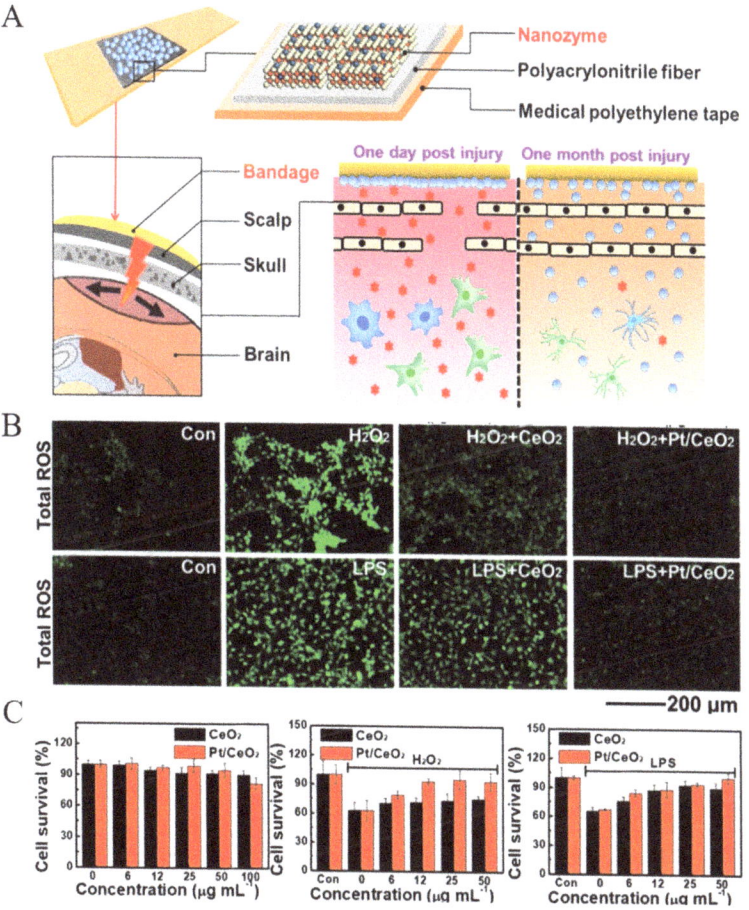

Figure 8. (**A**) Design principle of Pt@CeO_2 bandage. (**B**) ROS scavenging abilities of Pt/CeO_2 inside cells. (**C**) Alleviating cellular oxidative damage abilities of Pt/CeO_2 [105]. Copyright 2019, American Chemical Society.

In addition to the ability of SAzyme to simulate CAT, SOD, and GPx to alleviate cellular oxidative damage, Chen et al. [106] used electrochemical deposition to deposit Cu on g-C_3N_4 and obtained a kind of SAzyme in which 1 Cu atom was coordinated with four N atoms (denoted as Cu–SAs/CN). Cu–SAs/CN possessed ascorbate peroxidase (APX)-like activity, which can decompose H_2O_2 in the presence of AsA, thereby alleviating cellular oxidative damage. The Cu–SAs/CN had almost no cytotoxicity, and could alleviate H_2O_2-induced cell damage.

Although there are some reports on SAzymes that can scavenge ROS and alleviate cellular oxidative damage, they are limited to a few materials, so it is still necessary to expand material systems. At the same time, the intrinsic mechanisms of ROS scavenging for SAzymes are still relatively vague, and great efforts need to be paid in this direction.

5.2. SAzymes for Antibacterial

Pathogenic bacteria infection is a major threat to human health globally [107]. Over the past few decades, antibiotics, such as penicillin, have been widely used clinically as antibacterial agents [108]. In recent years, nanozymes with antibacterial activities are regarded as a novel bactericide, due to their negligible biotoxicities, no drug resistance, and broad-spectrum antibacterial performance [109]. SAzymes with highly efficient catalytic activities also play an important role in antibacterial treatments [22].

Xia et al. [110] successfully prepared atomic-level Ag-loaded MnO_2 porous hollow microspheres (Ag/MnO_2 PHMs) through the redox precipitation process, which exhibited superior photothermocatalytic inactivation of *E. coli* under solar light irradiation. On the one hand, atomic Ag with high conductivity increased the level of Mn^{3+} and oxygen vacancies to excite MnO_2, thus promoting the introduction of reactive species for photocatalysis. On the other hand, atomic Ag enhanced the photothermal conversion and lattice oxygen reducibility, thus promoting thermocatalysis.

Most SAzymes utilize their POD-like activities to generate toxic •OH, therefore achieving efficient sterilization. For instance, Xu et al. [47] fabricated the PMCS via an m-SiO_2-protected pyrolysis approach (Figure 9A). Owing to the high POD-like activity, PMCS showed outstanding antibacterial performance against *Pseudomonas aeruginosa* (Figure 9B). The wound caused by *Pseudomonas aeruginosa* healed well (Figure 9C,D), indicating that PMCS had good antibacterial properties.

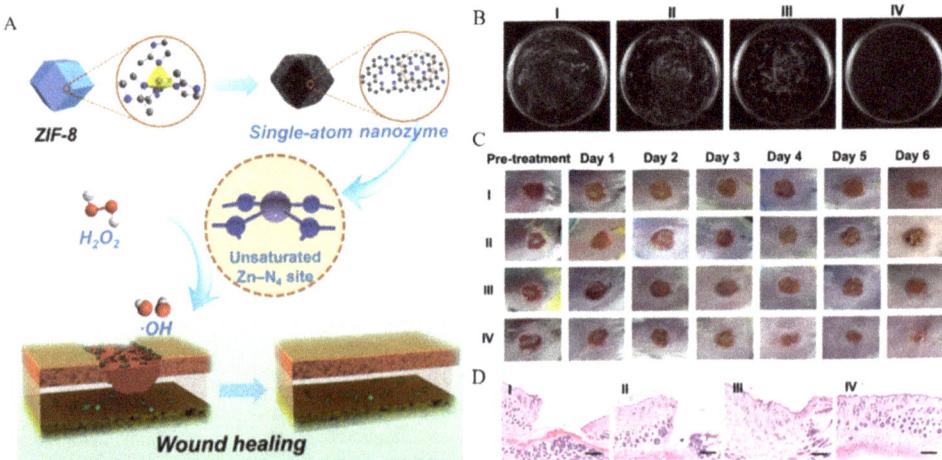

Figure 9. (**A**) Preparation of PMCS. (**B**) Antibacterial properties of PMSC. (**C**) Abilities of PMCS to promote wound healing. (**D**) Histologic analysis of the wounds (I: NaAc buffer, II: NaAc buffer + H_2O_2, III: PMCS, and IV: PMCS + H_2O_2) [47]. Copyright 2019, Wiley-VCH.

As reported by Huo et al. [111], nanocatalysts of single iron atoms anchored in nitrogen-doped amorphous carbon (SAF NCs) were synthesized via encapsulated-pyrolysis strategy. SAF NCs performed excellent POD-like activities in the presence of H_2O_2, producing toxic •OH to achieve high-efficiency sterilization effect against E. coli and Staphylococcus aureus (S. aureus). With the assistance of near-infrared light, antibacterial properties were further improved due to the intrinsic photothermal property of SAF NCs. Noticeably, the antibacterial mechanisms of crucial CM destruction induced by SAF NCs were also revealed. Wang et al. [112] prepared a novel Cu single-atom sites/N-doped porous carbon (Cu SASs/NPC) with POD-like activity by pyrolysis–etching–adsorption–pyrolysis strategy. The doping of Cu considerably enhanced POD-like activity and accelerated GSH-depleting and photothermal properties. The synergistic effect made Cu SASs/NPC exhibit excellent antibacterial performance against E. coli and methicillin-resistant S. aureus (MRSA). Remarkably, by reversing the thermal sintering process, Chen et al. [113] proposed the direct transformation of Pt NPs into Pt single atoms to gain Pt SAzyme (PtTS–SAzyme). It showed excellent POD-like catalytic activity, which was attributed to the unique structure with Pt_1–N_3PS active moiety. Compared with Pt NPs, PtTS–SAzyme exhibited highly efficient antibacterial performance and broad-spectrum antibacterial properties. In addition to POD-like activity, SAzymes with OXD-like activity were also used in antibacterial applications. Huang et al. [50] developed SAzymes with carbon nanoframe–confined FeN_5 active centers (FeN_5 SA/CNF), which showed effective antibacterial effects against E. coli and S. aureus.

Besides photothermal effect, Yu et al. [114] innovatively fabricated a red blood cell membrane modified Au nanorod-actuated single-atom-doped porphyrin metal–organic framework (denoted as RBC–HNTM–Pt@Au) with an excellent sonocatalytic activity. Under ultrasound, not only was the antibacterial activity of RBC–HNTM–Pt@Au greatly enhanced, but SAzymes were also directionally propelled, which played a significant part in the treatment of MRSA-infected osteomyelitis.

In summary, the oxidation effect of SAzymes, especially POD-like activity, may play a major role in antibacterial applications. The ROS, such as •OH, are extremely toxic to the bacteria cells usually by disrupting the integrity of the cell membrane. However, this effect is nonselective; thus, normal cells may also be damaged. To avoid such kind of side effect, the design of smart SAzymes whose activity only can be activated on the infection sites is significantly important. The whole applications mentioned in this section are summarized in Table 3.

Table 3. Summary of applications of SAzymes in ROS scavenging and antibacterial.

Applications	SAzymes	Enzyme-Like Activities	Ref.
ROS scavenging	Fe–SAs/NC	CAT, SOD	[103]
	Fe–N/C SACs	OXD, POD, CAT, GPx	[104]
	Pt@CeO$_2$	POD, CAT, SOD	[105]
	Co/PMCS	SOD, CAT, GPx	[46]
	Cu–SAs/CN	APX	[106]
Antibacterial	Ag/MnO$_2$ PHMS	/	[110]
	PMCS	POD	[47]
	SAF NCs	POD	[111]
	Cu SASs/NPC	POD	[112]
	PtTS–SAzyme	POD	[113]
	FeN$_5$ SA/CNF	OXD	[50]
	RBC–HNTM–Pt@Au	/	[114]

6. Summary and Outlook

SAzymes with excellent performance have been widely used in the field of biomedicine. Compared with ordinary nanozymes, they have defined active sites and coordination environments, which are important for understanding the relationship between their structures and activities. It is also beneficial for the research of the mechanism and the catalytic process in order to better mimic the natural enzyme. At the same time, atom utilization is greatly improved due to the atomic-level dispersion of active sites. In this review, we summarized the preparation and characterization of SAzymes, discussed their surface modification, and finally focused on their applications of ROS scavenging and antibacterial.

Although significant advances have been achieved in this area, challenges are still remaining. First of all, new fabrication strategies should always be pursued to obtain SAzymes with new structures and activities, especially those that have ROS scavenging activity. The preparation of SAzymes needs theoretical guidance. We can further combine theoretical calculation, big data, artificial intelligence, and other technologies to guide the design and preparation of SAzymes. Furthermore, the strategies which can combine the advantages of finely regulated structures and activity with large-scale and green production processes are highly welcomed. Moreover, the surface modification is necessary for SAzymes in biomedical applications; however, the basic knowledge of how different surface modifications would influence their catalytic activities is largely unknown. Finally, for the biomedical applications of SAzymes, their long-term in vivo biodegradability and toxicity should be carefully investigated, which is also crucial for their real applications. We believe these challenges can be addressed in the future through the collaborations of researchers from different disciplines, such as chemistry, material science, computer science, and biology, as well as medicine.

Author Contributions: Conceptualization, W.T. and H.S.; writing—original draft preparation, W.T., H.S. and M.Z.; writing—review and editing, W.T.; project administration, W.T.; funding acquisition, W.T. All authors have read and agreed to the published version of the manuscript.

Funding: This research was funded by the National Natural Science Foundation of China (22161132027, 51973187).

Institutional Review Board Statement: Not applicable.

Informed Consent Statement: Not applicable.

Data Availability Statement: Not applicable.

Conflicts of Interest: The authors declare no conflict of interest.

Abbreviations

SAzymes	Single-atom nanozymes
ROS	Reactive oxygen species
NPs	Nanoparticles
POD	Peroxidase
HRP	Horseradish peroxidase
SACs	Single-atom catalysts
FeOx	Iron oxide
AsA	Ascorbic acid
MOFs	Metal-organic frameworks
m-SiO$_2$	Mesoporous silica
SOD	Superoxide dismutase
CAT	Catalase
GPx	Glutathione peroxidase
FePc	Iron phthalocyanine
XANES	X-ray absorption near-edge spectroscopy
EXAFS	Extended X-ray absorption fine structure
EPR	Electron-paramagnetic resonance
Zr-MOFs	Zirconium-based metal-organic frameworks
TFA	Trifluoroacetate
PSE	Post-synthesis exchange
TGA	Thermogravimetric analysis
HAADF-STEM	High-angle annular dark-field scanning transmission electron microscopy
XAFS	X-ray absorption fine structure

FT-EXAFS	Fourier transform- extended X-ray absorption fine structure
WT-EXAFS	Wavelet transform- extended X-ray absorption fine structure
PEG	Polyethylene glycol
TPP	Triphenyl phosphorus
CA	Cinnamaldehyde
GSH	Glutathione
DOX	Doxorubicin
A549 CM	Human non-small cell lung cancer cell membrane
CM	Cell membrane
PM	Platelet membrane
CeNPs	Cerium oxide nanoparticles
TBI	Traumatic brain injury
LPS	Lipopolysaccharide
E. coli	*Escherichia coli*
APX	Ascorbate peroxidase
S. aureus	*Staphylococcus aureus*
MRSA	Methicillin-resistant *Staphylococcus aureus*

References

1. Breaker, R.R. DNA enzymes. *Nat. Biotechnol.* **1997**, *15*, 427–431. [CrossRef] [PubMed]
2. Wolfenden, R.; Snider, M.J. The Depth of Chemical Time and the Power of Enzymes as Catalysts. *Acc. Chem. Res.* **2001**, *34*, 938–945. [CrossRef] [PubMed]
3. Ma, L.; Jiang, F.; Fan, X.; Wang, L.; He, C.; Zhou, M.; Li, S.; Luo, H.; Cheng, C.; Qiu, L. Metal–Organic-Framework-Engineered Enzyme-Mimetic Catalysts. *Adv. Mater.* **2020**, *32*, 2003065. [CrossRef] [PubMed]
4. Gao, L.; Zhuang, J.; Nie, L.; Zhang, J.; Zhang, Y.; Gu, N.; Wang, T.; Feng, J.; Yang, D.; Perrett, S.; et al. Intrinsic peroxidase-like activity of ferromagnetic nanoparticles. *Nat. Nanotechnol.* **2007**, *2*, 577–583. [CrossRef]
5. Wu, J.; Wang, X.; Wang, Q.; Lou, Z.; Li, S.; Zhu, Y.; Qin, L.; Wei, H. Nanomaterials with enzyme-like characteristics (nanozymes): Next-generation artificial enzymes (II). *Chem. Soc. Rev.* **2019**, *48*, 1004–1076. [CrossRef]
6. Lin, Y.; Ren, J.; Qu, X. Catalytically Active Nanomaterials: A Promising Candidate for Artificial Enzymes. *Acc. Chem. Res.* **2014**, *47*, 1097–1105. [CrossRef]
7. Liang, M.; Wang, Y.; Ma, K.; Yu, S.; Chen, Y.; Deng, Z.; Liu, Y.; Wang, F. Engineering Inorganic Nanoflares with Elaborate Enzymatic Specificity and Efficiency for Versatile Biofilm Eradication. *Small* **2020**, *1*, 2002348. [CrossRef]
8. Duan, W.; Qiu, Z.; Cao, S.; Guo, Q.; Huang, J.; Xing, J.; Lu, X.; Zeng, J. Pd–Fe$_3$O$_4$ Janus nanozyme with rational design for ultrasensitive colorimetric detection of biothiols. *Biosens. Bioelectron.* **2022**, *196*, 113724. [CrossRef]
9. Sun, H.; Gao, N.; Dong, K.; Ren, J.; Qu, X. Graphene Quantum Dots-Band-Aids Used for Wound Disinfection. *ACS Nano* **2014**, *8*, 6202–6210. [CrossRef]
10. Ji, H.; Dong, K.; Yan, Z.; Ding, C.; Chen, Z.; Ren, J.; Qu, X. Bacterial Hyaluronidase Self-Triggered Prodrug Release for Chemo Photothermal Synergistic Treatment of Bacterial Infection. *Small* **2016**, *12*, 6200–6206. [CrossRef]
11. Gao, L.; Liu, Y.; Kim, D.; Li, Y.; Hwang, G.; Naha, P.C.; Cormode, D.P.; Koo, H. Nanocatalysts promote Streptococcus mutans biofilm matrix degradation and enhance bacterial killing to suppress dental caries in vivo. *Biomaterials* **2016**, *101*, 272–284. [CrossRef] [PubMed]
12. Singh, N.; Savanur, M.A.; Srivastava, S.; D'Silva, P.; Mugesh, G. A Redox Modulatory Mn$_3$O$_4$ Nanozyme with Multi-Enzyme Activity Provides Efficient Cytoprotection to Human Cells in a Parkinson's Disease Model. *Angew. Chem. Int. Ed.* **2017**, *56*, 14267–14271. [CrossRef]
13. Liu, Y.; Cheng, Y.; Zhang, H.; Zhou, M.; Yu, Y.; Lin, S.; Jiang, B.; Zhao, X.; Miao, L.; Wei, C.-W.; et al. Integrated cascade nanozyme catalyzes in vivo ROS scavenging for anti-inflammatory therapy. *Sci. Adv.* **2020**, *6*, eabb2695. [CrossRef] [PubMed]
14. Kim, C.K.; Kim, T.; Choi, I.-Y.; Soh, M.; Kim, D.; Kim, Y.-J.; Jang, H.; Yang, H.-S.; Kim, J.Y.; Park, H.-K.; et al. Ceria Nanoparticles that can Protect against Ischemic Stroke. *Angew. Chem. Int. Ed.* **2012**, *51*, 11039–11043. [CrossRef] [PubMed]
15. Huang, Y.; Liu, Z.; Liu, C.; Ju, E.; Zhang, Y.; Ren, J.; Qu, X. Self-Assembly of Multi-nanozymes to Mimic an Intracellular Antioxidant Defense System. *Angew. Chem. Int. Ed.* **2016**, *55*, 6646–6650. [CrossRef]
16. Zhu, L.; Liu, J.; Zhou, G.; Liu, T.-M.; Dai, Y.; Nie, G.; Zhao, Q. Remodeling of Tumor Microenvironment by Tumor-Targeting Nanozymes Enhances Immune Activation of CAR T Cells for Combination Therapy. *Small* **2021**, *17*, 2102624. [CrossRef]
17. Zhang, W.; Liu, J.; Li, X.; Zheng, Y.; Chen, L.; Wang, D.; Foda, M.F.; Ma, Z.; Zhao, Y.; Han, H. Precise Chemodynamic Therapy of Cancer by Trifunctional Bacterium-Based Nanozymes. *ACS Nano* **2021**, *15*, 19321–19333. [CrossRef]
18. Yuan, Z.; Liu, X.; Ling, J.; Huang, G.; Huang, J.; Zhu, X.; He, L.; Chen, T. In situ-transition nanozyme triggered by tumor microenvironment boosts synergistic cancer radio-/chemotherapy through disrupting redox homeostasis. *Biomaterials* **2022**, *287*, 121620. [CrossRef]
19. Cao, C.; Yang, N.; Su, Y.; Zhang, Z.; Wang, C.; Song, X.; Chen, P.; Wang, W.; Dong, X. Starvation, Ferroptosis, and Prodrug Therapy Synergistically Enabled by a Cytochrome c Oxidase like Nanozyme. *Adv. Mater.* **2022**, *34*, 2203236. [CrossRef]

20. Xiang, H.; Feng, W.; Chen, Y. Single-Atom Catalysts in Catalytic Biomedicine. *Adv. Mater.* **2020**, *32*, 1905994. [CrossRef]
21. Jiao, L.; Yan, H.; Wu, Y.; Gu, W.; Zhu, C.; Du, D.; Lin, Y. When Nanozymes Meet Single-Atom Catalysis. *Angew. Chem.* **2020**, *59*, 2565–2576. [CrossRef] [PubMed]
22. Zhang, X.; Li, G.; Chen, G.; Wu, D.; Zhou, X.; Wu, Y. Single-atom nanozymes: A rising star for biosensing and biomedicine. *Coord. Chem. Rev.* **2020**, *418*, 213376. [CrossRef]
23. Zandieh, M.; Liu, J. Surface Science of Nanozymes and Defining a Nanozyme Unit. *Langmuir* **2022**, *38*, 3617–3622. [CrossRef]
24. Qiao, B.; Wang, A.; Yang, X.; Allard, L.F.; Jiang, Z.; Cui, Y.; Liu, J.; Li, J.; Zhang, T. Single-atom catalysis of CO oxidation using Pt1/FeO$_x$. *Nat. Chem.* **2011**, *3*, 634–641. [CrossRef] [PubMed]
25. Li, Z.; Wang, D.; Wu, Y.; Li, Y. Recent advances in the precise control of isolated single-site catalysts by chemical methods. *Natl. Sci. Rev.* **2018**, *5*, 673–689. [CrossRef]
26. Wang, A.; Li, J.; Zhang, T. Heterogeneous single-atom catalysis. *Nat. Rev. Chem.* **2018**, *2*, 65–81. [CrossRef]
27. Chen, Y.; Ji, S.; Chen, C.; Peng, Q.; Wang, D.; Li, Y. Single-Atom Catalysts: Synthetic Strategies and Electrochemical Applications. *Joule* **2018**, *2*, 1242–1264. [CrossRef]
28. Wang, J.; Li, Z.; Wu, Y.; Li, Y. Fabrication of Single-Atom Catalysts with Precise Structure and High Metal Loading. *Adv. Mater.* **2018**, *30*, e1801649. [CrossRef]
29. He, J.; Li, N.; Li, Z.-G.; Zhong, M.; Fu, Z.-X.; Liu, M.; Yin, J.-C.; Shen, Z.; Li, W.; Zhang, J.; et al. Strategic Defect Engineering of Metal–Organic Frameworks for Optimizing the Fabrication of Single-Atom Catalysts. *Adv. Funct. Mater.* **2021**, *31*, 2103597. [CrossRef]
30. Fan, Y.; Liu, S.; Yi, Y.; Rong, H.; Zhang, J. Catalytic Nanomaterials toward Atomic Levels for Biomedical Applications: From Metal Clusters to Single-Atom Catalysts. *ACS Nano* **2021**, *15*, 2005–2037. [CrossRef]
31. Liu, G.; Gao, J.; Ai, H.; Chen, X. Applications and potential toxicity of magnetic iron oxide nanoparticles. *Small* **2013**, *9*, 1533–1545. [CrossRef] [PubMed]
32. Djurisic, A.B.; Leung, Y.H.; Ng, A.M.; Xu, X.Y.; Lee, P.K.; Degger, N.; Wu, R.S. Toxicity of metal oxide nanoparticles: Mechanisms, characterization, and avoiding experimental artefacts. *Small* **2015**, *11*, 26–44. [CrossRef] [PubMed]
33. Zhang, H.; Liu, G.; Shi, L.; Ye, J. Single-Atom Catalysts: Emerging Multifunctional Materials in Heterogeneous Catalysis. *Adv. Energy Mater.* **2018**, *8*, 1701343. [CrossRef]
34. Zhang, L.; Banis, M.N.; Sun, X.L. Single-atom catalysts by the atomic layer deposition technique. *Natl. Sci. Rev.* **2018**, *5*, 628. [CrossRef]
35. Wei, H.; Huang, K.; Wang, D.; Zhang, R.; Ge, B.; Ma, J.; Wen, B.; Zhang, S.; Li, Q.; Lei, M.; et al. Iced photochemical reduction to synthesize atomically dispersed metals by suppressing nanocrystal growth. *Nat. Commun.* **2017**, *8*, 1490. [CrossRef]
36. Liu, P.X.; Zhao, Y.; Qin, R.X.; Mo, S.G.; Chen, G.X.; Gu, L.; Chevrier, D.M.; Zhang, P.; Guo, Q.; Zang, D.D.; et al. Photochemical route for synthesizing atomically dispersed palladium catalysts. *Science* **2016**, *352*, 797–801. [CrossRef]
37. Peng, Y.; Lu, B.; Chen, S. Carbon-Supported Single Atom Catalysts for Electrochemical Energy Conversion and Storage. *Adv. Mater.* **2018**, *30*, 1801995. [CrossRef]
38. Wu, J.; Xiong, L.; Zhao, B.; Liu, M.; Huang, L. Densely Populated Single Atom Catalysts. *Small Methods* **2020**, *4*, 1900540. [CrossRef]
39. Zhu, D.; Chen, H.; Huang, C.; Li, G.; Wang, X.; Jiang, W.; Fan, K. H_2O_2 Self-Producing Single-Atom Nanozyme Hydrogels as Light-Controlled Oxidative Stress Amplifier for Enhanced Synergistic Therapy by Transforming "Cold" Tumors. *Adv. Funct. Mater.* **2022**, *32*, 2110268. [CrossRef]
40. Cheng, N.; Li, J.-C.; Liu, D.; Lin, Y.; Du, D. Single-Atom Nanozyme Based on Nanoengineered Fe–N–C Catalyst with Superior Peroxidase-Like Activity for Ultrasensitive Bioassays. *Small* **2019**, *15*, 1901485. [CrossRef]
41. Liu, J. Catalysis by Supported Single Metal Atoms. *ACS Catal.* **2016**, *7*, 34–59. [CrossRef]
42. Niu, X.; Shi, Q.; Zhu, W.; Liu, D.; Tian, H.; Fu, S.; Cheng, N.; Li, S.; Smith, J.N.; Du, D.; et al. Unprecedented peroxidase-mimicking activity of single-atom nanozyme with atomically dispersed Fe–Nx moieties hosted by MOF derived porous carbon. *Biosens. Bioelectron.* **2019**, *142*, 111495. [CrossRef] [PubMed]
43. Yang, M.; Zhao, Y.; Wang, L.; Paulsen, M.; Simpson, C.D.; Liu, F.; Du, D.; Lin, Y. Simultaneous detection of dual biomarkers from humans exposed to organophosphorus pesticides by combination of immunochromatographic test strip and ellman assay. *Biosens. Bioelectron.* **2018**, *104*, 39–44. [CrossRef] [PubMed]
44. Ethirajan, M.; Chen, Y.; Joshi, P.; Pandey, R.K. The role of porphyrin chemistry in tumor imaging and photodynamic therapy. *Chem. Soc. Rev.* **2011**, *40*, 340–362. [CrossRef]
45. Wang, S.; Shang, L.; Li, L.; Yu, Y.; Chi, C.; Wang, K.; Zhang, J.; Shi, R.; Shen, H.; Waterhouse, G.I.N.; et al. Metal–Organic-Framework-Derived Mesoporous Carbon Nanospheres Containing Porphyrin-Like Metal Centers for Conformal Phototherapy. *Adv. Mater.* **2016**, *28*, 8379–8387. [CrossRef]
46. Cao, F.; Zhang, L.; You, Y.; Zheng, L.; Ren, J.; Qu, X. An Enzyme-Mimicking Single-Atom Catalyst as an Efficient Multiple Reactive Oxygen and Nitrogen Species Scavenger for Sepsis Management. *Angew. Chem.* **2020**, *59*, 5108–5115. [CrossRef]
47. Xu, B.; Wang, H.; Wang, W.; Gao, L.; Li, S.; Pan, X.; Wang, H.; Yang, H.; Meng, X.; Wu, Q.; et al. A Single-Atom Nanozyme for Wound Disinfection Applications. *Angew. Chem. Int. Ed.* **2019**, *58*, 4911–4916. [CrossRef]
48. Wang, H.; Wang, Y.; Lu, L.; Ma, Q.; Feng, R.; Xu, S.; James, T.D.; Wang, L. Reducing Valence States of Co Active Sites in a Single-Atom Nanozyme for Boosted Tumor Therapy. *Adv. Funct. Mater.* **2022**, *32*, 2200331. [CrossRef]

49. Oprea, T.I.; Hummer, G.; García, A.E. Identification of a functional water channel in cytochrome P450 enzymes. *Proc. Natl. Acad. Sci. USA* **1997**, *94*, 2133–2138. [CrossRef]
50. Huang, L.; Chen, J.; Gan, L.; Wang, J.; Dong, S. Single-atom nanozymes. *Sci. Adv.* **2019**, *5*, eaav5490. [CrossRef]
51. Xu, B.; Li, S.; Zheng, L.; Liu, Y.; Han, A.; Zhang, J.; Huang, Z.; Xie, H.; Fan, K.; Gao, L.; et al. A Bioinspired Five-Coordinated Single-Atom Iron Nanozyme for Tumor Catalytic Therapy. *Adv. Mater.* **2022**, *34*, 2107088. [CrossRef] [PubMed]
52. Jiao, L.; Xu, W.; Zhang, Y.; Wu, Y.; Gu, W.; Ge, X.; Chen, B.; Zhu, C.; Guo, S. Boron-doped Fe-N-C single-atom nanozymes specifically boost peroxidase-like activity. *Nano Today* **2020**, *35*, 100971. [CrossRef]
53. Feng, M.; Zhang, Q.; Chen, X.; Deng, D.; Xie, X.; Yang, X. Controllable synthesis of boron-doped Zn–N–C single-atom nanozymes for the ultrasensitive colorimetric detection of p-phenylenediamine. *Biosens. Bioelectron.* **2022**, *210*, 114294. [CrossRef] [PubMed]
54. Baerlocher, C.; Xie, D.; McCusker, L.B.; Hwang, S.-J.; Chan, I.Y.; Ong, K.; Burton, A.W.; Zones, S.I. Ordered silicon vacancies in the framework structure of the zeolite catalyst SSZ-74. *Nat. Mater.* **2008**, *7*, 631–635. [CrossRef] [PubMed]
55. Xu, G.; Zhong, Z.; Bing, Y.; Ye, Z.G.; Shirane, G. Electric-field-induced redistribution of polar nano-regions in a relaxor ferroelectric. *Nat. Mater.* **2006**, *5*, 134–140. [CrossRef] [PubMed]
56. Wan, J.; Chen, W.; Jia, C.; Zheng, L.; Dong, J.; Zheng, X.; Wang, Y.; Yan, W.; Chen, C.; Peng, Q.; et al. Defect Effects on TiO_2 Nanosheets: Stabilizing Single Atomic Site Au and Promoting Catalytic Properties. *Adv. Mater.* **2018**, *30*, 1705369. [CrossRef]
57. Kitagawa, S.; Kitaura, R.; Noro, S.-I. Functional Porous Coordination Polymers. *Angew. Chem. Int. Ed.* **2004**, *43*, 2334–2375. [CrossRef]
58. Cavka, J.H.; Jakobsen, S.; Olsbye, U.; Guillou, N.; Lamberti, C.; Bordiga, S.; Lillerud, K.P. A New Zirconium Inorganic Building Brick Forming Metal Organic Frameworks with Exceptional Stability. *J. Am. Chem. Soc.* **2008**, *130*, 13850–13851. [CrossRef]
59. Taddei, M. When defects turn into virtues: The curious case of zirconium-based metal-organic frameworks. *Coord. Chem. Rev.* **2017**, *343*, 1–24. [CrossRef]
60. Mondloch, J.E.; Bury, W.; Fairen-Jimenez, D.; Kwon, S.; DeMarco, E.J.; Weston, M.H.; Sarjeant, A.A.; Nguyen, S.T.; Stair, P.C.; Snurr, R.Q.; et al. Vapor-Phase Metalation by Atomic Layer Deposition in a Metal–Organic Framework. *J. Am. Chem. Soc.* **2013**, *135*, 10294–10297. [CrossRef]
61. Burtch, N.C.; Jasuja, H.; Walton, K.S. Water Stability and Adsorption in Metal–Organic Frameworks. *Chem. Rev.* **2014**, *114*, 10575–10612. [CrossRef] [PubMed]
62. Hobday, C.L.; Marshall, R.J.; Murphie, C.F.; Sotelo, J.; Richards, T.; Allan, D.R.; Düren, T.; Coudert, F.-X.; Forgan, R.S.; Morrison, C.A.; et al. A Computational and Experimental Approach Linking Disorder, High-Pressure Behavior, and Mechanical Properties in UiO Frameworks. *Angew. Chem. Int. Ed.* **2016**, *55*, 2401–2405. [CrossRef] [PubMed]
63. Valenzano, L.; Civalleri, B.; Chavan, S.; Bordiga, S.; Nilsen, M.H.; Jakobsen, S.; Lillerud, K.P.; Lamberti, C. Disclosing the Complex Structure of UiO-66 Metal Organic Framework: A Synergic Combination of Experiment and Theory. *Chem. Mater.* **2011**, *23*, 1700–1718. [CrossRef]
64. Wu, H.; Chua, Y.S.; Krungleviciute, V.; Tyagi, M.; Chen, P.; Yildirim, T.; Zhou, W. Unusual and Highly Tunable Missing-Linker Defects in Zirconium Metal–Organic Framework UiO-66 and Their Important Effects on Gas Adsorption. *J. Am. Chem. Soc.* **2013**, *135*, 10525–10532. [CrossRef]
65. Fang, Z.; Bueken, B.; De Vos, D.E.; Fischer, R.A. Defect-Engineered Metal–Organic Frameworks. *Angew. Chem. Int. Ed.* **2015**, *54*, 7234–7254. [CrossRef]
66. Dissegna, S.; Epp, K.; Heinz, W.R.; Kieslich, G.; Fischer, R.A. Defective Metal-Organic Frameworks. *Adv. Mater.* **2018**, *30*, 1704501. [CrossRef]
67. Xiang, W.; Zhang, Y.; Chen, Y.; Liu, C.-J.; Tu, X. Synthesis, characterization and application of defective metal–organic frameworks: Current status and perspectives. *J. Mater. Chem. A* **2020**, *8*, 21526–21546. [CrossRef]
68. Li, T.; Bao, Y.; Qiu, H.; Tong, W. Boosted peroxidase-like activity of metal-organic framework nanoparticles with single atom Fe(III) sites at low substrate concentration. *Anal. Chim. Acta* **2021**, *1152*, 338299. [CrossRef]
69. Ye, G.; Gu, Y.; Zhou, W.; Xu, W.; Sun, Y. Synthesis of Defect-Rich Titanium Terephthalate with the Assistance of Acetic Acid for Room-Temperature Oxidative Desulfurization of Fuel Oil. *ACS Catal.* **2020**, *10*, 2384–2394. [CrossRef]
70. Wang, J.; Liu, L.; Chen, C.; Dong, X.; Wang, Q.; Alfilfil, L.; AlAlouni, M.R.; Yao, K.; Huang, J.; Zhang, D.; et al. Engineering effective structural defects of metal–organic frameworks to enhance their catalytic performances. *J. Mater. Chem. A* **2020**, *8*, 4464–4472. [CrossRef]
71. Xue, Z.; Liu, K.; Liu, Q.; Li, Y.; Li, M.; Su, C.-Y.; Ogiwara, N.; Kobayashi, H.; Kitagawa, H.; Liu, M.; et al. Missing-linker metal-organic frameworks for oxygen evolution reaction. *Nat. Commun.* **2019**, *10*, 5048. [CrossRef]
72. Zhang, X.; Zhang, Z.; Boissonnault, J.; Cohen, S.M. Design and synthesis of squaramide-based MOFs as efficient MOF-supported hydrogen-bonding organocatalysts. *Chem. Commun.* **2016**, *52*, 8585–8588. [CrossRef]
73. Cohen, S.M. The Postsynthetic Renaissance in Porous Solids. *J. Am. Chem. Soc.* **2017**, *139*, 2855–2863. [CrossRef]
74. Yang, P.; Mao, F.; Li, Y.; Zhuang, Q.; Gu, J. Hierarchical Porous Zr-Based MOFs Synthesized by a Facile Monocarboxylic Acid Etching Strategy. *Chem. Eur. J.* **2018**, *24*, 2962–2970. [CrossRef]
75. Chang, G.-G.; Ma, X.-C.; Zhang, Y.-X.; Wang, L.-Y.; Tian, G.; Liu, J.-W.; Wu, J.; Hu, Z.-Y.; Yang, X.-Y.; Chen, B. Construction of Hierarchical Metal-Organic Frameworks by Competitive Coordination Strategy for Highly Efficient CO_2 Conversion. *Adv. Mater.* **2019**, *31*, 1904969. [CrossRef]

76. Ma, X.; Wang, L.; Zhang, Q.; Jiang, H.-L. Switching on the Photocatalysis of Metal–Organic Frameworks by Engineering Structural Defects. *Angew. Chem. Int. Ed.* **2019**, *58*, 12175–12179. [CrossRef]
77. Zhang, J.; Wu, X.; Cheong, W.-C.; Chen, W.; Lin, R.; Li, J.; Zheng, L.; Yan, W.; Gu, L.; Chen, C.; et al. Cation vacancy stabilization of single-atomic-site Pt1/Ni(OH)$_x$ catalyst for diboration of alkynes and alkenes. *Nat. Commun.* **2018**, *9*, 1002. [CrossRef]
78. Liu, G.; Robertson, A.W.; Li, M.M.-J.; Kuo, W.C.H.; Darby, M.T.; Muhieddine, M.H.; Lin, Y.-C.; Suenaga, K.; Stamatakis, M.; Warner, J.H.; et al. MoS$_2$ monolayer catalyst doped with isolated Co atoms for the hydrodeoxygenation reaction. *Nat. Chem.* **2017**, *9*, 810–816. [CrossRef]
79. Liu, J. Aberration-corrected scanning transmission electron microscopy in single-atom catalysis: Probing the catalytically active centers. *Chin. J. Catal.* **2017**, *38*, 1460–1472. [CrossRef]
80. Sun, Z.; Liu, Q.; Yao, T.; Yan, W.; Wei, S. X-ray absorption fine structure spectroscopy in nanomaterials. *Sci. China Mater.* **2015**, *58*, 313–341. [CrossRef]
81. Ogino, I. X-ray absorption spectroscopy for single-atom catalysts: Critical importance and persistent challenges. *Chin. J. Catal.* **2017**, *38*, 1481–1488. [CrossRef]
82. Wu, Y.; Jiao, L.; Luo, X.; Xu, W.; Wei, X.; Wang, H.; Yan, H.; Gu, W.; Xu, B.Z.; Du, D.; et al. Oxidase-Like Fe-N-C Single-Atom Nanozymes for the Detection of Acetylcholinesterase Activity. *Small* **2019**, *15*, 1903108. [CrossRef] [PubMed]
83. Su, Y.; Wu, F.; Song, Q.; Wu, M.; Mohammadniaei, M.; Zhang, T.; Liu, B.; Wu, S.; Zhang, M.; Li, A.; et al. Dual enzyme-mimic nanozyme based on single-atom construction strategy for photothermal-augmented nanocatalytic therapy in the second near-infrared biowindow. *Biomaterials* **2022**, *281*, 121325. [CrossRef] [PubMed]
84. Zandieh, M.; Liu, J. Nanozyme Catalytic Turnover and Self-Limited Reactions. *ACS Nano* **2021**, *15*, 15645–15655. [CrossRef]
85. Liu, B.; Liu, J. Surface modification of nanozymes. *Nano Res.* **2017**, *10*, 1125–1148. [CrossRef]
86. Huo, M.; Wang, L.; Wang, Y.; Chen, Y.; Shi, J. Nanocatalytic Tumor Therapy by Single-Atom Catalysts. *ACS Nano* **2019**, *13*, 2643–2653. [CrossRef]
87. Wang, D.; Wu, H.; Phua, S.Z.F.; Yang, G.; Qi Lim, W.; Gu, L.; Qian, C.; Wang, H.; Guo, Z.; Chen, H.; et al. Self-assembled single-atom nanozyme for enhanced photodynamic therapy treatment of tumor. *Nat. Commun.* **2020**, *11*, 357. [CrossRef]
88. Gong, N.; Ma, X.; Ye, X.; Zhou, Q.; Chen, X.; Tan, X.; Yao, S.; Huo, S.; Zhang, T.; Chen, S.; et al. Carbon-dot-supported atomically dispersed gold as a mitochondrial oxidative stress amplifier for cancer treatment. *Nat. Nanotechnol.* **2019**, *14*, 379–387. [CrossRef]
89. Liu, Y.; Yao, M.; Han, W.; Zhang, H.; Zhang, S. Construction of a Single-Atom Nanozyme for Enhanced Chemodynamic Therapy and Chemotherapy. *Chemistry* **2021**, *27*, 13418–13425. [CrossRef]
90. Qi, P.; Zhang, J.; Bao, Z.; Liao, Y.; Liu, Z.; Wang, J. A Platelet-Mimicking Single-Atom Nanozyme for Mitochondrial Damage-Mediated Mild-Temperature Photothermal Therapy. *ACS Appl. Mater. Interfaces* **2022**, *14*, 19081–19090. [CrossRef]
91. Singh, S.; Dosani, T.; Karakoti, A.S.; Kumar, A.; Seal, S.; Self, W.T. A phosphate-dependent shift in redox state of cerium oxide nanoparticles and its effects on catalytic properties. *Biomaterials* **2011**, *32*, 6745–6753. [CrossRef] [PubMed]
92. Wang, S.; Kai, M.; Duan, Y.; Zhou, Z.; Fang, R.H.; Gao, W.; Zhang, L. Membrane Cholesterol Depletion Enhances Enzymatic Activity of Cell-Membrane-Coated Metal-Organic-Framework Nanoparticles. *Angew. Chem. Int. Ed.* **2022**, *61*, e202203115.
93. Wu, Y.; Wu, J.; Jiao, L.; Xu, W.; Wang, H.; Wei, X.; Gu, W.; Ren, G.; Zhang, N.; Zhang, Q.; et al. Cascade Reaction System Integrating Single-Atom Nanozymes with Abundant Cu Sites for Enhanced Biosensing. *Anal. Chem.* **2020**, *92*, 3373–3379. [CrossRef] [PubMed]
94. Wang, Y.; Qi, K.; Yu, S.; Jia, G.; Cheng, Z.; Zheng, L.; Wu, Q.; Bao, Q.; Wang, Q.; Zhao, J.; et al. Revealing the Intrinsic Peroxidase-Like Catalytic Mechanism of Heterogeneous Single-Atom Co–MoS$_2$. *Nano-Micro Lett.* **2019**, *11*, 102. [CrossRef]
95. Lu, X.; Gao, S.; Lin, H.; Shi, J. Single-Atom Catalysts for Nanocatalytic Tumor Therapy. *Small* **2021**, *17*, 2004467. [CrossRef]
96. He, H.; Fei, Z.; Guo, T.; Hou, Y.; Li, D.; Wang, K.; Ren, F.; Fan, K.; Zhou, D.; Xie, C.; et al. Bioadhesive injectable hydrogel with phenolic carbon quantum dot supported Pd single atom nanozymes as a localized immunomodulation niche for cancer catalytic immunotherapy. *Biomaterials* **2022**, *280*, 121272. [CrossRef]
97. Dickinson, B.C.; Chang, C.J. Chemistry and biology of reactive oxygen species in signaling or stress responses. *Nat. Chem. Biol.* **2011**, *7*, 504–511. [CrossRef]
98. Murphy, M.P. How mitochondria produce reactive oxygen species. *Biochem. J.* **2008**, *417*, 1–13. [CrossRef]
99. Dickinson, B.C.; Peltier, J.; Stone, D.; Schaffer, D.V.; Chang, C.J. Nox2 redox signaling maintains essential cell populations in the brain. *Nat. Chem. Biol.* **2011**, *7*, 106–112. [CrossRef]
100. Niethammer, P.; Grabher, C.; Look, A.T.; Mitchison, T.J. A tissue-scale gradient of hydrogen peroxide mediates rapid wound detection in zebrafish. *Nature* **2009**, *459*, 996–999. [CrossRef]
101. Yuan, A.; Xia, F.; Bian, Q.; Wu, H.; Gu, Y.; Wang, T.; Wang, R.; Huang, L.; Huang, Q.; Rao, Y.; et al. Ceria Nanozyme-Integrated Microneedles Reshape the Perifollicular Microenvironment for Androgenetic Alopecia Treatment. *ACS Nano* **2021**, *15*, 13759–13769. [CrossRef] [PubMed]
102. Wang, D.D.; Zhao, Y.L. Single-atom engineering of metal-organic frameworks toward healthcare. *CHEM* **2021**, *7*, 2635–2671. [CrossRef]
103. Ma, W.; Mao, J.; Yang, X.; Pan, C.; Chen, W.; Wang, M.; Yu, P.; Mao, L.; Li, Y. A single-atom Fe–N$_4$ catalytic site mimicking bifunctional antioxidative enzymes for oxidative stress cytoprotection. *Chem. Commun.* **2019**, *55*, 159–162. [CrossRef] [PubMed]
104. Lu, M.; Wang, C.; Ding, Y.; Peng, M.; Zhang, W.; Li, K.; Wei, W.; Lin, Y. Fe-N/C single-atom catalysts exhibiting multienzyme activity and ROS scavenging ability in cells. *Chem. Commun.* **2019**, *55*, 14534–14537. [CrossRef]

105. Yan, R.; Sun, S.; Yang, J.; Long, W.; Wang, J.; Mu, X.; Li, Q.; Hao, W.; Zhang, S.; Liu, H.; et al. Nanozyme-Based Bandage with Single-Atom Catalysis for Brain Trauma. *ACS Nano* **2019**, *13*, 11552–11560. [CrossRef]
106. Chen, Y.; Zou, H.; Yan, B.; Wu, X.; Cao, W.; Qian, Y.; Zheng, L.; Yang, G. Atomically Dispersed Cu Nanozyme with Intensive Ascorbate Peroxidase Mimic Activity Capable of Alleviating ROS-Mediated Oxidation Damage. *Adv. Sci.* **2022**, *9*, e2103977. [CrossRef]
107. Makvandi, P.; Wang, C.-Y.; Zare, E.N.; Borzacchiello, A.; Niu, L.-N.; Tay, F.R. Metal-Based Nanomaterials in Biomedical Applications: Antimicrobial Activity and Cytotoxicity Aspects. *Adv. Funct. Mater.* **2020**, *30*, 1910021. [CrossRef]
108. Hutchings, M.I.; Truman, A.W.; Wilkinson, B. Antibiotics: Past, present and future. *Curr. Opin. Microbiol.* **2019**, *51*, 72–80. [CrossRef]
109. Yang, D.; Chen, Z.; Gao, Z.; Tammina, S.K.; Yang, Y. Nanozymes used for antimicrobials and their applications. *Colloids Surf. B Biointerfaces* **2020**, *195*, 111252. [CrossRef]
110. Xia, D.; Liu, H.; Xu, B.; Wang, Y.; Liao, Y.; Huang, Y.; Ye, L.; He, C.; Wong, P.K.; Qiu, R. Single Ag atom engineered 3D-MnO$_2$ porous hollow microspheres for rapid photothermocatalytic inactivation of E. coli under solar light. *Appl. Catal. B Environ.* **2019**, *245*, 177–189. [CrossRef]
111. Huo, M.; Wang, L.; Zhang, H.; Zhang, L.; Chen, Y.; Shi, J. Construction of Single-Iron-Atom Nanocatalysts for Highly Efficient Catalytic Antibiotics. *Small* **2019**, *15*, 1901834. [CrossRef] [PubMed]
112. Wang, X.; Shi, Q.; Zha, Z.; Zhu, D.; Zheng, L.; Shi, L.; Wei, X.; Lian, L.; Wu, K.; Cheng, L. Copper single-atom catalysts with photothermal performance and enhanced nanozyme activity for bacteria-infected wound therapy. *Bioact. Mater.* **2021**, *6*, 4389–4401. [CrossRef] [PubMed]
113. Chen, Y.; Wang, P.; Hao, H.; Hong, J.; Li, H.; Ji, S.; Li, A.; Gao, R.; Dong, J.; Han, X.; et al. Thermal Atomization of Platinum Nanoparticles into Single Atoms: An Effective Strategy for Engineering High-Performance Nanozymes. *J. Am. Chem. Soc.* **2021**, *143*, 18643–18651. [CrossRef] [PubMed]
114. Yu, Y.; Tan, L.; Li, Z.; Liu, X.; Zheng, Y.; Feng, X.; Liang, Y.; Cui, Z.; Zhu, S.; Wu, S. Single-Atom Catalysis for Efficient Sonodynamic Therapy of Methicillin-Resistant Staphylococcus aureus-Infected Osteomyelitis. *ACS Nano* **2021**, *15*, 10628–10639. [CrossRef]

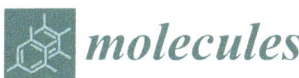

Article

Biodegradable Nanoparticles Loaded with Levodopa and Curcumin for Treatment of Parkinson's Disease

Bassam Felipe Mogharbel [1,†], Marco André Cardoso [1,2,†], Ana Carolina Irioda [1], Priscila Elias Ferreira Stricker [1], Robson Camilotti Slompo [1], Julia Maurer Appel [1], Nathalia Barth de Oliveira [1], Maiara Carolina Perussolo [1], Claudia Sayuri Saçaki [1], Nadia Nascimento da Rosa [1], Dilcele Silva Moreira Dziedzic [1], Christophe Travelet [2], Sami Halila [2], Redouane Borsali [2] and Katherine Athayde Teixeira de Carvalho [1,*]

[1] Advanced Therapy and Cellular Biotechnology in Regenerative Medicine Department, The Pelé Pequeno Príncipe Research Institute, Child and Adolescent Health Research & Pequeno Príncipe Faculties, Curitiba 80240-020, Brazil; bassamfm@gmail.com (B.F.M.); marcoacardoso@yahoo.com.br (M.A.C.); anairioda@gmail.com (A.C.I.); priscilaeferreira@gmail.com (P.E.F.S.); robsoncamilotti@gmail.com (R.C.S.); juliamappel@gmail.com (J.M.A.); nathybarth03@gmail.com (N.B.d.O.); perussolo10@gmail.com (M.C.P.); claudiasacaki@gmail.com (C.S.S.); nadianr@gmail.com (N.N.d.R.); dilceledz@gmail.com (D.S.M.D.)

[2] Centre de Recherches sur les Macromolécules Végétales (CERMAV), Centre National de la Recherche Scientifique (CNRS), Université Grenoble Alpes, F-38000 Grenoble, France; christophe.travelet@cermav.cnrs.fr (C.T.); sami.halila@cermav.cnrs.fr (S.H.); redouane.borsali@cermav.cnrs.fr (R.B.)

* Correspondence: katherinecarv@gmail.com; Tel.: +55-41-3310-1719
† These authors contributed equally to this work.

Abstract: Background: Parkinson's disease (PD) is the second most common age-related neurodegenerative disorder. Levodopa (L-DOPA) remains the gold-standard drug available for treating PD. Curcumin has many pharmacological activities, including antioxidant, anti-inflammatory, antimicrobial, anti-amyloid, and antitumor properties. Copolymers composed of Poly (ethylene oxide) (PEO) and biodegradable polyesters such as Poly (ε-caprolactone) (PCL) can self-assemble into nanoparticles (NPs). This study describes the development of NH_2–PEO–PCL diblock copolymer positively charged and modified by adding glutathione (GSH) on the outer surface, resulting in a synergistic delivery of L-DOPA curcumin that would be able to pass the blood–brain barrier. **Methods:** The NH_2–PEO–PCL NPs suspensions were prepared by using a nanoprecipitation and solvent displacement method and coated with GSH. NPs were submitted to characterization assays. In order to ensure the bioavailability, Vero and PC12 cells were treated with various concentrations of the loaded and unloaded NPs to observe cytotoxicity. **Results:** NPs have successfully loaded L-DOPA and curcumin and were stable after freeze-drying, indicating advancing into in vitro toxicity testing. Vero and PC12 cells that were treated up to 72 h with various concentrations of L-DOPA and curcumin-loaded NP maintained high viability percentage, indicating that the NPs are biocompatible. **Conclusions:** NPs consisting of NH_2–PEO–PCL were characterized as potential formulations for brain delivery of L-DOPA and curcumin. The results also indicate that the developed biodegradable nanomicelles that were blood compatible presented low cytotoxicity.

Keywords: nanoparticles; glutathione; Parkinson's disease; L-DOPA; curcumin

Citation: Mogharbel, B.F.; Cardoso, M.A.; Irioda, A.C.; Stricker, P.E.F.; Slompo, R.C.; Appel, J.M.; de Oliveira, N.B.; Perussolo, M.C.; Saçaki, C.S.; da Rosa, N.N.; et al. Biodegradable Nanoparticles Loaded with Levodopa and Curcumin for Treatment of Parkinson's Disease. *Molecules* 2022, 27, 2811. https://doi.org/10.3390/molecules27092811

Academic Editors: Wansong Chen and Jianhua Zhang

Received: 13 March 2022
Accepted: 23 April 2022
Published: 28 April 2022

Publisher's Note: MDPI stays neutral with regard to jurisdictional claims in published maps and institutional affiliations.

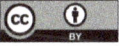

Copyright: © 2022 by the authors. Licensee MDPI, Basel, Switzerland. This article is an open access article distributed under the terms and conditions of the Creative Commons Attribution (CC BY) license (https://creativecommons.org/licenses/by/4.0/).

1. Introduction

Parkinson's disease (PD) is the second most common age-related neurodegenerative disorder and represents a growing healthcare concern with elderly populations. The disease is associated with a range of symptoms, including bradykinesia, rigidity, tremor, dementia, and depression [1]. Levodopa (L-DOPA) is the gold-standard drug for PD treatment, and its use results in a marked improvement in patient quality of life, but just for a limited period. L-DOPA shows tolerance and the development of induced dyskinesias during treatment. Fluctuations of L-DOPA blood levels are related to the intermittent stimulation of dopamine receptors, resulting in a discontinuous response with "On" and "Off" periods of action (wearing off) and disease progression [2]. Moreover, the metabolism of L-DOPA also generates a variety of free radicals that increase the loss of nigrostriatal dopaminergic neurons and the development of the disorder [3,4].

The blood–brain barrier (BBB) limits access to therapeutic molecules and macrostructures [5]. Brain-targeted drug delivery is a significant concern since the BBB permeability is crucial for nanoparticles (NPs) to exhibit a therapeutic effect. Thus, one great therapeutic challenge in PD treatment is developing an effective drug targeted system capable of improving the symptoms, extending the brain delivery of L-DOPA by crossing the BBB, avoiding fluctuations in its concentration, and reducing the rate of neurodegeneration.

Nanosized polymeric micelles formed by amphiphilic copolymers with A (hydrophilic)-B (hydrophobic) diblock structures could be employed as vehicles for drug administration to the brain once they can be designed to display different properties of targeting, pharmacokinetics, and cargo release of drugs, including insoluble or poorly soluble compounds and surmount the BBB [6].

Amphiphilic block copolymers composed of poly(ethylene oxide) (PEO) and biodegradable polyesters such as Poly(ε-caprolactone) (PCL), which can self-assemble into nanoparticles (NP) in aqueous medium, have gained much attention in the nanomedicine field. PEO is an FDA-approved biodegradable polymer and a common constituent for the hydrophilic outer shell of nanoparticles. It possesses a great number of useful physicochemical and biological properties, including hydrophilicity, solubility in water, lack of toxicity, and absence of antigenicity and immunogenicity [7]. PCL is one of the most widely used FDA-approved biodegradable polymers because of its biocompatibility, biodegradability, mechanical properties, non-toxicity, high drug permeability, and slow in vivo degradation properties. PCL has a wide spectrum of applications in the biomedical field, including formulations for drug delivery as nanocapsules capable of prolonging the drug release and enhancing the drug stability [8].

Therefore, to modify and improve pharmacological and therapeutic effects, drugs can be encapsulated in PEO/PCL-based NPs based in noncovalent interactions as hydrogen bonding and hydrophobic or ionic interactions and released by diffusion directly at a specific tissue or site of action [7]. Furthermore, NPs have also demonstrated the ability to deliver antioxidant compounds that reduce oxidative stress in various diseases, including PD [9,10].

Curcumin (CUR) is a natural low-molecular-weight hydrophobic polyphenolic phytoconstituent that is isolated from the perennial herb *Curcuma longa*, with various pharmacological properties [11,12]. The development of nanotechnology-based delivery systems of CUR demonstrated its neuroprotective effect in Parkinson's disease models [13,14].

The approaches for active targeting of NP to overcome the BBB involve different mechanism for the transport of macromolecules across the BBB, as the absorptive-mediated transcytosis (which comprises the use of positively charged moieties), the transporter-mediated transcytosis (correlated with nutrients or substrates, such as glutathione and glucose, among others), and the receptor-mediated transcytosis (associated with the facilitated passage of targeting ligands). Therefore, endocytic pathways can be activated by using direct moieties or ligands as vectors [15,16].

Glutathione (GSH) is a water-soluble endogenous tripeptide of glutamic acid, cysteine, and glycine that possesses antioxidant-like properties with an active uptake transporter highly expressed at the BBB. Once specific binding sites of BBB receptors for GSH are selective compared with other endogenous peptides, GSH can be used as a safe, effective, and specific ligand that can target and enhance drug delivery of NPs to the brain without toxicity. However, the detailed mechanisms of GSH as a ligand mediating endocytosis need to be elucidated [17,18].

More recent studies have also demonstrated that the use of GSH as a targeting ligand to deliver NPs inside the brain has enhanced their neuronal bioavailability and therapeutic effects, improving treatment outcomes and cellular internalization of different nanoformulations, including nanomedications undergoing clinical evaluation such as 2B3-101 [19–23].

This manuscript describes the development of NPs composed of NH_2–PEO–PCL diblock copolymer positively charged and modified by the addition of GSH on the outer surface, obtaining a dual functionalized system for a synergistic delivery of L-DOPA and CUR. This dual system would be able to pass the BBB, target the brain tissue, and provide a more sustained release of drugs for potential application in PD treatment.

2. Results and Discussion

2.1. Characterization of NH_2–PEO–PCL Nanoparticles

The NTA analysis, a technique that enables the visualization, sizing, and quantification of nanoparticles in suspension by using a highly sensitive video camera, demonstrated a narrow distribution of the NH_2–PEO–PCL NP and a size of 99.5 + 7.3 nm, smaller than those obtained by DLS (Figure 1).

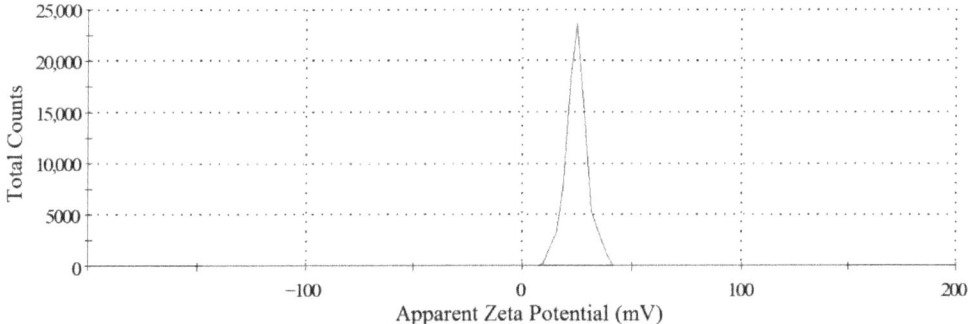

Figure 1. Surface zeta potential graph showing positive zeta potential value for NH_2-PEO-PCL nanoparticle.

The results show that the sizes of the reported NH_2–PEO–PCL NPs were bigger than those reported by Numata (2015) [24]. The NPs' formation during nanoprecipitation is primarily governed by the diffusion stranding phenomenon and the Marangoni effect. Thus, different preparation conditions and parameters on PCL NP preparation by solvent displacement can affect the nanoparticle size, as described by Badri et al. (2017) and Mora-Huertas et al. (2011) [25,26]. The physicochemical properties of solvents used in NP production, such as viscosity and water miscibility, are important factors that control the size and size distribution of the NP generated. Once THF is more viscous than acetone, the former can retard the diffusion of solute and solvent molecules during the mixing procedure of solvent displacement method and, thus, generate larger particles, in a similar way described by Tam et al. (2016) [27].

A further analysis of the DLS and SLS scattering data was performed. The shape factor, ρ, was obtained from the ratio $\rho = Dg/Dh$. The ρ values of 1.4 for NH_2–PEO–PCL NP fall between those of vesicles ($\rho = 1$) and rigid rods ($\rho \geq 2.0$), meaning that the overall shape of these NPs was spherical. According to Gross et al. (2016) [28], the shift in size could be explained because the size distributions obtained by DLS consist of weight distributions, whereas those obtained by NTA are number distributions.

The preparation method of nanoparticle aqueous suspensions formed by amphiphilic block copolymers, called nanoprecipitation or the solvent displacement technique, is the dissolution of the copolymer in a mixture of good solvents for both blocks, followed by the decrease of the organic solvent content by the injection of the solution in an excess of water. A further decrease in the content of the organic solvent, by evaporation or by dialysis of the solution against water, causes the collapse of hydrophobic cores, generating stable NPs [29].

The nanoprecipitation method described by Y. Numata et al. (2015) [24], with small modifications, was used for the preparation of NH_2–PEO–PCL NPs. In order to determine the minimization of the scattering intensity corresponding to the most dispersed polymer state in solution, the effect of the different organic solvent percentages (from 50% to 100% of THF in water) was studied in the polymer dissolution. The formation of NH_2–PEO–PCL aggregates formed in THF/water solutions decreased with the increasing percentage of THF, reaching a minimum at 90% of THF. Transmission electron microscopy determines the size of dry particles, while DLS determines the hydrodynamic diameter of particles in water. Because amphiphilic block polymeric micelles always have a loose structure in water, the particle size determined by DLS is always slightly more extensive than that determined by transmission electron microscopy [30]. TEM observed that the NH_2–PEO–PCL NP was the systems' spherical shape, as shown in Figure 2. Nanoparticles with a size less than 200 nm can be injected intravascularly, permeate and traffic through different tissues, bind to cell surface receptors, and enter to target cells for intracellular drug delivery [31]. This result demonstrates that the NH_2–PEO–PCL NPs are larger than the threshold for glomerular filtration in the kidney (Mw approximately 50 kDa) and smaller than 200 nm, increasing the blood circulation and the tissue targeting effect, especially to the brain [32].

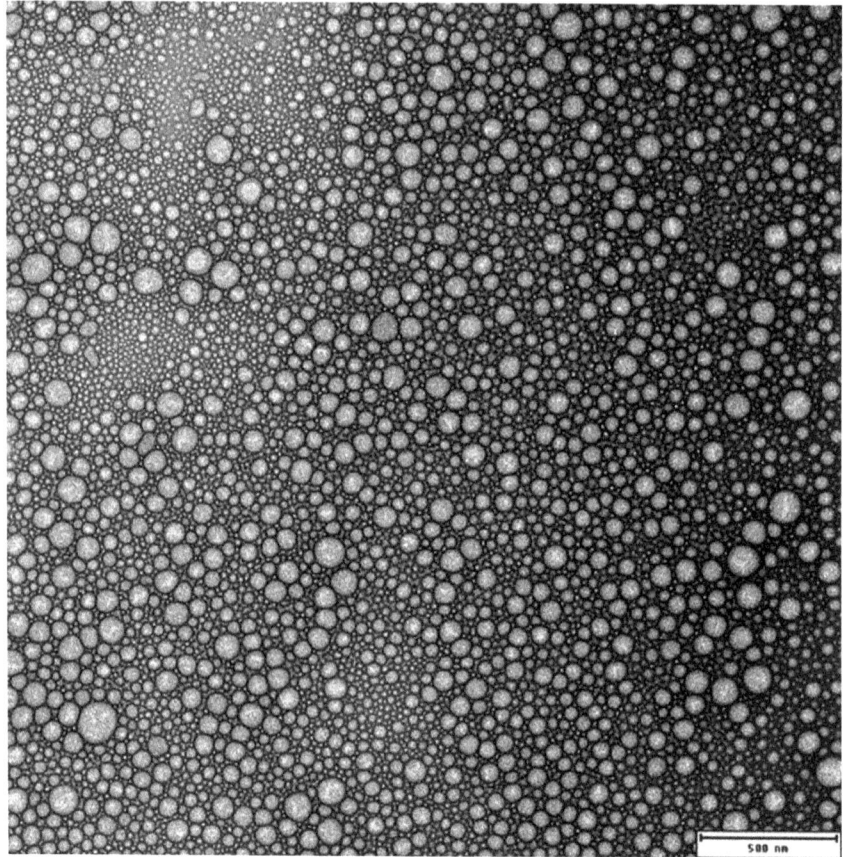

Figure 2. Transmission electron micrographs image of NH_2-PEO-PCL nanoparticles (bar 500 nm).

PDI is an indicative of the NPs size distribution, ranging from 0 to 1, and defines the dispersion homogeneity. Values close to 1 indicate heterogeneity and PDI values lower than

0.5 indicate NPs of better quality with a homogenous distribution of particle size [33,34]. All the NPs showed unimodal distribution, as indicated with PDI values of less than 0.35, suggesting a homogenous distribution under the preparation conditions.

Zeta potential (ZP) analysis can provide very useful information on the surface properties and stability of the NP system.

The ZP of the NH_2–PEO–PCL NPs was +25.6 + 0.5 mV (Table 1). This positive value is attributed to the formation of quaternary ammonium groups on NH_2–PEO chains generated by its protonation in aqueous medium and, as expected, suggest the orientation of the PEO chains to the outside of the micellar NPs. This absolute value of the ZP also implies a high stability of the NPs suspension once the repulsive forces generated by the positive charges surrounding the NPs prevent its aggregation and the chances of coalescence of NPs in the system [35].

Table 1. Physicochemical parameters of NH_2–PEO–PCL, GSH adsorbed and L-DOPA and curcumin-loaded nanoparticles in aqueous solution.

Sample	2 Rh (nm)	NTA (nm)	PDI	Zeta Potential (mV)
NH_2–PEO–PCL (UnNP)	$1.17 \times 10^2 \pm 8.4$	$9.95 \times 10 \pm 7.3$	0.22	$+25.6 \pm 0.45$
GSH NH_2–PEO–PCL (UnNP)	$1.28 \times 10^2 \pm 2.7$	$1.05 \times 10^2 \pm 1.8$	0.21	$+10.4 \pm 0.73$
L-DOPA + CUR NH_2–PEO–PCL (LdCurNP)	$1.33 \times 10^2 \pm 6.4$	$1.23 \times 10^2 \pm 4.0$	0.24	$+24.6 \pm 0.6$
GSH L-DOPA + CUR NH_2–PEO–PCL (LdCurNP)	$1.45 \times 10^2 \pm 3.2$	$1.34 \times 10^2 \pm 5.0$	0.30	$+6.4 \pm 0.53$

In addition, the ZP of NPs is an essential factor in determining the in vivo interactions of nanoparticles with the cell membrane. The positive charge of NP complexes can help the NPs bind tightly to the negatively charged cellular membrane, having a higher tendency to attach and internalize into the cells by endocytosis, compared to negatively or neutrally charged particles [36].

In order to evaluate the comportment of the ZP of the NH_2–PEO–PCL NPs in different ionic strengths, the NPs were submitted to a crescent NaCl concentration ranging from 1 mM to 2 M (Figure 3). WE observed a progressive drift toward neutral, or slightly negative, values for ZP that progressively neutralized the positive charges of NH_2–PEO–PCL NPs and confirmed its positive value.

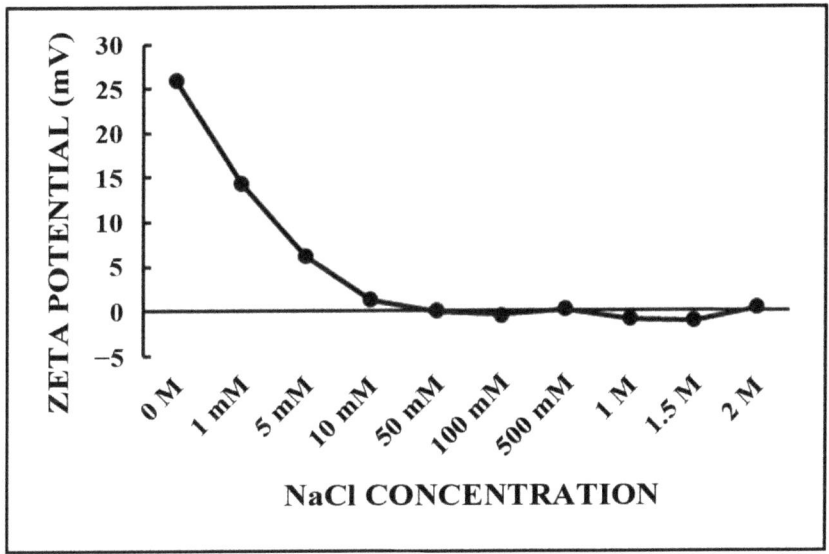

Figure 3. Zeta potential of NH_2-PEO-PCL nanoparticles as a function of NaCl concentration.

This implies that the presence of NaCl in the aqueous medium substantially influenced the properties of the NPs that were measurable by ZP and can be due to the electrostatic interactions after salt addition with the surface of the NPs, resulting in lower values of electrophoretic mobility [37].

The stability of NH_2–PEO–PCL NPs in diverse NaCl concentrations of the medium was also determined by measuring of the particle size by DLS. As depicted in Figure 3, the NH_2–PEO–PCL NPs were stable in a salt concentration superior to the physiological salt conditions (150 mM NaCl), showing just a slight variation in the size throughout all the salt concentrations evaluated. These results demonstrate the maintenance of NP suspensions in an aqueous medium, due to the steric repulsive forces of the NH_2–PEO corona and the hydrophobic interactions from the core of PCL, resulting in a stable system.

2.2. Curcumin (CUR) Encapsulation

A series of curcumin-loaded NPs formulated with different amounts of CUR (2, 3, 4, and 5 mg), added during the NPs preparation, were made in order to evaluate the CUR encapsulation efficiency. When the CUR-loaded micelles were prepared with 5 mg of CUR, the systems became instable, aggregating in a few minutes. On the other hand, at the drug-to-copolymer ratio ranging from 0.2 to 0.4 (2, 3, and 4 mg of CUR), no precipitate was detected, and the successful encapsulation was observed by the formation of a clear yellow solution of CUR loaded into micelles, as observed by Shao et al. (2011) [38], Wang et al. (2013) [30], and Scarano (2015) [39].

As described by Chow et al. (2015) [40], if the concentration of copolymer is low, relative to CUR in the organic phase, part of the hydrophobic CUR will be exposed to the external aqueous medium, due to an insufficient surface coverage of the NPs by the copolymer, resulting in particle aggregation, thus compromising the stability [40]. Moreover, the nanosuspension system prepared with a lower drug-to-copolymer ratio becomes more stable when the CUR-to-copolymer ratio decreases, and a more considerable amount of the copolymer covers the surfaces of the NP, increasing its steric stabilization [27]. After these results, the lowest tested CUR-to-copolymer ratio (0.2) was taken as the optimized formulation for the NP suspension preparation.

The drug loading and encapsulation efficiency of curcumin-loaded NPs, prepared with 2 mg of CUR, were 98.3% ± 0.9% and 19.8% ± 0.2%, respectively, in accordance with the results described by Gong et al. (2013) [11], Wang et al. (2013) [30], Mazzarino et al. (2014) [41], and Mogharbel et al. (2018) [42].

After the encapsulation, the size of the NPs increased as the CUR-to-copolymer ratio increased (129.3 + 6.5, 148.5 + 6.8, and 149.6 + 8.9 nm, to a copolymer/CUR ratio of 5, 3.3, and 2.5, respectively). This result was expected, because the incorporation of CUR into the hydrophobic cores increased the volume of the NPs [11,41,43], resulting in micelles with swollen cores forming spontaneously. The monodispersity was confirmed by polydispersity indices lower than 0.3 in all samples.

The CUR-loaded NP suspension was transparent and completely dispersed in aqueous media, with no aggregates, indicating full dispersibility of curcumin, while free CUR exhibited poor aqueous solubility, as described by Wang et al. (2013) [30]. Therefore, the encapsulation of CUR into polymeric micelles resulted in a homogenous and stable dosage form in aqueous solution with high drug loading and small particle size, making CUR administration possible.

As suggested by the results obtained by the determination of ZP, amphiphilic NH_2–PEO–PCL NPs were formed by a core–shell structure in water, constituted by the hydrophobic PCL chains in the core and the hydrophilic PEG chains oriented to the shell. Consequently, hydrophobic and water-insoluble drugs such as CUR can be encapsulated into the hydrophobic core by the hydrophobic interactions with PCL, and because of the surface hydrophilic shell of PEG, and became more useful in biological systems [43,44].

2.3. L-DOPA Encapsulation

The drug loading and encapsulation efficiency of L-DOPA-loaded NPs were 12% ± 1.4% and 3.6% ± 0.4%, respectively, which was reasonable considering the hydrophilic nature of dopamine. These values correlated with the results obtained by Arica et al. (2005) [45], with drug loading values ranging from 14% ± 1.2% to 20% ± 1.4%. Shin et al. (2014) [46] also published similar results for the drug loading of dopamine, the neurotransmitter originating from the decarboxylation of L-DOPA, with values ranging from 2.7% ± 1.8% to 18.6% ± 9.2%. No significant differences were observed for the size of unloaded and L-DOPA-loaded nanoparticles.

The advantages of PCL for drug release applications include its high permeability to drugs, slow and sustained release of entrapped therapeutic compounds, less acidic degradation products as compared to other types of aliphatic polyesters, and absence of systemic toxicity [8,47].

The results of L-DOPA encapsulation have demonstrated that NH_2–PEO–PCL NPs can encapsulate L-DOPA and, due to the PCL physicochemical characteristics, are also suitable for long-term sustained delivery of this bioactive agent. Consequently, it is expected that the developed NPs would be able to reduce the toxicity associated with L-DOPA; preserve the structural integrity of the encapsulated drug; enhance the drug stability, protecting it from rapid peripheral metabolism; and reduce the side effects associated with the L-DOPA treatment.

When loading both L-DOPA and curcumin (LdCurNP) in the same micelle, the drug loading and the encapsulation efficiency for L-DOPA were 10.4 ± 1.5% and 3.1 ± 0.5%; and for curcumin, they were 97.7 ± 1.0% and 19.5 ± 0.2%, respectively (Table 2).

Table 2. Drug loading and encapsulation efficiency of NH_2–PEO–PCL NPs loaded with curcumin, L-DOPA, or both.

Nanoparticle	Drug Loading	Encapsulation Efficiency
Curcumin-loaded NP	98.3% ± 0.9%	19.8% ± 0.2%
L-DOPA-loaded NP	12% ± 1.4%	3.6% ± 0.4%
L-DOPA and Curcumin-loaded NP (LdCurNP)	10.4 ± 1.5% (of L-DOPA)	3.1 ± 0.5% (of L-DOPA)
L-DOPA and Curcumin-loaded NP (LdCurNP)	97.7 ± 1.0% (of Curcumin)	19.5 ± 0.2% (of Curcumin)

2.4. GSH Coating of the NPs

Glutathione (GSH) coating promoted a slightly increase in the average size of the NH_2–PEO–PCL NPs, from 117.3 + 4.6 to 128.6 + 1.2. This is in agreement with the results reported previously by Mdzinarishvili et al. (2013) [48] and Geldenhuys (2011) [49], who used the same method for the functionalization of the NPs, as for the NPs produced by using chitosan conjugated with GSH for oral drug delivery proposed by Chronopoulou, et al. (2016) [50].

TEM observations of the GSH-coated NH_2–PEO–PCL NPs demonstrated that, after its functionalization, the system maintains the spherical shape, as shown in Figure 2.

The NTA analysis of the GSH-coated NH_2–PEO–PCL NPs demonstrated a size of 99.5 + 7.3 nm, smaller than those obtained by DLS (Figure 4).

This surface functionalization also gave rise to a significant decrease in the Zeta potential of the NP, from +25.6 + 0.5 to +11.0 + 0.4 mV, suggesting an effective masking effect on the exposed positively charged NH2- groups of PEO. This result was attributed to the formation of a coating of GSH adsorbed to the positively charged surface of NP, in a similar way described by Duxfield et al. (2016) [51].

The surface modification in our system was achieved by physical adsorption of GSH to the outside surface of NP; this is a simple approach that provides stability to the NP suspensions and sustains their bioactivity, due to ionic interaction between the positive charges of quaternary ammonium groups on NH_2–PEO chains outside of NP and the negative charge of GSH and reinforced by the hydrogen bonds between ether, hydroxyl, and amino groups from PEO and GSH.

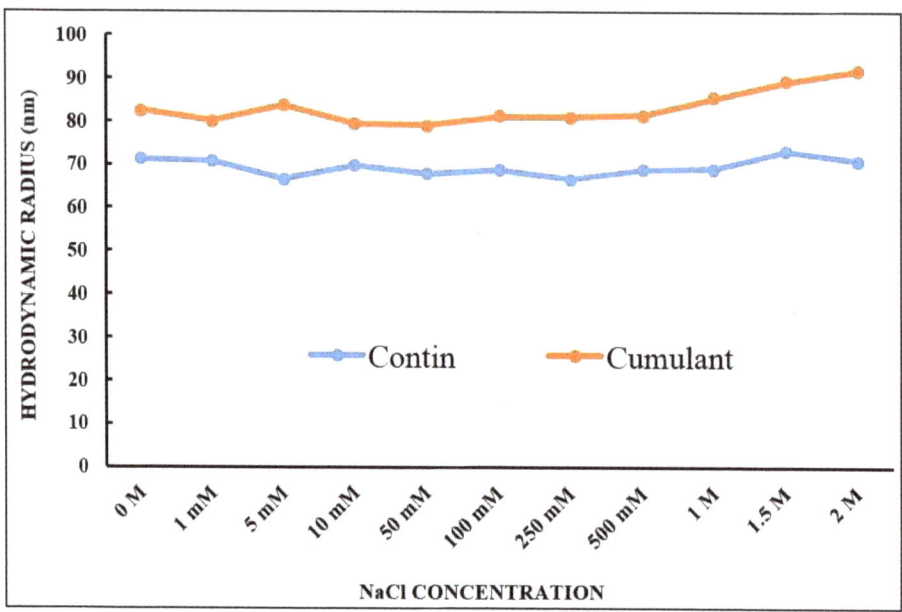

Figure 4. The hydrodynamic radius of NH$_2$-PEO-PCL nanoparticles as a function of NaCl concentration.

The GSH-adsorbed NPs were dialyzed against ultrapure water for two days by changing the water four times each day to evaluate the NPs' stability after their coating. It was observed that, after the dialysis, the ZP of the NPs remained unchanged (+11.2 + 1.6 mV), indicating that the interaction between the NPs surface and GSH is strong, making the functionalized system stable. This reveals that the GSH-coated NPs still retained a desirable positive charge at their surface.

No significant differences were observed for the unloaded and loaded GSH coated NP ZP values. GSH was coated onto the curcumin and L-DOPA NPs after their formation by the nanoprecipitation method coating the particles with GSH that would not modify the drug encapsulation.

Taking all of these results together, we hypothesized that the GSH-coated loaded NPs would be favorable for their transportation across the BBB by two different biological mechanisms.

First, the adhesion and transport properties of the NPs can be facilitated by the electrostatic attractions between the positively charged samples and the negatively charged cell membranes by adsorptive-mediated transcytosis (AMT). AMT is a vesicular transport route of cationic substances through the BBB, and, in contrast to receptor-mediated transcytosis, it does not require specific binding sites on cell surfaces but involves electrostatic interactions between polycationic substances and negative charges on the endothelial surface [52,53].

Second, GSH coating at loaded NPs can utilize the existing GSH transport mechanism in the BBB, contributing to the increase the permeability of positive charged NPs into the brain. GSH acts as an endogenous ligand for the NMDA and AMPA receptors present in the BBB, enabling the coated NPs to bind the NMDA receptor at glycine and glutamate site, enhancing the clathrin-mediated endocytosis-coated NP–NMDA receptor complex inside the cerebral cells.

Moreover, GSH glutathione-conjugated NPs could be recognized as endogenous units decreasing the clearance out of the brain and allowing the NPs to remain inside the brain for a longer time, enhancing its therapeutic effect [18,54]. In addition, authors have successfully demonstrated the delivery of GSH-conjugated NPs inside the brain as a safe, effective, and specific ligand for brain-targeted drug delivery systems that are capable of improving the transport of drugs across the blood–brain barrier [17,53,55].

2.5. Freeze-Drying Stability

After lyophilization, the observation of NH_2–PEO–PCL NPs revealed the formation of an intact cake occupying the same volume as the original frozen volume only in the samples which used hydroxypropyl-β-cyclodextrin (HPbCD) as a cryoprotectant.

The DLS analysis of the NPs submitted to lyophilization confirmed that, among all tested cryoprotectants, only HPbCD was capable of preserving the NPs during lyophilization. For the other protectants, the redispersed suspensions showed different extents of particle size and some visible precipitates.

The superior protectant performance of HPbCD relative to the other four protectants could be linked to its inherently non-crystalline nature and better adsorption onto the NPs surface during the sublimation of the aqueous phase. In addition, HPbCD is a collapse temperature modifier with a relatively high Tg' (i.e., the glass transition temperature of maximally cryo-concentrated solution), which renders it especially useful for raising the overall collapse temperature the nanoparticle formulation, as well as shortening the primary drying cycle. Moreover, HPbCD is an atoxic cyclic oligosaccharide used to improve the water-solubility and bioavailability of medicinal products currently found in marketed parenteral formulations [40].

One of the desired characteristics of the lyophilized NPs includes an intact cake occupying the same volume as the original frozen mass, which facilitates the rapid reconstitution of lyophilized product in a solvent system. A significant drop in volume may indicate formulation collapse, which is unacceptable from a gross macroscopic perspective. Apart from the lyophilization process, lyophilized cake formation is highly dependent on the composition of the formulation, including cryoprotectant [56]. Results obtained by other authors showed that HPbCD was also the most effective cryoprotectant among different sugars [40,57,58].

The reconstitution time of lyophilized NPs with HPbCD was practically instantaneous following the addition of water and gentle manual shaking by inversion. The NPs were readily dispersible, showing uniform distribution and no aggregation. The rehydration was achieved upon vortexing and sonication for the other collapsed formulations, which took a long reconstitution time.

The level of cryoprotection provided by sugars generally depends directly on their concentrations, meaning that, the higher the concentration of cryoprotectant, the better the stability of the nanoparticles. Moreover, it is essential to optimize the concentration of the used cryoprotectant, to use a minimum concentration while preserving all desirable characteristics [40].

As HPbCD was demonstrated to be the best protectant for the NPs during freeze-drying, eight different concentrations of HPbCD, ranging from 0.25 to 5% w/v, were tested. Precipitates were observed upon redispersion of the freeze-dried samples if the HPbCD concentration was below 2%. Then a minimum concentration of 2% of HPbCD was considered suitable for the reconstitution of lyophilized GSH-coated NH_2–PEO–PCL NPs. All the samples tested with concentrations of HPbCD ranging from 2 to 5% did not showed signs of aggregation and were easily reconstituted by manual shaking; in addition, the size measurement demonstrated an almost-identical mean particle size before and after freeze-drying. This result demonstrated no further enhancement of particle stability with higher HPbCD concentrations, as Chow et al. (2015) [40] presented.

After optimizing the lyophilization process and selecting the cryoprotectant, the results indicated that HPbCD at a concentration of 2% w/v was superior among all other sugars studied, resulting in desirable lyophilized NH_2–PEO–PCL NPs. The NPs' Zeta potential values were not statistically significant, confirming that the stabilization and NPs' outside charges were not affected.

2.6. Cytotoxicity Evaluations of the Loaded Nanoparticles

When evaluating the biocompatibility of newly designed nanoparticles, ensuring safety in vitro assays is necessary before advancing in preclinical/clinical trials [59]. This study performed three nanotoxicity assays: erythrocyte hemolysis, MTT, and the LIVE/DEAD® viability assay. The concentrations, ranging from 1 to 100 µM) of the L-DOPA and curcumin-loaded NH_2–PEO–PCL GSH-coated NPs (LdCurNP), applied in these studies were calculated based on the amount of loaded L-DOPA in nanoparticles, taking into account the encapsulation efficiency and drug loading previously described. Because of this difference, curcumin concentrations could be as high as five-fold the concentration of L-DOPA, and, thus, Supplementary Materials are available showing the assays using only curcumin-loaded nanoparticles (CurNP) ranging from 200 to 500 µM (Supplementary Figures S1–S4).

2.6.1. Erythrocyte Hemolysis Assay

In the present study, the centrifuged tubes demonstrated that none of the groups had similar hemolytic activity, as seen in the positive control sample (Figure 5A).

After calculating the hemolysis rate for each NP suspension concentration, it was detected that the hemolysis rate was lower than 5% for all concentration groups tested. Only a few concentrations were slightly over 2% in Sample 1 (Figure 5B and Table 3). In Sample 2, almost all the concentrations were above 2%, but none passed the threshold of 5% (Figure 5C and Table 3). Such results suggest that the unloaded and L-DOPA and curcumin-loaded NH_2–PEO–PCL GSH-coated NPs have good blood compatibility.

Table 3. Hemolysis assays of the L-DOPA and curcumin-loaded nanoparticles (LdCurNPs) and unloaded nanoparticles (UnNPs) results presented as mean ± standard error.

	% Hemolysis (LdCurNP)		% Hemolysis (UnNP)	
µM	Sample 1	Sample 2	Sample 1	Sample 2
1	−0.16 ± 0.11	2.68 ± 0.21	3.27 ± 0.26	2.50 ± 0.26
10	0.04 ± 0.32	2.61 ± 0.28	1.22 ± 0.13	2.31 ± 0.18
25	1.45 ± 0.14	2.00 ± 0.19	2.71 ± 0.58	1.43 ± 0.16
50	3.89 ± 0.22	2.62 ± 0.30	2.08 ± 0.39	2.59 ± 0.26
75	3.28 ± 0.14	2.43 ± 0.32	2.23 ± 0.34	2.62 ± 0.21
100	1.97 ± 0.15	2.98 ± 0.19	0.85 ± 0.09	2.93 ± 0.18

Since all administration routes of NPs lead to blood circulation, blood compatibility is one of the most important parameters when developing a new nanoparticle [60,61]. The standard ASTM-F765 [62] defines hemolytic rates of 0 to 2% as non-hemolytic, 2 to 5% as slightly hemolytic, and above 5% as hemolytic.

As a complement for the absorbance data, it is also important to record images of the centrifuged tubes for qualitative evaluation of the solutions in order to avoid false negatives [63].

The development of co-polymer NPs can be made within numerous combinations of different structures; this makes the comparison between them much more complex. It should consider the types of polymers that were used, if the NPs were coated, and if they were loaded or not with drugs.

Regarding all the differences between the NPs, it is essential to encounter a common ground between them. In the present study, the hemolytic results were validated by hemolysis assays for polymeric nanoparticles from Mazzarino et al. (2015) [64], who developed NPs with xyloglucan-block-polycaprolactone and also obtained good blood compatibility, and Fan et al. (2018) [65], who evaluated a co-polymeric curcumin-loaded NPs synthetized with poly (lactic-co-glycolic acid) and polyethylene glycol and also obtained good blood compatibility.

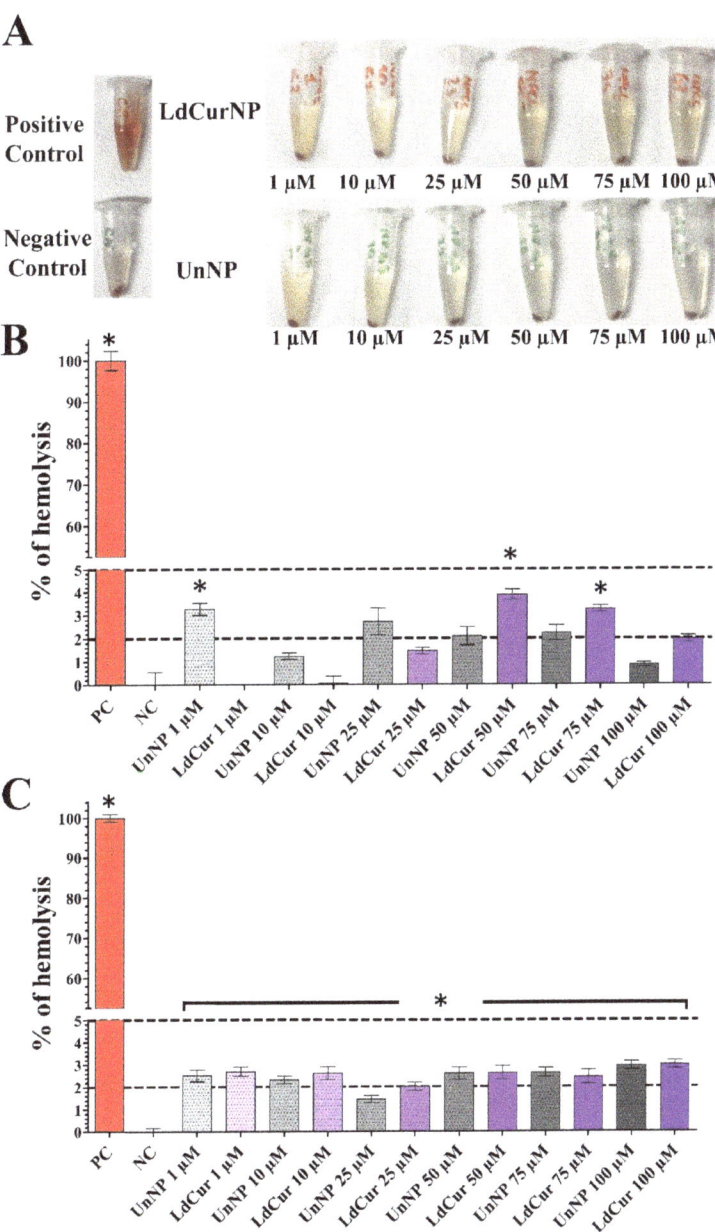

Figure 5. (**A**) Hemolysis assay microtubes after incubation with nanoparticles suspensions in different concentrations (1, 10, 25, 50, 75 and 100 μM) for 1 hour and centrifugation at 1500 G for 5 min. PC (Positive Control, distilled water), NC (Negative Control, saline), UnNPs (Unloaded Nanoparticles), LdCurNPs (L-DOPA and Curcumin- Loaded Nanoparticles). (**B**,**C**) The results presented are mean ± standard error of the hemolysis rate of samples 1 and 2, respectively. Dotted lines are the thresholds of 5% (slightly hemolytic) and 2% (non-hemolytic) hemolysis rate and * $p < 0.05$; n.s. $p > 0.05$ when compared with the negative control.

2.6.2. MTT Cytotoxicity Assay

The MTT assay is a widely used colorimetric experiment that evaluates the metabolic capacity of cells, more specifically, the capacity of oxidoreductases to split the tetrazolium ring into the purple-colored formazan [60,66,67].

In this assay, Vero and PC-12 cells were exposed to unloaded or L-DOPA and curcumin-loaded NH_2–PEO–PCL GSH NPs suspensions in different concentrations. The Vero cell line is often applied in general cytotoxic evaluations [42,68]; on the other hand, the PC-12 cell line, when differentiated, is mainly used when neuronal cytotoxicity needs to be observed [69,70].

In our findings related to the Vero cell line, at 24 h of incubation, only the concentration 10 µM of the LdCurNPs had a significant decrease in absorbance compared with the control.

However, at 48 and 72 h, both unloaded and loaded nanoparticles suspensions induced a decrease in the proportional absorbance compared to the control group in most of the concentrations tested, except UnNP at 48 h with 1 and 100 µM (Figure 6A, 48 and 72 h). A significant absorbance decrease was observed with Vero cells when comparing the unloaded versus the loaded nanoparticles (comparisons represented by # in Figure 6A), and this could be related with the slower drug delivery mechanism of nanoparticles. This decrease is also present in the assay with only curcumin-loaded nanoparticles (Supplementary Figure S2) and is corroborated with other authors that also applied the MTT assay and treating Vero cells with curcumin. Kong (2009) [71] observed a ratio decrease after 48 h of exposure of the Vero cells with curcumin at a concentration of 20 µM, and Prasetyaningrum (2018) [72] also reported a decrease in this same cell line, with around 30 µM of curcumin. Both studies used curcumin powder solubilized in DMSO, leading to an all-at-once exposure to these concentrations. When a drug is loaded into nanoparticles, the drug liberation is time-dependent, so it can be hypothesized that the curcumin liberation from the nanoparticles was sustained throughout the assay, maintaining a steady concentration.

Although there are reports in the literature that curcumin had no cytotoxicity effects in undifferentiated PC12 cells [73,74], some other studies have shown the opposite, [75–77]. Mendonça (2013) [76] also reported the cytotoxicity effects of curcumin in differentiated PC12 cells, but lower in undifferentiated cells.

Farani (2019) [78] tested a curcumin-loaded iron oxide G-NH_2 nanocarrier bonded with PEG in undifferentiated PC12 cells, with concentrations of the curcumin up to 134 µM and 48 h of incubation, and their results showed a cell viability above 80% even in higher concentrations.

Most of these studies treated cells with curcumin dissolved in DMSO solution and evaluated only 24 h of incubation before analysis. In the present study, we wanted to verify if long-term exposure (48 and 72 h) of L-DOPA and curcumin-loaded nanoparticles resuspended directly into the cell culture medium could somehow affect cells' viability.

When treating PC12 cells with L-DOPA (100 µM) for 24 h, studies have shown a decrease in viability when compared with the control group [79–81], thus corroborating our results.

It is also reasonable to consider that it is not entirely understood how suspended nanoparticles interact with cell membranes, organelles, and nuclei, and if such interactions can lead to cytotoxicity [82].

For the MTT assay, there is a significant difference when comparing the unloaded and the loaded nanoparticles in the Vero cell line; and this is accentuated in 48 and 72 h. These differences appear in fewer comparisons in the PC12 cell line (Figure 6B).

These considerations are important because there is a lack of works in the literature that report a longer exposure times of L-DOPA, and curcumin-loaded nanoparticles. Although the MTT analysis detected cytotoxicity, especially in longer exposure times (48 and 72 h), it is necessary to discuss that, besides being extensively used in cytotoxicity assays, this colorimetric assay has its flaws, such as over/underestimation of absorbance, susceptibility of microplate edge effect, particle-induced artifacts, and false positives [83–87].

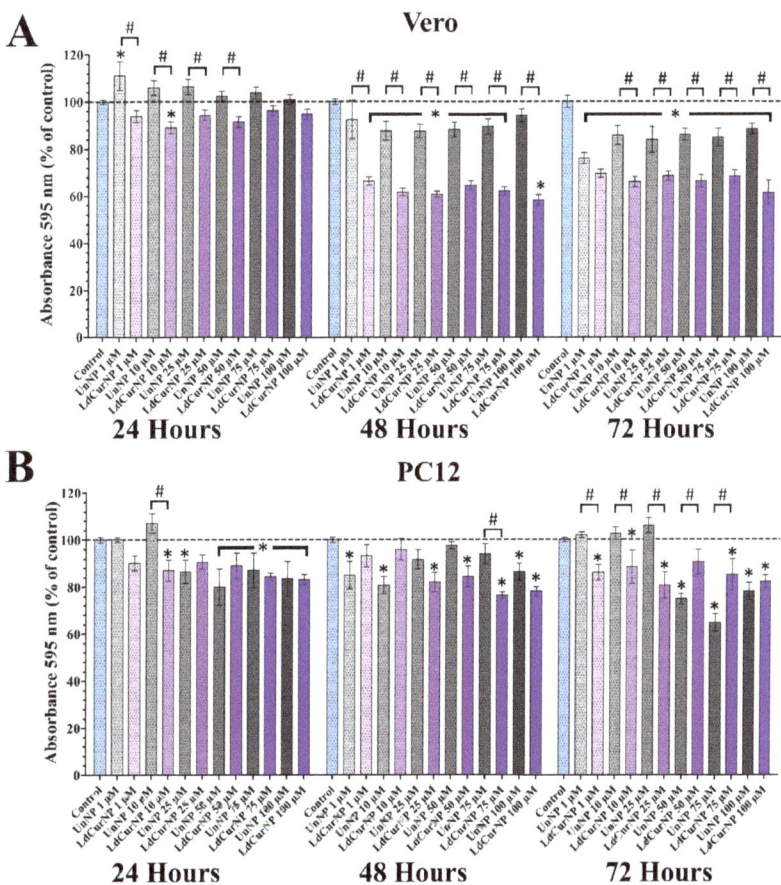

Figure 6. MTT assays of Vero and differentiated PC12 cells after 24, 48 and 72 h of incubation with the nanoparticles' suspensions in different concentrations. Absorbance was determined in spectrophotometer at wavelength of 595 nm and values are presented as mean ± standard error of the % of control group (* and # $p < 0.05$; n.s. $p > 0.05$). (**A**) Vero cells treated with L-DOPA and Curcumin-loaded nanoparticles (LdCurNP) and unloaded nanoparticles (UnNP) suspensions in concentration of 1, 10, 25, 50, 75 and 100 µM. (**B**) differentiated PC12 cells treated with LdCurNP and UnNP suspensions in concentration of 1, 10, 25, 50, 75 and 100 µM.

2.6.3. LIVE/DEAD Viability Assay

The LIVE/DEAD assay, together with high throughput microscopy, consisted of a more accurate representation of the cell population, regarding the viability, and can complement colorimetric assays. If cells are viable, they can convert, by intracellular esterases, the nonfluorescent calcein—AM into the green fluorescent calcein. Nevertheless, when cells are compromised and their cell membrane is damaged, the nuclei marker ethidium homodimer-1 binds with nuclei acids and emits a red fluorescence [67,88].

After analyzing the LIVE/DEAD viability assay of the Vero cell line treated with LdCurNP in different concentrations, it was observed that the viability was more than 95% in all concentrations and all time points. Although some concentrations had a significant difference compared with the control group, that cannot be biologically relevant (Figure 7B). An increase in cell number can also be observed between time points, suggesting that cells are viable and proliferating (Figure 7A).

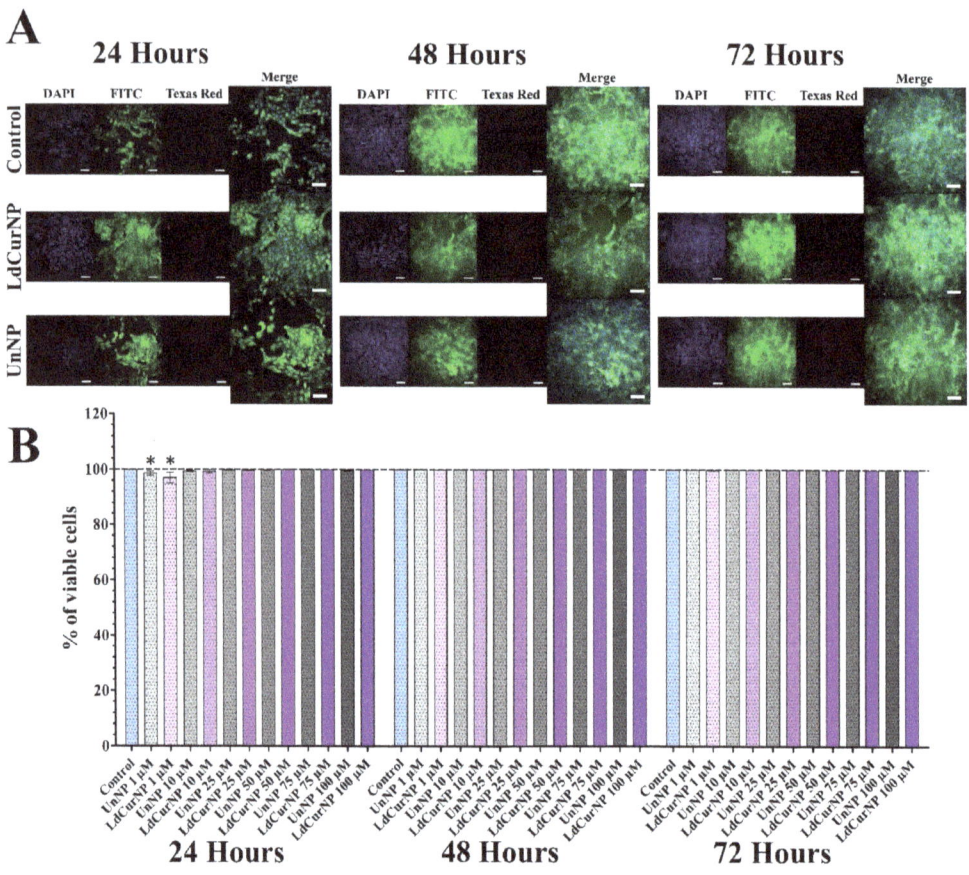

Figure 7. LIVE/DEAD viability assays of differentiated Vero cells after 24, 48 and 72 h of incubation with the nanoparticles' suspensions in different concentrations. (**A**) Representative images of control, L-DOPA and Curcumin-loaded nanoparticles (LdCurNP) 100 µM and unloaded nanoparticles (UnNP) 100 µM. Cells nuclei were stained with Hoechst 33342 and observed with the DAPI channel, live cells were stained with calcein and observed in the FITC channel, dead cells were stained with ethidium homodimer-1 and observed in the Texas Red channel. (Scale bar 100 µm). (**B**) LdCurNP and UnNP suspensions in concentration of 1, 10, 25, 50, 75 and 100 µM, Values were presented as mean ± standard error of the % of viable cells (* $p < 0.05$; n.s. $p > 0.05$).

Considering the analyzed LIVE/DEAD viability assay of PC12 cell line treated with LdCurNPs in different concentrations, it was observed that, in all concentrations and time points, the viability was above 95% (Figure 8B). Although some concentration had a significant difference compared with the control group, this difference cannot be considered biologically relevant. Because of the differentiation, the number of cells remained mostly equal in all time points (Figure 8A). The mechanism that the LIVE/DEAD employs to determine cytotoxicity differs from the colorimetric assays also performed in this paper. While colorimetric assays such as hemolysis, which quantifies the amount of hemoglobin solubilized after red blood cells lysis, or MTT, which quantifies the formazan produced by reduction of MTT by the oxidoreductases present in cells, the LIVE/DEAD assay can analyze the integrity of the cells by staining the cytoplasm if viable, or the nuclei if non-viable. High-throughput microscopy can transform a qualitative into a quantitative assay by analyzing the whole cell population.

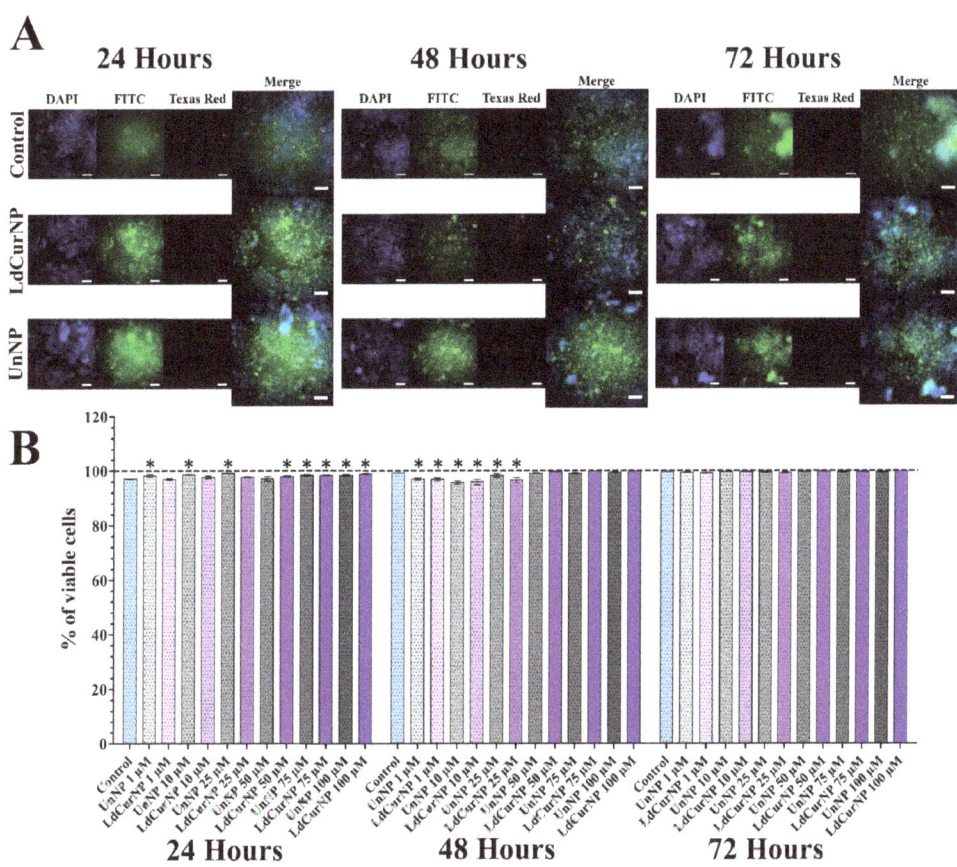

Figure 8. LIVE/DEAD viability assays of differentiated PC12 cells after 24, 48 and 72 h of incubation with the nanoparticles' suspensions in different concentrations. (**A**) Representative images of control, L-DOPA, and Curcumin-loaded Nanoparticles (LdCurNP) 100 µM and Unloaded Nanoparticles (UnNP) 100 µM. Cells nuclei were stained with Hoechst 33342 and observed with the DAPI channel, live cells were stained with calcein and observed in the FITC channel, dead cells were stained with ethidium homodimer-1 and observed in the Texas Red channel. (Scale bar 100 µm). (**B**) LdCurNP and UnNP suspensions in concentration of 1, 10, 25, 50, 75 and 100 µM, Values were presented as mean ± standard error of the % of viable cells (* $p < 0.05$; n.s. $p > 0.05$).

3. Material and Methods

3.1. Materials

The α-amino-ω-hydroxy-terminated (NH$_2$)-PEG-b-PCL used in this study was purchased from Polymer Source (Montreal, QC, Canada). The amphiphilic copolymer used had an average molar mass (Mn) of 5×10^3 g/mol for the PEG block and 10.5×10^3 g/mol for the PCL block (NH$_2$–PEO–PCL), and an Mw/number average molecular weight (Mn) ratio of 1.50. Curcumin and L-DOPA were purchased from Sigma-Aldrich Co., LLC (St. Louis, MO, USA).

3.2. Preparation of NH$_2$–PEO–PCL Nanoparticles

The NH$_2$–PEO–PCL nanoparticle suspensions were prepared by using a nanoprecipitation and solvent displacement method, similar to that described by Numata et al., 2015 [24]. Following this method, NH$_2$–PEO–PCL (10 mg) was dissolved in 0.5 mL of a mixture of THF/water 0.9/0.1 (v/v) and then stirred for 18 h. The polymer solution was then added in a drop-wise manner (5.0 mL/h) to ultrapure water, at room temperature (1 mL), under stirring (750 rpm). The remaining THF was rapidly eliminated by evaporation under reduced pressure at room temperature.

Curcumin and L-DOPA-loaded nanoparticles were prepared by cosolvent evaporation, as described above, except for dissolving curcumin and NH_2–PEO–PCL in a mixture of THF/water 0.9/0.1 (v/v), and adding the solution in a drop-wise manner to a solution of 3 mg/mL of L-DOPA in 0.01 M monobasic potassium phosphate, adjusted to pH 3.0 with phosphoric acid 85%.

Curcumin-loaded nanoparticles were prepared by cosolvent evaporation, as described above, except for dissolving curcumin and NH_2–PEO–PCL in a mixture of THF/water 0.9/0.1 (v/v). Then the nanoparticle suspension was centrifuged at 10,000 rpm for 5 min to remove the curcumin precipitate from the outside of the nanoparticles.

L-DOPA-loaded nanoparticles were prepared by cosolvent evaporation, as described above, except for adding the NH_2–PEO–PCL solution in a drop-wise manner to a solution of 3 mg/mL of L-DOPA in 0.01 M monobasic potassium phosphate, adjusted to pH 3.0 with phosphoric acid 85%.

3.3. Coating of the NPs

The coating of NH_2–PEO–PCL nanoparticle suspensions with glutathione (GSH) was prepared by using a method similar to Geldenhuys et al., 2015 [89]; 20 mg of glutathione was added to 1 mL of nanoparticle suspension in order to get a 2% w/v coating and allowed to sit at room temperature for at least 30 min before use in order to warrant a maximal GSH coating.

3.4. Characterization of NH_2–PEO–PCL Nanoparticles

3.4.1. Dynamic Light Scattering (DLS)

The size distribution, mean particle size, polydispersity index, and morphology of the nanoparticle suspensions in aqueous media were determined by using DLS at 25 °C by Static and Dynamic Light Scattering (SLS/DLS) with an ALV 5000 (ALV, Langen, Germany) providing a red helium–neon laser at a wavelength of 632.8 nm, utilizing 35 mW power. Then it was diluted in ultrapure water, and samples were placed in cylindrical measurement cells, which were immersed in a toluene bath at 25 °C. A very sensitive avalanche diode detected the scattered photons. In this study, the modulus of the scattering vector is denoted q and is equal to (4 pn/k)sin (h/2), where n represents the refractive index of pure water, h is the scattering angle, and k designates the light wavelength. Each experiment was performed during 120 s, and the scattered light was measured at different angles, ranging from 30° to 140°, with a 2.5° stepwise increase. The scattering intensity was corrected by considering the contributions of the solvent (water) and the toluene (standard), as well as the change of the scattering volume with the detection angle. The hydrodynamic radius (Rh) was determined by using the Stokes–Einstein equation, Rh = jBT/6 pgD, where jB is Boltzmann constant (in J/K), T is the temperature (in K), D is the diffusion coefficient, and g is the viscosity of the medium—pure water, in this case (g = 0.89 cP at 25 °C). Unloaded and loaded nanoparticle suspensions show no absorption at the wavelength used in light-scattering experiments. The data were acquired with the ALV correlator control software, and the distributions of the relaxation times, A(t), were obtained by using CONTIN analysis applied to the autocorrelation function, C(q, t).

3.4.2. Nanoparticles Tracking Analysis (NTA)

Nanoparticle Tracking Analysis (NTA) experiments were performed by analyzing with a digital microscope LM10 System (NanoSight, Salisbury, UK). The samples were diluted in ultrapure water and then introduced into the chamber with a syringe. Each sample was illuminated with a 405 nm blue laser and separated. The video images of particles were analyzed by the NTA analytical software version 2.1 (NanoSight, Salisbury,

UK). The particles were in movement under Brownian motion, and each video clip was captured over 60 s, at room temperature.

3.4.3. Transmission Electron Microscopy

The morphology of the NH$_2$–PEO–PCL nanoparticle was observed under a Philips CM200 microscope (Royal Philips, Amsterdam, Netherlands) operated at 120 kV. NH$_2$–PEO–PCL nanoparticles in aqueous media were released on a glow-discharge carbon-coated copper grid, staining negative with 2% (w/v) uranyl acetate to dry completely.

3.4.4. Zeta Potential Measurement

Nanoparticle samples were diluted in ultrapure water and placed in the electrophoretic cell, where a potential of ±150 mV was established. The laser-doppler anemometry with a Zetasizer Nano Series (Malvern Instruments, Worcestershire, UK) was used to determine the Zeta potential. The f potential values were used as the mean electrophoretic mobility calculated values, using Smoluchowski's equation.

3.5. Stability of the GSH-Coated Nanoparticles with Added Salt

At different concentrations of NaCl solutions, the GSH-coated and uncoated nanoparticle suspensions were diluted. The effects of salt addition on the particle size and Zeta potential were monitored by using DLS, as described above.

3.6. Determination of Drug Loading and Entrapment Efficiency

The amount of L-DOPA loading and entrapment efficiency was estimated after the determination of the drug concentration in the nanoparticle suspensions by UV–HPLC, according to the method described by Pereira et al. (2012) [90], using a PerkinElmer Lambda 10 UV/Vis spectrophotometer (PerkinElmer, Inc., Waltham, MA, USA) at 280 nm. The loading efficiency (%) was estimated as the difference between the total concentration of L-DOPA found in the solution used for the nanoprecipitation. Then the drug concentration in the supernatant was obtained by the suspension ultrafiltration/centrifugation procedure (13,000 rpm for 15 min), using Amicon Centrifugal Filter Devices with Ultracel-3000 membrane (3 kDa, Millipore Corp., Burlington, MA, USA), after the nanoprecipitation to separate the free drug in the supernatant from the L-DOPA-loaded nanoparticles. The amount of encapsulated L-DOPA was calculated from the calibration curve established, using standard solutions of L-DOPA in the same solvent. The loading and entrapment efficiencies of L-DOPA were calculated according to the following formulas:

$$\frac{Loading}{Efficiency} \% = \frac{LD\,in\,NPs - Free\,LD}{Total\,amount\,of\,LD} \times 100 \qquad (1)$$

$$\frac{Entrapment}{Efficiency} \% = \frac{LD\,in\,NPs - Free\,LD}{Total\,amount\,of\,NPs} \times 100 \qquad (2)$$

where LD = L-DOPA, and NPs = NH$_2$–PEO–PCL nanoparticles.

Curcumin (CUR) loading and entrapment efficiency in the nanoparticle suspension were calculated after the drug concentration in the nanoparticle suspensions by UV–HPLC, according to the method described by Monton et al. (2016) [91], at 425 nm. The loading efficiency (%) was estimated as being the difference between the total amount of CUR added to the formulations and the total concentration of curcumin found in the nanoparticle suspensions after their complete dissolution in acetonitrile, deducted from the concentration of the drug in the supernatant, obtained by the suspension ultrafiltration/centrifugation procedure, using Amicon Centrifugal Filter Devices with Ultracel-100 membrane (100 kDa, Millipore Corp., Burlington, MA, USA), as described by Mazzarino et al. (2012) [37] and Scarano et al. (2015) [39]). The amount of CUR calculated from the calibration curve was established by using standard solutions of curcumin in the same solvent. The loading and entrapment efficiencies of CUR were calculated according to the following formulas:

$$\frac{Loading}{Efficiency}\% = \frac{CURinNPs - FreeCUR}{Total\,amount\,of\,Cur} \times 100 \quad (3)$$

$$\frac{Entrapment}{Efficiency}\% = \frac{CURinNPs - FreeCUR}{Total\,amount\,of\,NPs} \times 100 \quad (4)$$

CUR = curcumin, and NPs = NH_2–PEO–PCL nanoparticles.

3.7. Freeze-Drying Stability

In order to minimize the physical changes of the NH_2–PEO–PCL NPs, lactose, mannitol, sucrose, trehalose, and hydroxypropyl-β-cyclodextrin (HPbCD) were tested as cryoprotectants. Aqueous solutions were made at various concentrations of cryoprotectants and mixed with aliquots of the NH_2–PEO–PCL NPs suspension before freeze-drying to obtain the final concentrations of cryoprotectant from 0.25 to 5%, w/v. The colloidal suspensions were placed inside a 1.5 mL microtube, frozen at −196 °C in liquid nitrogen, and then transferred immediately to a freeze dryer (Free Zone 6, Labconco, Kansas City, MO, USA) and lyophilized (−50 °C and 50 mbar) for 48 h. The freeze-dried cake was rehydrated by slowly injecting 1 mL ultrapure water onto the tube, stabilized for 5 min, and gently shaken to ensure complete disintegration and dissolution of the cake. The mean particle size of the original fresh nanoparticle was measured by DLS before (Si) and after (Sf) freeze-drying at 25 °C, and then it was compared and expressed as an Sf/Si % ratio.

3.8. Cytotoxicity Evaluations of the Loaded Nanoparticles

All cytotoxicity assays were performed by using drug concentrations of 1, 10, 25, 50, 75, and 100 µM.

3.8.1. Erythrocyte Hemolysis Assay

To perform the erythrocyte hemolysis assay, 2 mL of peripheral blood was collected from two healthy donors into tubes containing EDTA anticoagulant. The erythrocytes were washed by separating them with centrifugation at 1500 G for 5 min, the supernatant was removed with micropipette, and the erythrocytes were suspended with saline, and this process was repeated twice. After the removal of the supernatant, 1 mL of the washed erythrocytes was added to 9 mL of saline, referred to now as the stock solution of erythrocytes. In 1.5 mL microtubes, 50 µL of the stock solution of erythrocytes was added and treated with 950 µL of saline containing the NH_2–PEO–PCL NPs suspensions that were unloaded (UnNP) or loaded with curcumin and L-DOPA (LdCurNP) at a concentration of the drugs ranging from 1 to 100 µM (concentrations of the LdCurNPs), calculated regarding the drug L-DOPA. The negative control (established as 0% hemolysis) was treated with saline only, and the positive control (established as 100% hemolysis) was treated with distilled water only. The microtubes were homogenized and incubated in a shaker at 37 °C for 1 h. After the incubation time, the tubes were centrifuged 1500 G for 5 min, and the image of the tubes was recorded; the supernatant was collected and transferred to a 96-well plate and read at 405 nm wavelength in spectrophotometer. The hemolysis percentage was calculated according to the following formula:

$$Hemolysis\% = \frac{ABS - ABSnc}{ABSpc - ABSnc} \times 100 \quad (5)$$

where ABS = the observed absorbance of the samples, $ABSnc$ = the negative control absorbance, and $ABSpc$ = the positive control absorbance.

3.8.2. MTT Cytotoxicity Assay

Vero cells acquired from the Cell Bank of Rio de Janeiro (Duque de Caxias, RJ, Brazil) (BCRJ code: 0245/ATCC code: CCL-81) were cultivated with complete medium, DMEM-F12 supplemented with 10% fetal bovine serum, and 1% penicillin and streptomycin (100 U/mL and 100 µg/mL respectively), at 37 °C, with 5% CO_2. They were seeded in 96-well plates (seeding density of 2×10^3 cells per well). After 24 h, the medium was discarded, and the cells were treated with a complete medium containing the NH_2–PEO–PCL NP suspensions that were either unloaded (UnNP) or loaded with L-DOPA and curcumin (LdCurNP), at a concentration ranging from 1 to 100 µM, for 24, 48, and 72 h. After the incubation time, 20 µL of 3-(4,5-Dimethyl-2-thiazolyl)-2,5-diphenyl-2H-tetrazolium bromide (MTT) solubilized in DMEM was added to each well (final concentration of MTT for each well was 0.5 mg/mL). The plates were incubated for 3 h at 37 °C; after this period, the medium was removed with a micropipette, and 100 µL of DMSO was added. The plates were placed onto a shaker for at least 30 min to solubilize the formazan crystals and finally read with 595 nm wavelength in a spectrophotometer. Data collected from three individual experiments, each with quadruplicates samples, were presented as a percentage of the observed absorbance of the control group.

PC-12 cells acquired from the European Collection of Authenticated Cell Cultures (ECACC) (Porton Down, Wiltshire, UK) (Catalogue No.: 88,022,401) were previously cultivated in suspension with RPMI 1640 supplemented with 10% fetal horse serum, 5% fetal bovine serum, and 1% penicillin and streptomycin (100 U/mL and 100 µg/mL respectively), at 37 °C, with 5% CO_2. PC-12 cells can adhere to plastic pretreated with collagen type IV (Sigma Aldrich Catalogue Number C5533) (San Luis, MO, USA). The collagen coating was performed by adding 50 µL of a 0.01 mg/mL collagen solution in each well of a 96-well plate. Plates were left open in a laminar flow hood until total solvent evaporation. For sterilization, coated plates were exposed lidless to UV light for 1 h inside the laminar flow hood, sealed and maintained at 4 °C until use. PC-12 cells were seeded on a collagen type IV coated 96-well plate (seeding density of 2×10^3 cells per well) with neuronal differentiation medium, RPMI 1640 supplemented with 1% of fetal horse serum, and 100 ng/mL of Nerve Growth Factor-7S (Sigma Aldrich catalog number N05013) (San Luis, MO, USA) for 17 days. Three-quarters of the differentiation medium was replaced twice a week. After neuronal differentiation, the medium was replaced by a differentiation medium containing the NH_2–PEO–PCL NPs suspensions, followed by the same procedures described in this section.

3.8.3. LIVE/DEAD Viability Assay

Vero cells, previously cultivated as described above, were seeded in 96-well plates (seeding density of 5×10^3 per well). After 24 h, the medium was replaced, and the cells were treated with a complete medium containing the NH_2–PEO–PCL NPs suspensions that were either unloaded (UnNP) or loaded with curcumin and L-DOPA (LdCurNP), at a concentration ranging from 1 to 100 µM, for 24, 48, and 72 h. After the incubation time, 20 µL of Hoechst 33,342, calcein AM, and Ethidium Homodimer-1 solubilized in DMEM-F12 were added to each well (fluorescence markers' final concentration for each well was 2 µg/mL, 0.3 µM, and 0.6 µM, respectively). The plates were incubated for 30 min at 37 °C, and images were acquired with high-throughput microscopy (GE In Cell Analyzer 2000, Boston, MA, USA). The image acquisition protocol consisted of defined exposure time for each channel DAPI 650 ms, FITC 350 ms, and Texas Red 650 ms. These channels were used to observe the fluorescence of the Hoechst 33,342, calcein AM, and Ethidium Homodimer-1, respectively. In addition, each concentration having quadruplicate wells and images was acquired from four different fields in each well. Images were analyzed with an In Cell Analyzer Workstation v.3.7.3, using the cell nuclei for detection and the identification. Cell viability was determined by the positive staining with calcein, and cell death was marked with Ethidium Homodimer-1, respectively.

PC-12 cells were cultivated, seeded, and differentiated into neuron-like cells as described previously, followed by the same treatment and procedures described in this section.

4. Conclusions

In this study, NPs consisting of NH_2–PEO–PCL were characterized as potential formulations to pass across the BBB for brain delivery of both L-DOPA and curcumin, transporting these active compounds simultaneously.

It is the first time that both L-DOPA and curcumin were presented together in the same nanoparticle that can act in treating Parkinson's disease. L-DOPA is a dopamine precursor, and curcumin has antioxidant properties that could protect dopaminergic neurons.

The demonstrated results indicate that the developed biodegradable nanomicelles were blood compatible, with low cytotoxicity, and may be considered a promising novel therapy for treating Parkinson's disease. Such a therapy represents a promising approach for future clinical applications and constitutes an exciting drug delivery system, with desirable features for brain delivery of a neurotransmitter precursor associated with an antioxidant molecule capable of producing a synergistic therapeutic effect. The advantages of these nanoparticles are that the treatment could be applied with lower concentrations, with the possibility of new routes of administrations, such as nasal, allied with higher treatment tolerance, due to the reduction of unwanted collateral effects.

However, to evaluate the anti-parkinsonian effects, future in vivo studies should be carried on to verify if these nanocarriers can reduce the dopaminergic neuron degeneration or the motor symptoms related to Parkinson's disease.

Supplementary Materials: The following supporting information can be downloaded at: https://www.mdpi.com/article/10.3390/molecules27092811/s1, Figure S1: (A) Hemolysis assay microtubes after incubation with nanoparticles suspensions in different concentrations (200, 400 and 500 µM) for 1 h and centrifugation at 1500 G for 5 min Positive Control, distilled water (PC), Negative Control, saline (NC), Unloaded Nanoparticles (UnNPs), Curcumin-loaded Nanoparticles (CurNPs). (B,C) The results presented are mean ± standard error of the hemolysis rate of samples 1 and 2, respectively. Dotted lines are the thresholds of 5% (slightly hemolytic) and 2% (non-hemolytic) hemolysis rate and * $p < 0.05$; n.s. $p > 0.05$ when compared with the negative control; Figure S2: MTT assays of Vero and differentiated PC12 cells after 24, 48, and 72 h of incubation with the nanoparticles' suspensions in different concentrations. Absorbance was determined in a spectrophotometer at a wavelength of 595 nm, and values are presented as mean ± standard error of the % of the control group (* and # $p < 0.05$; n.s. $p > 0.05$); Figure S3: LIVE/DEAD viability assays of differentiated Vero cells after 24, 48, and 72 h of incubation with the nanoparticles' suspensions in different concentrations; Figure S4: LIVE/DEAD viability assays of differentiated PC12 cells after 24, 48 and 72 hours of incubation with the nanoparticles' suspensions in different concentrations.

Author Contributions: Conceptualization, K.A.T.d.C. and R.B.; methodology, B.F.M., M.A.C., A.C.I., P.E.F.S., R.C.S., M.C.P., N.B.d.O. and J.M.A.; validation, B.F.M., M.A.C. and A.C.I.; formal analysis, B.F.M., M.A.C., C.T., C.S.S., N.N.d.R. and S.H.; investigation, B.F.M., M.A.C. and S.H.; resources, K.A.T.d.C. and R.B.; data curation, B.F.M., M.A.C., R.B. and K.A.T.d.C.; writing—original draft preparation, B.F.M. and M.A.C.; writing—review and editing, B.F.M., S.H., D.S.M.D., R.B. and K.A.T.d.C.; visualization, B.F.M. and K.A.T.d.C.; supervision, K.A.T.d.C., S.H. and R.B.; project administration, K.A.T.d.C. and R.B.; funding acquisition, R.B. and K.A.T.d.C. All authors have read and agreed to the published version of the manuscript.

Funding: This research was funded by the financial support of Carnot Institute POLYNAT (France), CERMAV (France), and Coordination for the Improvement of Higher Education Personnel (CAPES), Finance Code 001 (Brazil).

Institutional Review Board Statement: Not applicable.

Informed Consent Statement: Not applicable.

Data Availability Statement: The data presented in this study are available in Supplementary Material.

Conflicts of Interest: This paper is entitled "Biodegradable Nanoparticles Loaded with Levodopa and Curcumin for Treatment of Parkinson's Disease"; the abstract of this paper was presented at the Conference Annual Meeting 2021, Coimbra Health School, as an online and oral presentation/conference talk with interim findings. The oral presentation's abstract was published as "Oral Abstracts" in *European Journal of Public Health*, Volume 31, Issue Supplement_2, August 2021, ckab120.070: Hyperlink with https://doi.org/10.1093/eurpub/ckab120.070 (accessed on 19 June 2021). The authors declare no conflict of interest.

References

1. Newland, B.; Newland, H.; Werner, C.; Rosser, A.; Wang, W. Prospects for polymer therapeutics in Parkinson's disease and other euro degenerative disorders. *Prog. Polym. Sci.* **2015**, *44*, 79–112. [CrossRef]
2. Leyva-Gómez, G.; Cortés, H.; Magaña, J.J.; Leyva-García, N.; Quintanar-Guerrero, D.; Florán, B. Nanoparticle technology for treatment of Parkinson's disease: The role of surface phenomena in reaching the brain. *Drug Discov. Today* **2015**, *20*, 824–837. [CrossRef] [PubMed]
3. Bisaglia, M.; Filograna, R.; Beltramini, M.; Bubacco, L. Are dopamine derivatives implicated in the pathogenesis of Parkinson's disease? *Ageing Res. Rev.* **2014**, *13*, 107–114. [CrossRef] [PubMed]
4. Goldstein, D.S.; Kopina, J.; Sharabi, Y. Catecholamine autotoxicity. Implications for pharmacology and therapeutics of Parkinson disease and related disorders. *Pharmacol. Ther.* **2014**, *144*, 268–282. [CrossRef]
5. Ross, K.A.; Brenza, T.M.; Binnebose, A.M.; Phanse, Y.; Kanthasamy, A.G.; Gendelman, H.E.; Salem, A.K.; Bartholomay, L.C.; Bellaire, B.H.; Narasimhan, B. Nano-enabled delivery of diverse payloads across complex biological barriers. *J. Control. Release* **2015**, *219*, 548–559. [CrossRef]
6. Mc Carthy, D.J.; Malhotra, M.; O'Mahony, A.M.; Cryan, J.F.; O'Driscoll, C.M. Nanoparticles and the blood-brain barrier: Advancing from in-vitro models towards therapeutic significance. *Pharm. Res.* **2015**, *32*, 1161–1185. [CrossRef]
7. Grossen, P.; Witzigmann, D.; Sieber, S.; Huwyler, J. PEG-PCL-based nanomedicines: A biodegradable drug delivery system and its application. *J. Control. Release* **2017**, *260*, 46–60. [CrossRef]
8. Dash, T.K.; Konkimalla, V.B. Poly-ε-caprolactone based formulations for drug delivery and tissue engineering: A review. *J. Control. Release* **2012**, *158*, 15–33. [CrossRef]
9. Richard, P.U.; Duskey, J.T.; Stolarov, S.; Spulber, M.; Palivan, C.G. New concepts to fight oxidative stress: Nanosized three-dimensional supramolecular antioxidant assemblies. *Expert. Opin. Drug Deliv.* **2015**, *12*, 1527–1545. [CrossRef]
10. Sandhir, R.; Yadav, A.; Sunkaria, A.; Singhal, N. Nano-antioxidants: An emerging strategy for intervention against neurodegenerative conditions. *Neurochem. Int.* **2015**, *89*, 209–226. [CrossRef]
11. Gong, C.; Deng, S.; Wu, Q.; Xiang, M.; Wei, X.; Li, L.; Gao, X.; Wang, B.; Sun, L.; Chen, Y.; et al. Improving antiangiogenesis and anti-tumor activity of curcumin by biodegradable polymeric micelles. *Biomaterials* **2013**, *34*, 1413–1432. [CrossRef] [PubMed]
12. Ghosh, S.; Banerjee, S.; Sil, P.C. The beneficial role of curcumin on inflammation, diabetes and neurodegenerative disease: A recent update. *Food Chem. Toxicol.* **2015**, *83*, 111–124. [CrossRef] [PubMed]
13. Ganesan, P.; Ko, H.M.; Kim, S.; Choi, D.K. Recent trends in the development of nanophytobioactive compounds and delivery systems for their possible role in reducing oxidative stress in Parkinson's disease models. *Int. J. Nanomed.* **2015**, *10*, 6757–6772. [CrossRef] [PubMed]
14. Hussain, Z.; Thu, H.E.; Amjad, M.W.; Hussain, F.; Ahmed, T.A.; Khan, S. Exploring Recent developments to improve antioxidant, anti-inflammatory and antimicrobial efficacy of curcumin: A review of new trends and future perspectives. *Mater. Sci. Eng. C* **2017**, *77*, 1316–1326. [CrossRef]
15. Cupaioli, F.A.; Zucca, F.A.; Boraschi, D.; Zecca, L. Engineered nanoparticles. How brain friendly is this new guest? *Prog. Neurobiol.* **2014**, *119–120*, 20–38. [CrossRef]
16. Saraiva, C.; Praça, C.; Ferreira, R.; Santos, T.; Ferreira, L.; Bernardino, L. Nanoparticle-mediated brain drug delivery: Overcoming blood-brain barrier to treat neurodegenerative diseases. *J. Control. Release* **2016**, *235*, 34–47. [CrossRef] [PubMed]
17. Patel, P.J.; Acharya, N.S.; Acharya, S.R. Development and characterization of glutathione-conjugated albumin nanoparticles for improved brain delivery of hydrophilic fluorescent marker. *Drug Deliv.* **2013**, *20*, 143–155. [CrossRef]
18. Lindqvist, A.; Rip, J.; Gaillard, P.J.; Björkman, S.; Hammarlund-Udenaes, M. Enhanced brain delivery of the opioid peptide damgo in glutathione pegylated liposomes: A microdialysis study. *Mol. Pharm.* **2013**, *10*, 1533–1541. [CrossRef]
19. Birngruber, T.; Raml, R.; Gladdines, W.; Gatschelhofer, C.; Gander, E.; Ghosh, A.; Kroath, T.; Gaillard, P.J.; Pieber, T.R.; Sinner, F. Enhanced doxorubicin delivery to the brain administered through glutathione PEGylated liposomal doxorubicin (2B3-101) as compared with generic Caelyx,®/Doxil®—A Cerebral open flow microperfusion pilot study. *J. Pharm. Sci.* **2014**, *103*, 1945–1948. [CrossRef]
20. Salem, H.F.; Ahmed, S.M.; Hassaballah, A.E.; Omar, M.M. Targeting brain cells with glutathione-modulated nanoliposomes: In vitro and in vivo study. *Drug Des. Dev. Ther.* **2015**, *9*, 3705–3727. [CrossRef]
21. Lin, K.H.; Hong, S.T.; Wang, H.T.; Lo, Y.L.; Lin, A.M.Y.; Yang, J.C.H. Enhancing anticancer Effect of gefitinib across the blood-brain barrier model using liposomes modified with one α-helical cell-penetrating peptide or glutathione and Tween 80. *Int. J. Mol. Sci.* **2016**, *17*, 1998. [CrossRef] [PubMed]

22. Maussang, D.; Rip, J.; van Kregten, J.; van den Heuvel, A.; van der Pol, S.; van der Boom, B.; Reijerkerk, A.; Chen, L.; de Boer, M.; Gaillard, P.; et al. Glutathione conjugation dose-dependently increases brain-specific liposomal drug delivery in vitro and in vivo. *Drug Discov. Today Technol.* **2016**, *20*, 59–69. [CrossRef] [PubMed]
23. Paka, G.D.; Ramassamy, C. Optimization of Curcumin-Loaded PEG-PLGA Nanoparticles by GSH Functionalization: Investigation of the internalization Pathway in Neuronal Cells. *Mol. Pharm.* **2017**, *14*, 93–106. [CrossRef] [PubMed]
24. Numata, Y.; Mazzarino, L.; Borsali, R. A slow-release system of bacterial cellulose gel and nanoparticles for hydrophobic active ingredients. *Int. J. Pharm.* **2015**, *486*, 217–225. [CrossRef]
25. Badri, W.; Miladi, K.; Nazari, Q.A.; Fessi, H.; Elaissari, A. Effect of process and formulation parameters on polycaprolactone nanoparticles prepared by solvent displacement. *Colloids Surf. A Physicochem. Eng. Asp.* **2017**, *516*, 238–244. [CrossRef]
26. Mora-Huertas, C.E.; Fessi, H.; Elaissari, A. Influence of process and formulation parameters on the formation of submicron particles by solvent displacement andmulsification-diffusion methods: Critical comparison. *Adv. Colloid Interface Sci.* **2011**, *163*, 90–122. [CrossRef]
27. Tam, Y.T.; To, K.K.W.; Chow, A.H.L. Fabrication of doxorubicin nanoparticles by controlled antisolvent precipitation fornhanced intracellular delivery. *Colloids Surf. B Biointerfaces* **2016**, *139*, 249–258. [CrossRef]
28. Gross, A.J.; Haddad, R.; Travelet, C.; Reynaud, E.; Audebert, P.; Borsali, R.; Cosnier, S. Redox-Active Carbohydrate-Coated Nanoparticles: Self-Assembly of a Cyclodextrin-Polystyrene Glycopolymer with Tetrazine-Naphthalimide. *Langmuir* **2016**, *32*, 11939–11945. [CrossRef]
29. Šachl, R.; Uchman, M.; Matějíček, P.; Procházka, K.; Štěpánek, M.; Špírková, M. Preparation and characterization of self-assembled nanoparticles formed by poly(ethylene oxide)-block-poly(ε-caprolactone) copolymers with long poly(ε-caprolactone) blocks in aqueous solutions. *Langmuir* **2007**, *23*, 3395–3400. [CrossRef]
30. Wang, B.L.; Shen, Y.M.; Zhang, Q.W.; Li, Y.L.; Luo, W.; Liu, Z.; Li, Y.; Qian, Z.Y.; Gao, X.; Shi, H.S. Codelivery of curcumin and doxorubicin by MPEG-PCL results in improved efficacy of systemically administered chemotherapy in mice with lung cancer. *Int. J. Nanomed.* **2013**, *8*, 3521–3531.
31. Hickey, J.W.; Santos, J.L.; Williford, J.M.; Mao, H.Q. Control of polymeric Nanoparticle size improved therapeutic delivery. *J. Control. Release* **2015**, *219*, 536–547. [CrossRef] [PubMed]
32. Kulkarni, S.A.; Feng, S.S. Effects of particle size and surface modification on cellular uptake and biodistribution of polymeric nanoparticles for drug delivery. *Pharm. Res.* **2013**, *30*, 2512–2522. [CrossRef] [PubMed]
33. Popiolski, T.M.; Otsuka, I.; Halila, S.; Muniz, E.C.; Soldi, V.; Borsali, R. Preparation of polymeric micelles of poly(ethylene oxide-b-lactic acid) and their encapsulation with lavender oil. *Mater. Res.* **2016**, *19*, 1356–1365. [CrossRef]
34. Mahmoudi Najafi, S.H.; Baghaie, M.; Ashori, A. Preparation and characterization of acetylated starch nanoparticles as drug carrier: Ciprofloxacin as a model. *Int. J. Biol. Macromol.* **2016**, *87*, 48–54. [CrossRef] [PubMed]
35. Mohamed, R.A.; Abass, H.A.; Attia, M.A.; Heikal, O.A. Formulation and evaluation of metoclopramide solid lipidanoparticles for rectal suppository. *J. Pharm. Pharmacol.* **2013**, *65*, 1607–1621. [CrossRef]
36. Gohulkumar, M.; Gurushankar, K.; Rajendra Prasad, N.; Krishnakumar, N. Enhanced cytotoxicity and apoptosis-induced anti cancer effect of silibinin-loaded nanoparticles in oral carcinoma (KB) cells. *Mater. Sci. Eng. C* **2014**, *41*, 274–282. [CrossRef]
37. Mazzarino, L.; Travelet, C.; Ortega-Murillo, S.; Otsuka, I.; Pignot-Paintrand, I.; Lemos-Senna, E.; Borsali, R. Elaboration of chitosan-coated Nanoparticles loaded with curcumin for mucoadhesive applications. *J. Colloidnterface Sci.* **2012**, *370*, 58–66. [CrossRef]
38. Shao, J.; Zheng, D.; Jiang, Z.; Xu, H.; Hu, Y.; Li, X.; Lu, X. Curcumin delivery by methoxy polyethylene glycol-poly(caprolactone)nanoparticles inhibits the growth of C6 glioma cells. *Acta Biochim. Biophys. Sin.* **2011**, *43*, 267–274. [CrossRef]
39. Scarano, W.; De Souza, P.; Stenzel, M.H. Dual-drug delivery of curcumin and platinum drugs in polymeric micelles enhances the synergistic effects: A double act for the treatment of multidrug-resistant cancer. *Biomater. Sci.* **2015**, *3*, 163–174. [CrossRef]
40. Chow, S.F.; Wan, K.Y.; Cheng, K.K.; Wong, K.W.; Sun, C.C.; Baum, L.; Chow, A.H.L. Development of highly stabilized curcumin nanoparticles by flash nanoprecipitation and lyophilization. *Eur. J. Pharm. Biopharm.* **2015**, *94*, 436–449. [CrossRef]
41. Mazzarino, L.; Otsuka Halila, S.; Bubniak, L.D.S.; Mazzucco, S.; Santos-Silva, M.C.; Lemos-Senna, E.; Borsali, R. Xyloglucan-block-poly(ε-caprolactone) copolymer nanoparticles coated with chitosan as biocompatible mucoadhesive drug delivery system. *Macromol. Biosci.* **2014**, *14*, 709–719. [CrossRef] [PubMed]
42. Mogharbel, B.F.; Francisco, J.C.; Rioda, A.C.; Dziedzic, D.S.M.; Ferreira, P.E.; de Souza, D.; de Souza, C.M.C.O.; Neto, N.B.; Guarita-Souza, L.C.; Franco, C.R.C.; et al. Fluorescence properties of curcumin-loaded nanoparticles for cell tracking. *Int. J. Nanomed.* **2018**, *13*, 5823–5836. [CrossRef] [PubMed]
43. Feng, R.; Song, Z.; Zhai, G. Preparation and in vivo pharmacokinetics of curcumin-loaded PCL-PEG-PCL triblock copolymeric nanoparticles. *Int. J. Nanomed.* **2012**, *7*, 4089–4098. [CrossRef] [PubMed]
44. Song, Z.; Zhu, W.; Song, J.; Wei, P.; Yang, F.; Liu, N.; Feng, R. Linear-dendrimer type methoxy-poly (ethylene glycol)-b-poly (ε-caprolactone) copolymer micelles for the delivery of curcumin. *Drug Deliv.* **2015**, *22*, 58–68. [CrossRef]
45. Arica, B.; Kas, H.S.; Moghdam, A.; Akalan, N.; Hincal, A.A. Carbidopa/levodopa-loaded biodegradable microspheres: In vivo evaluation on experimental Parkinsonism in rats. *J. Control. Release* **2005**, *102*, 689–697. [CrossRef]
46. Shin, M.; Kim, H.K.; Lee, H. Dopamine-loaded poly(D,L-lactic-co-glycolic acid) microspheres: New strategy for encapsulating small hydrophilic drugs with high efficiency. *Biotechnol. Prog.* **2014**, *30*, 215–223. [CrossRef]

47. Li, Z.; Tan, B.H. Towards the development of polycaprolactone based amphiphilic block copolymers: Molecular design, self-assembly and biomedical applications. *Mater. Sci. Eng. C* **2015**, *45*, 620–634. [CrossRef]
48. Mdzinarishvili, A.; Sutariya, V.; Talasila, P.K.; Geldenhuys, W.J.; Sadana, P. Engineering triiodothyronine (T3)nanoparticle for use in ischemic brain stroke. *Drug Deliv. Transl. Res.* **2013**, *3*, 309–317. [CrossRef]
49. Geldenhuys, W.; Wehrung, D.; Groshev, A.; Hirani, A.; Sutariya, V. Brain-targeted delivery of doxorubicin using glutathione-coated Nanoparticles for brain cancers. *Pharm. Dev. Technol.* **2015**, *20*, 497–506. [CrossRef]
50. Chronopoulou, L.; Nocca, G.; Castagnola, M.; Paludetti, G.; Ortaggi, G.; Sciubba, F.; Bevilacqua, M.; Lupi, A.; Gambarini, G.; Palocci, C. Chitosan based nanoparticles functionalized with peptidomimetic derivatives for oral drug delivery. *N. Biotechnol.* **2016**, *33*, 23–31. [CrossRef]
51. Duxfield, L.; Sultana, R.; Wang, R.; Englebretsen, V.; Deo, S.; Swift, S.; Rupenthal Al-Kassas, R. Development of gatifloxacin-loaded cationic polymeric nanoparticles for ocular drug delivery. *Pharm. Dev. Technol.* **2016**, *21*, 172–179. [CrossRef] [PubMed]
52. Trapani, A.; De Giglio, E.; Cafagna, D.; Denora, N.; Agrimi, G.; Cassano, T.; Gaetani, S.; Cuomo, V.; Trapani, G. Characterization and evaluation of chitosan nanoparticles for dopamine brain delivery. *Int. J. Pharm.* **2011**, *419*, 296–307. [CrossRef] [PubMed]
53. Raval, N.; Mistry, T.; Acharya, N.; Acharya, S. Development of glutathione-conjugated asiatic acid-loaded bovine serum albumin nanoparticles for brain-targeted drug delivery. *J. Pharm. Pharmacol.* **2015**, *67*, 1503–1511. [CrossRef] [PubMed]
54. Gaillard, P.J.; Appeldoorn, C.C.M.; Rip, J.; Dorland, R.; Van Der Pol, S.M.A.; Kooij, G.; De Vries, H.E.; Reijerkerk, A. Enhanced brain delivery of liposomal methylprednisolone improved therapeutic efficacy in a model of neuroinflammation. *J. Control. Release* **2012**, *164*, 364–369. [CrossRef] [PubMed]
55. Gaillard, P.J.; Appeldoorn, C.C.M.; Dorland, R.; Van Kregten, J.; Manca, F.; Vugts, D.J.; Windhorst, B.; Van Dongen, G.A.M.S.; De Vries, H.E.; Maussang, D.; et al. Pharmacokinetics, brain delivery, and efficacy in brain tumor-bearing mice of glutathione pegylated liposomal doxorubicin (2B3-101). *PLoS ONE* **2014**, *9*, e82331. [CrossRef] [PubMed]
56. Ayen, W.Y.; Kumar, N. A systematic study on lyophilization process of polymersomes for long-term storage using doxorubicin-loaded (PEG) 3-PLAanopolymersomes. *Eur. J. Pharm. Sci.* **2012**, *46*, 405–414. [CrossRef] [PubMed]
57. Vega, E.; Antònia Egea, M.; Calpena, A.C.; Espina, M.; Luisa García, M. Role of hydroxypropyl-β-cyclodextrin on freeze-dried and gamma-irradiated PLGA and PLGA-PEG diblock copolymer Nanospheres for ophthalmic flurbiprofen delivery. *Int. J. Nanomed.* **2012**, *7*, 1357–1371. [CrossRef]
58. Parra, A.; Clares, B.; Rosselló, A.; Garduño-Ramírez, M.L.; Abrego, G.; García, M.L.; Calpena, A.C. Ex vivo permeation of carprofen fromanoparticles: A comprehensive studyrough human, porcine and bovine skin as anti-inflammatory agent. *Int. J. Pharm.* **2016**, *501*, 10–17. [CrossRef]
59. Keene, A.M.; Bancos, S.; Tyner, K.M. *Handbook of Nanotoxicology, Nanomedicine and Stem Cell Use in Toxicology*; Sahu, S.C., Casciano, D.A., Eds.; Wiley: Hoboken, NJ, USA, 2014; pp. 35–63.
60. De Harpe, K.M.; Kondiah, P.P.D.; Choonara, Y.E.; Marimuthu, T.; Toit, L.C.; Pillay, V. The Hemocompatibility of Nanoparticles: A Review. *Cells* **2019**, *8*, 1029.
61. Matus, M.F.; Vilos, C.; Cisterna, B.A.; Fuentes, E. Nanotechnology and primary hemostasis: Differential effects of nanoparticles on platelet responses. *Vascul. Pharmacol.* **2018**, *101*, 1–8. [CrossRef]
62. *ASTM F756-00*; Standard Practice for Assessment of Hemolytic Properties of Materials. ASTM International: West Conshohocken, PA, USA, 2000; pp. 4–8.
63. Neun, B.W.; Ilinskaya, A.N.; Dobrovolskaia, M.A. Updated Method for In Vitro Analysis of Nanoparticle Hemolytic Properties. *Methods Mol. Biol.* **2018**, *1682*, 91–102. [PubMed]
64. Mazzarino, L.; Loch-Neckel, G.; Bubniak, L.D.S.; Mazzucco, S.; Santos-Silva, M.C.; Borsali, R.; Lemos-Senna, E. Curcumin-Loaded Chitosan-Coated Nanoparticles as a New Approach for the Local Treatment of Oral Cavity Cancer. *J. NanoSci. Nanotechnol.* **2015**, *15*, 781–791. [CrossRef] [PubMed]
65. Fan, S.; Zheng, Y.; Liu, X.; Fang, W.; Chena, X.; Liao, W.; Jing, X.; Lei, M.; Tao, E.; Ma, Q.; et al. Curcumin-loaded plga-peg nanoparticles conjugated with b6 peptide for potential use in alzheimer's disease. *Drug Deliv.* **2018**, *25*, 1044–1055. [CrossRef] [PubMed]
66. Mosmann, T. Rapid colorimetric assay for cellular growth and survival: Application to proliferation and cytotoxicity assays. *J. Immunol. Methods* **1983**, *65*, 55–63. [CrossRef]
67. Zanganeh, S.; Spitler, R.; Erfanzadeh, M.; Ho, J.Q.; Aieneravaie, M. Nanocytotoxicity. *Iron Oxide Nanopart. Biomed. Appl.* **2018**, 105–114. [CrossRef]
68. Zandi, K.; Ramedani, E.; Khosro, M.; Tajbakhsh, S.; Dailami Rastian, Z.; Fouladvand, M.; Yousefi, F.; Farshadpour, F. Natural Product Communications Evaluation of Antiviral Activities of Curcumin Derivatives. *Nat. Prod. Commun.* **2010**, *5*, 8–11.
69. Lee, M.Y.; Choi, E.J.; Lee, M.K.; Lee, J.J. Epigallocatechin gallate attenuates L-DOPA-induced apoptosis in rat PC12 cells. *Nutr. Res. Pract.* **2013**, *7*, 249–255. [CrossRef]
70. Chakraborty, S.; Karmenyan, A.; Tsai, J.W.; Chiou, A. Inhibitory effects of curcumin and cyclocurcumin in 1-methyl-4-phenylpyridinium (MPP+) induced neurotoxicity in differentiated PC12 cells. *Sci. Rep.* **2017**, *7*, 16978. [CrossRef]
71. Kong, Y.; Ma, W.; Liu, X.; Zu, Y.; Fu, Y.; Wu, N.; Liang, L.; Yao, L.; Efferth, T. Cytotoxic activity of curcumin towards CCRF-CEM leukemia cells and its effect on DNA damage. *Molecules* **2009**, *14*, 5328–5338. [CrossRef]
72. Prasetyaningrum, P.W.; Bahtiar, A.; Hayun, H. Synthesis and cytotoxicity evaluation of novel asymmetrical mono-carbonyl analogs of curcumin (AMACs) against vero, HeLa, and MCF7 cell lines. *Sci. Pharm.* **2018**, *86*, 25. [CrossRef]

73. Siddiqui, M.A.; Kashyap, M.P.; Kumar, V.; Tripathi, V.K.; Khanna, V.K.; Yadav, S.; Pant, A.B. Differential protection of pre-, co- and post-treatment of curcumin against hydrogen peroxide in PC12 cells. *Hum. Exp. Toxicol.* **2011**, *30*, 192–198. [CrossRef] [PubMed]
74. Fan, C.D.; Li, Y.; Xing, F.; Wu, Q.J.; Hou, Y.J.; Yang, M.F.; Sun, J.Y.; Fu, X.Y.; Zheng, Z.C.; Sun, B.L. Reversal of Beta-Amyloid-Induced Neurotoxicity in PC12 Cells by Curcumin, the important Role of ROS-Mediated Signaling and ERK Pathway. *Cell Mol. Neurobiol.* **2017**, *37*, 211–222. [CrossRef] [PubMed]
75. Mendonça, L.M.; dos Santos, G.C.; Antonucci, G.A.; dos Santos, A.C.; de Bianchi, M.L.P.; Antunes, L.M.G. Evaluation of the cytotoxicity and genotoxicity of curcumin in PC12 cells. *Mutat Res. Genet Toxicol. Environ. Mutagen* **2009**, *675*, 29–34. [CrossRef] [PubMed]
76. Mendonça, L.M.; da Silva Machado, C.; Correia Teixeira, C.C.; Pedro de Freitas, L.A.; de Pies Bianchi, M.L.; Greggi Antunes, L.M. Curcumin reduces cisplatin-induced neurotoxicity in NGF-differentiated PC12 cells. *Neurotoxicology* **2013**, *34*, 205–211. [CrossRef] [PubMed]
77. Chang, C.H.; Chen, H.X.; Yü, G.; Peng, C.C.; Peng, R.Y. Curcumin-protected PC12 cells against glutamate-induced oxidative toxicity. *Food Technol. Biotechnol.* **2014**, *52*, 468–478. [CrossRef]
78. Farani, M.R.; Parsi, P.K.; Riazi, G.; Ardestani, M.S.; Rad, H.S. Extending the application of a magnetic PEG three-part drug release device on a graphene substrate for the removal of gram-positive and gram-negative bacteria and cancerous and pathologic cells. *Drug Des. Devel. Ther.* **2019**, *13*, 1581–1591. [CrossRef]
79. Basma, A.N.; Morris, E.J.; Nicklas, W.J.; Geller, H.M. L-DOPA Cytotoxicity to PC12 Cells in Culture is via its Autoxidation. *J. Neurochem.* **1995**, *64*, 825–832. [CrossRef]
80. Jin, C.M.; Yang, Y.J.; Huang, H.S.; Kai, M.; Lee, M.K. Mechanisms of L-DOPA-induced cytotoxicity in rat adrenal pheochromocytoma cells: Implication of oxidative stress-related kinases and cyclic AMP. *Neuroscience* **2010**, *170*, 390–398. [CrossRef]
81. Zhang, M.; Lee, H.J.; Park, K.H.; Park, H.J.; Choi, H.S.; Lim, S.C.; Lee, M.K. Modulatory effects of sesamin on dopamine biosynthesis and l-DOPA-induced cytotoxicity in PC12 cells. *Neuropharmacology* **2012**, *62*, 2219–2226. [CrossRef]
82. Chatterjee, S.; Mankamna Kumari, R.; Nimesh, S. Nanotoxicology: Evaluation of toxicity potential of nanoparticles. *Adv. Nanomed. Deliv. Ther. Nucleic Acids* **2017**, *2010*, 188–201. [CrossRef]
83. Lundholt, B.K.; Scudder, K.M.; Pagliaro, L. A simple technique for reducing edge effect in cell-based assays. *J. Biomol. Screen* **2003**, *8*, 566–570. [CrossRef] [PubMed]
84. Funk, D.; Schrenk, H.H.; Frei, E. Serum albumin leads to false-positive results in the XTT and the MTT assay. *Biotechniques* **2007**, *43*, 178–186. [CrossRef] [PubMed]
85. Monteiro-Riviere, N.A.; Inman, A.O.; Zhang, L.W. Limitations and relative utility of screening assays to assess engineered nanoparticle toxicity in a human cell line. *Toxicol. Appl. Pharmacol.* **2009**, *234*, 222–235. [CrossRef] [PubMed]
86. Holder, A.L.; Goth-Goldstein, R.; Lucas, D.; Koshland, C.P. Particle-induced artifacts in the MTT and LDH viability assays. *Chem. Res. Toxicol.* **2012**, *25*, 1885–1892. [CrossRef] [PubMed]
87. Stepanenko, A.A.; Dmitrenko, V.V. Pitfalls ofhe MTT assay: Direct and off-target effects of inhibitors can result in over/underestimation of cell viability. *Gene* **2015**, *574*, 193–203. [CrossRef] [PubMed]
88. Gutiérrez, L.; Stepien, G.; Gutiérrez, L.; Pérez-Hernández, M.; Pardo, J.; Pardo, J.; Grazú, V.; de la Fuente, J.M. Nanotechnology in Drug Discovery and Development. *Compr. Med. Chem.* **2017**, *1–8*, 264–295.
89. Geldenhuys, W.; Mbimba, T.; Bui, T.; Harrison, K.; Sutariya, V. Brain-targeted delivery of paclitaxel using glutathione-coated nanoparticles for brain cancers. *J. Drug Target* **2011**, *19*, 837–845. [CrossRef]
90. Pereira, R.L.; Pain, C.S.; Barth, A.B.; Raffin, R.P.; Guterres, S.S.; Schapoval, E.E.S. Levodopa microparticles for pulmonary delivery: Photodegradation kinetics and LC stability-indicating method. *Pharmazie* **2012**, *67*, 605–610.
91. Monton, C.; Charoenchai, L.; Suksaeree, J.; Sueree, L. Quantitation of curcuminoid contents, dissolution profile, and volatile oil content of Turmeric capsules produced at some secondary government hospitals. *J. Food Drug Anal.* **2016**, *24*, 493–499. [CrossRef]

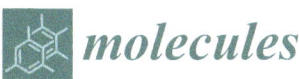 MDPI

Article

The Influence of Synthesis Conditions on the Antioxidant Activity of Selenium Nanoparticles

Aleksandra Sentkowska [1,*] and Krystyna Pyrzyńska [2]

1. Heavy Ion Laboratory, University of Warsaw, Pasteura 5A, 02-093 Warsaw, Poland
2. Department of Chemistry, University of Warsaw, Pasteura 1, 02-093 Warsaw, Poland; kryspyrz@chem.uw.edu.pl
* Correspondence: sentkowska@slcj.uw.edu.pl

Abstract: Selenium nanoparticles (SeNPs) have attracted great attention in recent years due to their unique properties and potential bioactivities. While the production of SeNPs has been long reported, there is little news about the influence of reaction conditions and clean-up procedure on their physical properties (e.g., shape, size) as well as their antioxidant activity. This study takes up this issue. SeNPs were synthesized by two methods using cysteine and ascorbic acid as selenium reductants. The reactions were performed with and without the use of polyvinyl alcohol as a stabilizer. After the synthesis, SeNPs were cleaned using various procedures. The antioxidant properties of the obtained SeNPs were investigated using DPPH and hydroxyl radical scavenging assays. It was found that their antioxidant activity does not always depend only on the nanoparticles size but also on their homogeneity. Moreover, the size and morphology of selenium nanoparticles are controlled by the clean-up step.

Keywords: selenium; selenium nanoparticles; antioxidant activities; clean-up procedure

Citation: Sentkowska, A.; Pyrzyńska, K. The Influence of Synthesis Conditions on the Antioxidant Activity of Selenium Nanoparticles. *Molecules* **2022**, *27*, 2486. https://doi.org/10.3390/molecules27082486

Academic Editor: Wansong Chen

Received: 2 March 2022
Accepted: 7 April 2022
Published: 12 April 2022

Publisher's Note: MDPI stays neutral with regard to jurisdictional claims in published maps and institutional affiliations.

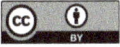

Copyright: © 2022 by the authors. Licensee MDPI, Basel, Switzerland. This article is an open access article distributed under the terms and conditions of the Creative Commons Attribution (CC BY) license (https://creativecommons.org/licenses/by/4.0/).

1. Introduction

Selenium is an essential trace element that supports many processes that occur in human body. The importance of selenium in the human diet comes from the fact that it is involved in protection of the cell from oxidative damage and plays a key role in decreasing lipid peroxidation [1,2]. Moreover, selenium is postulated to be useful for protection against various forms of cancer and many serious diseases, including cardiovascular disease, arthritis and muscular dystrophy [3,4]. For that reason, selenium dietary supplements generate considerable interest in pharmaceutical and food sciences [5]. Some of the selenium supplements, particularly the inorganic forms, have shown toxicity in higher nutritional doses. However, it is necessary to emphasize that the biological activity of the selenium depends on its chemical form and structure. In recent years, selenium nanoparticles (SeNPs) have attracted great attention due to their unique properties and potential bioactivities. The toxicity of SeNPs is significantly lower in comparison to that of inorganic and organic forms of selenium [6]. SeNPs offer great potential for several applications in the fields of medicine, diagnostics, therapeutics and toxicology [7–11]. On the other hand, due to their unique structural, optical and electronic properties, selenium nanomaterials also find applications in electronics and technology. The newest research shows great potential of SeNPs regarding their antimicrobial activity. Various mechanisms of their action were described, including the generation of radical oxygen species (ROS), interaction with cell barrier or inhibition of the synthesis of proteins and DNA [12]. The ROS species (e.g., hydroxyl radicals, superoxide anions, hydrogen peroxide) can inhibit DNA replication or amino acid synthesis, but they can also damage bacterial cell membranes. The potential of nanoparticles (NPs) as antimicrobial agents can be explained by their ability to simultaneously act through these multiple mechanisms. In such a situation, microbes are unable to develop resistance to these expressed mechanisms of action, contrary to the case for commercially available antibiotics [12]. The particle size, shape and surface morphology are important parameters determining the interaction of nanomaterials with bioorganisms. Due to these findings, the synthesis method is crucial when the obtained SeNPs are intended for use in the biomedical field.

Several chemical and physical methods have been proposed to prepare SeNPs. The main method of preparing nanoselenium is the chemical reduction of selenium salts [6,13–16]. Sodium selenite, sodium selenosulfate or selenious acid are examples of the precursors in the chemical synthesis of SeNPs. However, chemical methodologies are criticized due to the use of toxic chemicals in the synthesis protocol. Attempts have been made to use non-toxic reagents in the synthesis of SeNPs such as ascorbic acid [13,14,17,18] or sugars [13,18,19]; however, such actions are limited by the instability of the nanoparticles. This can be improved by adding stabilizers such as glucose, chitosan or polyvinyl alcohol (PVA) [13,14,20]. This is a very important aspect of nanoselenium synthesis because SeNPs are usually prone to agglomeration into large clusters in aqueous media, which results in a reduction in their bioactivity, biocompatibility and bioavailability [20]. On the other hand, some residuals of the used stabilizers limit the application of the obtained SeNPs in pharmaceutical and medicinal areas. Therefore, green synthesis methods of SeNPs preparation have recently garnered great attention [21–26]. These ecofriendly methods involve plant extracts or various microorganisms in their protocol. The main assumption of such methods is the use of naturally occurring substances in the extract as both stabilizers and reductants [13]. Many studies showed that SeNPs possesses higher antioxidant activity than the used plant extract itself [27,28]. It is known that particular synthesis conditions (e.g., concentration and type of selenium precursor and reductant, presence of stabilizer, temperature) affect the size, shape and stability of the obtained nanoparticles [6,14,29–31]. However, until now, it was not reported how the clean-up procedure of previously synthesized SeNPs affects their physical properties such as size and shape and, even more importantly, their antioxidant properties. Usually, the reaction protocols involve stirring of the reaction mixture for different time intervals and, in some cases, also heating at the desired temperature [30–32]. The most common way to purify and isolate NPs from surrounding liquid is centrifugation at different speeds and then washing with water [23,24,33–35]. However, the duration and speed of centrifugation (expressed as revolutions per minute (rpm)) are different in each study. In the research described by Sharma et al., SeNPs were centrifuged and precipitated at 15,000 rpm [34]. As a result, selenium nanoballs of a size of about 3–18 nm were obtained. Menon et al. centrifuged the reaction mixture at 10,000 rpm for 10 min and then washed three times with Mili-Q water [23]. As a result, shaped NPs in range 100–150 nm were obtained. SeNPs were also collected by centrifuging the solution at 12,000 rpm, and the pellet was resuspended in sterile double-distilled water before using in a bacterial experiment [35]. Centrifugation was also used by Chen et al. [36]. In this study, the post reaction solution was aged for 24 h followed by centrifugation at 9000 rpm for 30 min. Then, the precipitate was washed with twice with water and ethanol. At the end, the final product was redispersed in deionized water. In other studies, Chen et al. mentioned overnight dialysis against ultrapure water as a potential method for the purification of SeNPs [37,38]. This was a critical operation, due to the fact that, in the next stages of the research, the antioxidant properties of the SeNPs were tested. However, the impact of such a cleaning procedure on the physical properties of SeNPs was also not investigated. SeNPs have been considered as a potential anticancer and antioxidant agent. Before NPs can be used in treatment, they must undergo an entire clinical trial process similar to that of drugs [39]. One of the most challenging steps is the adaptation of the synthesis method from laboratory to industrial scale. The use of SeNPs in clinical trials depends on the approval of the production methods and quality assurance of the final product by the implementation and verification of good manufacturing practice (GMP). GMP is strictly connected with the quality assurance (QA) process, which should be implemented to guarantee that the obtained NPs follow the specifications and meet the required quality. Compliance with quality control (QC) requires SeNPs to be tested to confirm that they are of expected quality for the intended use. From the point of view of these regulations, it is obvious that the type and concentration of the used reductant must be characterized in detail, because it has enormous impact on the properties of the synthesized SeNPs. On the other hand, the very possibility of influencing the properties of SeNPs also at the purification stage gives enormous opportunities to improve some methods of SeNP synthesis so that they meet the requirements set by GMP and QC. Additionally, if they have such a large impact on the parameters of NPs, their optimization should be one of the points taken into account when developing GMP standards for SeNPs. It should be remembered that the methods of purifying NPs may not only improve their properties but also worsen them. Thus, there is the need to develop an optimal method for the purification of the synthesized NPs, as this step ultimately determines the quality of the obtained product. However, there is no comparison of the properties of NPs obtained with the same method but with different purification steps.

In this study, SeNPs were synthesized using two well-known chemical methods, involving ascorbic acid (AA) or cysteine (Cys) as the reductants and sodium selenite as the precursor. The syntheses were carried out in two variants: in the presence and without the use of polyvinyl alcohol (PVA) as a stabilizer. After each synthesis, SeNPs were cleaned by rinsing with water and centrifuging at different speeds (8000 and 12,000 rpm). The impact of additional post-synthesis heating on their physical properties was also investigated. The influence of all the above-mentioned factors on the antioxidant capacity of SeNPs has been evaluated. To the best of our knowledge, this has not been described so far. This step of SeNP synthesis is extremely important if the obtained SeNPs are intended for use in medicine, e.g., as a substitute for antibiotics [40].

The antioxidant properties of the synthesized SeNPs were examined using scavenging of the 2,2-diphenyl-1-picrylhydrazyl (DPPH) as well as hydroxyl (OH) radicals. The morphology of the SeNPs was compared using scanning electron microscopy (SEM) and transmission electron microscopy (TEM).

2. Results and Discussion

Syntheses of SeNPs were carried out in parallel by the reduction of sodium selenite using AA or Cys. Theoretically, the antioxidant properties of SeNPs can already be controlled at the stage of selecting the concentrations of the reactants for their synthesis. Li et al. [41] found that an excess of Cys to Se(IV) that was higher than 1:4 caused the aggregation of SeNPs. Such a process would be disadvantageous from the point of view of the antioxidant capacity of SeNPs. It has been proven that the antioxidant capacity of NPs increases with the decrease in their dimensions [42]. Therefore, a selenium to reductants ratio of 1:4 was selected for use. After mixing the reagents, the color of the product solutions gradually changed from colorless through light orange, to orange and brick red due to reduction of selenium ions, which confirmed SeNP formation (Figure 1).

The synthesis of SeNPs was also monitored by determining the decrease of the reagent's concentration in the supernatant using hydrophilic interaction chromatography coupled with mass spectrometry detection. For each compound used in the synthesis, the optimum conditions of MRM (multiple reaction mode) were determined. The obtained MS spectra are presented in Figure S1. Figure 2 shows the remaining concentration of selenium ions and AA or Cys at various time intervals during synthesis. The appropriate chromatograms as well as mass spectra of the reagents are shown in Figure S1. The obtained results a confirmed faster reaction rate with Cys. Its concentration decreased from an initial value of 4 to 0.07 mg L^{-1} after 5 min of reaction time; thus, the reduction of Se(IV) by Cys is almost instantaneous. In the presence of PVA as a stabilizer, this reaction is slightly slower. Cys was found in the reaction media at the level of 0.48 mg L^{-1} after 5 min of mixing with 88% synthesis yield. After 30 min of reaction with AA, the synthesis yields of SeNPs were found to be 68% and 77% in the absence and presence of PVA, respectively. Even after 60 min of intensive mixing with a stirring speed of 1000 rpm, there was still a small residue of both components in the reaction medium. The higher intensity of the transformation process using Cys was also confirmed on the basis of changes in the UV–Vis absorption spectra during the ongoing synthesis (Figure 3).

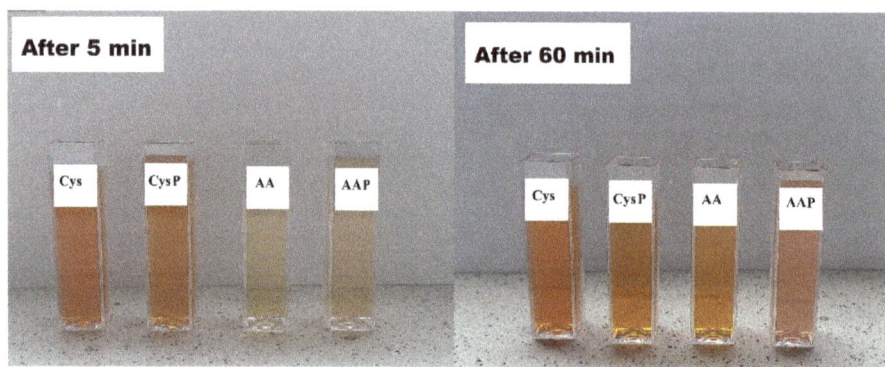

Figure 1. Color changes of product solutions upon synthesis of SeNPs (CysP or AAP—reductant in the presence of PVA).

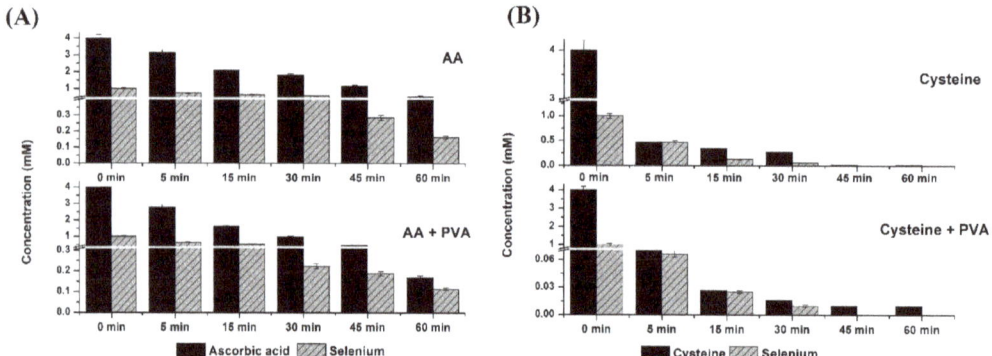

Figure 2. The changes in the concentration of selenium salt and reductants: (**A**) AA and (**B**) Cys as a function of synthesis time.

Lin et al. [43] postulated that the well-known belief that nano-Se is "red" is somewhat misleading. In fact, the color of the NPs' suspension strictly depends on their dimensions. These observations were the basis for the authors to develop a method for determining the size of SeNPs based on their UV–Vis spectra [43]. According to this method, the suspension of the SeNPs of 20 nm diameter had a yellowish-orange appearance and showed the absorption maximum below 250 nm. When the particle sizes increase, the characteristic red-shift of the absorbance peak maxima is observed. As result, SeNPs' suspension with diameters of about 100 nm was characterized by an absorption maximum below 350 nm, while for SeNPs' with diameters of 240 ± 32.2 nm, the absorbance maximum was observed at 680 nm. This method was also used in our study.

The obtained results indicate that the extension of the reaction time does not cause the changes in the spectra obtained for solutions of Cys as a reductant (Figure 3). This suggests that SeNPs obtained by this method do not change their dimensions with increasing mixing time. Therefore, they probably do not aggregate. Any change in the size of the obtained NPs would entail a change in the spectrum, which was not observed here. In the case of synthesis with Cys and CysP, the UV–Vis spectrum did not change within two hours from the end of the synthesis, and the stability of SeNPs was observed during this time interval. Based on the Lin et al. method [43], the predicted diameters of obtained Cys SeNPs were about 101 ± 9.8 nm. However, the shift of the maximum absorbance peak for the CysP suggests that SeNPs obtained this way are slightly smaller. This is in good accordance with our studies, in which size ranges equal to 108 ± 9.3 nm for Cys and 80 ± 5.1 nm for CysP were obtained. A totally different observation was made for the synthesis with the use of AA. In this case, changes in the location of the maximum absorbance peak were observed during the extension of the reaction time. This may be due to the slower reaction rate, which was confirmed by monitoring the decrease in the concentration of the reactants (Figure 2). As explained later in the publication, the process of NPs synthesis is a dynamic one, and depending on which mechanism prevails, changes in the size and structure of the NPs are observed. These changes are visible in the UV–Vis spectrum. For the synthesis with AA, the increasing absorbance of the peak located at 400 nm was observed, which suggests that larger of SeNPs are expected. Our research has proven the formation of SeNPs with the size of 193 ± 9.5 nm. The presence of a stabilizing agent greatly differentiates the sizes of NPs. The peak at 300 nm indicates the presence of particles of the size 70 ± 9.1 nm according to the Lin model and 90 ± 7.3 nm based on our studies. However, much bigger SeNPs can also be found—predicted to be 182.8 ± 33.2 nm and 189 ± 6.4 nm based on our study. It can be concluded that the use of a stabilizer does not always bring the desired effect. In the reaction with Cys, slightly lower dimensions of NPs were obtained when the PVA was used. However, in the synthesis with AA, the presence of PVA made the NPs less homogenous, with a predominance of larger particles.

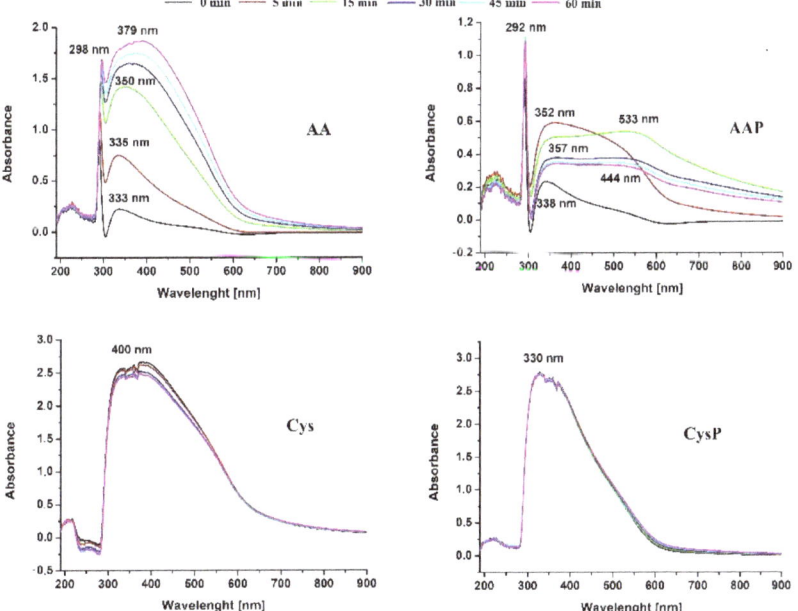

Figure 3. UV–visible spectra of SeNPs as a function of synthesis time.

It is worth noticing that the occurrence of the SeNPs' absorption spectra with maxima within visible and UV regions was often explained by the formation of surface plasma vibration on spherical NPs [13,22,24,33,44,45]. Probably, the authors of these works just copied it from reports on noble-metal NPs. Selenium, as a semiconductor, lacks free conduction electrons. The light irradiation of SeNPs can cause exciton resonance or transition to occur [46], determining the development of their unique optical properties.

In the past decade, prompted by rapid developments in nanotechnology, SeNPs have attracted extensive attention from researchers in biomedical fields [23,40]. SeNPs obtained by chemical synthesis should be cleaned first to be suitable for use in these applications, as residues of the reagents may be toxic or can block the desired effect of the nanomaterial. However, systematic studies on the impact of cleaning procedure on the properties of SeNPs are very rare. For evaluation of the antioxidant activity of SeNPs, an appropriate volume of the formed colloidal solution was just mixed with a given reagent [14,23,47]. In such a case, the presence of the used reductant residue could affect the results.

In our study, two centrifugation speeds 8000 and 12,000 rpm were used. The influence of the cleaning procedure on the properties of SeNPs can already be observed in the UV–Vis spectra of cleaned NPs (Figure 4). A wide band in the range of 350–550 nm was observed for AA SeNPs, which corresponds to the NPs in the size range 195 ± 5.0 nm. In the case of the AAP, the band at 382 nm exhibited lower intensity with a simultaneous increase in the intensity of the band at about 300 nm. This suggests that PVA prevents agglomeration of the resulting SeNPs, hence shifting the absorption maxima toward lower wavelengths. Moreover, the use of any purification method in the case of AA SeNPs led to a reduction in their size, as evidenced by the disappearance of the absorption band at 382 nm. It should be mentioned that other researchers have also reported a similar type of SeNP multimodal distribution [15,47,48]. Heating at different temperatures (70–120 °C) was also employed during the synthesis of SeNPs [32,48,49]. Zhang et al. found that heating treatment (1 h at 90 °C) caused aggregation of SeNPs into larger sizes and rods, which leads to a significant reduction of their bioactivity in mice [50]. In two synthesis methods using AA, heating of the post-reaction mixture led to an increase in peak intensity with an absorption maximum of 300 nm. This is a desirable effect, as this increases the formation intensity of NPs with dimensions of about 100 nm.

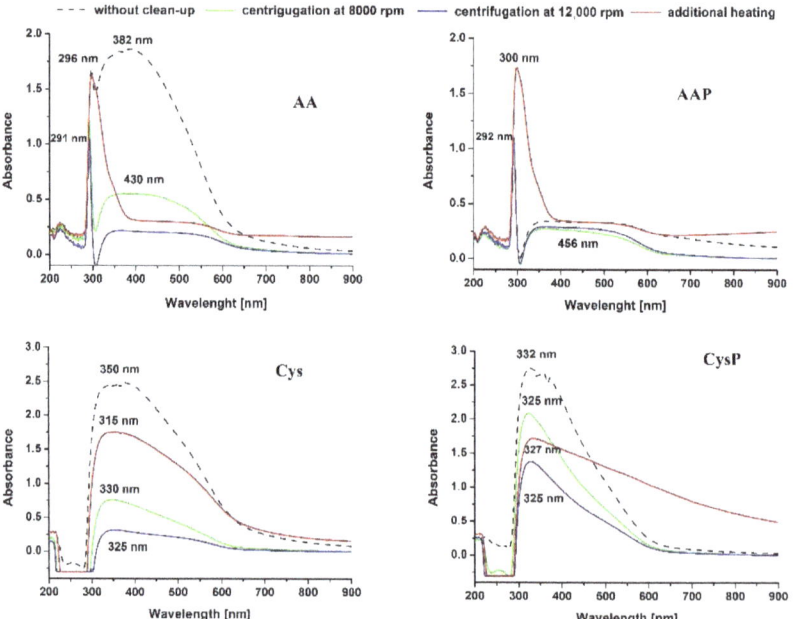

Figure 4. UV–visible spectra of SeNPs after the application of various cleaning procedures.

For synthesis conducted using Cys, the occurrence of a peak at 325–350 nm indicates the formation of SeNPs with lower diameters (108 ± 4.2 nm). The highest intensity was observed for NPs without a clean-up procedure, while the lowest observed for those centrifuged at high speed (12,000 rpm, 17,257 rcf), while tailoring the signal to higher wavelengths. This suggests that centrifugation does not prevent the aggregation of NPs but makes them less homogeneous with a predominance of NPs larger than 100 nm. It should be highlighted that heating the post-reaction mixture resulted in a reduction in the signal intensity of about 300 nm, and additionally, a significant tailing of the signal was observed, if PVA was used for synthesis. Surprisingly, none of the purification methods of SeNPs obtained from Cys synthesis seemed to improve their properties but rather favored their agglomeration.

According to previous reports, SeNPs are strong free radical scavengers that can be used as an active form of selenium in food supplements [14,23,24,45,47,51]. As mentioned before, the antioxidant capacity of NPs increases with the decrease in their dimensions [42]. This leads to the hypothesis that, since the cleaning procedure affects the size of the NPs, it also has an impact on their antioxidant capacity. However, the impact of these procedures on the antioxidant properties of SeNPs has not been reported on. Thus, we compared the free radical scavenging potential of SeNPs toward hydroxyl and DPPH radicals. Stable DPPH radicals are widely used to evaluate the antioxidant activity of NPs [52]. The scavenging of hydroxyl radicals is an important antioxidant activity because of the very high reactivity of the OH radical, enabling it to react with a wide range of molecules found in living cells. The applied cleaning procedure was not changed and involved centrifugation at two speeds (8000 and 12,000 rpm) or additional heating (1 h at 70 °C). The obtained results are presented in Figure 5.

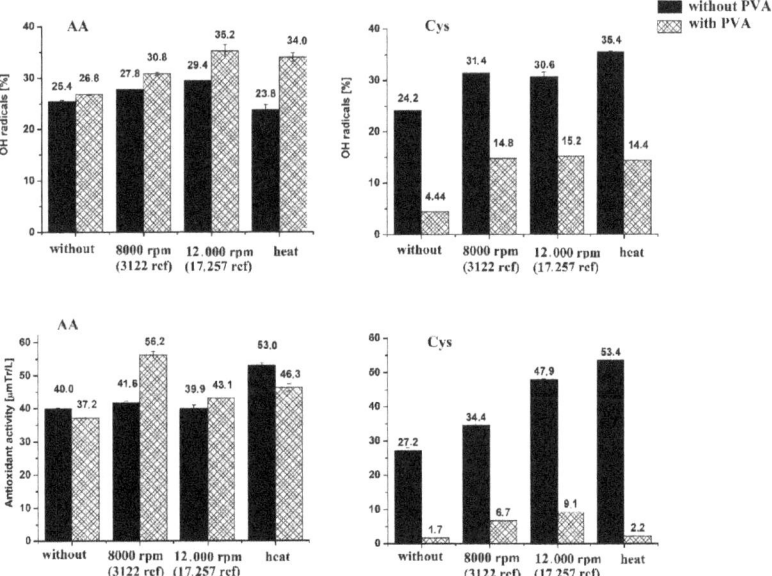

Figure 5. The antioxidant activity of the obtained SeNPs.

At the beginning, the antioxidant activity of the used reagents was established. In the DPPH assay, the antioxidant activity of AA (in the same concentration as in SeNP synthesis) was 1.15 ± 0.11 µmol TR L^{-1}. The addition of PVA did not change this value; in its presence, the value 1.16 ± 0.10 µmol TR L^{-1} was obtained. The same situation was observed for Cys, for which, the determined value of the antioxidant capacity was 1.11 ± 0.05 µmol TR L^{-1}. PVA itself shows a very low antioxidant capacity of 0.008 ± 0.0001 µmol TR L^{-1}. In the OH radical assay, the addition of PVA resulted in an increase in capacity, from 93.0% to 100% in case of Cys solution and from 33.3% to 98.1% for AA. This suggests a strong synergistic effect between the reactants. However, CysP SeNPs showed dramatically lower antioxidant capacity than those obtained from analogous synthesis but without the use of a stabilizer. Under these conditions, differences were obtained at a significant level ($p = 0.05$). Such differences were not observed in the case of synthesis with AA as a reductant. The use of any method of purification of NPs obtained with the use of AA did not significantly affect the antioxidant capacity they demonstrated. Only the heating of the reaction mixture increased these capabilities, but in this case, a higher effect was observed for the AA SeNPs. In the case of Cys SeNPs, applying any cleaning procedure increased their ability to scavenge DPPH radicals. As previously observed for the SeNPs from the synthesis with AA, the highest increase was observed for the synthesis protocol that involved heating. Such observations can suggest that the greater impact on the SeNPs' antioxidant activity was due to their homogeneity and not their size. If their dimensions were crucial, a significant increase in antioxidant capacity should have been observed when using high-speed centrifugation (12,000 rpm). Such a procedure prevents the aggregation of SeNPs, while heating makes them more spherical and homogeneous. The lowest results in the DPPH assay were obtained for CysP (1.7–9.1 µmol TR L^{-1}), which further confirmed our predictions as the stabilizer also prevents the aggregations of SeNPs, but the small dimensions of NPs are not the dominant factor affecting their antioxidant capacity.

The influence of the cleaning procedure for SeNPs on the scavenging of hydroxyl radicals was also positive. The highest ability to scavenge OH radicals was established for AAP SeNPs cleaned using high-speed centrifugation (35.2% ± 0.9%). This value was not statistically different from that obtained for Cys subjected to additional heating (35.4% ± 0.5%). Presence of the stabilizer during the synthesis of SeNPs with Cys, resulted in lower ability to scavenge the hydroxyl radicals; however, every cleaning procedure, applied just after the synthesis resulted in increased antioxidant capacity. For the synthesis of SeNPs with AA, the presence of a stabilizer resulted in a higher ability to scavenge OH radicals. Every clean-up procedure improved this ability, with the exception of additional heating of the post-reaction mixture without the stabilizer.

The morphology of synthesized SeNPs was evaluated by SEM analysis, and majority of them were found to be spherical (Figure 6). Only the Cys SeNPs centrifuged at high speed were nanorods. Similar shape of SeNPs was obtained with asparagines and polyvinylpyrrolidone [35]. Surprisingly, the highest antioxidant abilities were not determined for the most spherical SeNPs obtained for Cys. The highest ability to scavenge free radicals was found in SeNPs obtained without the use of PVA but subjected to additional heating; however, their average size increased at elevated temperature. This was caused by the aggregation of the NPs. A similar phenomenon was observed by others [31,48]. Literature reports indicate that smaller SeNPs exhibit higher antioxidant activity [34,50], but this correlation was observed only for AAP. Centrifugation reduced only reduced the size of AAP SeNPs, and these showed the highest ability to scavenge free radicals of all the protocols examined for synthesis involving AA. On the other hand, Zhang et al. demonstrated that SeNPs with different sizes (5–200 nm) have equal capacity in the induction of selenoenzymes in cultured cells and in mice [49]. Our results, rather, indicate that SeNPs with better homogeneity show higher scavenging activity toward free radicals. It should be recalled that synthesis of SeNPs is a dynamic process, which is controlled by both thermodynamics and kinetics. Thermodynamics deals with the driving force of a system moving from the initial state to the product state, whereas kinetics is concerned with the energy barriers of the specific pathways in this process [53]. Due to this fact, SeNPs are changing during synthesis to reach a relatively stable state. This can be explained by a well-known concept called Ostwald ripening. When the substrates used for synthesis are nearly depleted, some of the NPs can redissolve in the reaction solution. Such dissolved components can attach to the surface of the NPs, increasing their size. As a result, fewer but larger NPs are formed. Another phenomenon that can also take place during NPs synthesis is digestive ripening. In this process, larger NPs are transformed into smaller ones with a uniform monodisperse state by mixing NPs in a solution that contains digestive ripening ligands, e.g., PVA. The action of these two mechanisms is visible in the surface changes of NPs, as shown in Figure 6. When the results obtained for Cys are discussed, the larger SeNPs are broken up into smaller ones, which was induced by PVA. Then, these CysP were completely transformed into a nearly monodisperse form with an almost uniform size by centrifuging at 12,000 rpm. When centrifuging at 8000 rpm, monodisperse particles together with larger particles are formed. Thus, it can be inferred that digestive ripening is responsible for such an observation. On the other hand, probably due to the weak binding of PVA with SeNPs' surfaces, uniform SeNPs are transformed back to larger polyhedral particles as a result of heating, according to the mechanism of Ostwald ripening. Such a dynamic state is also observed for the SeNPs obtained via synthesis with AA. Using this phenomenon, the production of nanorods in the case of Cys centrifuged at 12,000 rpm can also be explained. Such nanostructures are synthesized in solution at low temperature mainly due to the wet-chemical reactions. The orientation and shape of nanorods can be controlled mostly by temperature, concentration of precursor and the length of the rod by the time of synthesis. In our case, only the method of cleaning previously formed SeNPs was changed. It can be assumed that centrifuging at high speed favors the process of Ostwald ripening. However, the mechanism in this case is different than for other cleaning procedures due to a combination of ligands that act as the shape-control agents and bond to different facets of the nanorod with different strengths. This allows different faces of the nanorod to grow at different rates, producing an elongated object.

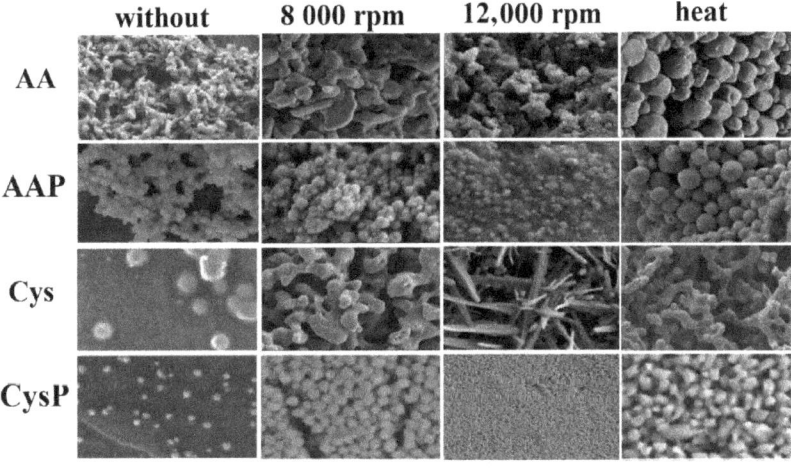

Figure 6. SEM images of the obtained SeNPs.

Figure 7 shows the TEM images of the obtained SeNPs. These results confirm that more spherical-shaped NPs were obtained without any purification procedure. Chen et al. found that the reaction temperature affects not only the size evolution of SeNPs but also their shape formation [48]. The TEM images were used for the construction of histograms of SeNP size distribution in each obtained sample. The results are presented in Figure S2. The obtained results confirmed the enormous influence of the cleaning procedure on the size of the NPs. In many cases, the applied procedure resulted in obtaining less-homogeneous particles of various sizes. This is especially evident when additional heating is used for AA and CysP. We previously linked the antioxidant capacity with the homogeneity of NPs. Referring to these results, this influence is particularly visible. A lower hydroxyl scavenging capacity was observed for the sample of AA subjected to heating than for the sample without the cleaning procedure. The use of heating also resulted in the reduction by half of the ability to neutralize hydroxyl radicals for CysP. On the other hand, it was observed that, for some samples with less homogeneity but with a predominance of smaller NPs, the antioxidant capacity was higher in comparison to that of the more homogeneous samples. Such a situation was observed for AA subjected to moderate-speed centrifugation (8000 rpm) or heating. This suggests that the antioxidant capacity of SeNPs is influenced by both size and homogeneity. Both these factors are important. Such relations can be also observed for the DPPH radical scavenging. For example, higher antioxidant activity was observed for the more homogenous sample of AAP, subjected to 8000 rpm, than for the sample without any cleaning procedure but with the predominance of smaller particles.

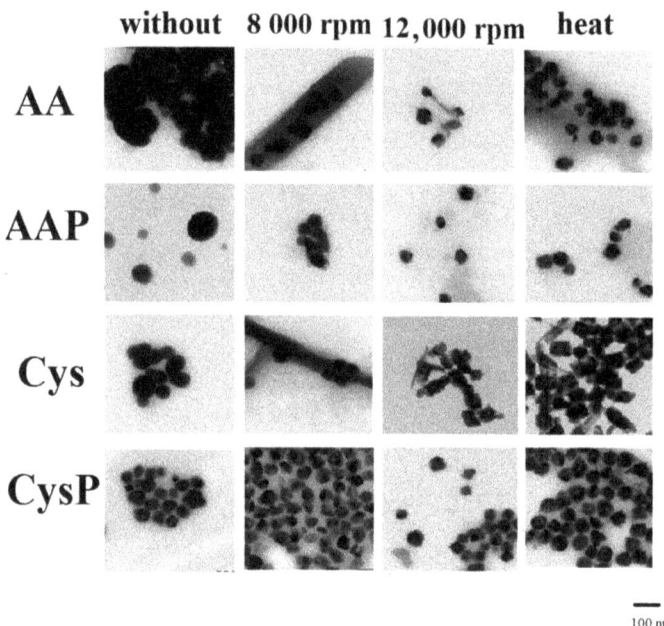

Figure 7. TEM images of the obtained SeNPs.

3. Materials and Methods

3.1. Reagents

The commercial standards of sodium selenite (Na_2SeO_3) as well as ascorbic acid (AA), L-cysteine (Cys) and polyvinyl alcohol (PVA) were purchased from Merck-Sigma (Steinheim, Germany). Ultrapure water from Milli-Q system (Millipore, Bedford, MA, USA) was used in all experiments.

3.2. Synthesis of Selenium Nanoparticles and Their Purification

SeNPs were synthesized via reduction of Na_2SeO_3 with ascorbic acid. The procedure was performed with and without polyvinyl alcohol (PVA) as a stabilizing agent. PVA is often used for this purpose [32]. Briefly, 20 mL of sodium selenite solution (5×10^{-3} mol L^{-1}) was placed in a beaker with a magnetic stirrer. Then, 10 mL of AA solution (40×10^{-3} mol L^{-1}) was added dropwise. After 60 min of stirring, 70 mL of Milli-Q water was added. In the second procedure of synthesis, PVA was added just after the first addition of AA in such amount that its final concentration was 1 mg L^{-1}.

SeNPs were also synthesized using Cys as the reductant. In detail, to 0.1 mol L^{-1} solution of Na_2SeO_3, Cys solution (50×10^{-3} mol L^{-1}) was added dropwise with vigorous stirring (stirring speed of 1000 rpm) for 60 min. In parallel, SeNPs were obtained using PVA as a stabilizing agent. In each method of synthesis, the final concentration of selenium was equal to 1×10^{-3} mol L^{-1}, and the reductants was equal to 4×10^{-3} mol L^{-1}.

After the synthesis, SeNPs were purified from the surrounding liquid containing dissolved substrate residuals using different procedures: (i) centrifugation for 10 min with two units of rotational speed 8000 rpm (3122 rcf) and 12,000 rpm (17,257 rcf), decantation and rising three times with 10 mL of deionized water; (ii) additional heating with magnetic stirring at 70 °C for 1 h, then rising three times with 10 mL of deionized water. Heating the reaction mixture is sometimes recommended in order to obtain more-homogeneous NPs [40]. The morphology and properties of SeNPs synthesized using these clean-up procedures were compared with those of SeNPs obtained directly by mixing reagents.

3.3. Characterization of Selenium Nanoparticles

The morphology and characterization of SeNPs were investigated using various methods. The size and shape of SeNPs were observed using transmission electron microscopy (TEM) with a TALOS F200 model (Thermo Fisher Scientific, Waltham, MA, USA) working at an accelerating voltage of 200 kV. A drop of bright red solution containing synthesized SeNPs was placed on copper grid and then air dried before examination. Scanning electron microscopy (SEM) was performed with a field-emission SEM (Merlin Zeiss) for images and morphology of SeNPs. Before measurements samples were plasma sputtered with a few-nanometer-thick Au/Pd layer. The obtained results were processed in the program iTEM, which is a part of the apparatus software. The histograms presented in the supplementary section were obtained based on the TEM images in the ImageJ program.

The UV–visible absorption spectra were recorded in the range of 250–900 nm using a Perkin Elmer model Lambda 20 spectrophotometer with cuvettes of 1 cm length.

Chromatographic analysis was performed to study the conversion of reagents at various time intervals by determining their remaining concentration in the supernatant. It was done with the Shimadzu LC system consisting of binary pumps LC20-AD, degasser DGU-20A5, column oven CTO-20AC, autosampler SIL-20AC and 8030 triple quadrupole mass spectrometer (Shimadzu, Japan) equipped with an ESI source operated in negative-ion mode for selenium or in positive mode for ascorbic acid and cysteine quantification. The ESI conditions were as follows: capillary voltage 4.5 kV, temperature 400 °C, source gas flow 3 L min^{-1} and drying gas flow 10 L min^{-1}. The separation was performed using a silica column Atlantis HILIC (100 × 2.1, 3 µm) from Phenomenex. The mobile phase consisted of methanol and water (85/15, v/v).

3.4. Antioxidant Activity

The hydroxyl radical scavenging activity of SeNPs was evaluated according to the method reported by Smirnoff and Cumbes [54]. The method involves the addition of 1 mL of SeNP solution to the reaction mixture containing: 1 mL iron sulfate (1.5×10^{-3} mol L^{-1}), 0.7 mL hydrogen peroxide (6×10^{-3} mol L^{-1}) and 0.3 mL sodium salicylate (2×10^{-2} mol L^{-1}). After 60 min of incubation at 37 °C, the absorbance was measured at 562 nm, and the percentage of hydroxyl radical scavenging inhibition was calculated.

The radical scavenging ability was also examined in vitro using DPPH radicals [36]. Briefly, 0.1 mL of a sample was added to 2.4 mL of DPPH solution (9×10^{-5} mol L^{-1} in methanol). After 30 min, the decrease in the absorbance was measured at 518 nm. Each sample was analyzed in triplicate, and the results are expressed as Trolox equivalent (TRE) in µM.

4. Conclusions

The potential of nanopharmaceuticals, such as the investigated SeNPs, is based on their morphology, size and shape, and those parameters are related to the applied purification method. Our results clearly showed that every procedure that is used on the purification step has a great impact on the properties of the final product. In fact, NPs synthesized by the same method, under the same conditions, by the same person but subjected to different cleaning methods will have different physical properties. This, in turn, has an impact on their properties, including the antioxidant properties. It can be assumed that depending on the applied cleaning method, the properties that can be used in medicine are also subject to major changes. Therefore, it should be also optimized as a separate step on the way to obtain SeNPs with desired shape and properties. Such an approach can maximize the potential of SeNPs in medicinal applications. Moreover, when the intention is to evaluate the antioxidant activity of the obtained SeNPs, the clean-up procedure is crucial. The results described in the paper are a good introduction to biomedical research. It is assumed that they will be continued in this direction.

Supplementary Materials: The following supporting information can be downloaded at https://www.mdpi.com/article/10.3390/molecules27082486/s1, Figure S1: The chromatograms of Se(IV) and ascorbic acid or cysteine in the function of synthesis time.; Figure S2: Particle size distribution histograms of selenium nanoparticles.

Author Contributions: A.S. and K.P.: research plan and methodology; A.S.: formal analysis and investigation; A.S. and K.P.: writing—original draft preparation; A.S.: writing—review and editing. All authors have read and agreed to the published version of the manuscript.

Funding: This research received no external funding.

Institutional Review Board Statement: Not applicable.

Informed Consent Statement: Not applicable.

Data Availability Statement: The data presented in this study are available on request from the corresponding author.

Conflicts of Interest: The authors declare no conflict of interest.

References

1. Rayman, M.P. Selenium intake, status, and health: A complex relationship. *Hormones* **2020**, *19*, 9–14. [CrossRef] [PubMed]
2. Kumar, A.; Prasad, K.S. Role of nano-selenium in health and environment. *J. Biotechnol.* **2020**, *325*, 152–163. [CrossRef] [PubMed]
3. Weekley, C.M.; Harris, H.H. Which form is that? The importance of selenium speciation and metabolism in the prevention and treatment of disease. *Chem. Soc. Rev.* **2013**, *42*, 8870–8894. [CrossRef] [PubMed]
4. Misra, S.; Boylan, M.; Selvan, A.; Spallholz, J.E.; Björnstedt, M. Redox-active selenium compounds from toxicity and cell death to cancer treatment. *Nutrients* **2015**, *7*, 3536–3556. [CrossRef] [PubMed]
5. Zakeri, N.; Kelishadi, M.R.; Asbaghi, O.; Naeini, F.; Afsharfar, M.; Mirzadeh, E.; Naserizadeh, S.K. Selenium supplementation and oxidative stress: A review. *Pharm. Nutr.* **2021**, *17*, 100263. [CrossRef]
6. Bhattacharjee, A.; Bastu, A.; Bhattacharya, S. Selenium nanoparticles are less toxic than inorganic and organic selenium in mice in vivo. *Nucleus* **2019**, *62*, 259–268. [CrossRef]
7. Chaudhary, S.; Umar, A.; Mehta, S.K. Selenium nanoparticles: A overview of recent developments in synthesis, properties and potential applications. *Prog. Mater. Sci.* **2016**, *83*, 270–329. [CrossRef]
8. Wang, X.; Zhang, D.; Pan, X.; Fahad, D.J.; Al-Misned, A.; Mortuza, M.G.; Gadd, G.M. Aerobic and anaerobic biosynthesis of nano-selenium for remediation of mercury contaminated soil. *Chemosphere* **2017**, *170*, 266–273. [CrossRef]
9. Khurana, A.; Tekula, S.; Saifi, M.A.; Venkatesh, P.; Godugu, C. Therapeutic applications of selenium nanoparticles. *Biomed. Pharm.* **2019**, *111*, 802–812. [CrossRef]
10. Gudkov, S.V.; Shafeev, G.A.; Glinushkin, A.P.; Shkirin, A.V.; Barmina, E.V.; Rakov, I.; Simakin, A.V.; Kislov, A.V.; Astashev, M.E.; Vodeneev, V.A.; et al. Production and use of selenium nanoparticles as fertilizers. *ACS Omega* **2020**, *5*, 17767–17774. [CrossRef]
11. Nayak, V.; Singh, K.R.B.; Singh, A.K.; Singh, R.P. Potentialities of selenium nanoparticles in biomedical science. *New J. Chem.* **2021**, *45*, 2849–2878. [CrossRef]
12. Filipović, N.; Usjak, D.; Milenković, M.T.; Zheng, K.; Liverani, L.; Boccaccini, A.R.; Stevanović, M.M. Comparative study of the antimicrobial activity of selenium nanoparticles with different surface chemistry and structure. *Front. Bioeng. Biotechnol.* **2021**, *8*, 1591. [CrossRef] [PubMed]
13. Bartosiak, M.; Giersz, J.; Jankowski, K. Analytical monitoring of selenium nanoparticles green synthesis using photochemical vapour generation coupled with MIP-OES and UV–Vis spectrophotometry. *Microchem. J.* **2019**, *145*, 1169–1175. [CrossRef]
14. Boroumand, S.; Safari, M.; Shaabani, E.; Shirzah, M.; Faridi-Majidi, R. Selenium nanoparticles: Synthesis, characterization and study of their cytotoxicity, antioxidant and antimicrobial activity. *Mater. Res. Exp.* **2019**, *6*, 0850d8. [CrossRef]
15. Guleria, A.; Neogy, S.; Raorane, B.S.; Adhikari, S. Room temperature ionic liquid assisted rapid synthesis of amorphous Se nanoparticles: Their prolonged stabilization and antioxidant studies. *Mater. Chem. Phys.* **2020**, *253*, 123369. [CrossRef]
16. Korany, M.; Marzook, F.; Mahmoud, B.; Ahmed, S.A.; Ayoub, S.M.; Sakr, T.M. Exhibiting the diagnostic face of selenium nanoparticles as a radio-platform for tumor imaging. *Bioorg. Chem.* **2020**, *100*, 103910. [CrossRef]
17. Hussein, H.H.; Darwesh, O.M.; Mekki, B.B. Environmentally friendly nano-selenium to improve antioxidant system and growth to groundnut cultivars under sandy soil conditions. *Biocat. Agric. Biotechnol.* **2019**, *18*, 101080. [CrossRef]
18. El Lateef Gharib, F.A.; Zaidi, I.M.; Ghazi, S.M.; Ahmed, E.Z. The response of cowpea (*Vigna unguiculata* L.) plants to foliar application of sodium selenate and selenium nanoparticles (SeNPs). *J. Nanomater. Mol. Nanotechnol.* **2019**, *8*, 4.
19. Nie, T.; Wu, H.; Wong, K.H.; Chen, T. Facile synthesis of highly uniform selenium nanoparticles using glucose as the reductant and surface decorator to induce cancer cell apoptosis. *J. Mater. Chem. B* **2016**, *4*, 23512358. [CrossRef]

20. Vieira, A.P.; Stein, E.M.; Andreguetti, D.X.; Cebrián-Torrejón, G.; Doménech-Carbó, A.; Colepicolod, P.; Ferreira, A.M.D. Sweet chemistry: A green way for obtaining selenium nanoparticles active against cancer cells. *J. Braz. Chem. Soc.* **2017**, *28*, 2021–2027. [CrossRef]
21. Husen, A.; Siddiqi, K.S. Plants and microbes assisted selenium nanoparticles: Characterization and application. *J. Nanobiotech.* **2014**, *12*, 28. [CrossRef] [PubMed]
22. Alipour, A.; Kalari, S.; Morowvat, M.H.; Sabahi, Z.; Dehshahri, A. Green synthesis of selenium nanoparticles by Cyanobacterium Spirulina platensis (abdf2224): Cultivation condition quality controls. *BioMed Res. Int.* **2021**, *2021*, 6635297. [CrossRef] [PubMed]
23. Menon, S.; Shrudhi, K.S.; Devi, H.; Agarwal, H.; Shanmugan, K. Efficacy of biogenic selenium nanoparticles from an extract of ginger towards evaluation on anti-microbial and anti-oxidant activities. *Colloid Interface Sci. Commun.* **2019**, *29*, 1–8. [CrossRef]
24. Gunti, L.; Dass, R.S.; Kalagatur, N.K. Phytofabrication of selenium nanoparticles from *Emblica officinalis* fruit extract and exploring its biopotential applications: Antioxidant, antimicrobial, and biocompatibility. *Front. Microbiol.* **2019**, *10*, 931. [CrossRef] [PubMed]
25. Alam, H.; Khatoon, N.; Khan, M.A.; Hussain, S.A.; Saravanan, M.; Sardar, M. Synthesis of selenium nanoparticles using probiotic bacteria Lactobacillus acidophilus and their enhanced antimicrobial activity against resistant bacteria. *J. Clust. Sci.* **2020**, *31*, 1003–1011. [CrossRef]
26. Pyrzynska, K.; Sentkowska, A. Biosynthesis of selenium nanoparticles using plant extracts. *J. Nanostr. Chem.* **2021**, 1–14. [CrossRef]
27. Vyas, J.; Rana, S. Antioxidants activity and green synthesis of selenium nanoparticles using *Allium sativum* extract. *Inter. J. Phytomed.* **2017**, *9*, 634–641. [CrossRef]
28. Wang, Y.Y.; Qiu, W.Y.; Sun, L.; Ding, Z.C.; Ya, J.K. Peparation, characterization, and antioxidant capacities of selenium nanoparticles stabilized using polysaccharide-protein complexes from *Corbicula fluminea*. *Food Biosen.* **2018**, *26*, 177–184. [CrossRef]
29. Zhang, W.; Zhang, J.; Ding, D.; Zhang, L.; Muehlmann, L.A.; Deng, S.; Wang, X.; Li, W. Synthesis and antioxidant properties of Lycium barbarom polysaccharides capped selenium nanoparticles using tea extract. *Art. Cells. Nanomed. Biotechnol.* **2018**, *46*, 1463–1470. [CrossRef]
30. Fardsadegh, B.; Vaghari, H.; Mohammad-Jafari, R.; Najian, Y.; Jafarizadeh-Malmiri, H. Biosynthesis, characterization and antimicrobial activities assessment of fabricated selenium nanoparticles using *Pelargonium zonale* leaf extract. *Green Proc. Synth.* **2019**, *8*, 191–198. [CrossRef]
31. Dumore, N.D.; Mukhopadhyay, M. Antioxidant of aqueous selenium nanoparticles (ASeNPs) and its catalysts activity for 1,1′-diphenyl-2-picrylhydrazyl (DPPH) reduction. *J. Mol. Struct.* **2020**, *1205*, 127637. [CrossRef]
32. Ingole, A.R.; Thakare, S.R.; Khati, N.T.; Wankhade, A.V. Green synthesis of selenium nanoparticles under ambient condition. *Chalcogenide Lett.* **2010**, *7*, 485–489.
33. Anu, K.; Devanesan, S.; Prasanth, R.; AlSalhi, M.S.; Ajithkumar, S.; Singaravelu, G. Biogenesis of selenium nanoparticles and their antileukemia activity. *J. King. Saud. Univ.* **2020**, *32*, 2520–2526. [CrossRef]
34. Sharma, G.; Sharma, A.R.; Bhavesh, R.; Park, J.; Ganbold, B.; Nam, J.S.; Lee, S.S. Biomolecule-mediated synthesis of selenium nanoparticles using dried Vitis vinifera (Raisin) extract. *Molecules* **2014**, *19*, 2761–2770. [CrossRef] [PubMed]
35. Vahdati, M.; Moghadam, T.T. Synthesis and characterization of selenium nanoparticles-lysozyme nanohybrid system with synergistic antibacterial properties. *Sci. Rep.* **2010**, *10*, 510. [CrossRef]
36. Chen, W.; Li, Y.; Yang, S.; Yue, L.; Jiang, Q.; Xia, W. Synthesis and antioxidant properties of chitosan and carboxymethyl chitosan-stabilized selenium nanoparticles. *Carbohydr. Polym.* **2015**, *132*, 574–581. [CrossRef]
37. Chen, W.; Yue, L.; Xia, W. Direct evidence of the OH scavenging activity of selenium nanoparticles. *Anal. Met.* **2018**, *10*, 3534. [CrossRef]
38. Chen, W.; Cheng, H.; Xia, W. Construction of Polygonatum sibiricum polysaccharide functionalized selenium nanoparticles for the enhancement of stability and antioxidant activity. *Antioxidants* **2022**, *11*, 240. [CrossRef]
39. Souto, E.B.; Silva, G.F.; Dias-Ferreira, J.; Zielinska, A.; Ventura, F.; Durazzo, A.; Lucarini, M.; Novellino, E.; Santini, A. Nanopharmaceutics: Part I—Clinical Trials Legislation and Good Manufacturing Practices (GMP) of Nanotherapeutics in EU. *Pharmaceutics* **2020**, *12*, 146. [CrossRef]
40. Geoffrion, L.D.; Hesabizadeh, T.; Medina-Cruz, D.; Kusper, M.; Taylor, P.; Vernet-Crua, A.; Chen, J.; Ajo, A.; Webster, T.J.; Guisbiers, G. Naked selenium nanoparticles for antibacterial and anticancer treatments. *ACS Omega* **2020**, *5*, 2660–2669. [CrossRef]
41. Li, Q.; Chen, T.; Yang, F.; Liu, J.; Zheng, W. Facile and controllable one-step fabrication of selenium nanoparticles assisted by L-cysteine. *Mater. Lett.* **2010**, *64*, 614–617. [CrossRef]
42. Shah, S.T.; Yehra, W.; Saad, O.; Simarani, S.; Chowdhury, Z.; Alhani, A.; Al-Ani, L.A. Surface functionalization of iron oxide nanoparticles with galic acid as potential antioxidant and antimicrobial agents. *Nanomaterials* **2017**, *7*, 306. [CrossRef] [PubMed]
43. Lin, Z.H.; Chris-Wang, C.R. Evidence on the size-dependent absorption spectral evolution of selenium nanoparticles. *Mater. Chem. Phys.* **2005**, *92*, 591–594. [CrossRef]
44. Mellinas, C.; Jiménez, A.; Garrigós, M.C. Microwave-assisted green synthesis and antioxidant activity of selenium nanoparticles using Theobroma cacao L. bean shell extract. *Molecules* **2019**, *24*, 4048. [CrossRef]
45. Alagesan, V.; Venugopal, S. Green synthesis of selenium nanoparticles using leaves extract of *Withania somnifera* and its biological applications and photocatalytic activities. *BioNanoScience* **2019**, *9*, 105–116. [CrossRef]

46. Kamnev, A.; Pamchenkova, P.V.; Dyatlova, Y.A.; Tugarova, A.V. FTIR spectroscopy studies of selenite reduction by cells of the rhizobacterium *Azospirillum brasilense* Sp7 and the formation of selenium nanoparticles. *J. Mol. Struct.* **2017**, *1140*, 106–112. [CrossRef]
47. Vyas, Y.; Rana, S. Antioxidant activity and biogenic synthesis of selenium nanoparticles using the leaf extract of *Aloe vera*. *Int. J. Curr. Pharm. Res.* **2017**, *9*, 147–152. [CrossRef]
48. Chen, W.; Yue, L.; Jiang, Q.; Liu, X.; Xia, W. Synthesis of varisized chitosan-selenium nanocomposites through heating treatment and evaluation of their antioxidant properties. *Inter. J. Biol. Macromol.* **2018**, *114*, 751–758. [CrossRef]
49. Zhang, J.; Wang, W.; Yongping, B.; Zhang, L. Nano red elemental selenium has no size effect in the induction of seleno-enzymes in both cultured cells and mice. *Life Sci.* **2004**, *75*, 237–244. [CrossRef]
50. Zhang, J.; Taylor, E.W.; Wan, X.; Peng, D. Impact of heat treatment on size, structure, and bioactivity of elemental selenium nanoparticles. *Int. J. Nanomed.* **2012**, *7*, 815–825. [CrossRef]
51. Yu, B.; You, P.; Song, M.; Zhou, Y.; Yu, F.; Zheng, W. A facile and fast synthetic approach to create selenium nanoparticles with diverse shapes and their antioxidant ability. *New J. Chem.* **2016**, *40*, 1118–1123. [CrossRef]
52. Pyrzynska, K.; Pękal, A. Application of free radical diphenylpicrylhydrazyl (DPPH) to estimate antioxidant capacity of food samples. *Anal. Meth.* **2013**, *55*, 4288–4295. [CrossRef]
53. Xu, L.; Liang, H.W.; Yang, Y.; Yu, S.H. Stability and reactivity: Positive and negative aspects for nanoparticle processing. *Chem. Rev.* **2018**, *118*, 3209–3250. [CrossRef] [PubMed]
54. Smirnoff, N.; Cumbes, Q.J. Hydroxyl radical scavenging activity of compatible solutes. *Phytochemistry* **1987**, *28*, 1057–1060. [CrossRef]

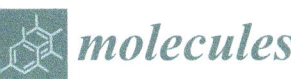

Article

Colorimetric and Electrochemical Methods for the Detection of SARS-CoV-2 Main Protease by Peptide-Triggered Assembly of Gold Nanoparticles

Yunxiao Feng [1], Gang Liu [2,3], Ming La [1,*] and Lin Liu [2,*]

1. College of Chemistry and Chemical Engineering, Pingdingshan University, Pingdingshan 467000, China; 2743@pdsu.edu.cn
2. Henan Province of Key Laboratory of New Optoelectronic Functional Materials, College of Chemistry and Chemical Engineering, Anyang Normal University, Anyang 455000, China; liugang08215@163.com
3. College of Chemistry and Chemical Engineering, Henan University of Technology, Zhengzhou 450011, China
* Correspondence: mingla2011@163.com (M.L.); liulin@aynu.edu.cn (L.L.)

Abstract: Severe acute respiratory syndrome coronavirus 2 (SARS-CoV-2) main protease (Mpro) has been regarded as one of the ideal targets for the development of antiviral drugs. The currently used methods for the probing of Mpro activity and the screening of its inhibitors require the use of a double-labeled peptide substrate. In this work, we suggested that the label-free peptide substrate could induce the aggregation of AuNPs through the electrostatic interactions, and the cleavage of the peptide by the Mpro inhibited the aggregation of AuNPs. This fact allowed for the visual analysis of Mpro activity by observing the color change of the AuNPs suspension. Furthermore, the co-assembly of AuNPs and peptide was achieved on the peptide-covered electrode surface. Cleavage of the peptide substrate by the Mpro limited the formation of AuNPs/peptide assembles, thus allowing for the development of a simple and sensitive electrochemical method for Mpro detection in serum samples. The change of the electrochemical signal was easily monitored by electrochemical impedance spectroscopy (EIS). The detection limits of the colorimetric and electrochemical methods are 10 and 0.1 pM, respectively. This work should be valuable for the development of effective antiviral drugs and the design of novel optical and electrical biosensors.

Keywords: SARS-CoV-2 main protease; colorimetry; electrochemical impedance spectroscopy; gold nanoparticles

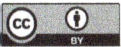

1. Introduction

The outbreak of pneumonia caused by the new coronavirus started from the beginning of 2020 in a global pandemic. The new coronavirus was defined as severe acute respiratory syndrome coronavirus 2 (SARS-CoV-2) by the International Committee on Taxonomy of Viruses and the pneumonia was named coronavirus disease 2019 (2019-nCoV) by the World Health Organization (WHO). The currently approved drugs for treating the infected patients show limited and toxic side effects. Thus, more effective antiviral drugs are still urgently desired [1–3]. The SARS-CoV-2 main protease (Mpro), also known as 3C-like protease (3CLpro), is involved in cleaving the viral polyprotein to produce the essential viral protein required for virus replication and pathogenesis. The protease plays a leading physiological role in the life cycle of the virus and has been regarded as one of the ideal targets for the design of antiviral drugs [4–8]. The commercial kits for the detection of the Mpro and the screening of its inhibitors mainly adopt the fluorescence resonance energy transfer (FRET) method, in which the Mpro catalyzes the hydrolysis of a double-labeled peptide substrate with an acceptor and donor couple [9,10]. Although the approach is sensitive and rapid, it requires the use of an expensive and complicated peptide substrate and advanced instruments [11]. For this reason, it is of importance to develop simple, sensitive, cost-efficient and high-throughput methods for the rapid detection of the Mpro and the screening of its potential inhibitors.

Gold nanoparticles (AuNPs) exhibit a high extinction coefficient and unique size-dependent optical properties. AuNPs-based colorimetric methods have been widely used in the field of biological analysis because of their simple sample processing and low instrument investment [12–15]. Peptides with cysteine and/or positively charged amino acid (e.g., Lys and Arg) residues can induce the aggregation of AuNPs through the Au-S and electrostatic interactions [16–22]. The protease-catalyzed cleavage of the peptide may regulate the aggregation of AuNPs, thus allowing for the detection of protease activity and the screening of its inhibitors. In the commercial kits, a double-labeled peptide with a sequence of acceptor–KTSAVLQSGFRKME–donor can be used as the substrate to monitor Mpro activity. When the substrate is cleaved into two short segments by the Mpro, the acceptor and donor labeled at the two ends of the peptide are separated, resulting in the fluorescence recovery of the donor. In the present work, we found that the label-free peptide with a sequence of RKTSAVLQSGFRK can induce the aggregation of AuNPs through the electrostatic interactions (Scheme 1A). Cleavage of the peptide by the Mpro inhibits the aggregation of AuNPs, thus allowing for the visual analysis of the Mpro by monitoring the color change of the AuNPs suspension. The AuNPs-based homogeneous method is simple, rapid, cost-efficient and high-throughput for monitoring Mpro activity and the screening of its inhibitors, but both the sensitivity and the anti-interference ability of the method for determining the Mpro in biological samples are poor. Electrochemical biosensors can sensitively monitor the cleavage event of the peptide at the liquid–solid interface. Recent studies have shown that the aggregation of nanoparticles induced by the targets can be initiated on the electrode surface, thus implanting one principle into another field [22–29]. Herein, we propose that the liquid phase analysis of the Mpro can be transformed into an electrochemical analysis by regulating the peptide-triggered assembly of AuNPs on the peptide-covered electrode surface (Scheme 1B). The resulting peptide/AuNPs networks can promote the electron transfer of $[Fe(CN)_6]^{3-/4-}$ due to the excellent conductivity and large specific surface area of AuNPs and the positive charges of the peptide framework [22,30]. However, when the peptide substrate immobilized on the electrode surface was cleaved by the Mpro, the assembly of AuNPs on the electrode surface would be prevented. The change of electron transfer resistance can be easily monitored by electrochemical impedance spectroscopy (EIS). The electrochemical method integrates the advantages of colorimetric analysis and surface-tethered biosensors. Finally, the colorimetric method was used to evaluate the activity of the Mpro in the absence and presence of inhibitors, and the electrochemical strategy was employed to determine the Mpro in biological samples.

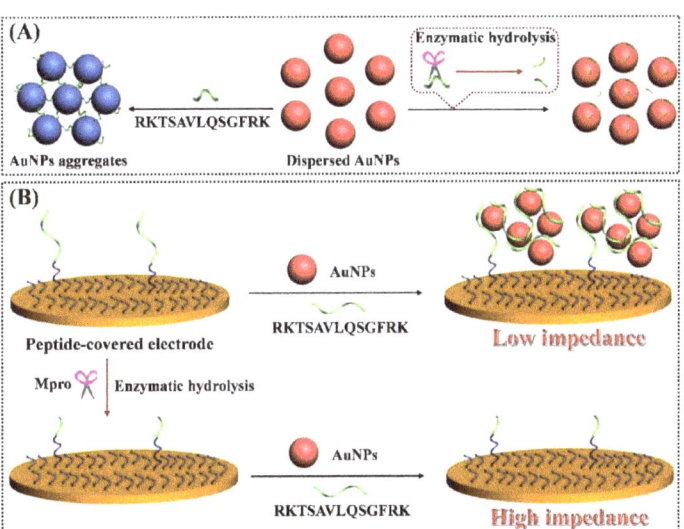

Scheme 1. Schematic illustration of colorimetric (**A**) and electrochemical (**B**) methods for Mpro detection based on the peptide-triggered assembly of AuNPs in solution and on electrode surface, respectively.

2. Results and Discussion

2.1. Feasibility for Colorimetric Analysis of Mpro

For the colorimetric analysis of Mpro activity, a label-free peptide substrate (RKT-SAVLQSGFRK) was designed according to the sequence of the commercial peptide substrate (acceptor–KTSAVLQSGFRKME–donor). The positively charged Lys and Arg residues at both ends can bind with AuNPs through the electrostatic interactions, thus leading to the aggregation of AuNPs. As shown in Figure 1A, the surface plasmon resonance bond of AuNPs changed from 520 nm to 585 nm with the addition of the peptide substrate (curves 1 and 2), which is accompanied by the change of the solution color from red to blue (tubes 1 and 2). The result demonstrated that the peptide can induce the aggregation of AuNPs, which is also confirmed by DLS analysis. Interestingly, when the peptide substrate was incubated with the Mpro for a given time, no apparent changes in the solution color and UV-Vis spectrum were observed (tube/curve 3), demonstrating that the cleavage of the peptide by the Mpro prevented the aggregation of AuNPs. Thus, the activity and concentration of the Mpro may be easily monitored by discriminating the solution color with the naked eye in a convenient and straightforward way. The peptide concentration is crucial for the aggregation of AuNPs. We found that the changes of the solution color and the UV-Vis spectrum were dependent upon the concentration of the peptide. The ratio of the absorbance at 585 nm and 520 nm (A_{585}/A_{520}) was used to evaluate the degree of AuNPs aggregates. The A_{585}/A_{520} was intensified with the increase of the peptide concentration in the range of 0.1~7.5 μM. Since a high concentration of the peptide substrate may decrease the sensitivity of the method, a compromised concentration of the peptide (5 μM) was used for the detection of the Mpro in the follow-up quantitative analysis.

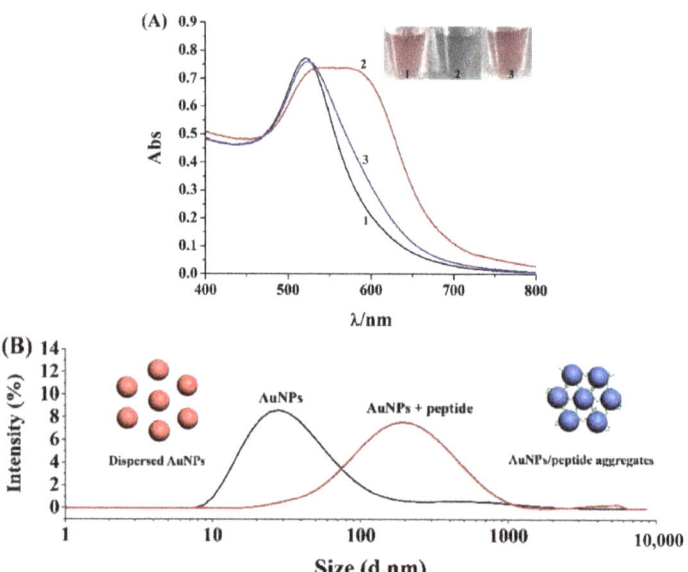

Figure 1. (**A**) UV-Vis spectra and photographs of AuNPs in the absence (curve/tube 1) and presence of peptide (curve/tube 2) or the mixture of peptide and Mpro (curve/tube 3). (**B**) DLS analysis for the peptide-triggered assembly of AuNPs.

2.2. Sensitivity for Colorimetric Analysis of Mpro

The sensitivity of the colorimetric method was evaluated by measuring different concentrations of the Mpro. As shown in Figure 2, the solution color gradually became purple and red from blue with the increase of the Mpro concentration, which was accompanied by the decrease of the absorption intensity at 585 nm. The A_{585}/A_{520} value decreased linearly with the Mpro concentration change from 0.01 to 0.5 nM. The linear equation can be expressed as A_{585}/A_{520} = 0.93–0.85 [Mpro] (nM). The lowest detectable concentration was comparable to that measured by the commercial fluorescence kit. However, the colorimetric method can be performed in a rapid and straightforward way and the peptide substrate is cheap and stable for long-term storage. To demonstrate the application of the method, the inhibitory effect of ebselen (a well-known Mpro inhibitor) was determined. As shown in Figure 3, the A_{585}/A_{520} value was intensified and the solution turned purple when the Mpro was incubated with increasing concentrations of ebselen, demonstrating that higher concentrations of ebselen could inhibit the Mpro activity more effectively. The half-maximum inhibition value (IC_{50}) was calculated according to the inhibition rate (%), described by the following equation:

$$\text{inhibition rate (\%)} = \frac{A^1 - A}{A^1 - A^0} \times \%$$

where A^0 and A^1 represent the A_{585}/A_{520} in the absence and presence of the Mpro at a fixed concentration; A represents the A_{585}/A_{520} in the presence of the Mpro and a given concentration of ebselen. Based on the relationship between the inhibitor rate and the ebselen concentration, the IC_{50} was found to be 7.6 nM, which is consistent with that obtained by the fluorescence kit. Thus, the colorimetric method can be employed to screen the potential Mpro inhibitors for the development of novel antiviral drugs.

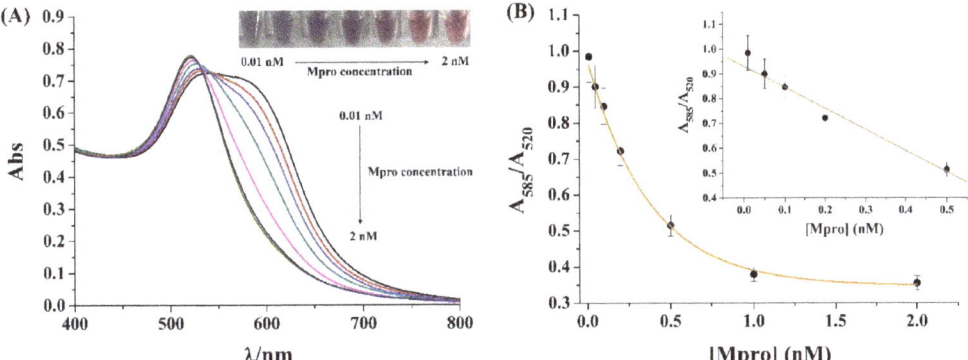

Figure 2. (**A**) UV-Vis spectra and photographs of AuNPs for the analysis of different concentrations of Mpro. (**B**) Dependence of A_{585}/A_{520} on the concentration of Mpro. The inset shows the linear portion of the curve.

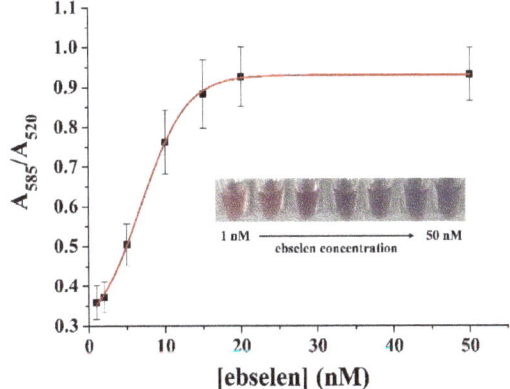

Figure 3. Dependence of A_{585}/A_{520} on the concentration of inhibitor ebselen. The inset shows the photographs for the assays of different concentrations of ebselen.

2.3. Feasibility for Electrochemical Detection of Mpro

Although the colorimetric method is simple and easy to operate, other components in biological samples may adsorb onto the surface of bare AuNPs [31], thus limiting its application for the determination of low concentrations of Mpro in biological matrixes. Based on the principle of the peptide-induced aggregation of AuNPs, we propose that AuNPs could be assembled on the peptide-covered electrode surface due to the similar environment of the gold electrode and AuNPs. The detection principle based on the co-assembly of peptide and AuNPs are illustrated in Scheme 1B. The peptide anchored on the electrode can capture AuNPs via the electrostatic interactions. Then, the captured AuNPs recruit the peptides (RKTSAVLQSGFRK) in the solution via the same interactions. The repeated recruitment of AuNPs and peptide will lead to the formation of peptide/AuNPs aggregates on the electrode surface, thus facilitating the electron transfer of $[Fe(CN)_6]^{3-/4-}$ due to the excellent conductivity and large specific surface area of AuNPs. Once the peptide-covered electrode was pre-incubated with the Mpro, the peptide on the electrode surface would be specifically recognized and cleaved, thus limiting the attachment of AuNPs and preventing the co-assembly of AuNPs and peptide on the electrode surface. As shown in Figure 4A, the electron transfer resistance (R_{et}) of the peptide-covered electrode (curve one) decreased after incubation with the mixture of AuNPs and peptide (curve two) or AuNPs (curve three). The R_{et} for the mixture is greatly lower than that for the AuNPs alone, and no significant change for the R_{et} was observed when the peptide-covered electrode was incubated with the peptide only (data not shown). The result indicated the decrease in the R_{et} (curve two) should be attributed to the co-assembly of AuNPs and peptide. When the peptide-covered electrode was treated by the Mpro, the R_{et} was intensified slightly (curve four), demonstrating that the direct EIS detection of the Mpro by the enzymatic hydrolysis of the peptide substrate on the electrode surface was less sensitive. When the Mpro-treated electrode was incubated with the mixture of AuNPs and peptide, no significant change in the R_{et} was observed (curve five). The result indicated that the cleavage of the peptide prevented the co-assembly of AuNPs and peptide on the electrode surface. The impedance change (ΔR_{et}) between curve two and curve five is greater than that between curve one and curve four, indicating that the sensitivity can be improved by simply treating the sensor electrode with the mixture of AuNPs and peptide. The results were also confirmed by cyclic voltammogram (CV). As depicted in Figure 4B, the incubation of the peptide-covered electrode (curve one) with AuNPs/peptide (curve two) or AuNPs alone (curve three) led to the increase of peak currents, confirming the capture and formation of the peptide/AuNPs networks. When the peptide-covered electrode was treated by the Mpro, the current decreased slightly (cf. curve one and curve four). No significant change was observed when the Mpro-treated sensing electrode was incubated with AuNPs/peptide (cf. curve four and curve five), indicating that the cleavage of the peptide substrate prevented the attachment of AuNPs and the follow-up formation of the AuNPs/peptide networks.

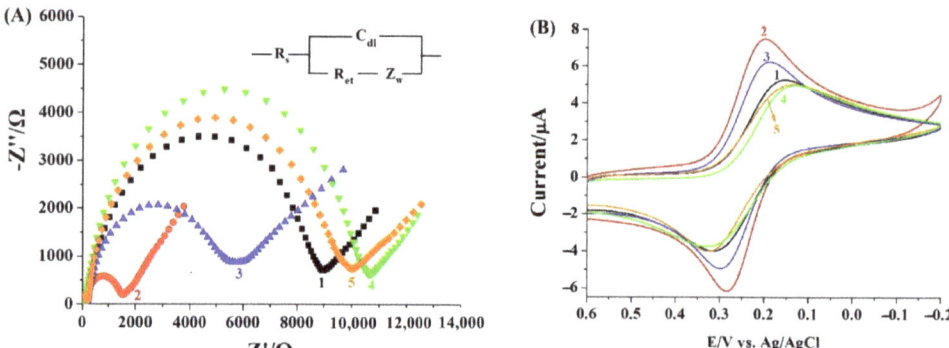

Figure 4. EIS (**A**) and CV (**B**) curves of the peptide-covered sensor electrode after treatment by different solutions: curve 1, buffer; curve 2, AuNPs/peptide; curve 3, AuNPs; curve 4, Mpro; curve 5, Mpro + AuNPs/peptide.

2.4. Sensitivity and Selectivity of the Electrochemical Method

The sensitivity of the electrochemical method was investigated by analyzing the different concentrations of the Mpro. As depicted in Figure 5, the R_{et} increased correspondingly with the increase of the Mpro concentration. A linear relationship was attained between the average ΔR_{et} value of three trails and the Mpro concentration in the range of 0.1~15 pM. The linear equation was found to be ΔR_{et} = 448.9 [Mpro] (pM) + 315.5 with a detection limit down to 0.1 pM. The value is lower than that of the above colorimetric method, demonstrating that the electrochemical method showed relatively higher sensitivity.

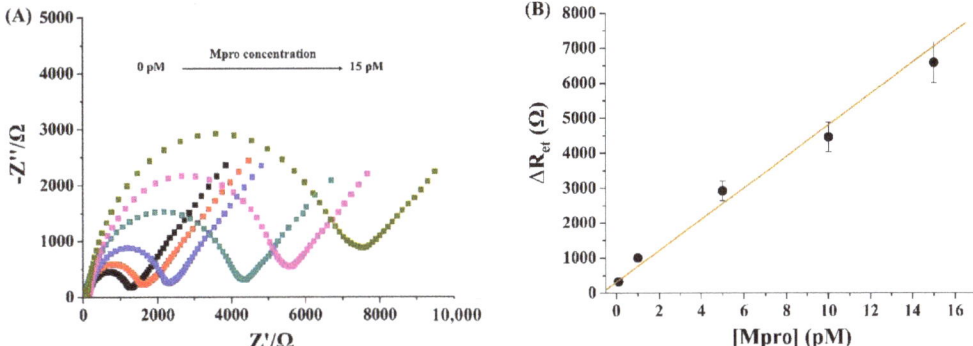

Figure 5. (**A**) EIS curves for the analysis of different concentrations of Mpro (0, 0.1, 1, 5, 10 and 15 pM). (**B**) Dependence of ΔR_{et} on the Mpro concentration.

The selectivity of the method was evaluated by testing BSA, IgG, thrombin and PKA. As shown in Figure 6, the ΔR_{et} value for the Mpro was significantly higher than that for the four proteins, even at a high concentration, demonstrating that the method exhibits excellent selectivity. Additionally, the anti-interference ability of the method was investigated by determining the Mpro in 10% serum. As a result, the ΔR_{et} for determining the Mpro in the serum is not significantly different from that in the buffer. This suggests that the electrochemical method exhibits great potential in biological sample analysis and clinical investigation.

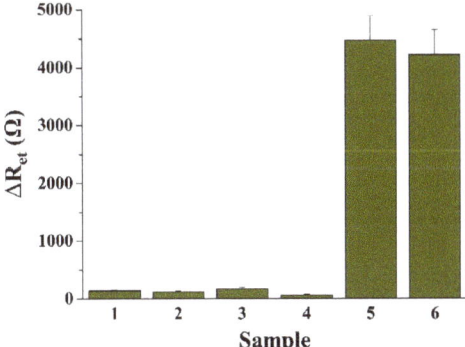

Figure 6. Selectivity of the method toward 0.1 μg/mL BSA (bar 1), 0.5 μg/mL IgG (bar 2), 10 ng/mL thrombin (bar 3), 100 U/mL PKA (bar 4) and 10 pM Mpro in the buffer (bar 5) or 10% serum (bar 6).

3. Materials and Methods

3.1. Chemicals and Reagents

Mpro kits were purchased from Beyotime Biotechnology (Shanghai, China). 11-Mercapto-1-undecanol (MUA), tris(2-carboxyethyl)phosphine (TCEP), bovine serum albumin (BSA), IgG, thrombin, protein kinase (PKA) and serum were purchased from Sigma-Aldrich (Shanghai, China). Chloroauric (III) acid, citrate, phosphate and other reagents were obtained from Aladdin Biochemical Technology Co., Ltd. (Shanghai, China). Peptides were prepared by the solid–solid phase synthesis method with a Focus XI peptide synthesizer.

3.2. Peptide-Triggered Aggregation of AuNPs

AuNPs with an average size of 13 nm were prepared through the citrate reduction method. The prepared AuNPs were diluted with 10 mM phosphate (pH 7.0) to a given concentration. Then, 50 μL of AuNPs suspension was added to 50 μL of peptide (RKTSAVLQS-

GFRK) at different concentrations. After incubation for 5 min, the change of solution color was observed by eyes and the UV-Vis spectra were collected on a Cary 50 spectrophotometer. The aggregation of AuNPs was confirmed by dynamic light scattering (DLS) analysis performed on a Zeta Sizer Nano ZS90 (Malvern Company, Worcestershire, England).

3.3. Colorimetric Assays of Mpro Activity

Mpro was diluted with phosphate buffer to different concentrations. Then, 25 μL of Mpro was mixed with 25 μL of RKTSAVLQSGFRK peptide in a centrifugal tube. After reaction at 37 °C for 30 min, 50 μL of AuNPs suspension was added to the mixture for 5 min incubation. After that, the color change was observed and the UV-Vis spectra were collected. For the inhibition analysis, 20 μL of 1 nM Mpro was first mixed with 5 μL of ebselen at different concentrations. After incubation for 10 min to inhibit the Mpro activity, 25 μL of peptide was added to the Mpro/ebselen mixed solution. The other procedures are similar to those for monitoring the activity of pure Mpro sample.

3.4. Preparation of Sensing Electrode

The gold electrode was incubated with piranha solution, rinsed with water and polished with 0.05 μm aluminum powder. After being washed in 50% ethanol under sonication, the electrode was electrochemically scanned in 0.5 M sulfuric acid. After being rinsed with water and dried with nitrogen, the cleaned electrode was immersed in the peptide solution (10 μM CPPPPKTSAVLQSGFRK and 0.5 mM TCEP in phosphate buffer) at 4 °C overnight. After that, the electrode was incubated with 10 mM MUA for 1 h to block the unreacted gold surface. Finally, the peptide-covered electrode was rinsed with 50% ethanol and used for the detection of Mpro. In this work, the CPPPP segment is an effective linker and spacer for peptide immobilization to attain high cleavage efficiency [32,33].

3.5. Electrochemical Detection of Mpro

For the electrochemical analysis of Mpro, the peptide-covered electrode was incubated with Mpro at a given concentration for 30 min to allow the hydrolysis of the peptide. Then, the electrode was incubated with 25 μL of AuNPs suspension, followed by the addition of 25 μL of RKTSAVLQSGFRK peptide. After being gently rinsed with water, the electrode was placed in 5 mM $[Fe(CN)_6]^{3-/4-}$ for EIS measurement.

4. Conclusions

In summary, this work indicated that the peptide substrate of the Mpro could induce the aggregation and color change of AuNPs. Cleavage of the peptide by Mpro prevented the aggregation of AuNPs and thus facilitated the development of a colorimetric method for the analysis of Mpro activity and the screening of its inhibitors. In contrast to the commercial fluorescence kit, the method features the advantages of being low cost, having good stability, facile operation and naked-eye readout. Furthermore, we developed a sensitive surface-tethered method for Mpro detection by implanting the principle of the colorimetric assay into the electrochemical field. In contrast to the colorimetric method, the electrochemical method showed a higher sensitivity and a better anti-interference ability and has been used for the assay of Mpro in a 10% human serum with a satisfactory result. The proposed approach based on the co-assembly of AuNPs and peptide on the electrode surface should be promising as a general strategy for the design of protease biosensors by matching the sequence of the peptide substrate and using appropriate types of nanomaterials.

Author Contributions: Conceptualization, M.L. and L.L.; methodology, Y.F.; investigation, Y.F. and G.L.; writing—original draft preparation, Y.F.; writing—review and editing, L.L; project administration, M.L.; funding acquisition, L.L. All authors have read and agreed to the published version of the manuscript.

Funding: This research was funded by the Program for Innovative Research Team of Science and Technology in the University of Henan Province (21IRTSTHN005) and the National Natural Science Foundation of China (U2004193).

Institutional Review Board Statement: Not applicable.

Informed Consent Statement: Not applicable.

Data Availability Statement: Not applicable.

Conflicts of Interest: The authors declare no conflict of interest.

Sample Availability: Not available.

References

1. Jin, Z.; Du, X.; Xu, Y.; Deng, Y.; Liu, M.; Zhao, Y.; Zhang, B.; Li, X.; Zhang, L.; Peng, C.; et al. Structure of Mpro from SARS-CoV-2 and discovery of its inhibitors. *Nature* **2020**, *582*, 289. [CrossRef] [PubMed]
2. Dai, W.; Zhang, B.; Jiang, X.-M.; Su, H.; Li, J.; Zhao, Y.; Xie, X.; Jin, Z.; Peng, J.; Liu, F.; et al. Structure-based design of antiviral drug candidates targeting the SARS-CoV-2 main protease. *Science* **2020**, *368*, 1331. [CrossRef] [PubMed]
3. Sarkar, A.; Mandal, K. Repurposing an antiviral drug against SARS-CoV-2 main protease. *Angew. Chem. Int. Ed.* **2021**, *60*, 23492. [CrossRef] [PubMed]
4. Zhang, L.; Lin, D.; Sun, X.; Curth, U.; Drosten, C.; Sauerhering, L.; Becker, S.; Rox, K.; Hilgenfeld, R. Crystal structure of SARS-CoV-2 main protease provides a basis for design of improved α α-ketoamide inhibitors. *Science* **2020**, *368*, 409. [CrossRef]
5. Olubiyi, O.O.; Olagunju, M.; Keutmann, M.; Loschwitz, J.; Strodel, B. High throughput virtual screening to discover inhibitors of the main protease of the coronavirus SARS-CoV-2. *Molecules* **2020**, *25*, 3193. [CrossRef]
6. Wang, J.; Lv, M.; Xia, H.; Du, J.; Zhao, Y.; Li, H.; Zhang, Z. Minimalist design for a hand-held SARS-Cov2 sensor: Peptide-induced covalent assembly of hydrogel enabling facile fiber-optic detection of a virus marker protein. *ACS Sens.* **2021**, *6*, 2465–2471. [CrossRef]
7. Chauhan, N.; Soni, S.; Gupta, A.; Jain, U. New and developing diagnostic platforms for COVID-19: A systematic review. *Expert. Rev. Mol. Diagn.* **2020**, *20*, 971. [CrossRef]
8. Soni, S.; Pudake, R.N.; Jain, U.; Chauhan, N. A systematic review on SARS-CoV-2-associated fungal coinfections. *J. Med. Virol.* **2022**, *94*, 99. [CrossRef]
9. Moore, C.; Borum, R.M.; Mantri, Y.; Xu, M.; Fajtová, P.; O'Donoghue, A.J.; Jokerst, J.V. Activatable carbocyanine dimers for photoacoustic and fluorescent detection of protease activity. *ACS Sens.* **2021**, *6*, 2356–2365. [CrossRef]
10. Brown, A.S.; Ackerley, D.F.; Calcott, M.J. High-throughput screening for inhibitors of the SARS-CoV-2 protease using a FRET-biosensor. *Molecules* **2020**, *25*, 4666. [CrossRef]
11. Cihlova, B.; Huskova, A.; Böserle, J.; Nencka, R.; Boura, E.; Silhan, J. High-throughput fluorescent assay for inhibitor screening of proteases from RNA viruses. *Molecules* **2021**, *26*, 3792. [CrossRef]
12. Liu, X.; Wang, Y.; Chen, P.; Wang, Y.; Zhang, J.; Aili, D.; Liedberg, B. Biofunctionalized gold nanoparticles for colorimetric sensing of botulinum neurotoxin a light chain. *Anal. Chem.* **2014**, *86*, 2345. [CrossRef]
13. Mauriz, E. Clinical applications of visual plasmonic colorimetric sensing. *Sensors* **2020**, *20*, 6214. [CrossRef]
14. Siddiquee, S.; Saallah, S.; Bohari, N.A.; Ringgit, G.; Roslan, J.; Naher, L.; Nudin, N.F.H. Visual and optical absorbance detection of melamine in milk by melamine-induced aggregation of gold nanoparticles. *Nanomaterials* **2021**, *11*, 1142. [CrossRef]
15. Guarise, C.; Pasquato, L.; Filippis, V.D.; Scrimin, P. Gold nanoparticles-based protease assay. *Proc. Natl. Acad. Sci. USA* **2006**, *103*, 3978. [CrossRef]
16. Chang, C.-C.; Chen, C.-P.; Wu, T.-H.; Yang, C.-H.; Lin, C.-W.; Chen, C.-Y. Gold nanoparticle-based colorimetric strategies for chemical and biological sensing applications. *Nanomaterials* **2019**, *9*, 861. [CrossRef]
17. Aldewachi, H.S.; Woodroofe, N.; Turega, S.; Gardiner, P.H.E. Optimization of gold nanoparticle-based real-time colorimetric assay of dipeptidyl peptidase IV activity. *Talanta* **2017**, *169*, 13. [CrossRef]
18. Chen, G.; Xie, Y.; Zhang, H.; Wang, P.; Cheung, H.-Y.; Yang, M.; Sun, H. A general colorimetric method for detecting protease activity based on peptide-induced gold nanoparticle aggregation. *RSC Adv.* **2014**, *4*, 6560. [CrossRef]
19. Kim, C.-J.; Lee, D.-I.; Kim, C.; Lee, K.; Lee, C.-H.; Ahn, I.-S. Gold nanoparticles-based colorimetric assay for Cathepsin B activity and the efficiency of its inhibitors. *Anal. Chem.* **2014**, *86*, 3825. [CrossRef]
20. Su, S.; Yu, T.; Hu, J.; Xianyu, Y. A bio-inspired plasmonic nanosensor for angiotensin-converting enzyme through peptide-mediated assembly of gold nanoparticles. *Biosens. Bioelectron.* **2022**, *195*, 113621. [CrossRef]
21. Xia, N.; Zhou, B.; Huang, N.; Jiang, M.; Zhang, J.; Liu, L. Visual and fluorescent assays for selective detection of beta-amyloid oligomers based on the inner filter effect of gold nanoparticles on the fluorescence of CdTe quantum dots. *Biosens. Bioelectron.* **2016**, *85*, 625. [CrossRef]
22. Xia, N.; Wang, X.; Yu, J.; Wu, Y.; Cheng, S.; Xing, Y.; Liu, L. Design of electrochemical biosensors with peptide probes as the receptors of targets and the inducers of gold nanoparticles assembly on electrode surface. *Sens. Actuat. B Chem.* **2017**, *239*, 834. [CrossRef]

23. Gu, Y.; Jiang, Z.; Ren, D.; Shang, Y.; Hu, Y.; Yi, L. Electrochemiluminescence sensor based on the target recognition-induced aggregation of sensing units for Hg^{2+} determination. *Sens. Actuat. B Chem.* **2021**, *337*, 129821. [CrossRef]
24. Liu, L.; Cheng, C.; Chang, Y.; Ma, H.; Hao, Y. Two sensitive electrochemical strategies for the detection of protein kinase activity based on the 4-mercaptophenylboronic acid-induced in situ assembly of silver nanoparticles. *Sens. Actuat. B Chem.* **2017**, *248*, 178. [CrossRef]
25. Wei, T.; Dong, T.; Wang, Z.; Bao, J.; Tu, W.; Dai, Z. Aggregation of individual sensing units for signal accumulation: Conversion of liquid-phase colorimetric assay into enhanced surface-tethered electrochemical analysis. *J. Am. Chem. Soc.* **2015**, *137*, 8880–8883. [CrossRef]
26. Xia, N.; Wang, X.; Zhou, B.; Wu, Y.; Mao, W.; Liu, L. Electrochemical detection of amyloid-beta oligomers based on the signal amplification of a network of silver nanoparticles. *ACS Appl. Mater. Interfaces* **2016**, *8*, 19303. [CrossRef]
27. Zhao, Y.; Cui, L.; Ke, W.; Zheng, F.; Li, X. Electroactive Au@Ag nanoparticle assembly driven signal amplification for ultrasensitive chiral recognition of D/LTrp. *ACS Sustain. Chem. Eng.* **2019**, *7*, 5157–5166. [CrossRef]
28. Zhou, M.; Han, L.; Deng, D.; Zhang, Z.; He, H.; Zhang, L.; Luo, L. 4-Mercaptobenzoic acid modified silver nanoparticles-enhanced electrochemical sensor for highly sensitive detection of Cu^{2+}. *Sens. Actuat B. Chem.* **2019**, *291*, 164. [CrossRef]
29. Han, Y.; Zhang, Y.; Wu, S.; Jalalah, M.; Alsareii, S.A.; Yin, Y.; Harraz, F.A.; Li, G. Co-assembly of peptides and carbon nanodots: Sensitive analysis of transglutaminase 2. *ACS Appl. Mater. Interfaces* **2021**, *13*, 36919–36925. [CrossRef] [PubMed]
30. Cao, Y.; Yu, J.; Bo, B.; Shu, Y.; Li, G. A simple and general approach to assay protease activity with electrochemical technique. *Biosens. Bioelectron.* **2013**, *45*, 1. [CrossRef] [PubMed]
31. Chang, C.-C.; Chen, C.-P.; Lee, C.-H.; Chen, C.-Y.; Lin, C.-W. Colorimetric detection of human chorionic gonadotropin using catalytic gold nanoparticles and apeptide aptamer. *Chem. Commun.* **2014**, *50*, 14443. [CrossRef]
32. Nowinski, A.K.; Sun, F.; White, A.D.; Keefe, A.J.; Jiang, S. Sequence, structure, and function of peptide self-assembled monolayers. *J. Am. Chem. Soc.* **2012**, *134*, 6000–6005. [CrossRef]
33. Xia, N.; Huang, Y.; Cui, Z.; Liu, S.; Deng, D.; Liu, L.; Wang, J. Impedimetric biosensor for assay of caspase-3 activity and evaluation of cell apoptosis using self-assembled biotin-phenylalanine network as signal enhancer. *Sens. Actuat. B Chem.* **2020**, *320*, 128436. [CrossRef]

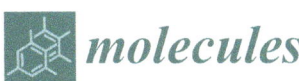

Review

Organic Nanoplatforms for Iodinated Contrast Media in CT Imaging

Peng Zhang [1,†], Xinyu Ma [2,†], Ruiwei Guo [2], Zhanpeng Ye [2], Han Fu [3], Naikuan Fu [1], Zhigang Guo [1], Jianhua Zhang [2,4,*] and Jing Zhang [1,*]

1. Department of Cardiology, Tianjin Chest Hospital, Tianjin University, Tianjin 300222, China; peng306588_0@163.com (P.Z.); cdrfnk@163.com (N.F.); zmedicalscience@163.com (Z.G.)
2. Key Laboratory of Systems Bioengineering of the Ministry of Education, Department of Polymer Science and Engineering, School of Chemical Engineering and Technology, Tianjin University, Tianjin 300350, China; 2019207009@tju.edu.cn (X.M.); rwguo@263.net (R.G.); yzphg@tju.edu.cn (Z.Y.)
3. Graduate School, Tianjin Medical University, Tianjin 300070, China; fuhan716@tmu.edu.cn
4. Tianjin Key Laboratory of Membrane Science and Desalination Technology, Tianjin University, Tianjin 300350, China
* Correspondence: jhuazhang@tju.edu.cn (J.Z.); zj2008tj@163.com (J.Z.)
† These authors contributed equally to this work.

Abstract: X-ray computed tomography (CT) imaging can produce three-dimensional and high-resolution anatomical images without invasion, which is extremely useful for disease diagnosis in the clinic. However, its applications are still severely limited by the intrinsic drawbacks of contrast media (mainly iodinated water-soluble molecules), such as rapid clearance, serious toxicity, inefficient targetability and poor sensitivity. Due to their high biocompatibility, flexibility in preparation and modification and simplicity for drug loading, organic nanoparticles (NPs), including liposomes, nanoemulsions, micelles, polymersomes, dendrimers, polymer conjugates and polymeric particles, have demonstrated tremendous potential for use in the efficient delivery of iodinated contrast media (ICMs). Herein, we comprehensively summarized the strategies and applications of organic NPs, especially polymer-based NPs, for the delivery of ICMs in CT imaging. We mainly focused on the use of polymeric nanoplatforms to prolong circulation time, reduce toxicity and enhance the targetability of ICMs. The emergence of some new technologies, such as theragnostic NPs and multimodal imaging and their clinical translations, are also discussed.

Keywords: biomedical imaging; iodinated contrast media; X-ray computed tomography; organic nanoparticles; iodinated polymers

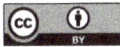

1. Introduction

Noninvasive in vivo bioimaging techniques are extremely valuable and useful for the visualization of an abnormal state within the body, the detection of the pathological situations of patients, assessment of the therapy efficacy and disease management [1,2]. According to the energy or signal sources to produce images, imaging modalities in the clinic are generally categorized using the following: ultrasound imaging (US), photoacoustic imaging (PA), positron emission tomography (PET), single-photon emission computed tomography (SPECT), fluorescence imaging (FI), luminescence imaging (LI), nuclear magnetic resonance imaging (MRI) and X-ray computed tomography (CT) [3]. Each imaging modality possesses its own unique advantages along with intrinsic limitations. US imaging offers real-time noninvasive imaging of soft tissue based on high-frequency sound waves. Its advantages include the fact that it is highly portable, has a low cost and is free of radiation risk, but its clinical applications are not suitable for adipose tissues and bones, and it can be strongly interfered with by air or gas and air-filled tissues [4]. PET and SPECT as high-resolution imaging modalities still suffer from the health hazard of radioactive components and extremely high costs [5]. The advantages of FI and LI imaging are their high sensitivity and high temporal resolution. Nevertheless, their clinical applications are severely impeded by the limited depth of light penetration through the tissues [6]. As a radiation-free and safe medical imaging technique, MRI can provide anatomical images of soft tissues, organs and blood vessels, but this expensive modality can be easily distorted by metal objects in the body [7].

Among all imaging modalities, computed tomography (CT) imaging has become one of the most powerful and popular imaging modalities for diseases diagnosis in modern clinical practice [1,8–10]. It can offer three-dimensional (3D) anatomic images with excellent spatial resolution based on X-ray attenuation. However, CT imaging can only offer superior images of electron-dense materials. To achieve high contrast within the body, it needs a very large difference between atomic weights or material densities within the patient. For example, due to the big difference between electron-dense bones and surrounding soft tissues, bone structures in the whole body can be visible using CT imaging under X-ray irradiation. However, for soft tissues with similar densities, their exquisite details cannot be distinguished clearly using CT imaging. Additionally, thus, to clearly delineate various tissues and detect subtle changes within tissues, the administration of exogenous contrast media is often required for most patients for effective CT imaging. Exogenous CT contrast media are distributed into different tissues, affording transient contrast enhancement in soft tissues under X-ray irradiation.

In current clinical practice, barium- and iodine-based compounds are routinely used as contrast media for in vivo CT imaging. Barium-based contrast media are restricted only to gastrointestinal tract imaging via oral route due to their inherent high toxicity. Therefore, iodinated contrast media (ICMs) have become the most prevalent intravenous media used for X-ray CT imaging. The yearly use of the ICMs was estimated to reach approximately 90 million doses worldwide.

2. Iodinated Contrast Media

For better visualization of soft tissues and especially for identifying the interface between two adjacent soft tissues, the presence of a great difference in X-ray attenuation around the lesion location is indispensable for CT imaging to achieve high contrast-to-noise ratios. The contrast media containing high-Z elements can enhance differentiation among different tissues, because the X-ray attenuation effect of a material generally increases with its atomic number [9,11]. Iodine has historically been the atom of choice for the applications of CT imaging, and now, small iodinated compounds predominantly dominate X-ray contrast media due to their high atomic number ($Z = 53$), high X-ray absorption coefficient and their great flexibility and versatility in chemical synthesis [12]. Water-soluble sodium iodide and potassium iodide are among the earliest contrast media, first used in 1924. However, at the concentrations necessary for imaging, inorganic iodine solutions exhibit high toxicity, which severely hinder their clinical applications. The development of ICMs rapidly moved from inorganic iodine to organic iodinated molecules. Some commercially available, clinically approved organic ICMs are summarized in Figure 1. Organic ICMs started as ionic mono-iodinated, di-iodinated and tri-iodinated molecules. As shown in Figure 1, ionic iodinated molecules mainly include Iothalamate, Uroselectan A, Uroselectan B and Diatrizoate, which are often the derivatives of iodine-containing benzoic acid [8,9,13,14]. These ionic iodinated molecules are high osmolar contrast materials, which are associated with some severe side effects.

Continuous efforts were directed toward minimizing risks of contrast reactions during the 1960s. Compared with ionic molecules, nonionic compounds do not dissociate in water and thus have much lower osmolality. Moreover, they have a lower tendency to interact with cell membranes, peptides and other biological structures. Therefore, the toxicity of nonionic compounds is significantly lower than that of ionic molecules. As a result, the exploitation of ICMs with improved imaging capabilities and reduced toxicity focused on the nonionic iodinated molecules. As presented in Figure 1, the nonionic iodinated contrast media mainly include Iohexol, Iopromide, Ioversol, Iomeprol, Iopamidol and Iopentol. Nearly all of them are tri-iodinated benzene derivatives with very similar structures. The benzene ring not only can offer a stable framework for the three adjacent iodine atoms, but also increase the effective molecular size and decrease the toxicity. Moreover, the other positions of the benzene ring are occupied by long side chains rich in hydroxy groups, ensuring high water solubility and low toxicity. In addition to iodinated monomers, ionic and nonionic dimers were also developed, such as Ioxaglate, Iotrolan and Iotrolan, as shown in Figure 2. Compared with monomers, dimers possess much lower osmolality, which can alleviate pain at the site of injection and decrease the renal injury and cardiovascular complications. However, the viscosity of nonionic dimers is much higher than that of monomers, often leading to a slower excretion and more painful injection compared with some monomeric agents [8,9,13,14].

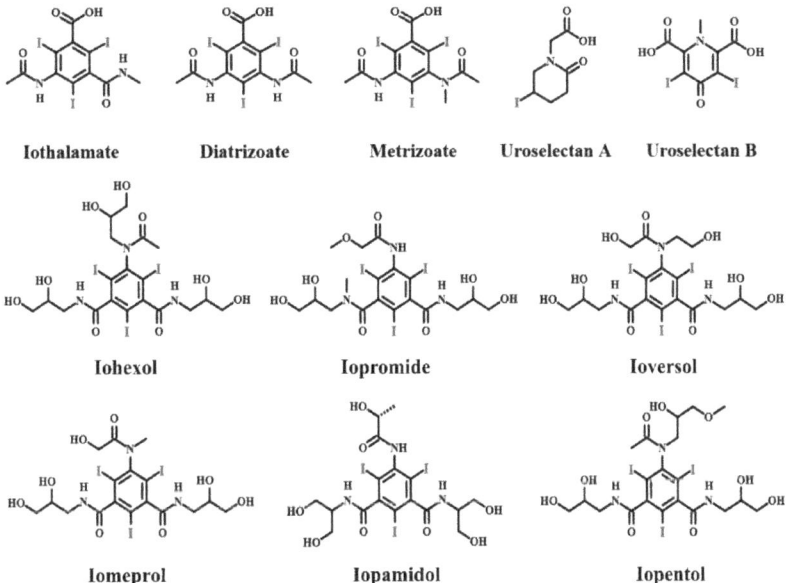

Figure 1. Ionic and nonionic iodinated contrast media.

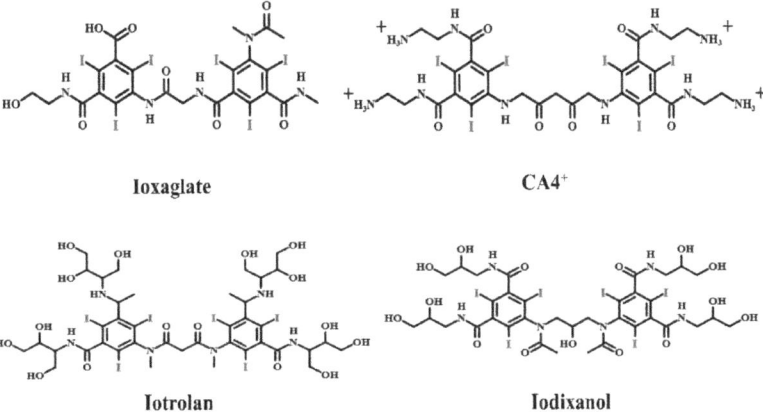

Figure 2. Ionic and nonionic dimers as iodinated contrast media.

3. Iodinated Macromolecular Contrast Media

The last several decades have witnessed tremendous progress in nonionic ICMs. However, their clinical applications are still hampered by some limitations: (1) rapid renal excretion and thus a very short circulation time [10,14,15]; (2) serious adverse effects, especially contrast-induced nephropathy (CIN), with potential life-threatening injuries [16,17]; (3) inefficient targetability and thus unclear CT imaging at target lesions [18,19]. In order to address these limitations, great efforts have been made to develop and optimize these small-molecule ICMs [8,9,20–23]. Due to their unique biocompatibility, designability, biodegradation, facile synthesis and modification capability, polymers have opened up a new avenue to enhance the delivery efficacy and biocompatibility of ICMs [24–35]. The applications of polymers for ICM delivery can be achieved using a combination of polymers and small iodinated compounds through various mechanisms. One of the most important approaches is the design and preparation of iodinated macromolecular contrast media. The main strategies based on polymerization technologies for combining polymer and ICMs to prepare macromolecular contrast media are shown in Figure 3. The macromolecular contrast media can be prepared by free radical polymerization, condensation polymerization or ring-opening polymerization of iodine-containing monomers [36–39]. For example, triiodobenzoate-containing vinylic monomers, such as 3-(methacryloy-lamidoacetamido)-2,4,6-triiodobenzoic acid (MABTIB) [40], 2-hydroxy-3-methacryloyloxypropyl (2,3,5-triiodobenzoate) (HMTIB) [41,42] and 2-methacryloyloxyethyl (2,3,5-triiodobenzoate) (MAOETIB) [36,43] were widely used to prepare radiopaque polymers by homo-polymerization or copolymerization with other vinylic monomers. It is worth pointing out that some iodine-containing vinylic monomers, such as triiodophenyl methacrylate, only can be used to obtain low molecular weight polymers (oligomers), due to the steric hinderance effect of the iodinated aromatic nucleus [44]. In addition, some iodine-containing diol monomers, such as 2,2-bis(iodomethyl)-1,3-propanediol [38] and 2,2-bis(hydroxymethyl)propane-1,3-diyl bis(2,3,5-triiodobenzoate) [45], were used to undergo condensation polymerization with diacids to prepare iodinated polyesters as a versatile platform for radiopaque biomaterials. Moreover, ring-opening polymerization also can be applied to prepare iodinated macromolecular contrast media. For example, a new iodine-functionalized trimethylene carbonate as monomer can be used in ring-opening polymerization using CH_3O-PEG-OH as an initiator and zinc bis[bis(trimethylsilyl) amide] as a catalyst to prepare iodinated polymer poly(ethylene glycol)-b-poly(iodine trimethylene carbonate) with an ultrahigh iodine content of 60.4 wt.% [30].

In addition, iodinated macromolecular contrast media can be also prepared via the modification or functionalization of polymer chains via iodination reaction, addition reaction and conjugation or graft reaction [46–48], as summarized in Figure 4. For example, polyvinyl phenol can be iodinated via aromatic electrophilic substitution, using sodium iodide (NaI) as an iodination reagent [46]. Iodic acid (HIO_3) was also used as an iodination reagent to prepare iodinated macromolecular contrast media [48]. In addition, the addition reaction between iodine and unsaturated carbon compounds was widely used as an effective approach to prepare diiodine compounds and iodinated polymers. For example, iodinated chitosan derivatives were prepared using the iodine addition reaction [49]. The most widely used strategy for the synthesis of iodinated polymers is chemical conjugation reaction. The chemical conjugation of iodinated compounds onto polymer backbones [50–53] or onto the surface of polymers including dendrimers [54–56] and star polyesters [45,57] was also widely used to prepare various macromolecular contrast media. Due to the high simplicity and versatility in preparation, the wide availability of starting materials and the extremely high reactivity with alcohols and phenols, or ammonia and amines, iodine-containing acyl chlorides (especially for 2,3,5-triiodobezoyl chloride) were widely conjugated onto various polymer chains, such as celluloses [58], chitosan [50,59] and polyvinyl alcohol [52], as well as dendrimers [54–56]. These results indicated that strategies based on iodinated macromolecular contrast media have great potential to overcome those intrinsic limitations of small molecular ICM compounds. In addition, it is worth pointing out that iodinated macromolecular contrast media often suffer from a relatively low iodine content. Nonetheless, macromolecular contrast media with tailored functionality have opened up new possibilities for precise imaging and diagnosis.

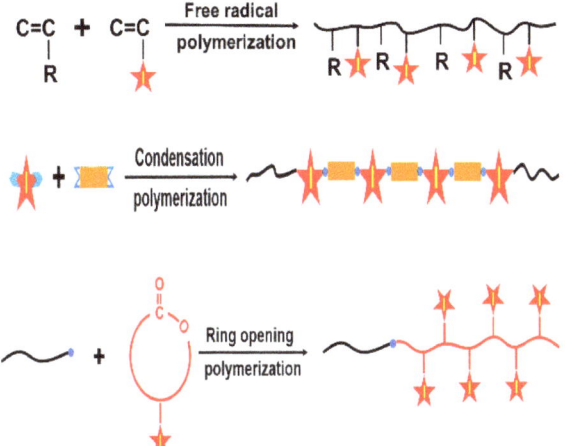

Figure 3. Polymerization strategies for combining polymer and ICMs to prepare iodinated macromolecular contrast media via free radical polymerization, condensation polymerization and ring opening polymerization of iodine-containing monomers, (Star refers to iodine-carrying groups or compounds).

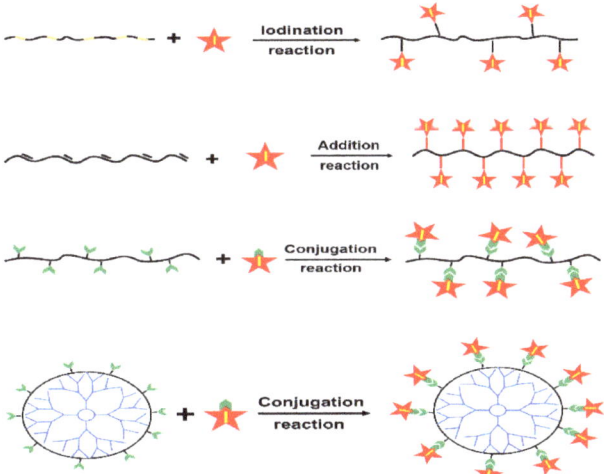

Figure 4. Reaction strategies for combining polymer and ICMs to prepare iodinated macromolecular contrast media via iodination reaction, iodine addition reaction and chemical conjugation of ICMs on polymer chains, the surface of dendrimers or hyperbranched polyesters, (Star refers to iodine-carrying groups or compounds).

Apparently, the strategies and applications of polymers to produce iodinated macromolecular contrast media can endow the unique advantages of polymers to small molecular ICMs, especially the ability of self-assembly into nanostructures, which will open a new avenue for the future design of biosafe and efficient CT contrast media. Moreover, both small molecular ICMs and iodinated macromolecular contrast media can also be loaded into various nanocarriers to form nanoscale contrast media, which can thoroughly improve the efficacy of ICMs' delivery and change their metabolic pathway, thus exhibiting great potential to address the abovementioned issues of traditional ICMs [1,8,20,60–64]. Nevertheless, an exhaustive discussion on the biomedical applications of organic nanoparticles (NPs) for delivering ICMs is currently missing in the literature. Herein we comprehensively summarize the strategies and applications of organic NPs, including liposomes, nanoemulsions, micelles, polymersomes, dendrimers, polymer conjugates and polymeric particles, for the efficient delivery of small molecular ICMs and iodinated macromolecular contrast media. We mainly focus on the use of polymeric nanoplatforms to prolong circulation time, reduce toxicity and enhance the targetability of ICMs. The emergence of some new technologies, such as theragnostic NPs and multimodal imaging and their clinical translations, are also discussed.

4. Organic Nanoparticles for ICMs Delivery
4.1. Nanoparticles for Biomedical Applications

In the past several decades, nanoparticulate systems have gained a great amount of attention as one of the most promising biomedical materials, due to their unique physicochemical properties, nano-sized characteristics, controlled shape and versatile modification possibilities, as well as well-defined multifunctionalities. A wide variety of nanomaterials, such as carbon-based NPs, silica-based and other inorganic NPs, semiconductor NPs, metal and metal oxide NPs, as well as organic NPs (e.g., liposomes, nanoemulsions and polymer-based NPs, including micelles and nanogels, polymersomes, dendrimer, polymer-drug conjugations and protein NPs) have been developed and employed in a diverse array of biomedical fields, as shown in Figure 5. These nanomaterials provide a powerful platform for the site-specific and controllable delivery of drugs, genes, proteins and contrast agents; some of them exhibit noticeable antibacterial, antiviral and antifungal activities. Some inorganic and metal NPs with unique physicochemical properties can be used for photoacoustic, photothermal or photodynamic as well as hyperthermal therapy. In addition, some functional NPs can find wide applications in a new generation of intelligent biosensing, bioseparation, cell labeling, bioimaging and diagnosing.

The in vivo transportation behavior and metabolic processes of NPs are different from traditional small molecular compounds. After invading a biological milieu, NPs will inevitably make contact with a huge variety of biomolecules in body fluids or blood, such as sugars, proteins and lipids, leading to the formation of the so-called "protein corona" and clearance via the reticuloendothelial system (RES) and/or mononuclear phagocytic system (MPS). Undoubtedly, the circulation behavior and time in blood of NPs are critical for their biodistribution and metabolism, accumulation in targeted tissues and thus therapeutic and diagnostic efficacy. As is well known, the in vivo behaviors of NPs are dictated by their physicochemical properties, such as hydrophilic–lipophilic properties, surface feature and surface charge, particle size and particle shape. For example, the hydrophilicity of NPs can impede aggregation and opsonization in water or serum and prolong the circulation time of NPs. Surface charge is another important factor that can definitely affect the fate of NPs administered in biological systems. Positively charged NPs have higher affinity with negatively charged cell membrane but often suffer from serious aggregation and rapid clearance after injection due to nonspecific interactions with blood components. The size and shape of NPs also contribute significantly to their biodistribution in circulation and interaction with tissues and cells. Generally, the ideal size of NPs for long circulation is in the range of 20–200 nm. The size of NPs should be larger than 20 nm in diameter in order to avoid filtration via the kidney and smaller than 200 nm to avoid specific sequestration via fenestra of liver and sinusoids in spleen. Spherical NPs can be more efficiently taken up by cells than non-spherical NPs with similar sizes and under the same conditions. Nevertheless, non-spherical NPs exhibit superior properties to their spherical counterparts in terms of escaping from phagocytosis and circulating in blood. In sum, the effect of the physicochemical properties of NPs on biological systems is very complicated and unclear, which should be fully demonstrated prior to the widespread application of NPs in pharmaceutical, biomedical and diagnostic fields.

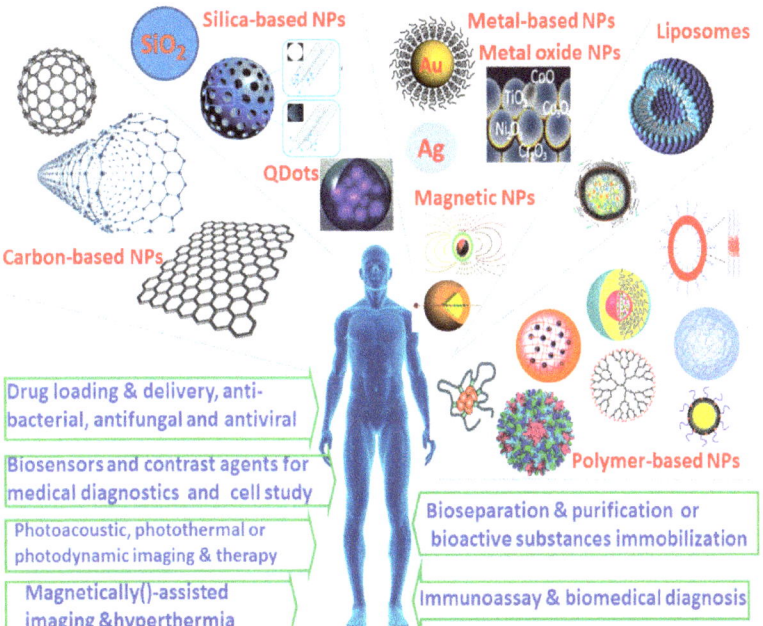

Figure 5. Types of nanoplatforms currently described in biomedical fields [65]. Reprinted with permission from ref. [65], Copyright 2015 MDPI.

As mentioned above, iodine-based contrast media have shown a very high potential for CT diagnostic applications. However, some inherent drawbacks, such as the short circulation time, poor biocompatibility and inefficient targeting capability, inhibited the more widespread application of such media. To meet increasingly rigorous requirements for clinical use, a great number of approaches have been explored to effectively surmount these drawbacks [8,9,21–23,61,62,66,67]. The strategies and applications of organic NPs with desirable functions and excellent performances for medical imaging have gained an enormous amount of attention [3,32–34,38,68–76]. This is due to the fact that organic NPs possess a great number of desirable physicochemical properties, such as simplicity for drug loading, high biocompatibility, desirable biodegradation, facile synthesis, low cost as well as great flexibility and versatility in modification or functionalization [28,34,61,62,65,72–82]. Apparently, the applications of organic NPs and especially polymeric NPs for ICMs' delivery offer an excellent improvement in X-ray imaging and medical diagnosis [33,34,83]. A variety of organic NPs, such as PEGylated liposomes, nanoemulsions, micelles, polymersomes, dendrimers and natural NPs, have been explored in the development of functionalized contrast media with better biocompatibility, longer circulation time or more efficient targeting capability [8,33,34,64,76,83]. Different types of organic NPs for ICMs' delivery are described below.

4.2. Liposomes for ICMs Delivery

As mentioned above, small iodinated compounds are widely used as injectable CT contrast media in the clinic. However, because small ICMs can be rapidly cleared from the bloodstream through the kidney, one of the long-standing challenges for their application is their inherently short circulation time, leading to a very narrow window for imaging after injection and serious side effects in the excretion pathway [8,10,60]. Great effort has been made to develop long-acting forms of ICMs. As one of the earliest and most widespread nanotechnologies for drug delivery, liposomes have been widely used for ICMs' delivery [82,84–87]. As shown in Figure 6, liposomes consist of an aqueous core enclosed by a lipid bilayer of natural phospholipids, which can be used to encapsulate hydrosoluble ICMs such as Iopamidol and Iodixanol in an aqueous core and load iodinated oils within the hydrophobic bilayer [88]. Due to their high biocompatibility from the innocuous nature of phospholipids, the first batch of liposomal formulations containing contrast agents was reported in the 1980s, which achieved enhanced vascular and hepatic imaging [89–91]. However, these liposomes can be rapidly recognized and cleaned by the immune system.

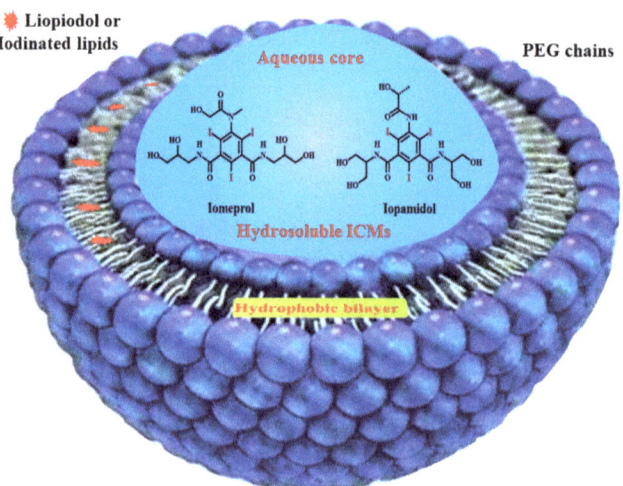

Figure 6. Liposomes structure for ICMs' delivery. Hydrophobic ICMs loaded within bilayer; hydrosoluble ICMs encapsulated in aqueous core.

Some hydrophilic polymers have been proved to be able to prolong the blood circulation time of drug delivery systems. Among them, polyethylene glycol (PEG) and PEG-containing polymers are the most commonly employed in biological and pharmaceutical fields for the development of long-circulating drug delivery systems [92–94]. This is due to the fact that the PEG chain provides a high hydration level, big hydrodynamic size and strong steric hindrance, which can not only enhance in vivo stability, but also prevent the attachment of serum proteins and impede uptake by the reticuloendothelial system, leading to a significant decrease in the clearance rate from circulation. As a result, the modification of liposomal surfaces with PEG was widely applied to formulate long-circulating liposomes with improved pharmacodynamic properties for a variety of pharmaceutical, biomedical and bioimaging applications. For example, PEG phospholipids, such as 1, 2-distearoyl-sn-glycero-3-phosphoethanolamine-poly(ethylene glycol) (DSPE-PEG), were widely used and successfully demonstrated to be able to enhance stability, improve encapsulation efficiency and prolong the blood circulation time of liposomes [95,96]. Water-soluble ICMs, such as Iohexol [97] or Iodixanol [98], were encapsulated into the core of PEG-coated liposomes as effective blood pool contrast media for use in long-term imaging of pulmonary arteries. Iodixanol-loaded liposomes can maintain contrast enhancement over several hours in rabbits. On the contrary, Iodixanol is rapidly cleared from the body within minutes [98]. Moreover, renal filtration was found to be a non-dominant approach for liposome clearance from blood, which can decrease the risk of contrast-induced nephrotoxicity.

In addition to rapid clearance via kidney, the inefficient targetability of ICMs delivery is another key issue yet to be resolved, as small molecular ICMs are nonspecific compounds. After intravascular injection, they are mainly distributed within the extracellular fluid compartment and then rapidly cleared from human blood via kidney filtration and clearance, which not only results in a short timeframe for CT imaging and undesirable renal toxicity, but also impedes the specific visualization and detection of target tissues [14,99,100]. Delivery systems for liposomal ICMs have attracted significant research interest and demonstrated targeted imaging of tumor tissues, cardiovascular diseases and lymph nodes, as liposomes can deliver both drug molecules and contrast media via passive targeting [14]. Generally, one of the main mechanisms of passive delivery is the reticuloendothelial system (RES)—recognized accumulation [101–103]. After intravenous injection, exogenous nanoparticles are rapidly recognized and sequestered by RES and hepatocytes in spleen and liver, especially for non-PEGylated (i.e., non-stealth) nanoparticulate drug delivery systems. In addition, even PEGylated long-circulating nanoparticles can also gradually accumulate in the liver via RES and hepatocytes. This kind of phenomena has initiated a surge of development in the passively targeted delivery of X-ray contrast media to spleen and liver. For example, some studies have demonstrated that the non-PEGylated iodinated liposomes specifically accumulated in the spleen and liver [104,105]. For example, Kweon et al. reported a kind of liposome that simultaneously loaded water-soluble iodinated compound (Iopamidol) and an iodinated ethyl ester of poppy seed oil (Lipiodol) via the modified reverse-phase evaporation method. Compared with free liposomes or liposomes loaded with Iopamidol alone, liposomes coloaded with Iopamidol/Lipiodol after intravenous injection into rats produced more pronounced contrast enhancement and more significant persistence in RES-rich organs, such as the liver and spleen. These results indicated that liposomes can serve as an RES-targeted contrast agent for targeted CT imaging [106].

The other main mechanism of passive delivery is the accumulation of delivery systems for nanoparticulate ICMs through the enhanced permeation and retention (EPR) effect. The EPR effect is a property where there is a significantly higher accumulation of macromolecules and nanoparticles with appropriate nanoscale size in tumor tissues than in normal tissues [107–109]. In normal tissues, the tight junctions of endothelial cells prevent the transport of nanoparticles. In contrast, due to the leakage of tumor vasculature and poor lymphatic drainage, tumor tissues can selectively accumulate and retain macromolecular drugs and nanoparticles, especially for PEGylated long-circulating nanomedicines. Therefore, the EPR effect has become an important guiding principle for the development of nanomedicines and nanoparticulate contrast media for cancer treatment and diagnosis [18,85,95]. The Allen group tried to longitudinally quantify and visualize the biodistribution of Iohexol-containing PEGylated liposomes in various body compartment volumes over a 14-day period in VX2 sarcoma-bearing New Zealand White rabbits using volumetric high-resolution CT imaging [110]. The results indicated that liposomes can be passively accumulated at tumor sites through the EPR effect. Other PEGylated liposomes, including Iopamidol-loaded liposome [95] and Iodixanol-loaded liposome [111], also achieved a prolonged blood pool contrast enhancement and an increased accumulation of iodinated liposomes in tumor tissues via the EPR effect.

It is well known that each imaging modality has its own unique advantages and intrinsic limitations. Imaging modalities with high resolution often suffer from relatively low sensitivity resolution, while those with high sensitivity have relatively poor resolution. Recently, to resolve this problem, the use of multimodal imaging, i.e., combining two or more imaging modalities into one system, has gained significant attention, because this synergistic method of imaging can overcome the limitations and take advantage of the strengths of each modality [1,112–115]. For example, imaging modalities with high spatial resolution (such as CT imaging) are frequently combined with other imaging modalities with high sensitivity (PET, optical, etc.). A complementary combination of CT imaging with high resolution and fluorescence (FL) imaging with high sensitivity has exhibited some desirable advantages in cancer diagnostics. Recently, Xu et al. reported a kind of PEGylated liposome that co-encapsulated clinically approved Iodixanol as ICMs and hydrophilic meso-tetrakis(4-sulphonatophenyl) porphine (TPPS$_4$) as a photosensitizer for concurrent CT and

FL imaging-guided cancer theragnostics [116], as shown in Figure 7A. Liposomes with sizes of about 100 nm were found to have an enhanced passive tumor uptake via the EPR effect, along with insignificant accumulation in the liver and other organs. Their highly tumor-specific biodistribution was manifested using both FL (Figure 7B) and CT imaging (Figure 7C), which can demonstrate the applicability of liposomes as contrast agents for bimodal tumor imaging and the imaging-guided treatment of cancer.

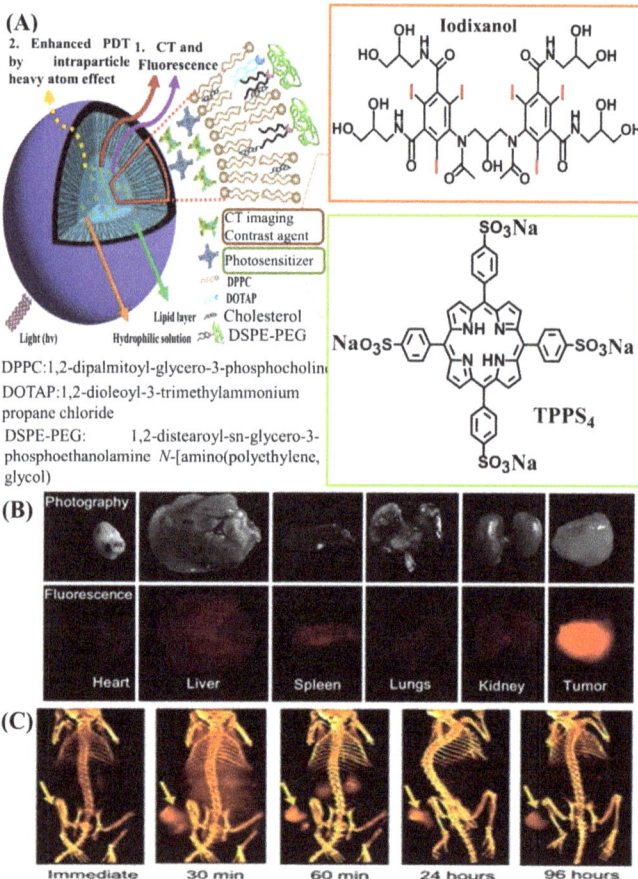

Figure 7. Liposomes co-encapsulating Iodixanol TPPS$_4$ for concurrent CT and FL imaging [116]. (A) Schematic diagram illustrating the structure and composition of liposomes; (B) photography and fluorescence images of the major organs resected from mouse after 96 h injection; (C) CT images at different time after injection; Reprinted with permission from ref. [116], Copyright 2021 Ivyspring. Although liposomes, especially PEG-coated liposomes, used for ICMs delivery can prolong the blood circulation time, increase targetability via the EPR effect and enhance sensitivity via multimodal imaging, they still suffer from a variety of challenges. In addition to the complexity of the formulation processes and very low drug loading, the stability of liposomes is one of their main disadvantages. Liposomes can be degraded through various physicochemical processes, such as auto-oxidation, hydrolysis, destabilization by dilution, self-aggregation and coalescence, often leading to premature ICMs leakage during storage and a strong ICMs burst release in blood. More research from various fields is needed to truly exploit the clinical experience of liposomes in combination with ICMs toward more capable imaging.

4.3. Nanoemulsions for ICMs Delivery

In addition to liposomes, significant progress was recently observed in exploiting the ICMs-loaded nanoemulsions as an effective contrast agent with improved performance [117]. The nanoemulsions-based contrast media were generally a colloidal dispersion form of ICMs with diameters ranging from 20 to 200 nm. The ICMs-loaded nanoemulsions generally consisted of water-insoluble iodinated oil and different types of lipids as the oily phase and PEGylated surfactants or PEG-containing block polymers as dispersion stabilizers in an aqueous medium [118–123]. As shown in Figure 8, after mixing the organic iodinated oil into the aqueous solution of PEGylated nonionic surfactants, the lipophilic molecules in the form of nanoscale droplets were immediately stabilized by the surfactant molecules, leading to the formation of an iodinated oily core surrounded by a hairy layer of the PEG moiety from nonionic surfactant. For nanoemulsions, the dispersion stabilizers are very important to govern the phase behavior of nanoemulsions and inhibit the occurrence of the flocculation, coalescence and sedimentation of nanoemulsions. Moreover, the presence of free surfactants had a significant impact in regard to the elimination, pharmacokinetics and biodistribution of nanoemulsions [121].

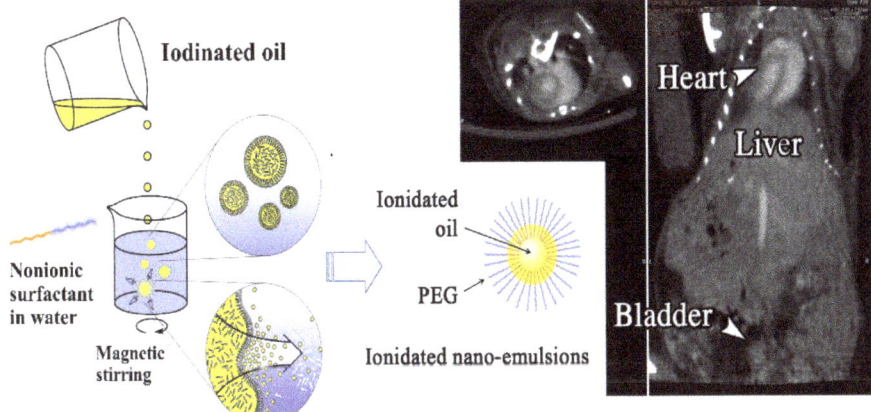

Figure 8. Schematic representation of the formation process of iodinated nanoemulsions and application for CT imaging [121]. Reprinted with permission from ref. [121], Copyright 2013 Elsevier.

Some ICMs-loaded nanoemulsions are commercially available, such as Fenestra®, which consists of poly-iodinated triglyceride (ITG) and phospholipids and cholesterol as a dispersion stabilizer [124]. These iodinated nanoemulsions are mainly used for blood pool or liver/spleen preclinical imaging and found an important place in the market of preclinical CT contrast agents. However, their iodine content is relatively low and thus the injection of a relatively large volume must be required, often leading to a non-negligible toxicity of the product. To decrease the toxicity even more, Attia et al. used the PEGylated nonionic surfactant, PEG-35 castor oil (trade name Kolliphor® ELP), to develop PEGylated nanoemulsions with iodinated monoglyceride and iodinated castor oil [118]. The obtained PEGylated nanoemulsions not only were endowed with very high iodine concentration, leading to a very strong X-ray attenuation property, but also achieved a very high contrast enhancement in blood with a half-life around 6 h. In addition, PEG-containing block polymers were demonstrated to be able to more effectively stabilize the nanoemulsions. Vries et al. synthesized three hydrophobic iodinated oils for use as the oily phase, based on the 2,3,5-triiodobenzoate moiety [119]. These new iodinated oils have a very high iodine content over 50%. In addition, then, poly(ethylene glycol)-b-poly(propylene glycol)-b-poly(ethylene glycol)(PEG-PPG-PEG, Pluronic F68) and poly(butadiene)-b-poly(ethylene glycol) (PBD-PEG) were used as dispersion stabilizers to prepare long-circulating blood pool contrast media. Compared with the commercial formulations (Fenestra®), the PBD-PEG stabilized nanoemulsions could exhibit much lower in vivo toxicity and achieved a longer blood circulation time, exhibiting great potential for use as blood pool agents in contrast-enhanced CT imaging. In addition, due to their excellent biocompatibility and biodegradability, a PEG-polyester, such as diblock copolymer poly(ethylene glycol)-b-polycaprolactone (PEG-PCL), was also used as a dispersion stabilizer to prepare ICMs-loaded nanoemulsions [125].

Compared with liposomal formulations, nanoemulsions actually have many more advantages. Firstly, the stability of nanoemulsions is much higher. They are relatively stable against dilution and under heating. In addition, their formulation and fabrication are much simpler and cheaper, especially for the fabrication process of nanoemulsion droplets. Moreover, nanoemulsions exhibited higher encapsulation efficacy of ICMs and had a higher loading capacity for water-insoluble ICMs or hydrophobic drugs than liposomes. Finally, PEG or specific ligands can be more easily introduced onto the droplets' surface, conferring them strong stealth properties or targetability [88,124]. Apparently, nanoemulsions and liposomes have exhibited great potential for efficient ICMs delivery. However, these nanocarriers still suffer from the leakage of internal payloads and very low drug loading capacity.

4.4. Polymeric Nanoparticles for ICMs Delivery

Over the past several decades, polymers and their related nanomaterials have gained great attention and exhibited great potential for biomedical and pharmaceutical applications due to their unique biocompatibility, designability, biodegradation, facile synthesis and modification capability. According to their morphology and composition in the core and periphery, polymeric NPs can be mainly categorized as micelles, solid NPs, nanogels, polymersomes, polyplexes and dendrimers, as shown in Figure 9. These polymeric NPs can be incorporated with drugs or ICMs via encapsulation or conjugation, which have opened up a new avenue to improve the biocompatibility, delivery efficacy and diagnosis sensitivity of ICMs [24–35].

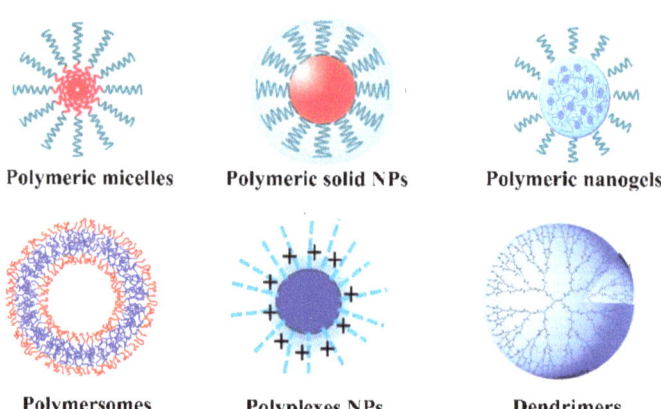

Figure 9. Schematic illustration of typical polymeric nanoparticles.

4.4.1. Polymeric Micelles

Polymeric micelles, a kind of aggregation colloid derived from the self-assembly of amphiphilic polymers in water, have been demonstrated as an effective approach to address the issues related to the delivery and release of drug or diagnostic agents [32,33,86,126]. Micelles are a kind of unique core–shell nanostructure. Their hydrophilic shells are mainly composed of PEG or similar hydrophilic polymers, such as polyvinyl pyrrolidone (PVP), polyvinyl alcohol (PVA), dextran, chitosan, hyaluronic acid, polyacrylic acid (PAA) as well as polyelectrolytes and zwitterionic polymers. Hydrophilic polymers on the shells provide stability to the cores in water. The hydrophobic cores are generally derived from the aggregations of hydrophobic chains or the co-assembly of lipophilic chains and hydrophobic drugs due to the hydrophobic interactions. Due to their excellent biocompatibility and biodegradability, polyesters, including poly(caprolactone) (PCL), poly(lactide) (PLA), poly(lactide-co-glycolide) (PLGA) and poly(amino acids), were widely accepted as hydrophobic polymers for the construction of micelles for pharmaceutical applications. The hydrophilic and hydrophobic chains can be easily tailor-made by changing the number of structural repeating units and the chain composition in each polymeric chain.

The superior flexibilities in structure, composition and functionalization made polymeric micelles attractive for their use in of drug delivery, especially for hydrophobic drugs. Generally, drugs can be loaded in polymeric micelles via physical encapsulation to prepare polymeric drug delivery systems. However, it was ineffective and very difficult for common micelles to encapsulate ICMs via hydrophobic interactions. On the one hand, ICMs are typically water-soluble ionic or nonionic iodinated molecules, or water-insoluble iodinated oil. On the other hand, different from liposomes with an internal aqueous core and nanoemulsions with an internal oily core, polymeric micelles with aggregation-forming hydrophobic cores were not suitable for loading water-soluble molecules or lipophilic oil. Therefore, one of the main strategies for the fabrication of iodinated micelles is via the covalent linkage of ICMs to the hydrophobic tails of amphiphiles, and then self-assembly of the iodinated moieties into the center of the micelles. For example, the Torchilin group has developed a kind of amphiphilic block copolymer (mPEG-PA-PLL) by conjugating a hydrophilic PEG chain with 12-repeat-unit polylysine. Then, 2,4,6-triiodobenzoic acid was conjugated to the amine groups of the mPEG-PA-PLL chain to prepare iodinated amphiphilic block copolymer (ICPM-forming copolymer) [34,53], as shown in Figure 10A. The ICPM-forming copolymer possessed the ability of forming polymeric micelles with iodine content of about 17.7% by weight. A strong contrast of over 50 HU could still be observed in the heart, liver and spleen after injection in rat for 2 h (Figure 10B). This kind of iodinated polymeric micelle exhibited great potential for long-lasting blood pool contrast [34,53,124].

In addition, based on the self-assembly of amphiphilic polymers into micelles, amphiphilic macromolecular ICMs (PEG-PHEMA-I) were prepared via the atom transfer radical polymerization (ATRP) polymerization of 2-hydroxyethyl methacrylate (HEMA) in the presence of macro-ATRP initiator (PEG-Br) and subsequent esterification reaction with 2,3,5-triiodobenzoic acid to introduce iodine onto the side chain of PHEMA [127]. The obtained PEG-PHEMA-I can self-assemble into iodinated polymeric micelles. Moreover, to overcome the barriers of encapsulating ICMs into micelles, co-assembly between iodinated polymers and amphiphilic polymers was also widely used to prepare iodinated micelles. In this strategy, iodinated macromolecular contrast agents were prepared firstly as shown in Figures 3 and 4, and then iodinated macromolecular contrast media were used as a building block to co-assemble with amphiphilic polymers or surfactant to form micelles, as shown in Figure 11. For example, Balegamire et al. prepared a kind of iodinated polymer (TIB-PVAL) via the attachment of tri-iodobenzoyl to the PVAL backbone. Then, TIB-PVAL was co-assembled with poly(caprolactone)-b-poly(ethylene glycol) (PCL-b-PEG) to form polymeric micelles with diameters of about 150 nm (Figure 11A). The intravenous injection of polymeric micelles into rats resulted in a clear visualization of the cardiovascular system over several hours [52]. Di-iodinated polyvinyl phenol was prepared via aromatic electrophilic substitution using sodium iodide (Figure 11B). Then, di-iodinated polyvinyl phenol was co-assembled with polystyrene-b-polyethylene glycol (PS-b-PEG) to produce micelles with iodine loadings up to 45 wt.% [46]. In addition, macromolecular ICMs poly(MAOTIB) was prepared via the free radical polymerization of MAOTIB (Figure 11C). Poly(MAOTIB) can be co-assembled with PEGylated surfactant PEG-35 castor oil [27]. The obtained micelles can be formulated with a size of about 140–200 nm, exhibiting a very strong X-ray attenuation capacity for blood pool. As shown in Figure 11D, a variety of iodinated aliphatic polyesters with high biocompatibility and biodegradability, as well as tunable thermal and mechanical properties, were prepared. Then, the co-assembly of thermosets with PEG-monostearate and lecithin was used to obtain iodinated micelles. The initial studies indicated that these micelles show good continual contrast without uptake into the kidneys [38]. These results indicate that the co-assembly strategies show great potential for the fabrication of iodinated polymer micelles for CT imaging.

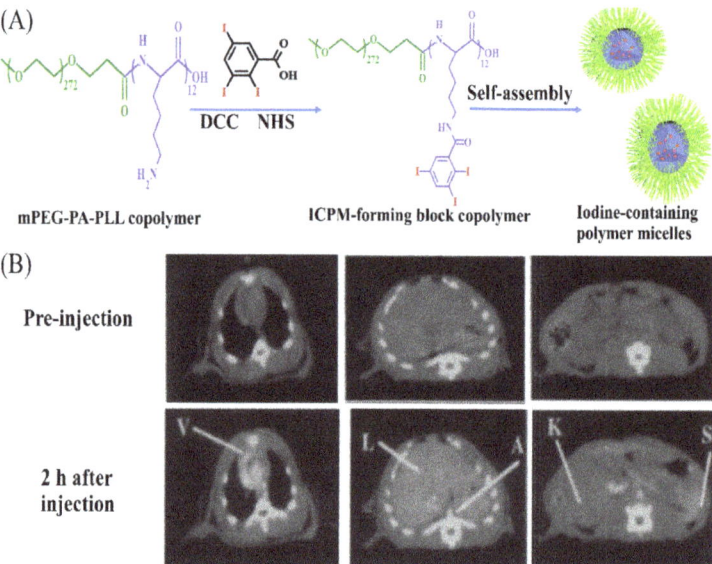

Figure 10. Micelles formed from iodinated amphiphilic block copolymer for CT imaging. (A) Schematic depiction of preparation process and chemical structure of ICPM-forming copolymer. (B) Micelles formed from ICPM-forming copolymer for CT imaging of a rat [126]. Reprinted with permission from ref. [126], Copyright 2013 Wiley.

It is well known that each imaging modality has its own unique advantages and intrinsic limitations. Thus, a single imaging modality can no longer satisfy the rapidly growing demand for the more reliable and accurate detection of disease sites. Recently, to resolve this problem, the use of multimodal imaging, i.e., combining two or more imaging modalities into one system, has gained significant attention, because this synergistic imaging can overcome the limitations and take advantage of the strengths of each modality [1,112–115]. Co-assembly strategies have also been used to prepare multimodal iodinated micelles. For example, Zhou et al. reported novel iodine-rich semiconducting polymer-based multimodal iodinated micelles for use as contrast agents for CT and fluorescence dual-modal imaging [127]. The combination of CT and fluorescence imaging is due to the fact that the fluorescence imaging has relatively high sensitivity, which can compensate for the low sensitivity of CT imaging. Iodine-grafted amphiphilic copolymer (PEG-PHEMA-I) was firstly prepared via a combination of atom transfer radical polymerization of 2-hydroxyethyl methacrylate (HEMA) and esterification with 2,3,5-triiodobenzoic acid. Then, the semiconducting polymer (PCPDTBT) as the source of NIR fluorescence signal and the photosensitizer was used to co-assemble with PEG-PHEMA-I to form multimodal iodinated micelles in aqueous solution, as shown in Figure 12A. Multimodal iodinated micelles with sizes of about 50 nm not only have a high density of iodine to provide a high X-ray attenuation coefficient for CT imaging, but also possess a high content of PCPDTBT with high fluorescence quantum yields for fluorescence imaging. The performance of in vivo CT/fluorescence imaging for SPN-I was investigated using tumor bearing c57b1/6 male mice. After the injection of SPN-I, both CT and fluorescence signals in the tumor area were observed to gradually increase with time. These results indicated that SPN-I could passively accumulate in a tumor via the EPR effect and successfully detect a xenograft tumor both via CT and fluorescence imaging. Moreover, due to enhanced photosensitization via the iodine-induced heavy-atom effect, multimodal iodinated micelles have an improved $^1O_2$ quantum yield, which can be used for efficient photodynamic therapy (Figure 12B). In vivo antitumor studies confirmed that photodynamic therapy achieves a significant tumor inhibition rate (98.7%).

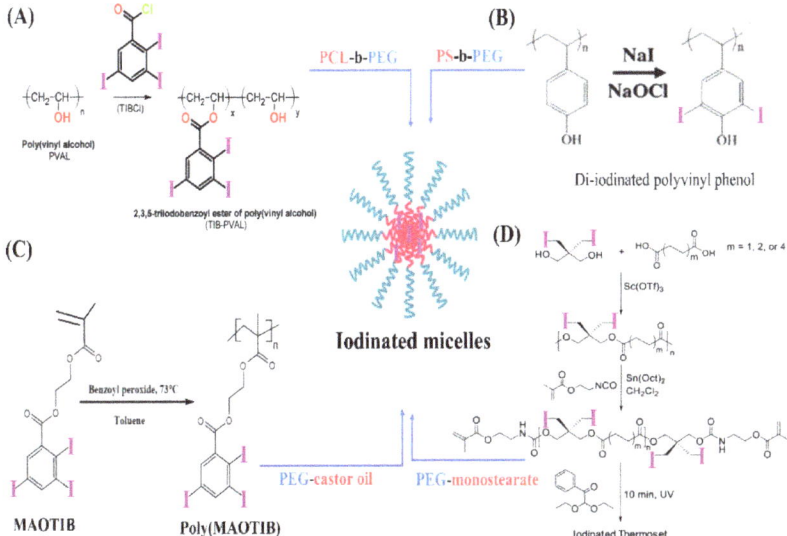

Figure 11. Iodinated macromolecular contrast agents for construction of micelles by co-assembly for CT imaging. (**A**) TIB-PVAL co-assembly with PCL-b-PEG [52]; Reprinted with permission from ref. [52], Copyright 2020 Royal Society of Chemistry; (**B**) di-iodinated polyvinyl phenol co-assembly with PS-b-PEG [46]; Reprinted with permission from ref. [46] Copyright 2018 Wiley; (**C**) poly(MAOTIB) co-assembly with PEG-35 castor oil [27]; Reprinted with permission from ref. [27], Copyright 2017 Elsevier; (**D**) iodinated thermoset co-assembly with PEG-monostearate [38]. Reprinted with permission from ref. [38], Copyright 2017 Wiley.

4.4.2. Polymersomes

Polymersomes, types of self-assembled vesicular structures of amphiphilic block copolymers, consist of a bilayer shell of amphiphilic copolymers and an aqueous core [128,129]. Apparently, the structures of polymersomes are different from the structure of micelles but very similar to liposomes. However, compared with liposomes, polymersomes have exhibited some significant advantages, such as higher stability in vivo circulation, tunable membrane property and versatility in chemical synthesis, which make them an attractive option for application in the encapsulation and delivery of various drugs [130–132].

Similar with polymer micelles, polymersomes are also not suitable for encapsulating and delivering small molecular ICMs, and no reports on this topic can be found. However, some iodine-containing amphiphilic copolymers can be assembled into iodinated polymersomes. For example, the group of Du recently designed and synthesized a kind of biodegradable, iodinated amphiphilic block copolymer poly(ethylene oxide)-block-poly(triiodobenzoic chlorideconjugated polylysine-stat-phenylboronic acid pinacol ester-conjugated polylysine) (PEO_{45}-b-P[(Lys-IBC$)_{45}$-stat-(Lys-PAPE$)_{15}$]), which can self-assemble into renoprotective angiographic polymersomes [31], as shown in Figure 13. Polymersomes can be used as renoprotective blood pool CT contrast media due to rationally chosen repeat units. Firstly, PEO (i.e., PEG) can not only stabilize the formed polymersomes in water with a high concentration, but also endow polymersomes with a stealth function when circulating in blood. Second, Lys-IBC with high content iodine can possess a concentration-dependent X-ray attenuation capability. In addition, considering that the generation of reactive oxygen species (ROS) within the kidneys contributes to CIN pathology, Lys-PAPE with an ROS-scavenging ability was introduced into polymersomes. PAPE can scavenge ROS due to the oxidization and hydrolysis of aryl boronic ester groups. In vivo experiments indicated that the use of polymersomes as a renoprotective angiographic contrast agent can markedly reduce the risk of CIN in mice with kidney injury.

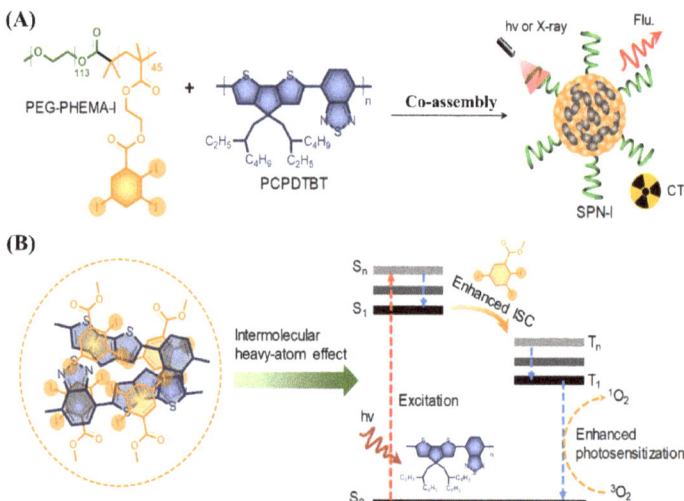

Figure 12. Schematic illustration of multimodal iodinated micelles for CT/fluorescence dual-modal imaging [127]. (**A**) Co-assembly of iodinated polymer PEG-PHEMA-I and semiconducting polymer PCPDTBT; (**B**) enhanced photosensitization by iodine-induced heavy-atom effect. Reprinted with permission from ref. [127], Copyright 2020 Wiley.

To improve tumor accumulation and retention rates, some researchers designed and developed some active targeting polymersomes. Recently, the group of Zhong designed and developed a kind of cyclic RGD-directed, disulfide crosslinked iodine-rich biodegradable polymersome (cRGD-XIP), as shown in Figure 14. The cRGD-XIPs were prepared via the co-assembly of poly(ethylene glycol)-b-poly(dithiolane trimethylene carbonate-co-iodinated trimethylene carbonate) copolymer (PEG-P(DTC-IC)) and cRGD functionalized PEG-P(DTC-IC) (cRGD-PEG-P(DTC-IC)) [133]. These novel theranostic polymersomes with size of about 90 nm exhibited a very high content of iodine (55.5 wt.%). Moreover, the cRGD-XIPs achieved a high loading content of doxorubicin (15.3 wt.%) via the pH-gradient method. Moreover, the polymersomes cRGD-XIPs and doxorubicin-loaded cRGD-XIPs (cRGD-XIPs-Dox) possessed superior colloidal stability during blood circulation due to the disulfide-crosslinked nanostructure but underwent fast drug release within tumor cells in response to the reductive microenvironment. Moreover, cRGD can act as an active targeting ligand to $\alpha_v\beta_3$ integrin on overexpressed cancer cells. Thus, cRGD-targeted polymersomes can actively deliver and preferentially accumulate in tumor tissues. Compared with Iohexol, in vivo CT imaging of cRGD-XIP-treated mice presented much stronger tumor contrast. These results demonstrated that cRGD-XIPs can serve as a robust, non-toxic and smart theranostic agent with the ability to significantly enhance CT imaging of tumors. Moreover, cRGD-XIPs-Dox displayed an enhanced targetability to tumors and achieved an elevated accumulation in tumors, which was significantly effective in inhibiting the growth of B16 melanoma model. Similarly, they also reported a kind of tumor-targeted biodegradable polymersome derived from the self-assembly of iodinated amphiphilic polyesters (cRGD-PEG-b-PIC and PEG-b-PIC), which possessed not only an ultrahigh iodine content, but also an excellent ability to target neovascular and $\alpha_v\beta_3$ integrin due to the presence of cRGDfK cyclic peptide [30]. They first synthesized the iodinated amphiphilic polyester PEG-b-PIC and cRGDfK cyclic peptide (cRGD) functionalized polyester (cRGD-PEG-b-PIC) via ring-opening polymerization of a new iodine-functionalized trimethylene carbonate (IC) monomer using mPEG-OH and NHS-PEG-OH as initiator, respectively. The co-assembly of cRGD-PEG-b-PIC and PEG-b-PIC can form stable polymersomes with a small hydrodynamic size of about 100 nm. The obtained polymersomes were demonstrated to have an unprecedented iodine content (about 60 wt.%), low viscosity, and iso-osmolality, as well as long circulating property. In $\alpha_v\beta_3$ integrin-overexpressing B16 melanoma xenografted mice, the cRGD-targeted polymersomes achieved a significantly higher tumor accumulation and yielded more a sufficient contrast of tumors at 6–8 h after administration when compared to Iohexol and nontargeted polymersomes groups. This kind of targeted polymersome showed great potential for application in high-performance targeted CT imaging.

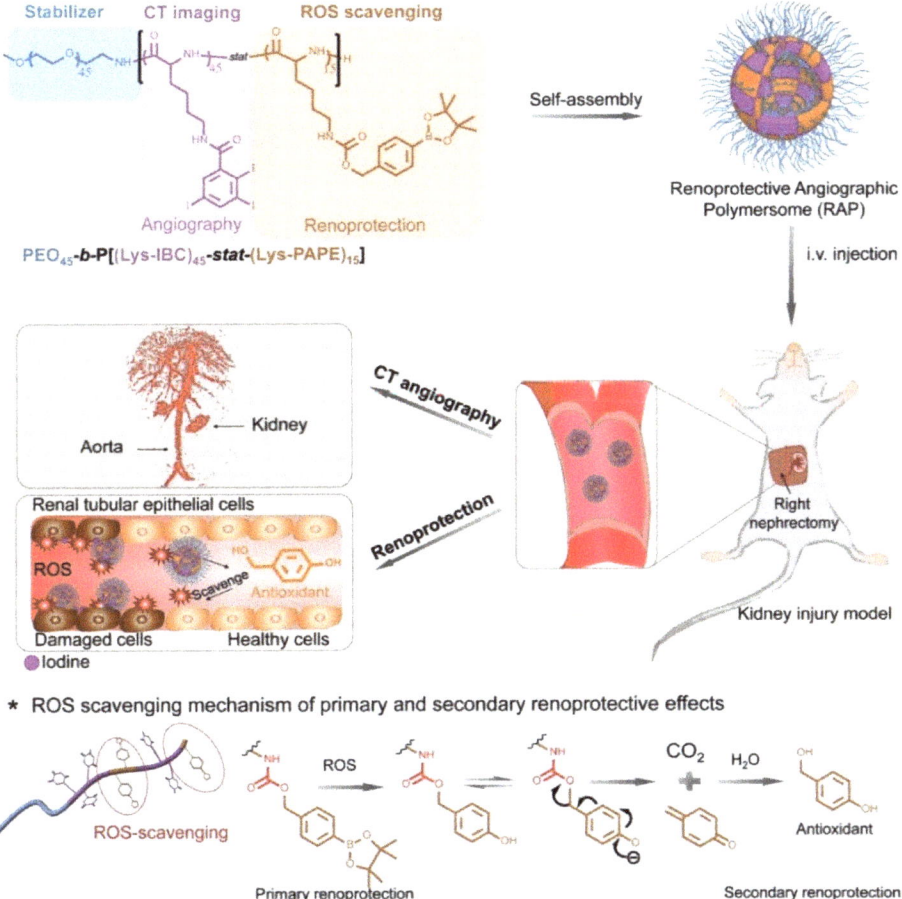

Figure 13. Schematic illustration of preparation process of renoprotective angiographic polymersome, the renoprotection behavior by ROS scavenging and ROS scavenging mechanism [31]. Reprinted with permission from ref. [31], Copyright 2020 Wiley.

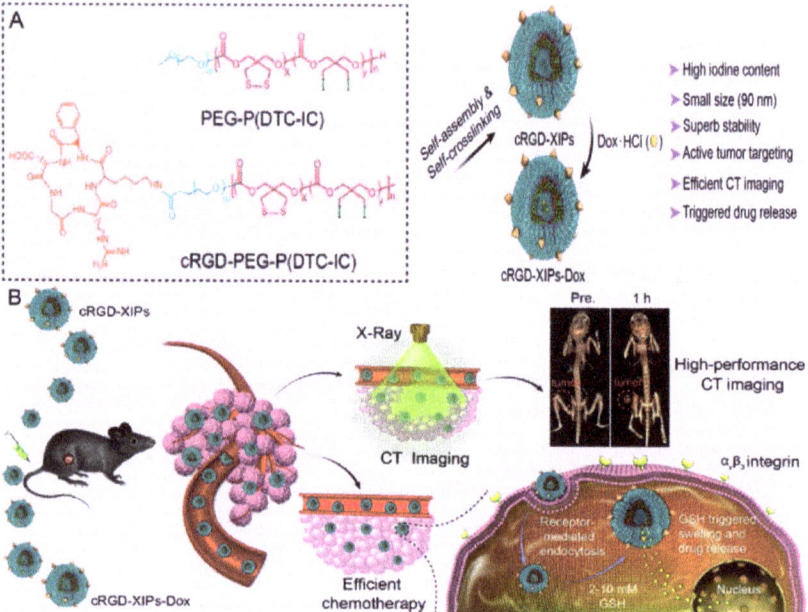

Figure 14. cRGD-targeted biodegradable polymersomes [133]. (**A**) Co-assembly of cRGD-PEG-b-PIC and PEG-b-PIC to prepare cRGD-targeted polymersomes (cRGD-XIPs and cRGD-XIPs-Dox); (**B**) cRGD-XIPs for enhanced in vivo CT imaging of tumor and cRGD-XIPs-Dox for targeted chemotherapy. Reprinted with permission from ref. [133], Copyright 2019 Ivyspring.

To meet the demand of high sensitivity and high-spatial resolution diagnosis of tumors, the group of Zhong recently developed a kind of iodine-rich polymersome (I-PS) and then, the I-PS was labeled with radioiodine (^{125}I and ^{131}I) [25], as shown in Figure 15. ^{125}I and ^{131}I have been demonstrated to be able to be used for imaging and radioisotope therapy, respectively. ^{125}I-PS with size of about 100 nm exhibited not only a prolonged circulation, but also an obviously enhanced distribution in tumors and the reticuloendothelial system. Meanwhile, ^{131}I-PS used for radioisotope therapy could significantly inhibit the growth of $4T_1$ breast tumors and effectively prolong mice survival time. More importantly, the ^{125}I-labeled I-PS was demonstrated to be able to effectively achieve high-efficiency CT imaging and SPECT imaging as multimodal contrast agent for breast cancer in vivo. This study provided a robust and versatile platform for dual-modal imaging and targeted radioisotope therapy.

4.4.3. Dendrimers

Dendrimers are another very important and stable nanoplatform for the development of polymer-based contrast media for use in computed tomography [134,135]. Dendrimers represent a versatile and well-defined nanoscale architecture, which are a class of unique polymeric molecules. They are synthesized in a step-wise fashion, generally starting from a multifunctional core of the dendrimer and then outwards, growing by the layer-by-layer addition of monomeric units. With the increase in the generation, the morphological structure of dendrimers will turn into a globular shape. These hyperbranched macromolecules are often monodispersed but have a highly branched and tree-like molecular architecture with uniform composition, well-defined geometry and abundant terminal functional groups. Especially, abundant terminal functional groups can not only provide many sites for functionalization at the ends of the branches, but also offer many reactive groups for the conjugation of drugs at the available termini of the molecules. Compared with linear polymers, dendrimers often have a higher solubility in various solvents and show much lower viscosity under the same conditions. In addition to their nanometric size range, permeability across the biological membrane and a relatively high biocompatibility, dendrimers have displayed significant potential as a versatile delivery system for drugs and diagnostic agents [69,136,137].

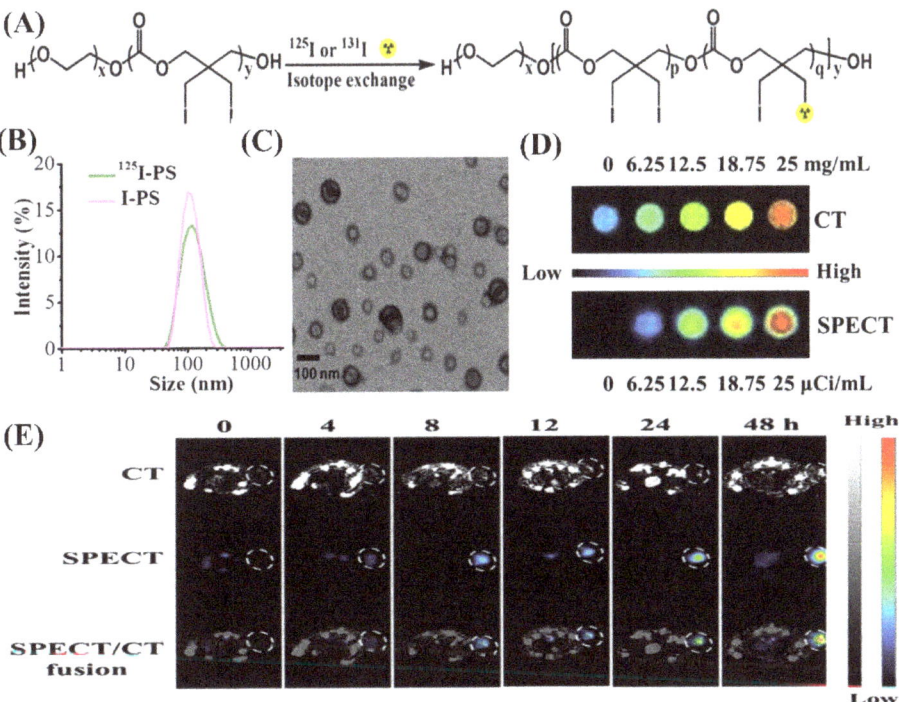

Figure 15. Radiolabeled iodine-rich polymersomes as multimodal contrast agent for SPECT/CT imaging [25]. (**A**) Synthesis of PEG-PIC (^{125}I) and PEG-PIC (^{131}I) by isotopic exchange; (**B**) size distribution profiles of I-PS and ^{125}I-PS; (**C**) morphology of ^{125}I-PS; (**D**) phantom reconstructions of ^{125}I-PS measured at different polymer concentrations; (**E**) coronal section of in vivo CT, SPECT, and fusion images of mice. Reprinted with permission from ref. [25], Copyright 2019 American Chemical Society.

As a typical dendrimer, poly(amido amine) (PAMAM) consists of an ethylenediamine core, tertiary amine branches, and alkyl amide spacers, which allows for functionalization and drug conjugation through amine groups on its outer surface. PAMAM has been widely used to load and deliver ICMs to increase imaging time, decrease rental toxicity and improve specificity. For example, amine-terminated fourth-generation (G4) PAMAM dendrimers were used as a multifunctional platform to conjugate a small iodinated compound 3-N-[(N,N-dimethylaminoacetyl) amino]-a-ethyl-2,4,6-triiodobenzenepropanoic acid. The obtained iodinated dendritic nanoparticles [G-4-(DMAA-IPA)$_{37}$] with a hydrodynamic radius of 2.4 nm can achieve 33% iodine content by weight and retain their high water solubility [138]. Amine-terminated third- and fourth-generation PAMAM dendrimers with ethylenediamine cores were also conjugated with tetraiodobenzene derivatives to prepare blood pool contrast media for use in CT imaging [56], as shown in Figure 16. The obtained unimolecular dendritic contrast media with the size of 13–22 nm are water soluble and exhibited high contrast enhancement in the blood pool and effectively extended their blood half-lives. Fu et al. synthesized a series of paired, symmetrical dendritic polylysines initiated from a large PEG core (3000–12,000 g/mol). Then, triiodophthalamide molecules were conjugated onto the amine termini of these dendrimers. The in vivo enhancement for CT contrast in a rat model was evaluated. The results indicated that the iodinated PEG-core dendrimer conjugates achieve high X-ray attenuation intensity, high water solubility, good chemical stability and persistent intravascular enhancement, with a blood half-life of about 35 min [55].

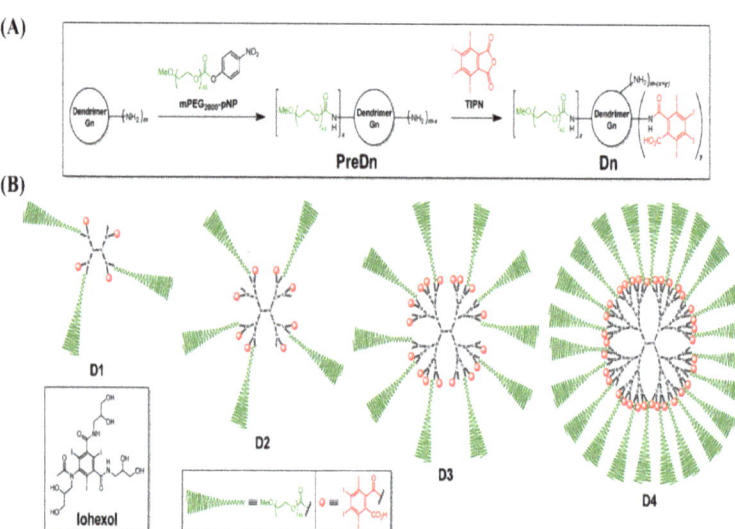

Figure 16. Synthesis process of iodinated dendritic nanoparticles [56]. (A) Synthetic process; (B) dendritic CT contrast agents. Reprinted with permission from ref. [56], Copyright 2016 Elsevier.

4.4.4. Polymeric Solid Nanoparticles

Although polymeric micelles and polymersomes have been demonstrated to have significant potential for improving the delivery efficiency and circulation time of ICMs, their intrinsic instability limits their wider applications [32,33,126]. Therefore, developing polymeric NPs with high stabilities is highly demanded. Polymeric solid nanoparticles (SNPs) with stable core structures due to crosslinking or multiple interactions can serve as an excellent platform for ICMs delivery. For example, some core-crosslinked polymeric SNPs were designed and developed for the delivery of contrast agents. Ding et al. reported a one-pot strategy for the synthesis of core-crosslinked Iohexol nanoparticles (INPs) on a large scale for CT imaging [139]. They used Iohexol acrylate as a crosslinking agent via polymerization-induced self-assembly to achieve the high stability and good dispersion of INPs even in an extremely high concentration. INPs can not only have lower toxicity and a longer circulation time, but also exhibit strong imaging capability and prominent accumulation in tumors when compared with Iohexol. Hainfeld et al. reported a kind of PEG-coated core-crosslinked polymer iodinated nanoparticle with a size of about 20 nm [140]. Iodine SNPs are a polymerized triiodobenzene compound coated with PEG, which were demonstrated to not only have an extraordinarily long blood half-life (40 h) for better tumor uptake, but also to be non-toxic after an intravenous dose of 4 g iodine/kg. These iodine SNPs may serve as an X-ray contrast agent with novel properties for cancer therapy and vascular imaging.

Similarly, the Cheng group developed a kind of poly(iohexol) SNP by using the addition reaction between hexamethylene diisocyanate and Iohexol with multiple hydroxyl groups as a comonomer [141], as shown in Figure 17A. After nanoprecipitation with mPEG-polylactide (mPEG-PLA), poly(iohexol) SNPs with sizes of about 150 nm in diameter with narrow size distributions were obtained (Figure 17B). PEGylated poly(iohexol) SNPs exhibited remarkable stability without any significant size changes or premature release of

Iohexol in PBS and human serum buffer, as the crosslinked core could prevent disassembly against dilutions upon administration (Figure 17C). The potential of poly(iohexol) SNPs for in vivo CT diagnosis was evaluated and is shown in Figure 17D. The results indicated that poly(iohexol) SNPs with high stability exhibited a substantial improvement in tissue retention and CT contrast (a 36-fold increase in CT contrast 4 h post injection).

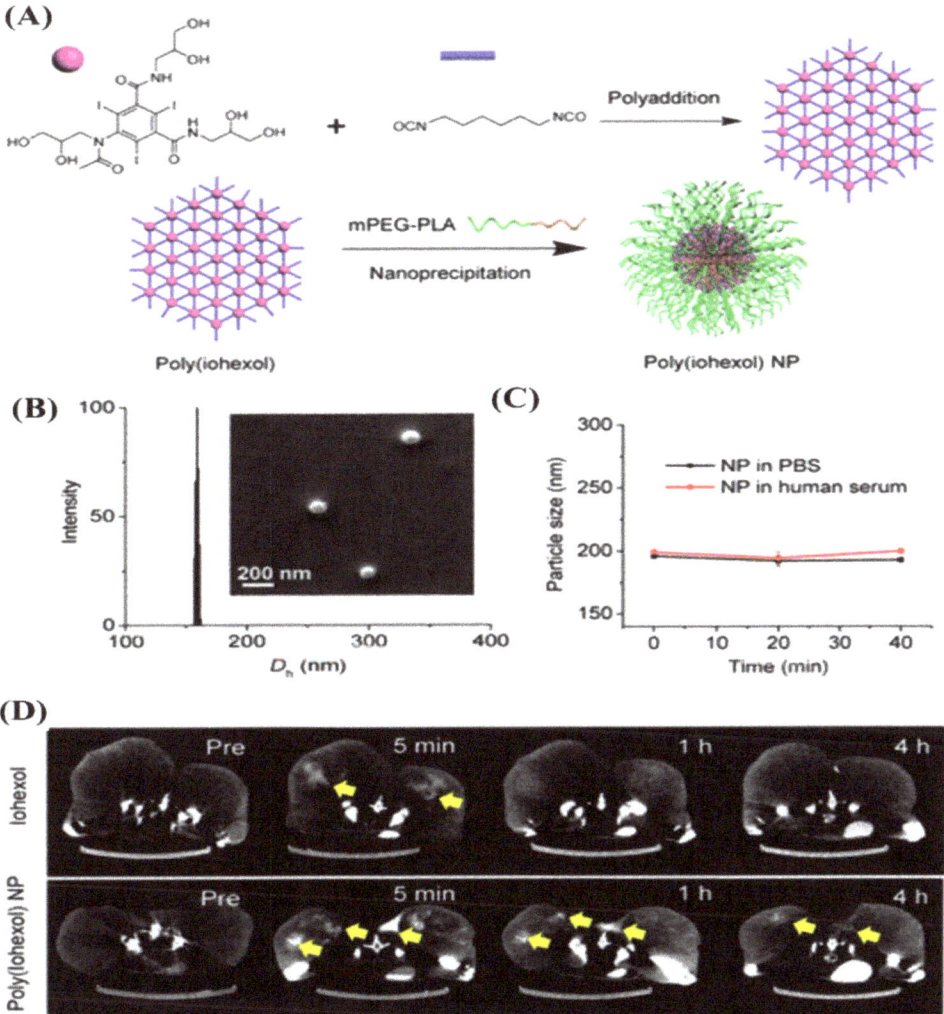

Figure 17. Synthesis and structure of core-crosslinked poly(iohexol) SNPs [141]. (**A**) Synthetic illustration of preparing cross-linked poly(iohexol) and PEGylated poly(iohexol) SNPs; (**B**) size and morphology; (**C**) stability in PBS or human serum buffer for different times; (**D**) serial axial CT images of the MCF-7 tumors in mice after intratumoral injection Iohexol and poly(iohexol) SNPs. Reprinted with permission from ref. [141], Copyright 2013 American Chemical Society.

Considering their endogenous origin, nonimmunogenic, biocompatible and biodegradable nature as well as relatively high stability, lipoproteins, including low-density lipoproteins (LDL) and high-density lipoproteins (HDL) as natural SNPs, have been demonstrated to be highly suitable as a platform for delivering imaging agents [28,75,142]. For example, the radio-iodine as radiotracers, including iodine-131 (^{131}I) and iodine-125 (^{125}I), were used to label LDL. The obtained radio-iodinated LDL SNPs were used to image and characterize tumor accumulation within animals for over several decades [143]. Zheng et al. incorporated poly-iodinated triglyceride into LDL for the delivery of a CT contrast agent [144], achieving an enhancement on CT imaging via LDL-induced RES targeting. Radiopaque iodinated copolymeric SNPs with sizes ranging between 30 and 350 nm were prepared via the emulsion copolymerization of MAOETIB and glycidyl methacrylate (GMA) in the presence of sodium dodecyl sulfate as a surfactant and potassium persulfate as an initiator. The obtained P(MAOETIB-GMA) SNPs with high iodine contents of 58% possess a significant radiopaque nature. In vivo CT imaging was performed in a dog model. The results indicated that the obtained P(MAOETIB-GMA) SNPs can achieve significant enhanced visibility of the liver, spleen and lymph nodes of model animals by RES-selective uptake [43].

Recently, Krafft et al. reported a series of stable iodinated coordination polymer SNPs with the ability to carry a very high payload of iodine (over 60 wt.%) [145]. As shown in Figure 18A, 2,3,5,6-tetraiodo-1,4-benzenedicarboxylic acid (I_4-BDC-H_2) as bridging ligands and CuII or ZnII metal as connecting points were used to synthesize five new coordination polymer SNPs. Scanning electron microscopy images confirmed that the formed iodinated coordination polymer SNPs, typically polymer (3), are plate-like particles, 50 nm thick and with a diameter of 300 nm and (Figure 18B). This is due to the fact that each CuII center can coordinate to two water molecules and three carboxylate oxygen atoms in a square pyramidal geometry. They also conducted phantom studies on the obtained polymer SNPs to evaluate their potential for use as CT contrast media. As shown in Figure 18C, the coordination polymer SNPs show a very high X-ray attenuation coefficient, which can be comparable to that of the molecular contrast agent (Iodixanol). These new nanomaterials can deliver high payloads of iodine, which shows that they have great potential for the development of efficient CT contrast media without the inherent drawbacks of small-molecule ICMs.

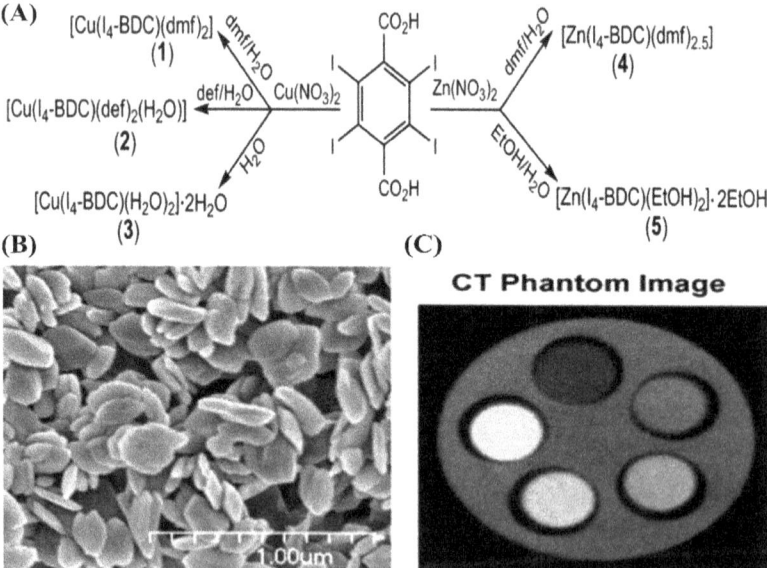

Figure 18. Iodinated coordination polymer SNPs with high payload of iodine [145]. (**A**) Synthesis process; (**B**) Typical morphology of iodinated coordination polymer SNPs; (**C**) CT phantom images. Reprinted with permission from ref. [145], Copyright 2009 Wiley.

To further achieve targeted CT imaging on tumors, Gao et al. firstly synthesized a kind of methacrylated Iopamidol (MAI) monomer, and then, MAI was polymerized to obtain poly(methacrylated Iopamidol) (PMAI) SNPs via a precipitation polymerization method [146], as shown in Figure 19. Subsequently, PMAI SNPs were PEGylated via the introduction of PEG chains, and then, the targeting ligand cRGD peptide was conjugated onto the outer surface to obtain poly(methacrylated iopamidol)-polyethylene glycol-cRGD (PMAI-PEG-RGD) SNPs with sizes of about 150 nm and iodine contents of about 30 wt.%. The X-ray attenuation capability of PMAI-PEG-RGD SNPs was detected. Compared with Iopamidol, the stronger X-ray attenuation effect of PMAI-PEG-RGD SNPs was demonstrated. These results indicated that PMAI-PEG-RGD SNPs can act as a promising contrast agent for X-ray CT imaging. More importantly, PMAI-PEG-RGD SNPs were endowed with tumor-targeting ability due to the presence of cRGD ligand with a specific affinity for $\alpha_v\beta_3$ integrin overexpressed on cancer cells. In vivo CT imaging indicated that PMAI-PEG-RGD SNPs can show greatly enhanced CT imaging efficacy, confirming their more efficient tumor accumulation due to the cRGD peptide-mediated active targeting effect.

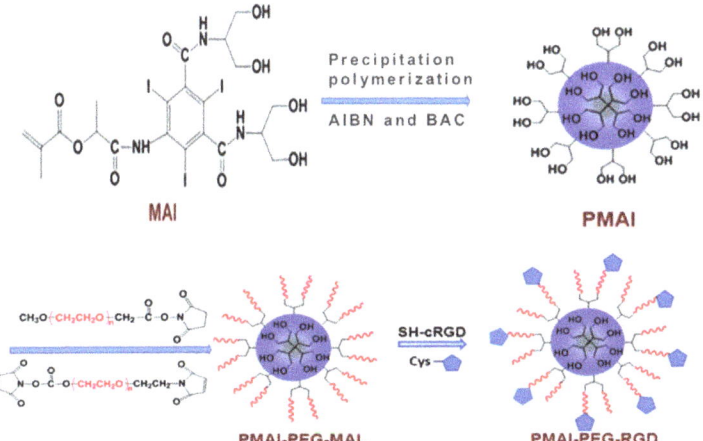

Figure 19. Synthesis process of poly(methacrylated iopamidol)-polyethylene glycol-cRGD (PMAI-PEG-RGD) SNPs [146]. Reprinted with permission from ref. [146], Copyright 2020 Royal Society of Chemistry.

Hyaluronic acid (HA), as a highly water-soluble, negatively charged polysaccharide, was widely used to increase stability in aqueous solution and prolong the circulation time of nanoparticles in vivo. More importantly, HA, as a specific ligand for CD44 often overexpressed on tumor cells, was also applied for the tumor-targeted delivery of anticancer drugs and imaging contrast media [147]. Liu et al. recently reported a facile but effective approach to synthesize multifunctional HA-coated iodinated SNPs with Au nanoshells (PMATIB/PEI/Au nanoshell/HA) [26]. They first prepared iodinated crosslinked SNPs (PMATIB) via the precipitation polymerization of 2-methacryl(3-amide-2,4,6-triiodobenzoic acid) (MATIB) using N,N-methylenebis-(acrylamide) (MBAAm) as a cross-linker. Subsequently, PMATIB SNPs were modified with PEI and ultrafine Au NPs through the electrostatic interaction. Finally, HA was coated on the outer surface to obtain PMATIB/PEI/Au nanoshell/HA SNPs with sizes of about 200 nm and excellent dispersibility in aqueous solution. After intravenous injection into MCF-7 tumor-bearing mice, PMATIB/PEI/Au nanoshell/HA SNPs could efficiently be accumulated in the tumor and significantly enhance CT imaging of the tumor. Pan et al. presented a novel approach based on a soft, radio-opaque, and vascular-constrained colloidal particle, which can improve targeting specificity for intraluminal thrombus [148]. In this study, the amphiphilic diblock copolymer, polystyrene-b-polyacrylic acid (PS-b-PAA) was used to encapsulate ethiodized oil (a mixture of iodostearic acid ethyl ester and ethyldiiodostearate with 37 wt.% of total iodine content). Then, the particles were crosslinked via carbodiimide-mediated intramolecular cross-linking and then conjugated with biotin hydrazide as the targeting ligand on the surface of cross-linked particle, which finally obtained the soft type, vascularly constrained, stable colloidal radio-opaque iodinated polymeric SNPs (iodinated-cROMP-Biotin). The carboxylic acid groups throughout the nanoparticle shell led to a significant enhancement on stability. Moreover, the biotinylated cROMP particles were demonstrated to be able to effectively target to acellular fibrin clot phantoms with classic avidin–biotin interactions.

Single CT imaging modality often cannot satisfy the rapidly growing demand for the more reliable and accurate detection of disease sites, due to its low sensitivity. The combination of two or more imaging modalities into one system can overcome the limitations and take advantage of the strengths of each modality [1,112–115]. Polymeric SNPs were also designed for multimodal imaging. For example, the group of Whittaker designed and synthesized a kind of multifunctional, crosslinked hyperbranched polymer SNP containing iodine and fluorine, which can be used as bimodal imaging contrast media for use in CT/19F MRI imaging [149]. The hyperbranched iodopolymer (HBIP) was first synthesized via the reversible addition–fragmentation chain transfer polymerization of poly(ethylene glycol) methyl ether methacrylate (PEGMA), 2-(2′,3′,5′-triiodobenzoyl)ethyl methacrylate (TIBMA), and a degradable crosslinker bis-(2-methacryloyl)oxyethyl disulfide (DSDMA). Then, hyperbranched iodopolymers containing 19F (HBIPFs) with different contents of iodine and fluorine were prepared via the chain-extension reaction between the HBIP with PEGMA and 2,2,2-trifluoroethyl acrylate (TFEA). After the direct dissolution of HBIPFs in water, HBIPF SNPs with diameters of 10–15 nm were obtained. The radio-opacity of HBIPF SNPs in water was investigated using 19F MRI and CT imaging. The results indicated that HBIPF SNPs are attractive multimodal imaging contrast media for use in CT/19F MRI bimodal imaging.

Due to its high safety, low cost and portability, ultrasound (US) imaging has been widely utilized in clinical diagnosis. However, US imaging often suffers from very low resolution. The combination of high-resolution CT imaging with US imaging has significant merits for the development of multimodal imaging. To obtain real-time imaging and additional anatomic information about a tumor, Choi et al. synthesized a kind of iodine containing diatrizoic acid (DTA)-conjugated glycol chitosan (GC) SNP, which was used to physically encapsulate a US imaging agent (perfluoropentane, PFP) via the O/W emulsion method to prepare GC-DTA-PFP nanoparticles [59]. The in vitro and in vivo X-ray CT/US dual-modal imaging efficacy of GC-DTA-PFP SNPs was evaluated. The results indicated that as imaging contrast agents, GC-DTA-PFP SNPs presented very strong X-ray CT and US signals in phantom tests. Moreover, after intravenous injection, GC-DTA-PFP SNPs can be effectively accumulated on the tumor site by EPR effects, which thus could be used in X-ray CT/US dual-modal imaging to provide comprehensive and accurate diagnostic information about a tumor. In sum, due to their high stability, excellent biocompatibility, multifunctionality and flexibility in modification, polymeric SNPs provide a variety of multifunctional platforms for not only improved ICMs delivery, but also the development of multimodal contrast media for multimodal imaging.

Photoacoustic (PA) imaging is a type of biomedical imaging based on laser-generated ultrasound. As a new and hybrid modality, PA imaging integrates the high spatial resolution and deep penetration of ultrasound imaging with the high-contrast and specificity of optical imaging [150]. Polyaniline (PANi), with intense near-infrared (NIR) absorbance and a stable light-to-heat conversion capacity, has exhibited excellent imaging capability as a PA contrast agent [151]. To design multimodal contrast media for CT/PA-guided therapy, recently, Fu et al. rationally designed and developed a kind of iodinated polyaniline (LC@I-PANi) SNP via the simultaneous iodination and chemical oxidation polymerization of aniline in one system [48], as shown in Figure 20. LC@I-PANi SNPs with sphere-like morphologies and around 170 nm diameters have excellent colloidal stability and high biocompatibility. Furthermore, in vitro and in vivo experiments confirmed that LC@I-PANi SNPs possess favorable CT and PA imaging performance and good photothermal performance under NIR laser irradiation, providing a promising multifunctional therapeutic nanoplatform.

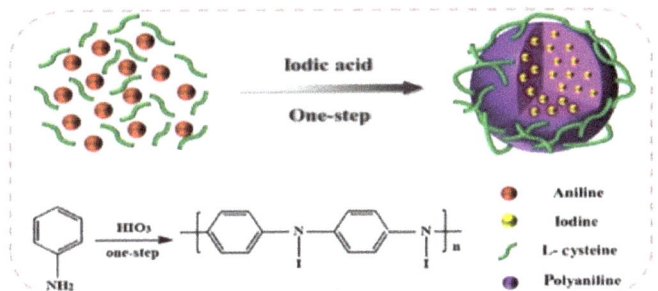

Figure 20. Schematic illustration of the preparation process of LC@I-PANi SNPs as multimodal contrast agent for CT/PA dual-modal imaging [48]. Reprinted with permission from ref. [48], Copyright 2021 Elsevier.

5. Conclusions

The clinical applications of X-ray CT imaging in medical diagnosis are still limited by the intrinsic drawbacks of iodine-based contrast media. Small molecular ICMs, used as the main contrast media in clinic, still suffer from fast renal clearance and serious adverse effects, especially the acute renal toxicity and inefficient targetability as well as low sensitivity. Due to their unique advantages, organic NPs, especially polymeric NPs, have exhibited great potential for the development of next-generation drug delivery systems with desirable properties. In this review, we comprehensively summarized the strategies and applications of organic NPs for ICMs delivery. Undoubtedly, these nanocarriers can significantly prolong blood circulation time, decrease renal toxicity, enhance delivery targetability and improve the sensitivity.

Despite the tremendous progress, the use of organic NPs for ICMs delivery is still far from applicable to clinical practice at the moment. Many challenges, such as batch-to-batch reproducibility, long-term biocompatibility, specific delivery, in vitro/in vivo stability and desirable pharmacokinetics need to be urgently overcome. As a result, tremendous efforts are still needed to develop efficient organic NPs for ICMs delivery. First, the scale-up preparation of organic NPs with controlled and uniform morphology is still a big challenge. With regard to nanomedicines and nanoimaging agents, the uniformity in nanostructure, the stability in physicochemical property and therapeutic performance, especially the controllability in the preparation process and the reproducibility in product quality are very important requirements for pharmaceutical and biomedical applications. However, due to the heterogeneity in the raw materials and the complexity and extremely high variability in the preparation process, the biomedical applications of organic NPs need to address the scalable production and batch-to-batch reproducibility. Thus, it is imperative to develop an effective approach to fabricate organic NPs with precise sizes, nanostructures and geometries in a scalable process, achieving high uniformity, reproducibility and thus high-performance. Second, ICMs were loaded into various organic NPs, often leading to a relatively low iodine content. As a result, a massive dose of contrast agents often necessitates the need for clear CT imaging, which will always pose a risk of renal toxicity and cytotoxicity. In addition, the in vivo degradation behaviors or decomposition product of organic NPs remain unclear, and thus thorough toxicological evaluations will be needed to confirm the biocompatibility of organic NPs for ICMs delivery. In addition, the delivery of sufficient amounts of contrast media in the targeted disease site is indispensable for successful imaging. Therefore, how to avoid fast clearance from the system but achieve the high accumulation of ICMs in malignant tissues is a key issue yet to be resolved, especially for the preoperative and intraoperative identification of tumors as well as intraoperative image-guided surgery. Significant efforts have been focused on improving the ability to target the delivery of ICMs via use of active and passive targeting strategies. However, the sophisticated pathophysiological barriers from the injection site to the site of action and the unsatisfying targetability of nanocarriers result in a very low delivery efficiency. Despite the enormous progress in nanomedicines, the design and development of advanced nanocarriers that can simultaneously meet the contradictory requirements to successively overcome each of the biological barriers is still a key issue to be addressed. Finally, we are witnessing a paradigm shift from conventional therapy to a more personalized, customized treatment model based on theragnosis. As a result, theragnostic agents must synergistically integrate multiple functions, including the therapeutic efficacy of drugs, disease recognition via imaging and targeted delivery to disease sites, leading to a formidable challenge in the fabrication of theragnostic agents. Organic NPs have been demonstrated to be a promising platform for theragnostic agents but are still in their infancy.

In sum, various organic NPs have exhibited significant advantages for ICMs delivery, opening up some new avenues in the search for optimal ICMs for use in CT imaging with maximum sensitivity, minimal toxicity, improved specificity and biodistribution.

Author Contributions: P.Z. and X.M. contributed equally to this work. P.Z. and X.M.: literature search, writing the first draft and preparation of figures; R.G., Z.Y., H.F., N.F. and Z.G.: literature search, organizing and writing Sections 4.4.2–4.4.4; J.Z. (Jianhua Zhang) and J.Z. (Jing Zhang): supervising the project and editing the whole manuscript. All authors have read and agreed to the published version of the manuscript.

Funding: This research was funded by Natural Science Foundation of Tianjin City (19JCYBJC17200), Tianjin Haihe Medical Scholar and the Tianjin Municipal Health and Family Planning Commission (14KG124).

Data Availability Statement: Not applicable.

Conflicts of Interest: The authors declare no conflict of interest.

References

1. Lee, D.E.; Koo, H.; Sun, I.C.; Ryu, J.H.; Kim, K.; Kwon, I.C. Multifunctional nanoparticles for multimodal imaging and theragnosis. *Chem. Soc. Rev.* **2012**, *41*, 2656–2672. [CrossRef]
2. Tempany, C.M.C.; McNeil, B.J. Advances in biomedical imaging. *J. Am. Med. Assoc.* **2001**, *285*, 562–567. [CrossRef]
3. Wallyn, J.; Anton, N.; Akram, S.; Vandamme, T.F. Biomedical imaging: Principles, technologies, clinical aspects, contrast agents, limitations and future trends in nanomedicines. *Pharm. Res.* **2019**, *36*, 78. [CrossRef] [PubMed]
4. Moran, C.M.; Thomson, A.J.W. Preclinical ultrasound imaging—A review of techniques and imaging applications. *Front. Phys.* **2020**, *8*, 124. [CrossRef]
5. Armana, R.; Habibb, Z. PET versus SPECT: Strengths, limitations and challenges. *Nucl. Med. Commun.* **2008**, *29*, 193–207. [CrossRef]
6. Leeuwen, F.W.B.V.; Hardwick, J.C.H.; Erkel, A.R.V. Luminescence-based imaging approaches in the field of interventional molecular imaging. *Radiology* **2015**, *276*, 12–29. [CrossRef] [PubMed]
7. Kumar, V.; Gu, Y.; Basu, S.; Berglund, A.; Eschrich, S.A.; Schabath, M.B.; Forster, K.; Aerts, H.J.W.L.; Dekker, A.; Fenstermacher, D.; et al. Radiomics: The process and the challenges. *Magn. Reson. Imaging* **2012**, *30*, 1234–1248. [CrossRef]
8. Lee, N.; Choi, S.H.; Hyeon, T. Nano-sized CT contrast agents. *Adv. Mater.* **2013**, *25*, 2641–2660. [CrossRef] [PubMed]
9. Lusic, H.; Grinstaff, M.W. X-ray-computed tomography contrast agents. *Chem. Rev.* **2013**, *113*, 1641–1666. [CrossRef]
10. LIU, Y.; AI, K.; LU, L. Nanoparticulate X-ray computed tomography contrast agents: From design validation to in vivo applications. *Acc. Chem. Res.* **2012**, *45*, 1817–1827. [CrossRef] [PubMed]
11. De La Vega, J.C.; Hafeli, U.O. Utilization of nanoparticles as X-ray contrast agents for diagnostic imaging applications. *Contrast. Media Mol. I* **2015**, *10*, 81–95. [CrossRef]
12. Gignac, P.M.; Kley, N.J.; Clarke, J.A.; Colbert, M.W.; Morhardt, A.C.; Cerio, D.; Cost, I.N.; Cox, P.G.; Daza, J.D.; Early, C.M.; et al. Diffusible iodine-based contrast-enhanced computed tomography (diceCT): An emerging tool for rapid, high-resolution, 3-D imaging of metazoan soft tissues. *J. Anat.* **2016**, *228*, 889–909. [CrossRef]
13. Koc, M.M.; Aslan, N.; Kao, A.P.; Barber, A.H. Evaluation of X-ray tomography contrast agents: A review of production, protocols, and biological applications. *Microsc. Res. Techniq.* **2019**, *82*, 812–848. [CrossRef]
14. Li, X.; Anton, N.; Zuber, G.; Vandamme, T. Contrast agents for preclinical targeted X-ray imaging. *Adv. Drug Deliv. Rev.* **2014**, *76*, 116–133. [CrossRef]
15. Thomsen, H.S. Gadolinium-or iodine-based contrast media: Which choice? *Acta. Radiol.* **2014**, *55*, 771–775. [CrossRef] [PubMed]

16. Seeliger, E.; Sendeski, M.; Rihal, C.S.; Persson, P.B. Contrast-induced kidney injury: Mechanisms, risk factors, and prevention. *Eur. Heart. J.* **2012**, *33*, 2007–2015. [CrossRef]
17. Ronco, C.; Stacul, F.; McCullough, P.A. Subclinical acute kidney injury (AKI) due to iodine-based contrast media. *Eur. Radiol.* **2013**, *23*, 319–323. [CrossRef]
18. Meng, X.; Wu, Y.; Bu, W. Functional CT contrast nanoagents for the tumor microenvironment. *Adv. Healthc. Mater.* **2021**, *10*, 2000912. [CrossRef] [PubMed]
19. Krause, W. Delivery of diagnostic agents in computed tomography. *Adv. Drug Deliv. Rev.* **1999**, *37*, 159–173. [CrossRef]
20. Kim, D.; Kim, J.; Park, Y.I.; Lee, N.; Hyeon, T. Recent development of inorganic nanoparticles for biomedical imaging. *ACS Cent. Sci.* **2018**, *4*, 324–336. [CrossRef] [PubMed]
21. Ehlerding, E.B.; Grodzinski, P.; Cai, W.; Liu, C.H. Big potential from small agents: Nanoparticles for imaging-based companion diagnostics. *ACS Nano.* **2018**, *12*, 2106–2121. [CrossRef]
22. Annapragada, A. Advances in nanoparticle imaging technology for vascular pathologies. *Annu. Rev. Med.* **2015**, *66*, 177–193. [CrossRef]
23. Zhang, X.; Dai, Z. Advances in multifunctional nano-sized CT contrast agents. *Chinese Sci. Bull.* **2015**, *60*, 3424–3437. [CrossRef]
24. Mulder, W.J.M.; van Leent, M.M.T.; Lameijer, M.; Fisher, E.A.; Fayad, Z.A.; Perez-Medina, C. High-density lipoprotein nanobiologics for precision medicine. *Acc. Chem. Res.* **2018**, *51*, 127–137. [CrossRef]
25. Cao, J.; Wei, Y.; Zhang, Y.; Wang, G.; Ji, X.; Zhong, Z. Iodine-rich polymersomes enable versatile SPECT/CT imaging and potent radioisotope therapy for tumor in vivo. *ACS Appl. Mater. Interfaces* **2019**, *11*, 18953–18959. [CrossRef] [PubMed]
26. Liu, X.; Gao, C.; Gu, J.; Jiang, Y.; Yang, X.; Li, S.; Gao, W.; An, T.; Duan, H.; Fu, J.; et al. Hyaluronic acid stabilized iodine-containing nanoparticles with Au nanoshell coating for X-ray CT imaging and photothermal therapy of tumors. *ACS Appl. Mater. Interfaces* **2016**, *8*, 27622–27631. [CrossRef]
27. Wallyn, J.; Anton, N.; Serra, C.A.; Bouquey, M.; Collot, M.; Anton, H.; Weickert, J.L.; Messaddeq, N.; Vandamme, T.F. A new formulation of poly(MAOTIB) nanoparticles as an efficient contrast agent for in vivo X-ray imaging. *Acta. Biomater.* **2018**, *66*, 200–212. [CrossRef] [PubMed]
28. Thaxton, C.S.; Rink, J.S.; Naha, P.C.; Cormode, D.P. Lipoproteins and lipoprotein mimetics for imaging and drug delivery. *Adv. Drug Deliv. Rev.* **2016**, *106*, 116–131. [CrossRef]
29. Attia, M.F.; Brummel, B.R.; Lex, T.R.; Van Horn, B.A.; Whitehead, D.C.; Alexis, F. Recent advances in polyesters for biomedical imaging. *Adv. Healthc. Mater.* **2018**, *7*, 1800798. [CrossRef]
30. Zou, Y.; Wei, Y.; Wang, G.; Meng, F.; Gao, M.; Storm, G.; Zhong, Z. Nanopolymersomes with an ultrahigh iodine content for high-performance X-ray computed tomography imaging In vivo. *Adv. Mater.* **2017**, *29*, 1603997. [CrossRef]
31. Liu, D.; Cornel, E.J.; Du, J. Renoprotective angiographic polymersomes. *Adv. Funct. Mater.* **2020**, *31*, 2007330. [CrossRef]
32. Torchilin, V.P. PEG-based micelles as carriers of contrast agents for different imaging modalities. *Adv. Drug Deliv. Rev.* **2002**, *54*, 235–252. [CrossRef]
33. Trubetskoy, V.S. Polymeric micelles as carriers of diagnostic agents. *Adv. Drug Deliv. Rev.* **1999**, *37*, 81–88. [CrossRef]
34. Torchilin, V.P. Polymeric contrast agents for medical imaging. *Curr. Pharm. Biotechnol.* **2000**, *1*, 183–215. [CrossRef]
35. Tian, L.; Lu, L.; Feng, J.; Melancon, M.P. Radiopaque nano and polymeric materials for atherosclerosis imaging, embolization and other catheterization procedures. *Acta. Pharm. Sin. B* **2018**, *8*, 360–370. [CrossRef] [PubMed]
36. Galperin, A.; Margel, D.; Baniel, J.; Dank, G.; Biton, H.; Margel, S. Radiopaque iodinated polymeric nanoparticles for X-ray imaging applications. *Biomaterials* **2007**, *28*, 4461–4468. [CrossRef]
37. Jin, E.; Lu, Z.R. Biodegradable iodinated polydisulfides as contrast agents for CT angiography. *Biomaterials* **2014**, *35*, 5822–5829. [CrossRef] [PubMed]
38. Houston, K.R.; Brosnan, S.M.; Burk, L.M.; Lee, Y.Z.; Luft, J.C.; Ashby, V.S. Iodinated polyesters as a versatile platform for radiopaque biomaterials. *J. Polym. Sci. Pol. Chem.* **2017**, *55*, 2171–2177. [CrossRef]
39. El Habnouni, S.; Blanquer, S.; Darcos, V.; Coudane, J. Aminated PCL-based copolymers by chemical modification of poly(α-iodo-ε-caprolactone-co-ε-caprolactone). *J. Polym. Sci. Pol. Chem.* **2009**, *47*, 6104–6115. [CrossRef]
40. Horák, D.; Metalová, M.; Rypáček, F. New radiopaque polyHEMA-based hydrogel particles. *J Biomed. Mater. Res.* **1997**, *34*, 183–188. [CrossRef]
41. Davy, K.W.M.; Anseau, M.R.; Berry, C. Iodinated methacrylate copolymers as X-ray opaque denture base acrylics. *J. Dent.* **1997**, *25*, 499–505. [CrossRef]
42. He, J.; Vallittu, P.K.; Lassila, L.V. Preparation and characterization of high radio-opaque e-glass fiber-reinforced composite with iodine containing methacrylate monomer. *Dent. Mater.* **2017**, *33*, 218–225. [CrossRef]
43. Aviv, H.; Bartling, S.; Kieslling, F.; Margel, S. Radiopaque iodinated copolymeric nanoparticles for X-ray imaging applications. *Biomaterials* **2009**, *30*, 5610–5616. [CrossRef] [PubMed]
44. Jayakrishnan, A.; Thanoo, B.C. Synthesis and polymerization of some iodine- containing monomers for biomedical applications. *J. Appl. Polym. Sci.* **1992**, *44*, 743–748. [CrossRef]
45. Rode, C.; Schmidt, A.; Wyrwa, R.; Weisser, J.; Schmidt, K.; Moszner, N.; Gottlöber, R.-P.; Heinemann, K.; Schnabelrauch, M. Synthesis and processability into textile structures of radiopaque, biodegradable polyesters and poly(ester-urethanes). *Polym. Int.* **2014**, *63*, 1732–1740. [CrossRef]

46. Tang, C.; York, A.W.; Mikitsh, J.L.; Wright, A.C.; Chacko, A.-M.; Elias, D.R.; Xu, Y.; Lim, H.-K.; Prud'homme, R.K. Preparation of PEGylated iodine- loaded nanoparticles via polymer-directed self-assembly. *Macromol. Chem. Phys.* **2018**, *219*, 1700592. [CrossRef]
47. Zou, Q.; Huang, J.; Zhang, X. One-step synthesis of iodinated polypyrrole nanoparticles for CT imaging guided photothermal therapy of tumors. *Small* **2018**, *14*, 1803101. [CrossRef] [PubMed]
48. Fu, L.; Yang, S.; Jiang, S.; Zhou, X.; Sha, Z.; He, C. One-step synthesis of multifunctional nanoparticles for CT/PA imaging guided breast cancer photothermal therapy. *Colloid. Surface B* **2021**, *201*, 111630. [CrossRef]
49. Ghosh, P.; Das, M.; Rameshbabu, A.P.; Das, D.; Datta, S.; Pal, S.; Panda, A.B.; Dhara, S. Chitosan derivatives cross-linked with iodinated 2,5-dimethoxy-2,5-dihydrofuran for non-invasive imaging. *ACS Appl. Mater. Interfaces* **2014**, *6*, 17926–17936. [CrossRef]
50. Lim, C.K.; Shin, J.; Kwon, I.C.; Jeong, S.Y.; Kim, S. Iodinated photosensitizing chitosan: Self-assembly into tumor-homing nanoparticles with enhanced singlet oxygen generation. *Bioconjugate Chem.* **2012**, *23*, 1022–1028. [CrossRef]
51. Revel, D.; Chambon, C.; Havard, P.; Dandis, G.; Canet, E.; Corot, C.; Amiel, M. Iodinated polymer as blood-pool contrast agent computed tommography evaluation in rabbits. *Invest. Radiol.* **1991**, *26*, 57–59. [CrossRef]
52. Balegamire, J.; Vandamme, M.; Chereul, E.; Si-Mohamed, S.; Azzouz Maache, S.; Almouazen, E.; Ettouati, L.; Fessi, H.; Boussel, L.; Douek, P.; et al. Iodinated polymer nanoparticles as contrast agent for spectral photon counting computed tomography. *Biomater. Sci.* **2020**, *8*, 5715–5728. [CrossRef]
53. True3etskoy, V.S.; Gazelle, G.S.; Wow, G.L.; Torchilin, V.I.P. Block-copolymer of polyethylene glycol and polylysine as a carrier of organic iodine: Design of long-circulating particulate contrast medium for X-ray computed tomography. *J. Drug Target.* **1997**, *4*, 381–388. [CrossRef] [PubMed]
54. Zhao, L.; Zhu, J.; Cheng, Y.; Xiong, Z.; Tang, Y.; Guo, L.; Shi, X.; Zhao, J. Chlorotoxin-conjugated multifunctional dendrimers jlabeled with radionuclide 131I for single photon emission computed tomography imaging and radiotherapy of gliomas. *ACS Appl. Mater. Interfaces* **2015**, *7*, 19798–19808. [CrossRef]
55. Fu, Y.; Nitecki, D.E.; Maltby, D.; Simon, G.H.; Berejnoi, K.; Raatschen, H.-J.; Yeh, B.M.; Shames, D.M.; Brasch, R.C. Dendritic iodinated contrast agents with PEG- cores for CT imaging: synthesis and preliminary characterization. *Bioconjugate Chem.* **2006**, *17*, 1043–1056. [CrossRef]
56. You, S.; Jung, H.Y.; Lee, C.; Choe, Y.H.; Heo, J.Y.; Gang, G.T.; Byun, S.K.; Kim, W.K.; Lee, C.H.; Kim, D.E.; et al. High-performance dendritic contrast agents for X-ray computed tomography imaging using potent tetraiodobenzene derivatives. *J. Control Release* **2016**, *226*, 258–267. [CrossRef] [PubMed]
57. Sun, Y.; Hu, H.; Yu, B.; Xu, F.J. PGMA-based cationic nanoparticles with polyhydric iodine units for advanced gene vectors. *Bioconjugate Chem.* **2016**, *27*, 2744–2754. [CrossRef] [PubMed]
58. Mottu, F.; Ruufenacht, D.A.; Laurentc, E.D. Iodine-containing cellulose mixed esters as radiopaque polymers for direct embolization of cerebral aneurysms and arteriovenous malformations. *Biomaterials* **2002**, *23*, 121–131. [CrossRef]
59. Choi, D.; Jeon, S.; You, D.G.; Um, W.; Kim, J.Y.; Yoon, H.Y.; Chang, H.; Kim, D.E.; Park, J.H.; Kim, H.; et al. Iodinated echogenic glycol chitosan nanoparticles for X-ray CT/US dual imaging of tumor. *Nanotheranostics* **2018**, *2*, 117–127. [CrossRef]
60. Padmanabhan, P.; Kumar, A.; Kumar, S.; Chaudhary, R.K.; Gulyas, B. Nanoparticles in practice for molecular-imaging applications: An overview. *Acta. Biomater.* **2016**, *41*, 1–16. [CrossRef] [PubMed]
61. Cormode, D.P.; Jarzyna, P.A.; Mulder, W.J.; Fayad, Z.A. Modified natural nanoparticles as contrast agents for medical imaging. *Adv. Drug Deliv. Rev.* **2010**, *62*, 329–338. [CrossRef] [PubMed]
62. Janib, S.M.; Moses, A.S.; MacKay, J.A. Imaging and drug delivery using theranostic nanoparticles. *Adv. Drug Deliv. Rev.* **2010**, *62*, 1052–1063. [CrossRef] [PubMed]
63. Jakhmola, A.; Anton, N.; Vandamme, T.F. Inorganic nanoparticles based contrast agents for X-ray computed tomography. *Adv. Healthc. Mater.* **2012**, *1*, 413–431. [CrossRef]
64. Hahn, M.A.; Singh, A.K.; Sharma, P.; Brown, S.C.; Moudgil, B.M. Nanoparticles as contrast agents for in-vivo bioimaging: Current status and future perspectives. *Anal. Bioanal. Chem.* **2011**, *399*, 3–27. [CrossRef] [PubMed]
65. Zhao, F.; Yao, D.; Guo, R.; Deng, L.; Dong, A.; Zhang, J. Composites of polymer hydrogels and nanoparticulate systems for biomedical and pharmaceutical applications. *Nanomaterials* **2015**, *5*, 2054–2130. [CrossRef]
66. Sun, Z.; Chen, W.; Sun, W.; Yu, B.; Zhang, Q.; Lu, L. Nanoparticles: Untying the gordian knot in conventional computed tomography imaging. *CCS Chem.* **2021**, *3*, 1242–1257. [CrossRef]
67. Rosen, J.E.; Yoffe, S.; Meerasa, A.; Verma1, M.; Gu, F.X. Nanotechnology and diagnostic imaging: New advances in contrast agent technology. *J. Nanomedic. Nanotechnol.* **2011**, *2*, 1000115. [CrossRef]
68. Elsabahy, M.; Wooley, K.L. Design of polymeric nanoparticles for biomedical delivery applications. *Chem. Soc. Rev.* **2012**, *41*, 2545–2561. [CrossRef]
69. Stiriba, S.-E.; Frey, H.; Haag, R. Dendritic polymers in biomedical applications: From potential to clinical use in diagnostics and therapy. *Angew. Chem. Int. Ed.* **2002**, *41*, 1329–1334. [CrossRef]
70. Shim, M.S.; Kwon, Y.J. Stimuli-responsive polymers and nanomaterials for gene delivery and imaging applications. *Adv. Drug Deliv. Rev.* **2012**, *64*, 1046–1059. [CrossRef] [PubMed]
71. Papadimitriou, S.A.; Salinas, Y.; Resmini, M. Smart polymeric nanoparticles as emerging tools for imaging-the parallel evolution of materials. *Chemistry* **2016**, *22*, 3612–3620. [CrossRef] [PubMed]
72. Duncan, R. The dawning era of polymer therapeutics. *Nat. Rev. Drug Discov.* **2003**, *2*, 347–360. [CrossRef] [PubMed]

73. Kim, J.-H.; Park, K.; Nam, H.Y.; Lee, S.; Kim, K.; Kwon, I.C. Polymers for bioimaging. *Prog. Polym. Sci.* **2007**, *32*, 1031–1053. [CrossRef]
74. Nottelet, B.; Darcos, V.; Coudane, J. Aliphatic polyesters for medical imaging and theranostic applications. *Eur. J. Pharm. Biopharm.* **2015**, *97*, 350–370. [CrossRef] [PubMed]
75. Skajaa, T.; Cormode, D.P.; Falk, E.; Mulder, W.J.; Fisher, E.A.; Fayad, Z.A. High-density lipoprotein-based contrast agents for multimodal imaging of atherosclerosis. *Arteriocl. Throm. Vas.* **2010**, *30*, 169–176. [CrossRef]
76. Shilo, M.; Reuveni, T.; Motiei, M.; Popovtzer, R. Nanoparticles as computed tomography contrast agents: Current status and future perspectives. *Nanomedicine* **2012**, *7*, 257–269. [CrossRef]
77. Zhu, C.; Liu, L.; Yang, Q.; Lv, F.; Wang, S. Water-soluble conjugated polymers for imaging, diagnosis, and therapy. *Chem. Rev.* **2012**, *112*, 4687–4735. [CrossRef]
78. Nair, L.S.; Laurencin, C.T. Biodegradable polymers as biomaterials. *Prog. Polym. Sci.* **2007**, *32*, 762–798. [CrossRef]
79. Guan, Y.; Sun, T.; Ding, J.; Xie, Z. Robust organic nanoparticles for noninvasive long-term fluorescence imaging. *J. Mater. Chem. B* **2019**, *7*, 6879–6889. [CrossRef]
80. Margulis-Goshen, K.; Magdassi, S. Organic nanoparticles from microemulsions: Formation and applications. *Curr. Opin. Colloid Interface Sci.* **2012**, *17*, 290–296. [CrossRef]
81. Palazzolo, S.; Bayda, S.; Hadla, M.; Caligiuri, I.; Corona, G.; Toffoli, G.; Rizzolio, F. The clinical translation of organic nanomaterials for cancer therapy: A focus on polymeric nanoparticles, micelles, liposomes and exosomes. *Curr. Med. Chem.* **2018**, *25*, 4224–4268. [CrossRef] [PubMed]
82. Al-Jamal, W.T.; Kostarelos, K. Liposomes: From a clinically established drug delivery system to a nanoparticle platform for theranostic nanomedicine. *Acc. Chem. Res.* **2011**, *44*, 1094–1104. [CrossRef]
83. Boase, N.R.B.; Blakey, I.; Thurecht, K.J. Molecular imaging with polymers. *Polym. Chem.* **2012**, *3*, 1384–1389. [CrossRef]
84. Krause, W.; Leike, J.; Sachse, A.; Schuhmann-Giampieri, G. Characterization of iopromide liposomes. *Invest. Radiol.* **1993**, *28*, 1028–1032. [CrossRef] [PubMed]
85. Silindir, M.; Erdogan, S.; Ozer, A.Y.; Dogan, A.L.; Tuncel, M.; Ugur, O.; Torchilin, V.P. Nanosized multifunctional liposomes for tumor diagnosis and molecular imaging by SPECT/CT. *J. Liposome Res.* **2013**, *23*, 20–27. [CrossRef] [PubMed]
86. Torchilin, V.; Babich, J.; Weissig, V. Liposomes and micelles to target the blood pool for imaging purposes. *J. Liposome. Res.* **2000**, *10*, 483–499. [CrossRef]
87. Xu, H.; Ohulchanskyy, T.Y.; Qu, J.; Yakovliev, A.; Ziniuk, R.; Yuan, Z.; Qu, J. Co-encapsulating indocyanine green and CT contrast agent within nanoliposomes for trimodal imaging and near infrared phototherapy of cancer. *Nanomedicine* **2020**, *29*, 102269. [CrossRef]
88. Anton, N.; Vandamme, T.F. Nanotechnology for computed tomography: A real potential recently disclosed. *Pharm. Res.* **2014**, *31*, 20–34. [CrossRef]
89. Ryan, P.J.; Davis, M.A.; DeGaeta, L.R.; Woda, B.; Melchior, D.L. Liposomes loaded with contrast material for image enhancement in computed tomography. Work in progress. *Radiology* **1984**, *152*, 759–762. [CrossRef]
90. Havron, A.; Seltzer, S.E.; Davis, M.A.; Shulkin, P. Radiopaque liposomes: A promising new contrast material for computed tomography of the spleen. *Radiology* **1981**, *140*, 507–511. [CrossRef]
91. Benita, S.; Poly, P.A.; Puisieux, F.; Delattre, J. Radiopaque liposomes: Effect of formulation conditions on encapsulation efficiency. *J. Pharm. Sci.* **1984**, *73*, 1751–1755. [CrossRef]
92. Knop, K.; Hoogenboom, R.; Fischer, D.; Schubert, U.S. Poly(ethylene glycol) in drug delivery: Pros and cons as well as potential alternatives. *Angew. Chem. Int. Ed.* **2010**, *49*, 6288–6308. [CrossRef] [PubMed]
93. Otsuka, H.; Nagasaki, Y.; Kataoka, K. PEGylated nanoparticles for biological and pharmaceutical applications. *Adv. Drug Deliv. Rev.* **2012**, *64*, 246–255. [CrossRef]
94. Hoang Thi, T.T.; Pilkington, E.H.; Nguyen, D.H.; Lee, J.S.; Park, K.D.; Truong, N.P. The importance of poly(ethylene glycol) alternatives for overcoming PEG immunogenicity in drug delivery and bioconjugation. *Polymers* **2020**, *12*, 298. [CrossRef] [PubMed]
95. Samei, E.; Saunders, R.S.; Badea, C.T.; Ghaghada, K.B.; Hedlund, L.W.; Qi, Y.; Yuan, H.; Bentley, R.C.; Jr, S.M. Micro-CT imaging of breast tumors in rodents using a liposomal, nanoparticle contrast agent. *Int. J. Nanomed.* **2009**, *4*, 277–282. [CrossRef]
96. Ghaghada, K.B.; Badea, C.T.; Karumbaiah, L.; Fettig, N.; Bellamkonda, R.V.; Johnson, G.A.; Annapragada, A. Evaluation of tumor microenvironment in an animal model using a nanoparticle contrast agent in computed tomography imaging. *Acad. Radiol.* **2011**, *18*, 20–30. [CrossRef]
97. Mukundan, S., Jr.; Ghaghada, K.B.; Badea, C.T.; Kao, C.Y.; Hedlund, L.W.; Provenzale, J.M.; Johnson, G.A.; Chen, E.; Bellamkonda, R.V.; Annapragada, A. A liposomal nanoscale contrast agent for preclinical CT in mice. *Am. J. Roentgenol.* **2006**, *186*, 300–307. [CrossRef] [PubMed]
98. Burke, S.J.; Annapragada, A.; Hoffman, E.A.; Chen, E.; Ghaghada, K.B.; Sieren, J.; Beek, E.J.R.v. Imaging of pulmonary embolism and t-PA therapy effects using MDCT and liposomal iohexol blood pool agent: Preliminary results in a rabbit model. *Acad. Radiol.* **2007**, *14*, 355–362. [CrossRef] [PubMed]
99. Choi, H.S.; Kim, H.K. Multispectral image-guided surgery in patients. *Nat. Biomed. Eng.* **2020**, *4*, 245–246. [CrossRef]
100. Koudrina, A.; DeRosa, M.C. Advances in medical imaging: Aptamer-and peptide-targeted MRI and CT contrast agents. *ACS Omega.* **2020**, *5*, 22691–22701. [CrossRef] [PubMed]

101. Bertrand, N.; Wu, J.; Xu, X.; Kamaly, N.; Farokhzad, O.C. Cancer nanotechnology: The impact of passive and active targeting in the era of modern cancer biology. *Adv. Drug Deliv. Rev.* **2014**, *66*, 2–25. [CrossRef]
102. Lammers, T.; Kiessling, F.E.; Hennink, W.; Storm, G. Drug targeting to tumors: Principles, pitfalls and (pre-) clinical progress. *J. Control Release* **2012**, *161*, 175–187. [CrossRef]
103. Moghimi, S.M.; Hunter, A.C.; Murray, J.C. Long-circulating and target-specific nanoparticles: Theory to practice. *Pharmacol. Rev.* **2001**, *53*, 283–318.
104. Gazelle, G.S.; Wolf, G.L.; McIntire, G.L.; Bacon, E.R.; Na, G.; Halpern, E.E.; Toner, J.L. Hepatic imaging with iodinated nanoparticles: A comparison with iohexol in rabbits. *Acad. Radiol.* **1995**, *2*, 700–704. [CrossRef]
105. Desser, T.S.; Rubin, D.L.; Muller, H.; McIntire, G.L.; Bacon, E.R.; Toner, J.L. Blood pool and liver enhancement in CT with liposomal Iodixanol: Comparison with Iohexol. *Acad. Radiol.* **1999**, *6*, 176–183. [CrossRef]
106. Kweon, S.; Lee, H.-J.; Hyung, W.J.; Suh, J.; Lim, J.S.; Lim, S.-J. Liposomes coloaded with iopamidol/lipiodol as a RES-targeted contrast agent for computed tomography imaging. *Pharm. Res.* **2010**, *27*, 1408–1415. [CrossRef] [PubMed]
107. Shi, Y.; Meel, R.v.d.; Chen, X.; Lammers, T. The EPR effect and beyond: Strategies to improve tumor targeting and cancer nanomedicine treatment efficacy. *Theranostics* **2020**, *10*, 7921–7924. [CrossRef]
108. Overchuk, M.; Zheng, G. Overcoming obstacles in the tumor microenvironment: Recent advancements in nanoparticle delivery for cancer theranostics. *Biomaterials* **2018**, *156*, 217–237. [CrossRef] [PubMed]
109. Wilhelm, S.; Tavares, A.J.; Dai, Q.; Ohta, S.; Audet, J.; Dvorak, H.F.; Chan, W.C.W. Analysis of nanoparticle delivery to tumours. *Nat. Rev. Mater.* **2016**, *1*, 16014. [CrossRef]
110. Zheng, J.; Jaffray, D.; Allen, C. Quantitative CT imaging of the spatial and temporal distribution of liposomes in a rabbit tumor model. *Mol. Pharm.* **2009**, *6*, 571–580. [CrossRef]
111. Ghaghada, K.B.; Sato, A.F.; Starosolski, Z.A.; Berg, J.; Vail, D.M. Computed tomography imaging of solid tumors using a liposomal-iodine contrast agent in companion dogs with naturally occurring cancer. *PLoS. ONE* **2016**, *11*, e0152718. [CrossRef]
112. Kim, J.; Piao, Y.; Hyeon, T. Multifunctional nanostructured materials for multimodal imaging, and simultaneous imaging and therapy. *Chem. Soc. Rev.* **2009**, *38*, 372–390. [CrossRef] [PubMed]
113. Louie, A. Multimodality imaging probes: Design and challenges. *Chem. Rev.* **2010**, *110*, 3146–3195. [CrossRef]
114. Tsang, M.-K.; Wong, Y.-T.; Hao, J. Cutting-edge nanomaterials for advanced multimodal bioimaging applications. *Small Methods* **2018**, *2*, 1700265. [CrossRef]
115. Rieffel, J.; Chitgupi, U.; Lovell, J.F. Recent advances in higher- order, multimodal, biomedical imaging agents. *Small* **2015**, *11*, 4445–4461. [CrossRef]
116. Xu, H.; Ohulchanskyy, T.Y.; Yakovliev, A.; Zinyuk, R.; Song, J.; Liu, L.; Qu, J.; Yuan, Z. Nanoliposomes co-encapsulating CT imaging contrast agent and photosensitizer for enhanced, imaging guided photodynamic therapy of cancer. *Theranostics* **2019**, *9*, 1323–1335. [CrossRef]
117. Jenjob, R.; Phakkeeree, T.; Seidi, F.; Theerasilp, M.; Crespy, D. Emulsion techniques for the production of pharmacological nanoparticles. *Macromol. Biosci.* **2019**, *19*, 1900063. [CrossRef]
118. Attia, M.F.; Anton, N.; Chiper, M.; Akasov, R.; Anton, H.; Messaddeq, N.; Fournel, S.; Klymchenko, A.S.; Mély, Y.M.; Vandamme, T.F. Biodistribution of X-ray iodinated contrast agent in nano-emulsions is controlled by the chemical nature of the oily core. *ACS Nano* **2014**, *8*, 10537–10550. [CrossRef] [PubMed]
119. de Vries, A.; Custers, E.; Lub, J.; van den Bosch, S.; Nicolay, K.; Grull, H. Block-copolymer-stabilized iodinated emulsions for use as CT contrast agents. *Biomaterials* **2010**, *31*, 6537–6544. [CrossRef]
120. Li, X.; Anton, N.; Zuber, G.; Zhao, M.; Messaddeq, N.; Hallouard, F.; Fessi, H.; Vandamme, T.F. Iodinated alpha-tocopherol nano-emulsions as non-toxic contrast agents for preclinical X-ray imaging. *Biomaterials* **2013**, *34*, 481–491. [CrossRef]
121. Hallouard, F.; Briancon, S.; Anton, N.; Li, X.; Vandamme, T.; Fessi, H. Iodinated nano-emulsions as contrast agents for preclinical X-ray imaging: Impact of the free surfactants on the pharmacokinetics. *Eur. J. Pharm. Biopharm.* **2013**, *83*, 54–62. [CrossRef]
122. Attia, M.F.; Anton, N.; Akasov, R.; Chiper, M.; Markvicheva, E.; Vandamme, T.F. Biodistribution and toxicity of X-ray iodinated contrast agent in nano-emulsions in function of their size. *Pharm. Res.* **2016**, *33*, 603–614. [CrossRef]
123. Hallouard, F.; Anton, N.; Zuber, G.; Choquet, P.; Li, X.; Arntz, Y.; Aubertin, G.; Constantinesco, A.; Vandamme, T.F. Radiopaque iodinated nano-emulsions for preclinical X-ray imaging. *RSC Adv.* **2011**, *1*, 792–801. [CrossRef]
124. Hallouard, F.; Anton, N.; Choquet, P.; Constantinesco, A.; Vandamme, T. Iodinated blood pool contrast media for preclinical X-ray imaging applications-a review. *Biomaterials* **2010**, *31*, 6249–6268. [CrossRef]
125. Hallouard, F.; Briancon, S.; Anton, N.; Li, X.; Vandamme, T.; Fessi, H. Influence of diblock copolymer PCL-mPEG and of various iodinated oils on the formulation by the emulsion-solvent diffusion process of radiopaque polymeric nanoparticles. *J. Pharm. Sci.* **2013**, *102*, 4150–4158. [CrossRef] [PubMed]
126. Cormode, D.P.; Naha, P.C.; Fayad, Z.A. Nanoparticle contrast agents for computed tomography: A focus on micelles. *Contrast. Media Mol. I* **2014**, *9*, 37–52. [CrossRef]
127. Zhou, W.; Chen, Y.; Zhang, Y.; Xin, X.; Li, R.; Xie, C.; Fan, Q. Iodine-rich semiconducting polymer nanoparticles for CT/fluorescence dual-modal imaging-guided enhanced photodynamic therapy. *Small* **2020**, *16*, 1905641. [CrossRef] [PubMed]
128. Discher, B.M.; Won, Y.-Y.; Ege, D.S.; Lee, J.C.-M.; Bates, F.S.; Discher, D.E.; Hammer, D.A. Polymersomes: Tough vesicles made from diblock copolymers. *Science* **1999**, *284*, 1143–1146. [CrossRef]
129. Discher, D.E.; Ahmed, F. Polymersomes. *Annu. Rev. Biomed. Eng.* **2006**, *8*, 323–341. [CrossRef]

130. Pawar, P.V.; Gohil, S.V.; Jain, J.P.; Kumar, N. Functionalized polymersomes for biomedical applications. *Polym. Chem.* **2013**, *4*, 3160–3176. [CrossRef]
131. Thevenot, J.; Oliveira, H.; Lecommandoux, S. Polymersomes for theranostics. *J. Drug Deliv. Sci. Technol.* **2013**, *23*, 38–46. [CrossRef]
132. Leong, J.; Teo, J.Y.; Aakalu, V.K.; Yang, Y.Y.; Kong, H. Engineering polymersomes for diagnostics and therapy. *Adv. Healthc. Mater.* **2018**, *7*, 1701276. [CrossRef] [PubMed]
133. Zou, Y.; Wei, Y.; Sun, Y.; Bao, J.; Yao, F.; Li, Z.; Meng, F.; Hu, C.; Storm, G.; Zhong, Z. Cyclic RGD-functionalized and disulfide-crosslinked iodine-rich polymersomes as a robust and smart theranostic agent for targeted CT imaging and chemotherapy of tumor. *Theranostics* **2019**, *9*, 8061–8072. [CrossRef] [PubMed]
134. Yu, M.; Jie, X.; Xu, L.; Chen, C.; Shen, W.; Cao, Y.; Lian, G.; Qi, R. Recent advances in dendrimer research for cardiovascular diseases. *Biomacromolecules* **2015**, *16*, 2588–2598. [CrossRef]
135. Mignani, S.; Rodrigues, J.; Tomas, H.; Caminade, A.-M.; Laurent, R.; Shi, X.; Majoral, J.-P. Recent therapeutic applications of the theranostic principle with dendrimers in oncology. *Sci. China. Mater.* **2018**, *61*, 1367–1386. [CrossRef]
136. Qiao, Z.; Shi, X. Dendrimer-based molecular imaging contrast agents. *Prog. Polym. Sci.* **2015**, *44*, 1–27. [CrossRef]
137. Kesharwani, P.; Jain, K.; Jain, N.K. Dendrimer as nanocarrier for drug delivery. *Prog. Polym. Sci.* **2014**, *39*, 268–307. [CrossRef]
138. Yordanov, A.T.; Lodder, A.L.; Woller, E.K.; Cloninger, M.J.; Patronas, N.; Milenic, D.; Brechbiel, M.W. Novel iodinated dendritic nanoparticles for computed tomography (CT) imaging. *Nano. Lett.* **2002**, *2*, 595–599. [CrossRef]
139. Ding, Y.; Zhang, X.; Xu, Y.; Cheng, T.; Ou, H.; Li, Z.; An, Y.; Shen, W.; Liu, Y.; Shi, L. Polymerization-induced self-assembly of large-scale iohexol nanoparticles as contrast agents for X-ray computed tomography imaging. *Polym. Chem.* **2018**, *9*, 2926–2935. [CrossRef]
140. Hainfeld, J.F.; Ridwan, S.M.; Stanishevskiy, Y.; Smilowitz, N.R.; Davis, J.; Smilowitz, H.M. Small, Long blood half-life iodine nanoparticle for vascular and tumor imaging. *Sci. Rep.* **2018**, *8*, 13803. [CrossRef]
141. Yin, Q.; Yap, F.Y.; Yin, L.; Ma, L.; Zhou, Q.; Dobrucki, L.W.; Fan, T.M.; Gaba, R.C.; Cheng, J. Poly(iohexol) nanoparticles as contrast agents for in vivo X-ray computed tomography imaging. *J. Am. Chem. Soc.* **2013**, *135*, 13620–13623. [CrossRef] [PubMed]
142. Cormode, D.P.; Skajaa, T.; Schooneveld, M.M.V.; Koole, R.; Jarzyna, P.; Lobatto, M.E.; Calcagno, C.; Barazza, A.; Gordon, R.E.; Zanzonico, P.; et al. Nanocrystal core high-density lipoproteins: A multimodality contrast agent platform. *Nano. Lett.* **2008**, *8*, 3715–3723. [CrossRef]
143. Ng, K.K.; Lovell, J.F.; Zheng, G. Lipoprotein-inspired nanoparticles for cancer theranostics. *Acc. Chem. Res.* **2011**, *44*, 1105–1113. [CrossRef]
144. Hill, M.L.; Corbin, I.R.; Levitin, R.B.; Cao, W.; Mainprize, J.G.; Yaffe, M.J.; Zheng, G. In vitro assessment of poly-iodinated triglyceride reconstituted low-density lipoprotein: Initial steps toward CT molecular imaging. *Acad. Radiol.* **2010**, *17*, 1359–1365. [CrossRef] [PubMed]
145. deKrafft, K.E.; Xie, Z.; Cao, G.; Tran, S.; Ma, L.; Zhou, O.Z.; Lin, W. Iodinated nanoscale coordination polymers as potential contrast agents for computed tomography. *Angew. Chem. Int. Ed.* **2009**, *48*, 9901–9904. [CrossRef] [PubMed]
146. Gao, C.; Zhang, Y.; Zhang, Y.; Li, S.; Yang, X.; Chen, Y.; Fu, J.; Wang, Y.; Yang, X. cRGD-modified and disulfide bond-crosslinked polymer nanoparticles based on iopamidol as a tumor-targeted CT contrast agent. *Polym. Chem.* **2020**, *11*, 889–899. [CrossRef]
147. Mizrahy, S.; Peer, D. Polysaccharides as building blocks for nanotherapeutics. *Chem. Soc. Rev.* **2012**, *41*, 2623–2640. [CrossRef]
148. Pan, D.; Williams, T.A.; Senpan, A.; Allen, J.S.; Scott, M.J.; Gaffney, P.J.; Wickline, S.A.; Lanza, G.M. Detecting vascular biosignatures with a colloidal, radio-opaque polymeric nanoparticle. *J. Am. Chem. Soc.* **2009**, *131*, 15522–15527. [CrossRef]
149. Wang, K.; Peng, H.; Thurecht, K.J.; Puttick, S.; Whittaker, A.K. Multifunctional hyperbranched polymers for CT/19F MRI bimodal molecular imaging. *Polym. Chem.* **2016**, *7*, 1059–1069. [CrossRef]
150. Attia, A.B.E.; Balasundaram, G.; Moothanchery, M.; Dinish, U.S.; Bi, R.; Ntziachristos, V.; Olivo, M. A review of clinical photoacoustic imaging: Current and future trends. *Photoacoustics* **2019**, *16*, 100144. [CrossRef]
151. Zhou, Y.; Hu, Y.; Sun, W.; Zhou, B.; Zhu, J.; Peng, C.; Shen, M.; Shi, X. Polyaniline-loaded gamma-polyglutamic acid nanogels as a platform for photoacoustic imaging-guided tumor photothermal therapy. *Nanoscale* **2017**, *9*, 12746–12754. [CrossRef] [PubMed]

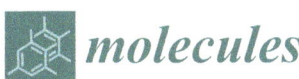

Review

Nanomaterials for Modulating the Aggregation of β-Amyloid Peptides

Yaliang Huang [1,2], Yong Chang [2], Lin Liu [2,*] and Jianxiu Wang [1,*]

[1] Hunan Provincial Key Laboratory of Micro & Nano Materials Interface Science, College of Chemistry and Chemical Engineering, Central South University, Changsha 410083, China; 182301010@csu.edu.cn
[2] Henan Province of Key Laboratory of New Optoelectronic Functional Materials, College of Chemistry and Chemical Engineering, Anyang Normal University, Anyang 455000, China; 7180610011@stu.jiangnan.edu.cn
* Correspondence: liulin@aynu.edu.cn (L.L.); jxiuwang@csu.edu.cn (J.W.)

Abstract: The aberrant aggregation of amyloid-β (Aβ) peptides in the brain has been recognized as the major hallmark of Alzheimer's disease (AD). Thus, the inhibition and dissociation of Aβ aggregation are believed to be effective therapeutic strategies for the prevention and treatment of AD. When integrated with traditional agents and biomolecules, nanomaterials can overcome their intrinsic shortcomings and boost their efficiency via synergistic effects. This article provides an overview of recent efforts to utilize nanomaterials with superior properties to propose effective platforms for AD treatment. The underlying mechanisms that are involved in modulating Aβ aggregation are discussed. The summary of nanomaterials-based modulation of Aβ aggregation may help researchers to understand the critical roles in therapeutic agents and provide new insight into the exploration of more promising anti-amyloid agents and tactics in AD theranostics.

Keywords: Alzheimer disease's; amyloid-β; nanomaterials; photothermal therapy; photodynamic therapy

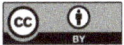

1. Introduction

Abnormal changes in protein spatial structure can lead to the occurrence of protein conformational diseases [1]. For example, the precipitation and aggregation of protein amyloid fibers in neurons or brain parenchyma can induce cytotoxicity and eventually lead to neurodegenerative diseases, such as Alzheimer's disease (AD), amyotrophic lateral sclerosis (ALS), Huntington's disease (HD) and Parkinson's disease (PD) [2–5]. As the most common form of dementia, AD affects about 40 million people worldwide [6]. Although the pathogenesis of AD is multifactorial [7–11], the abnormal aggregation of β-amyloid (Aβ) peptides is still considered the most salient feature in AD. Aβ peptides consisting of 39–43 amino acid residues are the proteolytic cleavage products of the β-amyloid precursor protein (APP) [12,13]. Aβ$_{1-40}$ and Aβ$_{1-42}$ are two major abundant types in amyloid plaques [14]. Aβ monomers can assemble into β-sheet-rich oligomers with different sizes and form into long fibrils. Recent studies revealed that extracellular soluble Aβ oligomers and fibrils exhibit strong neurotoxicity, which may be the potential targets for AD treatment [15]. Oxidative stress maybe the potential mechanism that explains the neurotoxicity induced by Aβ aggregates [16]. Thus, the inhibition of Aβ fibrillogenesis and the disassembly of Aβ aggregates are considered to be important treatment strategies for AD.

Prompted by the need to pursue effective treatment of AD, many inhibitors against Aβ aggregation and cytotoxicity were explored, including small molecules, peptides [17–19], proteins [20–22] and antibodies [23]. For example, we demonstrated that 5,10,15,20-tetrakis(N-methyl-4-pyridyl)-porphyrin (TMPyP), a water-soluble porphyrin, can inhibit Aβ aggregation, disintegrate the preformed Aβ aggregates and alleviate Aβ-induced cytotoxicity [24]. Peptides with a special sequence that is homologous to Aβ can keep it from aggregating through hydrophobic, hydrogen, covalent or electrostatic interactions, which are known as β-sheet breaker peptides, including LPFFD, KLVFFAE, CGGGGGIGLMVG and LVFFARK (LK7). It was suggested that denaturation of native Aβ to oxygenated forms via photooxygenation could slow Aβ aggregation and neurotoxicity [25]. Thus, various photosensitizers were explored for light-induced preclusion of Aβ aggregation, such as methylene blue, porphyrins and riboflavin [26–29]. However, significant shortcomings limit the further application of these reagents, such as low solubility andpoor stability in physiological conditions. Moreover, the low permeability of the blood-brain barrier (BBB) also renders these inhibitors unsuitable for the treatment of AD [30]. Therefore, the demand is still urgent to develop effective drugs that target Aβ aggregation with great clinical application potential.

With the development of nanotechnology in the past decades, numerous nanomaterials have been designed, synthesized and applied in different fields, such as physics, environmental science and biosensors. Due to the superb biocompatibility, stable physiochemical properties and synthesis and modification flexibility, nanomaterials-based approaches offer enormous potential to overcome the challenges in current therapeutic/diagnostic bio-reagents applications. In this regard, great efforts have been committed to discussing solutions from the nanomaterials perspective for improving AD treatment efficiency. Based on the characteristics of nanomaterials, traditional small molecule inhibitors can get across the BBB by being encapsulated into or modified with nanomaterials, such as mesoporous nano-selenium [31]. Furthermore, nanomaterials can be conjugated with target ligands, such as folate, polysaccharides, cell-penetrating peptidesand antibodies, to improve the bioavailability in brain regions and the efficiency of intracellular particles delivery [32,33]. Although there are a lot of studies that utilized different nanomaterials to inhibit the aggregation of the Aβ peptide, their effects on peptide fibrillation still need to be investigated [34].

In this review, we focused on recent progress in nanomaterials-based methodology for inhibiting Aβ aggregation. Meanwhile, we also paid close attention to novel strategies that use photo-sensitive or enzyme-mimicking properties inAD treatment.

2. Nanomaterials

According to the main composition and dimensions, the types of nanomaterialsfor modulating the aggregation of β-amyloid peptidesare various, including gold, carbon, transition oxide, two-dimensional (2D) nanomaterials, metal-organic framework (MOF) and self-assembled nanomaterials (Scheme 1).

2.1. Gold-Based Nanomaterials

Gold-based nanomaterials have the strengths ofbeing chemically inert, having tunable local surface plasmon resonance (LSPR) absorption and good conductivity. The LSPR absorption can be tuned by varying the size, shape, surrounding environment and dispersion state [35]. Owing to their unique properties and easeof manipulation, gold-based nanomaterials have broad applications in drug delivery, disease diagnosis and illness treatment, including central nervous system diseases [36]. The main category of gold nanomaterials that are used for treating AD includes bare gold nanoparticles (AuNPs) and gold nanocomposites modified with peptides or other molecules.

AuNPs were reported by many researchers as having functions of penetrating through the BBB, inhibiting Aβ peptide from aggregation [37] and degrading Aβ aggregates based on their size, surface charge, shape, functionality and even concentration [38–41]. For example, Ma et al. found that the negatively charged citrate-capped AuNPs could induce Aβ peptides to quickly form short protofibrils, subsequently causing them to assemble into short fibril bundles or even bundle conjunctions [42]. Wang and co-workers investigated the effect of AuNPs with different shapes on the aggregation of $Aβ_{1-40}$ peptides (Figure 1A) [43]. Moreover, because of the high degree of surface atomic unsaturation to adsorb $Aβ_{1-40}$ peptides with high affinity, Au nanospheres exhibited a more significant increase of the fibrillation process than Au nanocubes. Liu et al. investigated the size effect of gold nanorods (AuNRs) on modulating the kinetic process of Aβ aggregation (Figure 1B) [44]. They found that the inhibition efficiency of larger AuNRs is better than that of smaller AuNRs and the rate constant was a quadratic function of the diameters or lengths. Liao et al. studied the effect of the surface charge of AuNPs on Aβ aggregation [41]. As shown in Figure 1C, the negatively charged AuNPs could not only inhibit Aβ fibrillization to form fragmented fibrils and spherical oligomers but also remodel preformed fibrils into smaller and ragged Aβ species. Furthermore, by means of enhanced sampling molecular dynamics simulations, the interactions between Aβ peptides and Au nanomaterials with various sizes and morphologies are well characterized, which is helpful for understanding the inhibition mechanism and explore new strategies for AD treatment [45,46].

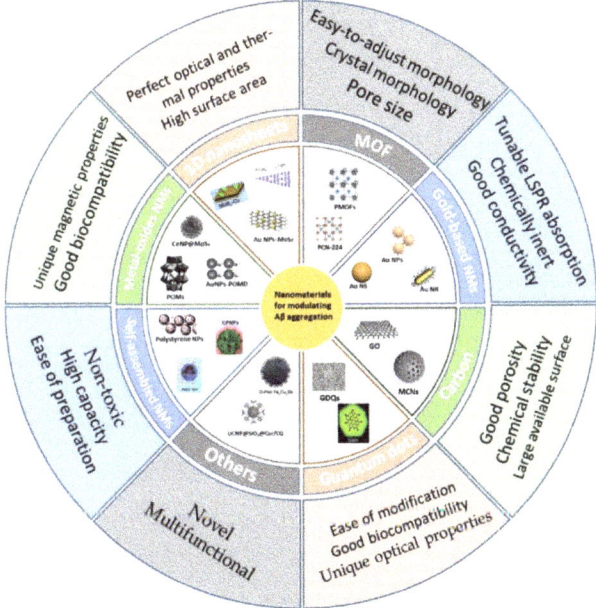

Scheme 1. A graphic summary with the important characteristics of nanomaterials discussed in this article.

Small molecules and peptides can be conjugated on the surface of nanomaterials to improve the properties and efficiency of both the modifiers and the nanomaterials [47]. For example, Palmal et al. prepared curcumin-functionalized AuNPs and found that water-soluble AuNPs with multiple curcumin moieties on the surface could inhibit Aβ fibrillation and dissolve Aβ fibrils without using other external agent or force [48]. β-Sheet breaker peptides can also be integrated with Au nanomaterials. Xiong et al. designed a branched dual-inhibitor sequence (VVIACLPFFD) for inhibiting Aβ aggregation and cytotoxicity, whose inhibitory effects were greatly enhanced due to its special surface orientation and conformation (Figure 2A) [49]. However, it was also reported that N-methylated peptides (CGGIGLMVG and CGGGGGIGLMVG) exhibit less effective inhibition of Aβ fibril than free peptides because β-sheet N-methylated peptides, with their more ordered arrangement on the surface, show weak affinity toward Aβ in solution. In contrast, CLPFFD peptides modified on the nanoparticle surface can improve the stability of NPs, reduce the effect on cell viability and increase the delivery efficiency to the brain [50,51]. Moreover, the sequence of the peptide has an influence on the conjugation and stability of AuNPs and the affinity ability for Aβ fibrils [52].

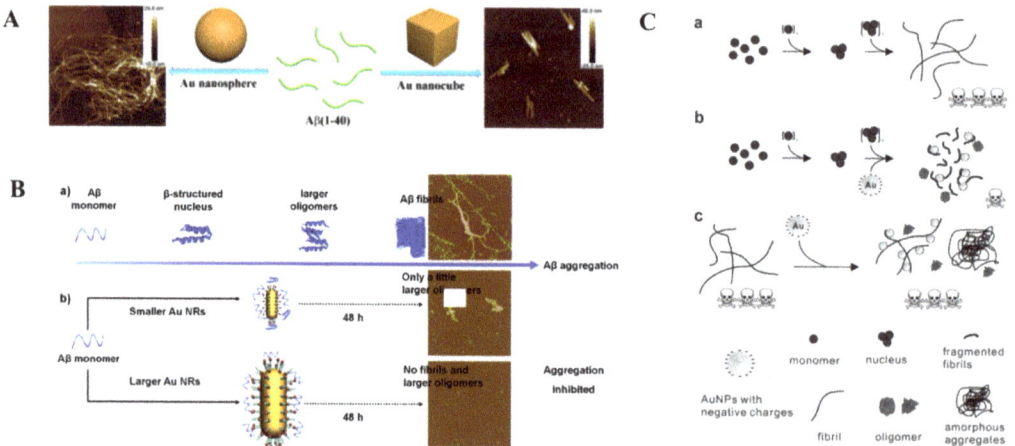

Figure 1. (**A**) Schematic of effects of gold nanospheres and nanocubes on Aβ$_{1-40}$ peptide fibrillation. Reprinted with permission from reference [43]. Copyright 2019 American Chemical Society. (**B**) Schematic of (a) the process of Aβ aggregation and (b) The schematic of CTAB-stabilized AuNRs with different sizes inhibiting Aβ peptides fibrillation [44]. Copyright 2019 Elsevier. (**C**) Diagram of Aβ fibrillization pathways influenced by negatively charged AuNPs. (a) Aβ monomers assemble into mature amyloid fibrils and cause neurotoxicity. (b) Aβ monomers incubated with the AuNPs possessing negative surface potential lead to formation of short and fragmented fibrils along with spherical oligomers. The alteration rescues the toxicity generated from mature Aβ fibrils. (c) AuNPs addition to preformed Aβ fibrils induces ragged fibrils and amorphous aggregates without changing the toxicity level [41]. Copyright 2012 Wiley-VCH.

Aβ aggregation can be disintegrated via local heat generation. Kogan et al. found that AuNPs modified with Cys-PEP peptides and CLPFFD can selectively attach to the Aβ fibrils and prefibrillar intermediate amyloidogenic aggregates (PIAA) (Figure 2B) [53,54]. Then, microwave irradiation generated local heat using nanoparticles to dissolve Aβ aggregates. In photothermal therapy (PTT), light can be converted into heat with the aid of molecules or nanomaterialsthat display photothermal conversion ability. PTT was shown to be a promising strategy for the treatment of various diseases due to its remarkable advantages of site- and time-specificity, non-invasiveness and targeting selectivity. Owing to the extinction coefficient of theLSPR, Au nanomaterials can cause the photothermal ablation of amyloid peptide aggregates using laser irradiation [50,55,56]. As shown in Figure 2C, using penetratin peptide (Pen)-modified Au nanostars as part of an NIR photothermal method could be activated using ultralow irradiation to treat AD [57]. Due to the irregular morphology, Au nanostars possessed a high NIR absorption-scattering ratio and large specific surface area. Pen peptides can enhance the travel across the BBB and the cellular internalization of nanomaterials. The Pen-Au nanostars not only inhibited the formation of Aβ fibrils but also disassembled the preformed Aβ fibrils under the NIR irradiation. Moreover, a fluorescent ruthenium complex was loaded on the nanostars for tracking the drug delivery. To shorten the laser irradiation time, Lin et al. applied an NIR femtosecond laser for the destruction of the preformed AuNR-modified Aβ fibrils (Aβ fibrils@AuNRs) (Figure 2D) [58]. The results showed that in the presence of AuNRs, the femtosecondlaser irradiation could efficiently dissociate the Aβ fibrils into small fragments with a non-β-sheet structure in 5 min at a safe energy level and the morphology of AuNRs was transformed into amorphous shapes. However, there was no obvious destruction effect on the Aβ fibrils or Aβ fibrils@Au nanospheres under the laser irradiation.

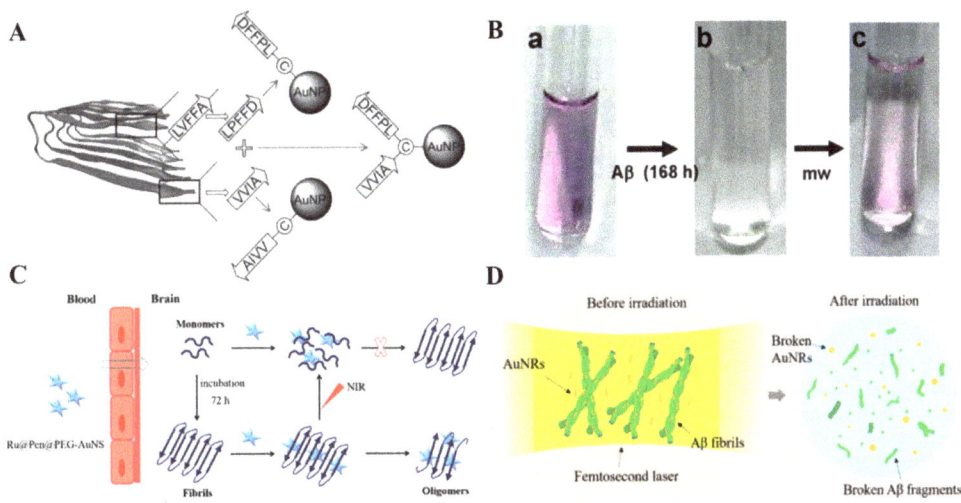

Figure 2. (**A**) Schematic of the design of peptide hybrid-functionalized AuNPs. Reprinted with permission from reference [49]. Copyright 2017 Wiley-VCH. (**B**) Schematic of remote dissolution of Aβ$_{1-42}$ precipitates. (a) AuNPCys-PEP solution mixed with Aβ$_{1-42}$ before the incubation. UVvis absorption peak at 527 nm. (b) After incubation of AuNPCys-PEP with Aβ$_{1-42}$ for 7 days at 37 °C. No UV-vis absorption peak. (c) Irradiation of B for 8 h with 0.1 W and 12 GHz microwave field. UV-vis absorption peak at 527 nm. Reprinted with permission from reference [53]. Copyright 2006 American Chemical Society. (**C**) Schematic of Pen-modified Au nanostars for the NIR photothermal treatment of AD. Reprinted with permission from reference [57]. Copyright 2019 American Chemical Society. (**D**) Schematic of highly efficient destruction of amyloid-β fibrils by femtosecond laser-induced nanoexplosion of gold nanorods. Reprinted with permission from reference [58]. Copyright 2016 American Chemical Society.

Metal ions, such as Zn^{2+} and Cu^{2+}, were shown to participate in the pathology of AD [59,60]. A metal chelator can capture metal ions, hamper ROS formation and inhibit metal ion-induced Aβ aggregation [61]. However, they have some disadvantages, such as poor permeability of the BBB and limited ability to distinguish toxic metal ions related to Aβ aggregates from those associated with normal biological homeostasis [62,63]. Inspired by stimuli-responsive controlled-release drug delivery systems, the controllable release of chelators from "containers" may avoid this problem. Shi et al. reported a dual-responsive "caged metal chelator" release system based on NIR-absorbing Au nanocages [64]. As illustrated in Figure 3A, the chelator of clioquinol (CQ) was encapsulated in Au nanocages and the pore was blocked by human IgG via the redox- and thermal-sensitive arylboronic ester bond. Over-produced H_2O_2 that was induced by deviant Aβ-metal ions aggregates would initiate the degradation of arylboronic ester and the subsequent release of CQ. Moreover, Au nanocages with NIR light could generate local heat to break the bond, thus enhancing the CQ release and dissolving Aβ deposits via noninvasive remote control.

Unlike AuNPs, gold nanoclusters (AuNCs) consist of several to dozens of atoms that have excellent optical properties of intense fluorescence and high photostability. As shown in Figure 3B, Hao et al. found that AuNCs modified with CLVFFA via Au-S bonds showed improved inhibitory ability [65]. The results exhibited that AuNCs-CLVFFA could block the fibrillogenesis of Aβ$_{1-40}$ and the prolongation of fibrils and disaggregate the mature fibrils into oligomers. Zhang et al. found that Cys-Arg (CR) dipeptide-caped Au$_{23}$(CR)$_{14}$ NCs could completely dissolve exogenous mature Aβ fibrils and endogenous Aβ plaques and restore the natural unfolded state of Aβ peptide from a β-sheet structure [66].

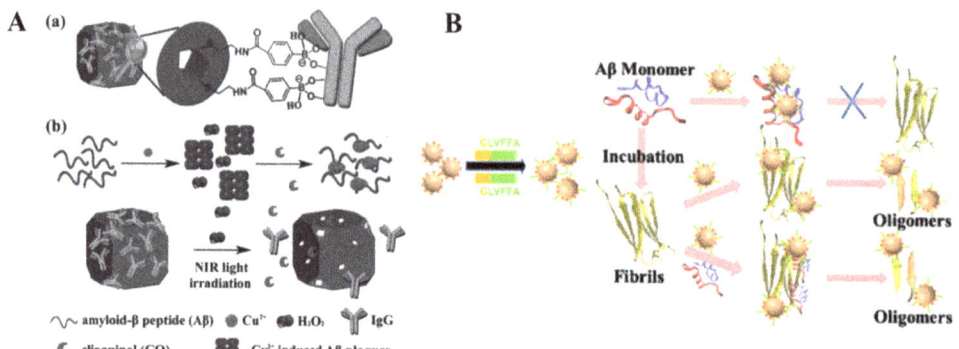

Figure 3. (**A**) (a) Illustration of IgG capped Au nanocages. (b) Schematic representation of H_2O_2-triggered and photothermal-responsive release of chelator CQ from IgG capped Au nanocages [64]. Copyright 2013 Wiley-VCH. (**B**) Schematic of CLVFFA-functionalized AuNCs for the inhibition of Aβ fibrillation. Reprinted with permission from reference [65]. Copyright 2019 American Chemical Society.

2.2. Carbon

Carbon nanomaterials, including carbon nanotubes, graphene, fullerene, carbon nanospheres and carbon dots, have received great attention in the biological field due to their unique physical and chemical features. Carbon nanomaterials with hydrophobic surfaces can interact with various biomolecules, such as DNA, proteins and amyloid nanostructures. Moreover, when entering into a living organism, they may disturb the self-assembly processes of peptides or proteins.

2.2.1. Graphene-Based Materials

Owing to the large available surface and hydropathy, graphene oxide (GO) was applied to modulate the aggregation of Aβ via the adsorption of amyloid monomers and decreasing the kinetic reaction [67–69]. Yang et al. found that pristine graphene and GO could inhibit Aβ peptide fibrillation and clear mature amyloid fibrils through experimental and computational investigation [70]. Mahmoudi et al. found that the formation of a protective protein corona on GO sheets could further enhance the inhibition effect [71]. The size effect of GO on modulating Aβ aggregation was also investigated by Wang and co-workers [72]. Surface chirality was also shown to play an important role in protein adsorption dynamics and cell behaviors. As shown in Figure 4A, Qing et al. studied the chiral effect on amyloid formation by using cysteine-enantiomer-modified GO as a platform [73]. The result showed that R-cysteine-modified GO suppressed the absorption, nucleation and fiber elongation processes of $Aβ_{1-40}$, thus leading to a remarkable inhibition rate of amyloid fibril formation. However, s-cysteine-modified GO accelerated these processes. The stereoselective interaction between chiral moieties and Aβ peptides caused the enrichment of oligomers on the GO surface, but the distance between them should be short enough (1–2 nm). This work provided novel insights into understanding the key roles of biological membranes on protein amyloidosis.

Based on its high optical absorption in the NIR region, graphene has been widely explored in biomedical applications. In 2012, Li et al. first reported the photothermal treatment of AD by using thioflavin-S (ThS)-modified GO (Figure 4B) [74]. The ThS-modified GO can produce local heat to dissociate Aβ fibrils under low-power NIR laser irradiation with improved selectivity because of the specific targeting of ThS toward amyloid. Moreover, the Aβ morphology change during the photothermal treatment can be monitored in real time by recording the increased fluorescence of ThS in the complex of ThS and Aβ fibrils. Taking advantage of the permeation and disruption of the cellular membrane by Aβ oligomers, Xu et al. developed an oligomer-self-triggered and NIR-enhanced system based on the lipid-bilayer-coated graphene (GMS-Lip) [75]. Dyes and drugs were co-loaded within GMS-Lip, which could be released by the amyloid oligomers. In addition, thermal-sensitive Lip could be further destroyed by the heat produced by graphene under an NIR laser to ensure the release efficiency. Moreover, the NIR-assisted release could be initiated locally by tracking the fluorescence.

GO can hybridize with other nanomaterials to achieve improved inhibition performance based on the synergistic effect. Moreover, the decoration of nanomaterials on GO can avoid the easy agglomeration and restacking of GO. For instance, GO/AuNPs nanocompositeswere prepared using pulsed laser ablationin water to reduce Aβ aggregation, which produced an enhanced effect compared with using GO or AuNPsalone [76]. Due to the hydrophobic interactions between the nanocomposites with hydrophobic amino acids of Aβ$_{1-42}$, the nucleation process was significantly disturbed and the fibrillation was subsequently slowed. The result showed that the GO/AuNPs nanocomposites not only reduced Aβ$_{1-42}$ aggregation and cytotoxicity but also led to the deploymerization of amyloid fibrils and inhibition of their cellular cytotoxicity. In addition, Ahmad et al. reported that a GO–Fe$_4$O$_4$ nanocomposite showed the enhanced inhibitory effect of Aβ$_{1-42}$ peptides and depolymerized Aβ$_{1-42}$ fibrils (Figure 4C) [77].

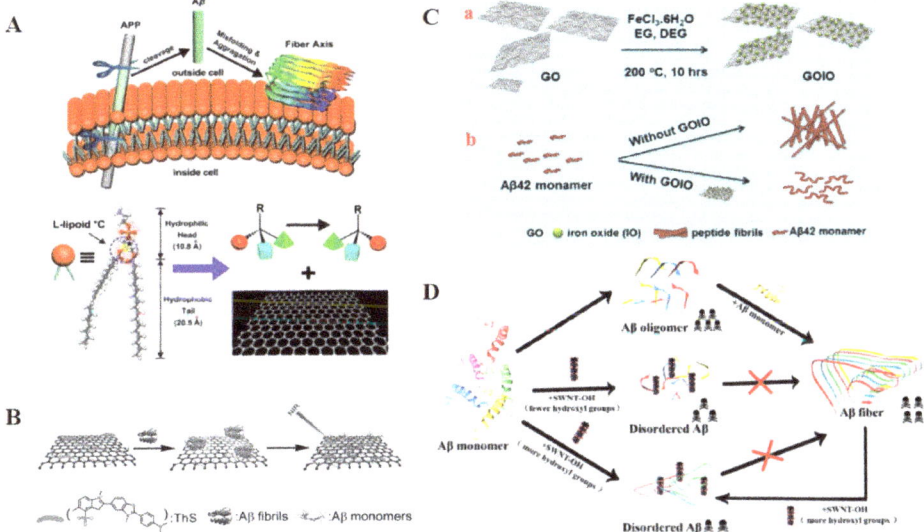

Figure 4. (**A**) Schematic representation of the chiral effect at the protein/graphene interface to understand amyloid formation. Reprinted with permission from reference [73]. Copyright 2014 American Chemical Society. (**B**) Schematic representation of ThS-modified GO with high NIR absorbance used for AD treatment. Reprinted with permission from reference [74]. Copyright 2012 Wiley-VCH. (**C**) Schematic representation of the (a) preparation of GOIO and (b) modulation of Aβ$_{1-42}$ aggregation using GOIO. Reprinted with permission from reference [77]. Copyright 2012 Elsevier. (**D**) Schematic representation of the effect of SWNT-OH on Aβ aggregation. Reprinted with permission from reference [78]. Copyright 2019 American Chemical Society.

2.2.2. Carbon Nanotubes (CNTs)

CNTs are tubular structures of rolled-up sheets of graphene, including single-wall (SWCNTs) and multi-wall (MWCNTs) species. CNTs can be exploited for biosensing, tissue engineering and drug delivery due to their chemical stability, good porosity and high surface area. Moreover, SWCNTs were shown to shuttle drugs into a wide range of cell types [79,80]. Luo et al. found that SWNTs can induce Aβ peptides to form β-sheet-rich yet non-amyloid fibrils, and Aβ peptidescan reduce the toxicity of SWNTs [80]. However, the poor dispersibility of pristine SWNTs in solution greatly decreased the inhibition efficiency. Functionalization of SWNTs with hydrophilic groups may increase their dispersibility. Liu et al. investigated the inhibitory effect of SWNT-OH on $A\beta_{1-42}$ fibrillogenesis [78]. As shown in Figure 4D, the percentage of hydroxyl groups in SWNT-OH was crucial for their inhibition capacity against $A\beta_{1-42}$ aggregation. Moreover, SWNT-OH could transform the mature fibrils into smaller granular aggregates but not oligomers. Xie et al. revealed that the electrostatic, hydrophobic and aromatic stacking interactions between hydroxylated SWCNT and $A\beta_{16-22}$ not only inhibit the $A\beta_{16-22}$ fibrillization but also shifted the conformations of oligomers from the ordered β-sheet-rich structures into the disordered coil aggregates [81].

2.2.3. Carbon Nanospheres

Phototherapy, including photothermal therapy (PTT) and photodynamic therapy (PDT), is generally activated by visible or first NIR-I light. However, it has limited tissue penetration through dense skull and scalp and may cause damage to nearby normal tissues. Thus, utilizing excitation light at second near-infrared light (NIR-II, 1000–1700 nm) is a more attractive option for deeper tissue penetration and a lower signal-to-noise ratio. Ma et al. designed $A\beta$ targeting, N-doped three-dimensional mesoporous carbon nanospheres (KD8@N-MCNs) for NIR-II PTT of AD (Figure 5A) [82]. KLVFFAED (KD8) was used as the target of $A\beta$ and receptor of the advanced glycation end-products (AGEs). N-MCN was selected as the NIR-II photothermal agent due to its excellent photothermal effect and superoxide dismutase (SOD) and catalase (CAT)-like activities. Combining the above advantages, KD8@N-MCNs can dissolve $A\beta_{1-42}$ aggregates under NIR-II illumination, scavenge intracellular ROS and alleviate neuroinflammation in vivo. Moreover, KD8@N-MCNs can efficiently cross the BBB due to the modification of KD8 on the nanosphere's surface.

2.2.4. Fullerene

Fullerene possesses the advantages of strong hydrophobicity and high electrophilicity, which endow it with the potential ability to inhibit the aggregation of $A\beta$ peptides [83]. For example, Xie et al. investigated the molecular mechanism of fullerene-based inhibition, which could be attributed to the strong hydrophobic and aromatic-stacking interactions between the fullerene hexagonal rings and the Phe rings of $A\beta_{16-22}$ peptide [84]. Moreover, Kim et al. reported that a C_{60} derivate (1,2-dimethoxymethanofullerene) could bind to the central motif, namely, $A\beta_{16-20}$ (KLVFF), based on the strong hydrophobic interaction and inhibit the aggregation of $A\beta$ peptides at the early stage [85]. After that, other C_{60} derivates were also synthesized and applied for inhibiting the aggregation of $A\beta$ peptides, including hydroxylated fullerene and sodium fullerenolate $Na_4[C_{60}(OH)_{\sim 30}]$ [86–90].

C_{60} could produce reactive oxygen species (ROS) via the photo-excitation of C_{60} and O_2 to stimulate DNA and protein photocleavage [91,92]. Ishida et al. employed a C_{60}–sugar hybrid to inhibit $A\beta$ aggregation and degrade $A\beta$ oligomers under long-wavelength UV radiation and neutral conditions [93]. Besides the hydrophobic interaction between $A\beta$ and C_{60}, the hydrophilic sugar can interact with the hydrophilic N-terminal of $A\beta_{1-42}$ through the formation of hydrogen bonds. Aiming to improve the solubility, C_{60} was functionalized with a sulfo or amino group [94]. These two hydrophilic groups could further strongly interact with the termini of $A\beta_{1-42}$ through the ionic interactions and/or hydrogen bonds.

In addition to generating ROS under photo-excitation, C_{60} can be used as a ROS scavenger in the dark. Du et al. designed a NIR-switchable nanoplatform for synergy therapy of AD based on the ROS-generating and -quenching properties of C_{60} [95]. As shown in Figure 5B, UCNPs were conjugated with C_{60} and the $A\beta$-target peptide KLVFF. Under NIR irradiation, C_{60} was photo-sensitized using UCNPs through FRET to produce ROS, leading to the oxygenation of $A\beta$ and inhibition of its aggregation. In the dark, C_{60} could eliminate the overproduced ROS to protect the cell from oxidative stress.

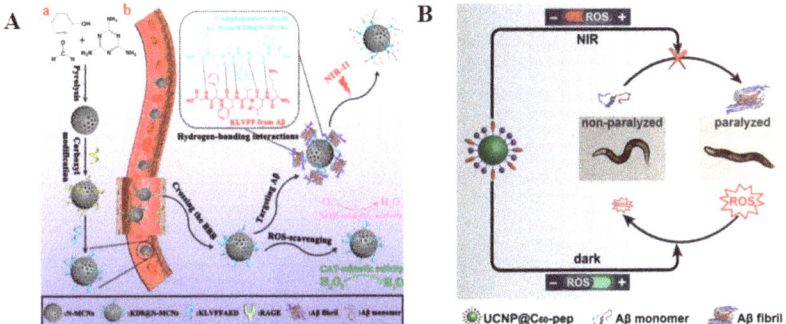

Figure 5. (**A**) (a) Schematic chart of KD8@N-MCNs synthesis and (b) schematic diagram of the KD8@N-MCNs mechanism of action. Reprinted with permission from reference [82]. Copyright 2020 American Chemical Society. (**B**) Schematic of UCNP@C_{60}-PEP inhibiting Aβ aggregation in vivo and attenuating the oxidative stress to prolong the lifespan of the CL2006 strain. Reprinted with permission from reference [95]. Copyright 2018 Wiley-VCH.

2.2.5. Carbon Dots

Since being accidentally discovered as byproducts during the purification of SWCNTs, carbon dots (CDs) have received growing interest in biomedical and biosensing fields [96]. As a potential alternative to semiconductor QDs, CDs have prominent characteristics, such as their low cost, ease of synthesis, good biocompatibility and intrinsic fluorescence. Moreover, the absorption and emission spectra can be tuned by adjusting the degree of carbonization and the percentage of surface moieties.

CDs generally have abundant functional groups on their conjugated aromatic core, such as hydroxyl, amino and carboxyl groups. They can interact with Aβ peptides and aggregates through electrostatic, hydrogen bonding, π-π stacking and hydrophobic interactions because of their abundant surface chemical properties and small size (generally less than 10 nm). Liu et al. demonstrated that graphene quantum dots (GQDs) can inhibit A$β_{1-42}$ peptide aggregation, mainly via hydrophobic interactions, and rescue A$β_{1-42}$ oligomer-induced cytotoxicity [97]. The surface chirality of nanoparticles also has an influence on the inhibition efficiency against Aβ aggregation [98]. L-Lys-CDs were reported to exhibit a higher affinity toward A$β_{1-42}$ peptides than D-Lys-CDs and could remodel the A$β_{1-42}$ secondary structure and fibril morphologies [99]. CDs can cross the BBB because of their small size, which allows them to be utilized as nano-carriers to transport functional molecules to the brain. Thus, GQDs conjugated with an endogenous neuroprotective glycine-proline-glutamate peptide showed an enhanced neuroprotective effect and improved learning and memory capability of APP/PS1 mice [100]. CDs can also be used as fluorescent nanoprobes for biological imaging. Among them, CDs with red fluorescence possess several advantages of low biological fluorescence background signal and high tissue penetration ability. Recently, Gao et al. discovered new functions of nitrogen-doped carbonized polymer dots (CPDs) to target Aβ aggregation [101]. The non-covalent interactions between Aβ aggregates and CPDs limited the molecular vibration and rotation of CPDs, resulting in the red emission. As shown in Figure 6A, after interacting with Aβ fibrils, CPDs emitted an increased red fluorescence signal, indicating that CPDs can be utilized as a multifunctional therapeutic agent for disintegrating and monitoring Aβ fibrils.

Photoexcited CDs can generate reactive oxygen species (ROS) through energy-transfer and electron-transfer pathways, which endows them with the ability to denature toxic biomolecules. For example, branched polyethylenimine-passivated CDs (bPEI@CDs) were reported as photosensitizers that inhibit the self-assembly of Aβ peptide and disassemble preformed Aβ aggregates upon light irradiation (Figure 6B) [102]. Photoactivated bPEI@CDs produced ROS to oxygenate and break β-sheet-rich Aβ aggregates into smaller fragments. Meanwhile, it was more efficient for reducing Aβ-mediated toxicity compared with bPEI@CDs under dark conditions. However, the UV-to-Vis dependent photoexcitation is a potential obstacle to the use of bPEI@CDs. To improve the effectiveness of photoexcitation of CDs and grant the ability to target Aβ, red-light-responsive DNA aptamer-functionalized CDs (Apta@CDs) were designed for the Aβ-targeting spatiotemporal suppression of Aβ aggregation [103]. As shown in Figure 6C, Apta@CDs could specifically bind to Aβ aggregates in the 5xFAD (five familial Azheimer's) mouse brain. Photoexcited Apta@CDs under red LED (617 nm) light can generate $^1O_2$, denature the Aβ peptide, slow the formation of β-sheet-rich aggregates and alleviate the Aβ-associated cytotoxicity.

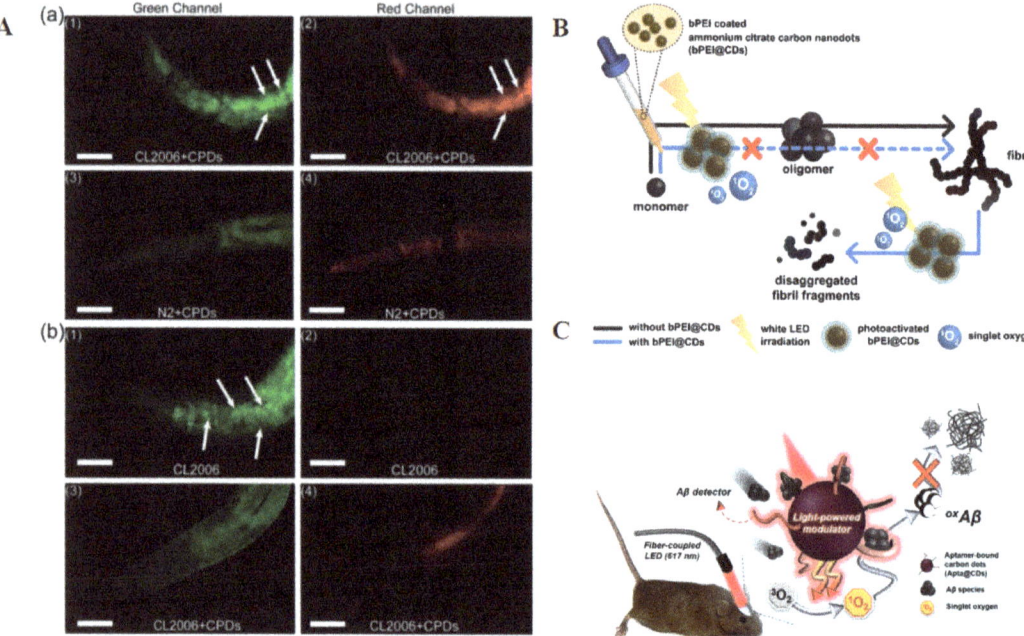

Figure 6. (**A**) In vivo assays with C. elegans (CL2006 and N2). (a) Fluorescence images of CL2006 (a1,a2) and N2 (a3,a4) nematodes that were co-stained with ThT and CPDs. (b) Fluorescent images of inhibiting Aβ deposits after treating without (b1,b2) or with (b3,b4) CPDs in CL2006 nematodes. Reprinted with permission from reference [101]. Copyright 2020 Wiley-VCH. (**B**) Schematic of bPEI@CDs' capabilities regarding inhibiting Aβ assembly and disaggregating preformed fibrillar aggregates. Reprinted with permission from reference [102]. Copyright 2017 Wiley-VCH. (**C**) Schematic of Aβ-targeting, CD-mediated photomodulation modality for the spatiotemporal inhibition of Aβ aggregation in vivo. Reprinted with permission from reference [103]. Copyright 2020 American Chemical Society.

2.3. Metal-Oxide Nanomaterials

2.3.1. Magnetic Nanoparticle (MNPs)

MNPs have the advantages of good biocompatibility and unique magnetic properties. They were deemed as therapeutics and imaging agents in the treatment of brain diseases. Mahmoudi et al. investigated the physicochemical effects (size, charge and surface treatment) of coated superparamagnetic iron oxide nanoparticles (SPIONs) on Aβ aggregation (Figure 7A) [104]. They found that the size and surface area have significant effects on Aβ fibrillation. Lower concentrations of SPIONs inhibited the fibrillation and higher concentrations promoted the rate, reversely. Furthermore, the positively charged SPIONs promoted fibrillation at significantly lower particle concentrations. In addition, peptide- and antibody-modified MNPs also significantly inhibited Aβ fibrillation [105,106].

MNP-based targeted tissue drug delivery was shown to be a promising therapeutic approach because MNPs can be directed toward a specific site in disease tissue locations by a magnetic force. Mesoporous silica-coated MNPs (MMSNPs) were utilized as smart vehicles to encapsulate quercetin (QC) with anti-amyloid and antioxidant properties, overcoming the limitations of poor solubility and bioavailability (Figure 7B) [107]. They found that biophenols QC can bind with Aβ monomers and oligomers to block the fibril formation [108]. Moreover, the released QCs could decrease the Aβ-related cytotoxicity and minimize the Aβ-induced ROS. Li et al. designed light-responsive magnetic nanoparticle prochelator conjugates for inhibiting metal-induced Aβ aggregation [109]. In this complex, Fe_3O_4 NPs were utilized to cage CQ through a photoactive o-nitrobenzyl bromide (ONB) linkage and the conjugates did not interact with Cu^{2+} in the prochelator form. After the photolytic cleavage under UV radiation at 365 nm, the caged CQ was liberated from the NPs, efficiently preventing metal-induced Aβ aggregation, decreasing cellular reactive oxygen species (ROS) and protecting cells against Aβ-related toxicity.

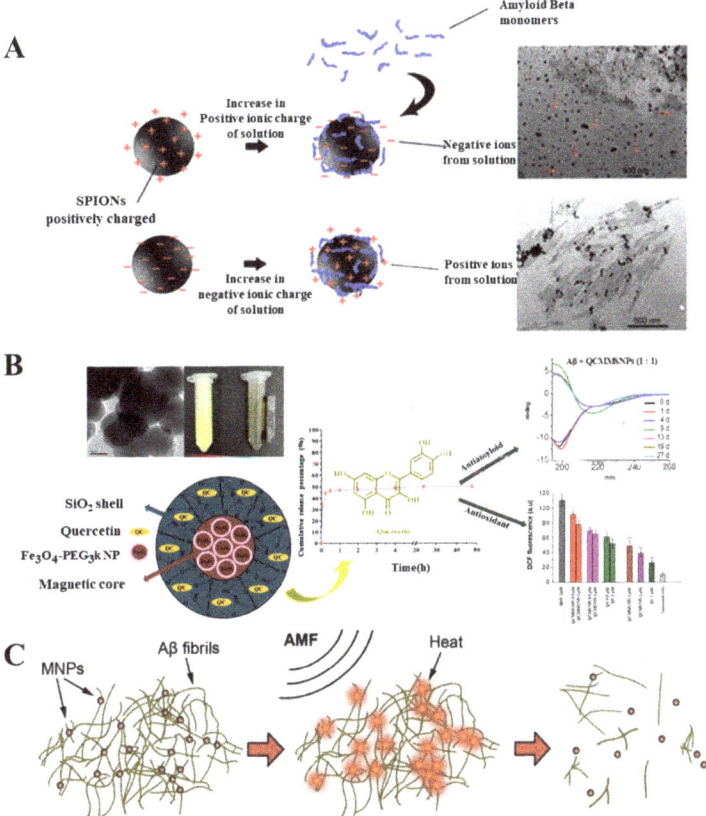

Figure 7. (**A**) Schematic of the influence of the physiochemical properties of SPIONs on Aβ fibrillation in solution. Reprinted with permission from reference [104]. Copyright 2013 American Chemical Society. (**B**) Schematic of the encapsulation of QC in MMSNPs, which enhances its aqueous solubility and its effect on Aβ aggregation. Reprinted with permission from reference [107]. Copyright 2020 Elsevier. (**C**) Schematic of a method for remote protein disaggregation using AMF and MNPs. Reprinted with permission from reference [110]. Copyright 2012 American Chemical Society.

Previous studies indicated that MNPs can effectively improve the local temperature in the area extremely close to the MNPs (about 5 nm) through alternating the magnetic field, which reduces the penetration depth limit and damage to the neighboring tissues [111,112].

Therefore, it is a non-invasive strategy for clearing Aβ aggregates by using MNPs/AMF hyperthermia [113]. For instance, Loynachan et al. used LPFFD-functionalized PEG-coated MNPs for the remote magnetothermal disruption of Aβ aggregates under a high-frequency alternating magnetic field (AMF) (Figure 7C) [110]. They found that the local heat dissipated by targeted MNPs could dramatically decrease the size of Aβ aggregates from microns to tens of nanometers upon exposure to a physiologically safe AMF, which is attributed to the dissociation of Aβ deposits. The reduced Aβ cytotoxicity due to the magnetothermal disruption was confirmed in primary hippocampal neuronal cultures. Moreover, for simultaneous diagnosis and treatment, an Aβ oligomer-sensitive naphthalimide-based fluorescent probe (NFP) was loaded on the KLVFF-conjugated MNPs [114].

2.3.2. Polyoxometalates (POMs)

Polyoxometalates (POMs) are early-transition-metal-oxygen-anion clusters that usually include the d^0 species V(V), Nb(V), Ta(V), Mo(VI) and W(VI) with versatile structures. They have been widely explored in recent years for biomedical applications [115] and showed remarkable effects against acquired immune deficiency syndrome (AIDS) [116]. Because of the similarity to water-solubilized fullerene derivatives, POMs can be utilized as Aβ aggregation inhibitors. For example, Li et al. identified four POMs with the size-dependent ability of inhibiting Aβ peptide aggregation via a high-throughput screening method, in which $K_8[P_2CoW_{17}O_{61}]$ with a Wells–Dawson structure exhibits the highest inhibition (Figure 8A) [117]. They also found that POMs electrostatically bind to the cationic His_{13}–Lys_{16} cluster (HHQK) of Aβ peptides. Zhou et al. demonstrated that two POMs with the wheel-shaped Preyssler structure and the Keggin-type structure could interact with $Aβ_{1-40}$ and inhibit its fibrillization [118]. To suppress the peroxidase-like activity of Aβ-hemin, POM-Dawson was further functionalized with transition metal ions of various histidine-chelating metals. These transition metalPOMs not only specifically targeted the HHQK in Aβ peptides but also showed a stronger inhibition effect on Aβ-hemin formation [119]. After that, organoplatinum-substituted POMs were reported to inhibit Aβ aggregation [120]. Moreover, POMs can also significantly inhibit metal-ion-induced $Aβ_{1-40}$ aggregation because POMs with high negative charges show strong interactions with Zn^{2+} and Cu^{2+} [121].

POMs have been broadly used for homogeneous photocatalysis in water to produce ROS and oxidize various substrates, including pyrimidine bases [122,123]. Inspired by this fact, Li et al. demonstrated that POMs can photodegrade Aβ monomers and even oligomers under photoirradiation conditions [124]. At a low concentration, POMs still showed a high inhibition efficiency under UV irradiation. To disaggregate the neurotoxic Aβ fibrils, Li et al. further developed a redox-activated NIR-responsive reduced POMs (rPOM)-based agent for the photothermal treatment of AD (Figure 8B) [125]. In this work, mesoporous silica nanoparticles (MSNs) were used to load rPOM and thermally responsive copolymer poly(N-isopropylacrylamide-co-acrylamide) was employed to cap the pores of MSNs to prevent rPOMs leakage and ensure they remained intact. When being irradiated by an 808 nm laser, rPOMs with strong NIR absorption produced local hyperthermia to melt the shell away from the channels, which would inhibit Aβ aggregation and disaggregate Aβ fibrils by local heat. Moreover, rPOM could act as antioxidants to clear ROS and the product of POMs can inhibit Aβ aggregation.

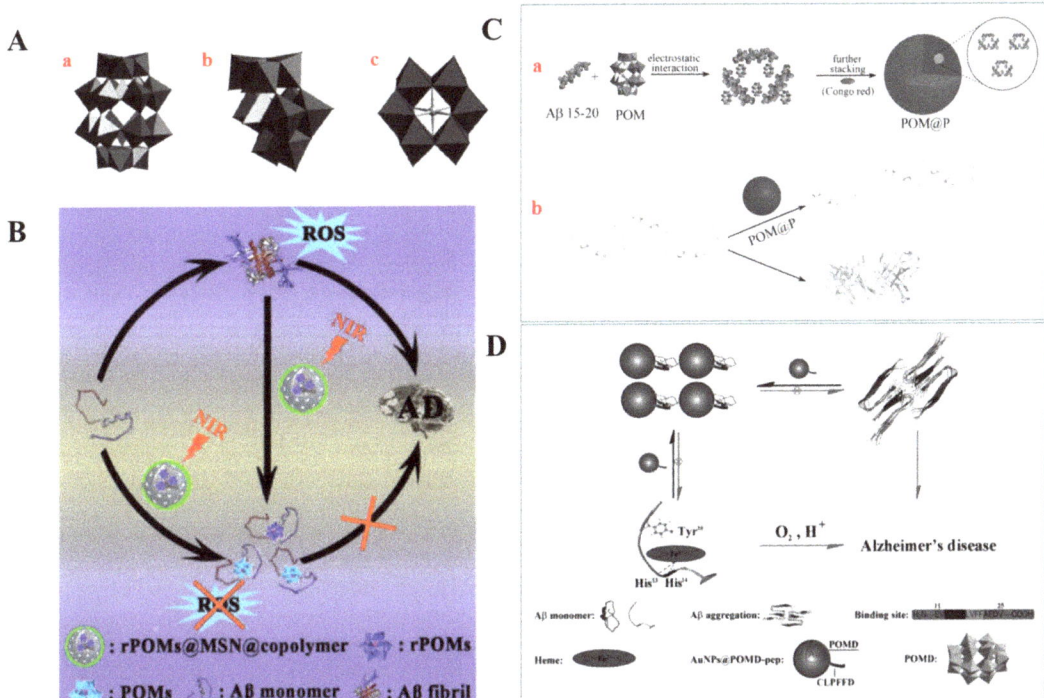

Figure 8. (**A**) Schematic of the structures of typical polyoxometalates: (a) Wells–Dawson structure, $K_8[P_2CoW_{17}O_{61}]$; (b) trivacant Keggin structure, $\alpha\text{-}Na_9H\text{-}[SiW_9O_{34}]$; (c) Anderson structure, $Na_5[IMo_6O_{24}]$. Reprinted with permission from reference [117]. Copyright 2011 Wiley-VCH. (**B**) Schematic of the NIR-responsive rPOMDs@MSNs@copolymer acting as a multifunctional photothermal agent for the treatment of AD. Reprinted with permission from reference [125]. Copyright 2018 Wiley-VCH. (**C**) Schematic of the peptide–POM conjugates used for AD treatment. (a) The schematic illustration of self-assembly of Aβ15-20 and POM to hybrid spheres. (b) The assembled peptide and POM nanoparticles can effectively inhibit Aβ$_{1-40}$ aggregation. Reprinted with permission from reference [126]. Copyright 2013 Wiley-VCH. (**D**) Schematic of the Aβ pathway influenced by AuNPs@POMD–peptide. Reprinted with permission from reference [127]. Copyright 2015 Wiley-VCH.

POMs can be employed as inorganic nanobuilding blocks to fabricate organic–inorganic assembly nanoarchitectures with the aid of peptide or protein building blocks. POM–peptide (POM@P) hybrid particles were synthesized as two-in-one bifunctional particles through the self-assembly of these dual inhibitors (Figure 8C) [126]. Aβ$_{15-20}$ peptides (Ac–QKLVFF–NH$_2$) with a high local density can not only bind the homologous sequence in Aβ peptides and disrupt their aggregation but also enhance the targeting inhibition efficiency. Moreover, congo red (CR), which is a clinically used Aβ fibril-specific staining dye, was loaded into the nanospheres for real-time monitoring of the inhibition process of POM@P. To develop novel drugs with multiple functions against AD, Gao et al. synthesized AuNPs@POM–peptide as a novel multifunctional Aβ inhibitor (Figure 8D) [127]. In this hybrid, AuNPs were utilized to carry two inhibitors (POMs and LPFFD peptides) to efficiently cross the BBB. In addition to the inhibition of Aβ aggregation and the dissociation of Aβ fibrils, AuNPs@POMD–peptides also decreased Aβ–heme peroxidase activity and Aβ-induced cytotoxicity via synergistic effects. Based on a similar principle, AuNRs with a high NIR absorption property were used instead of AuNPs for the hyperthermia-induced disassembly of Aβ fibrils [128]. Moreover, due to the shape and size-dependent optical properties, AuNRs could also be used to sensitively detect the Aβ aggregates.

2.3.3. Cerium Oxide Nanoparticles (CNPs)

Owing to their rapid transformation between Ce^{4+} and Ce^{3+} at physiological pH, CeO_2 NPs can act as free radical scavengers and protect cells from oxidative stress. CeO_2 NPs possess powerful multienzyme activity, including superoxide oxidase, catalase and oxidase [129]. Although CeO_2 NPs exhibit no obvious inhibition effect on Aβ aggregation, it is usually utilized to eliminate over-expressed ROS produced by Aβ-Cu^{2+} and protect against neurodegeneration [130,131]. To realize the targeted delivery of AD therapeutic agents, Li et al. designed a double delivery platform for AD treatment based on the H_2O_2-responsive release of antioxidant CeO_2 NPs and the metal chelator clioquinol (CQ) [132]. In this study, CQ was entrapped into the phenylboronic-acid-modified MSN (MSN-BA) and glucose-coated CeO_2 was used as the gatekeeper via the formation of cyclic boronate moieties. H_2O_2 could induce the breakage of arylboronic esters, thus resulting in the release of CeO_2 NPs and CQ. Finally, the two-in-one bifunctional nanoparticles effectively inhibited Aβ aggregation, reduced intracellular ROS and rescued cells from Aβ-related toxicity. To treat AD in multiple pathways, Guan et al. prepared CeO_2 NPs with a functional $MnMoS_4$ shell (CeNPs@$MnMoS_4$-n; n = 1–5), as displayed in Figure 9A [133]. $MnMoS_4$ could eliminate intracellular toxic Cu^{2+} through ion exchange. In turn, the release of Mn^{2+} promoted neurite outgrowth. Moreover, CeNPs@$MnMoS_4$-3 with the SOD activity decreased the oxidative stress.

According to previous reports, POMs as a class of artificial proteases have the ability to hydrolyze peptides [134]. Cerium dioxide/POMs (CeONP@POMs) mixed nanoparticles were used to mimic metallopeptidase for the treatment of the neurotoxicity caused by Aβ (Figure 9B) [135]. The mixed NPs with peptide hydrolysis and superoxide dismutase activity efficiently degraded Aβ aggregates and decreased cellular ROS. Moreover, in addition to promoting PC12 cell proliferation and crossing the BBB, CeONP@POMs inhibited Aβ-induced BV2 microglial cell activation. Kim et al. designed an extracorporeal strategy for cleansing blood Aβ by using core/shell structured multifunctional magnetite/ceria nanoparticle assemblies (MCNAs) [136]. As shown in Figure 9C, the nano-assemblies were further conjugated with antifouling polyethylene glycol (PEG) and Aβ antibodies for the specific capture of Aβ peptides. The MNPs enabled the magnetic separation of the captured Aβ peptides by applying an external magnetic field. The ceria NPs alleviated oxidative stress by scavenging the ROS generated by the immune response during the process. The blood-cleansing treatment of 5xFAD transgenic mice demonstrated that the levels of Aβ in the blood and brain were effectively reduced and the spatial working memory deficit was rescued.

2.4. 2D Nanosheets

2.4.1. Black Phosphorus

As a new member of 2D layered semiconductor nanomaterials, black phosphorus (BP) has attracted broad attention because of its perfect optical and thermal properties. Moreover, BP can degrade into nontoxic phosphate and phosphite anions under physiological conditions. In 2019, Lim et al. synthesized titanium sulfonate ligand (TiL_4)-modified BP nanosheets and BP quantum dots and reported for the first time that they could inhibit $Aβ_{1-40}$ to form fibrils by adsorbing the monomers [137]. To further improve the stability of BP, Yang et al. constructed an inhibitor (LK7)-coupled and polyethylene glycol (PEG)-stabilized BP-based nano-system (PEG-LK7@BP) (Figure 10A) [138]. Besides the enhanced electrostatic and hydrophobic interactions, LK7 with a high local concentration on the BP surface could enhance the affinity between the Aβ species and the BP. Based on the synergistic effect, PEG-LK7@BP prevented the conformational shift of $Aβ_{1-42}$ to a β-sheet structure, suppressed $Aβ_{1-42}$ aggregation and attenuated the toxicity of $Aβ_{1-42}$.

BP with a thickness-dependent energy bandgap from 0.3 eV (bulk) to 2.0 eV (monolayer) has broad absorption across the ultraviolet and entire visible light regions. BP, including the bulk material and ultrathin nanosheets, was found to be an effective photosensitizer for the generation of $^1O_2$ under the entire visible light region and was applied in the fields of catalysis and PDT [139]. Interestingly, BP QDs, BP NPs and BP NSs have been reported to possess NIR photothermal properties for PTT [140–142]. Li et al. employed BP nanosheets as the NIR-activated photosensitizer to generate $^1O_2$ and oxidize Aβ peptide in vitro and in vivo (Figure 10B) [143]. BP nanosheets were modified with 4-(6-methyl-1,3-benzothiazol-2-yl) phenylamine (BTA) to increase the stability and endowed BP with Aβ binding selectivity. Moreover, the BP@BTA could reduce the Aβ-induced cytotoxicity and show neuroprotection to the transgenic strain Caenorhabditis elegans CL2006.

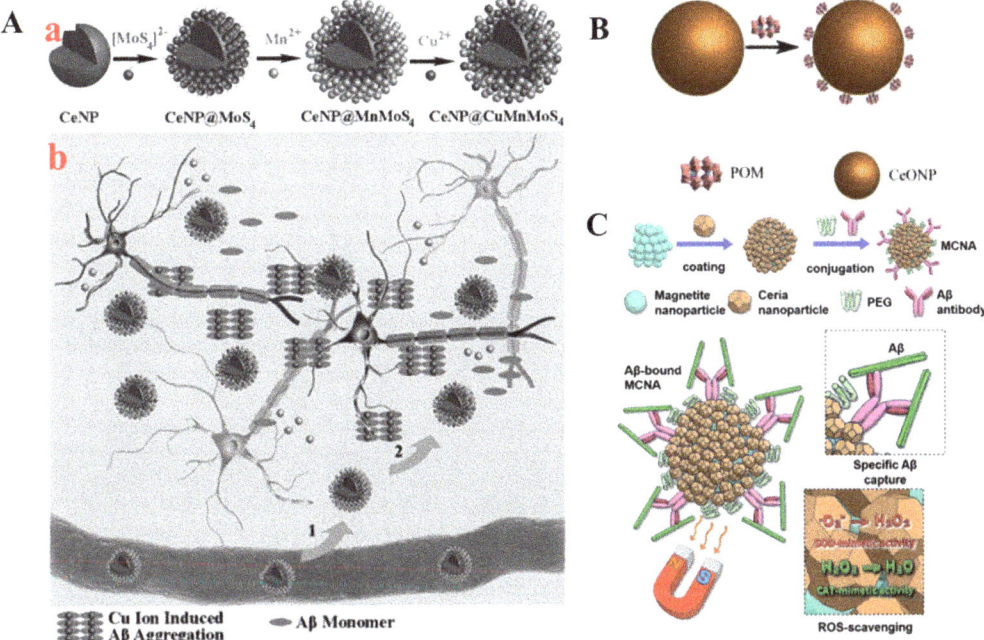

Figure 9. (**A**) Schematic of (a) the preparation of CeNP@MnMoS$_4$-n with a MnMoS$_4$ shell; (b) schematic interpretation of CeNP@MnMoS$_4$-n in vivo. Reprinted with permission from reference [133]. Copyright 2016 Wiley-VCH. (**B**) Schematic drawing of the synthesis of CeONP@POMs. Reprinted with permission from reference [135]. Copyright 2016 Elsevier. (**C**) Schematic of the synthesis and characterization of magnetite/ceria nanoparticle assemblies. Reprinted with permission from reference [136]. Copyright 2019 Wiley-VCH.

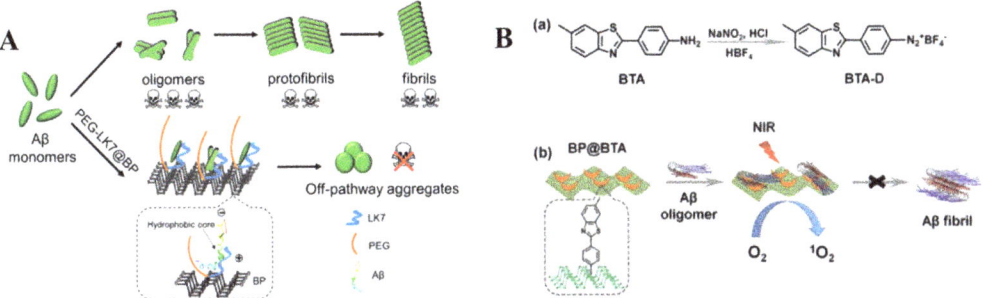

Figure 10. (**A**) Schematic of the Aβ$_{1-42}$ aggregation pathways influenced by PEG-LK7@BP. Reprinted with permission from reference [138]. Copyright 2020 American Chemical Society. (**B**) (a) Schematic illustration of the fabrication of BTA-D from BTA. (b) Schematic illustration of BP@BTA producing $^1O_2$ under NIR to inhibit Aβ aggregation. Reprinted with permission from reference [143]. Copyright 2019 Wiley-VCH.

2.4.2. Transition Metal Dichalcogenides

Transition metal dichalcogenides (TMDs) have attracted worldwide attention in the areas of nanoelectronics, optoelectronics and electrocatalysis. They are always used for drug delivery and tissue ablation. The basal plane of TMD NSs can adsorb or conjugate various aromatics (e.g., pyridine and purine) and other compounds. Mudedla et al. investigated the interaction between Aβ fibrils and MoS$_2$-based materials and found that MoS$_2$ nanotubes could inhibit the aggregation of smaller protofibrils to matured fibrils and bust the preformed fibrils [144]. Wang et al. confirmed the inhibition effect of monolayer MoS$_2$ on the Aβ$_{33-42}$ aggregation [145]. Liu et al. reported the concentration-dependent contradictory effect of AuNP-decorated MoS$_2$ nanocomposites on Aβ$_{1-40}$ aggregation [146]. As displayed in Figure 11A, a low concentration of AuNP-MoS$_2$ nanocomposite could act as the nuclei to accelerate the nucleus formation and fibrillation of Aβ$_{1-40}$, but a high concentration of nanocomposites could limit the structural flexibility of Aβ$_{1-40}$, leading to the inhibition of nucleus formation and aggregation.

The 2D TMDs analogous to graphene exhibit excellent properties, such as high colloidal stability in aqueous media and a high mass extinction coefficient at 800 nm [147]. Li et al. first reported that WS$_2$ could adsorb Aβ$_{1-40}$ monomers on the surface through van der Waals and electrostatic interactions, effectively inhibiting Aβ aggregation and dissociating the preformed Aβ fibrils via photothermal ablation upon NIR irradiation [148]. To further enhance the inhibition ability, Wang et al. prepared multifunctional MoS$_2$/AuNR nanocomposites with high stability and good biocompatibility through electrostatic self-assembly [149]. This nanocomposite with high NIR absorption can modulate the aggregation of Aβ peptides, disrupt mature fibrils under low laser power NIR irradiation and alleviate Aβ-induced ROS against neurotoxicity.

Artificial Aβ-degrading enzymes were designed for the efficient cleavage of Aβ [150,151]. However, the specific hydrolysis sites are always embedded inside the β-sheet structure, hindering the access and hydrolysis efficiency. Therefore, Ma et al. developed a NIR (near-IR) controllable artificial metalloprotease (MoS$_2$–Co), combining MoS$_2$ and a cobalt complex of 1,4,7,10-tetraazacyclododecane-1,4,7,10-tetraacetic acid (Codota) (Figure 11B) [152]. MoS$_2$–Co can inhibit the formation of a β-sheet structure and shorten the distance between Aβ peptides and MoS$_2$–Co. Moreover, under NIR irradiation, MoS$_2$–Co can produce local heat to disintegrate Aβ aggregates and facilitate the hydrolysis activity of Codota toward Aβ peptides.

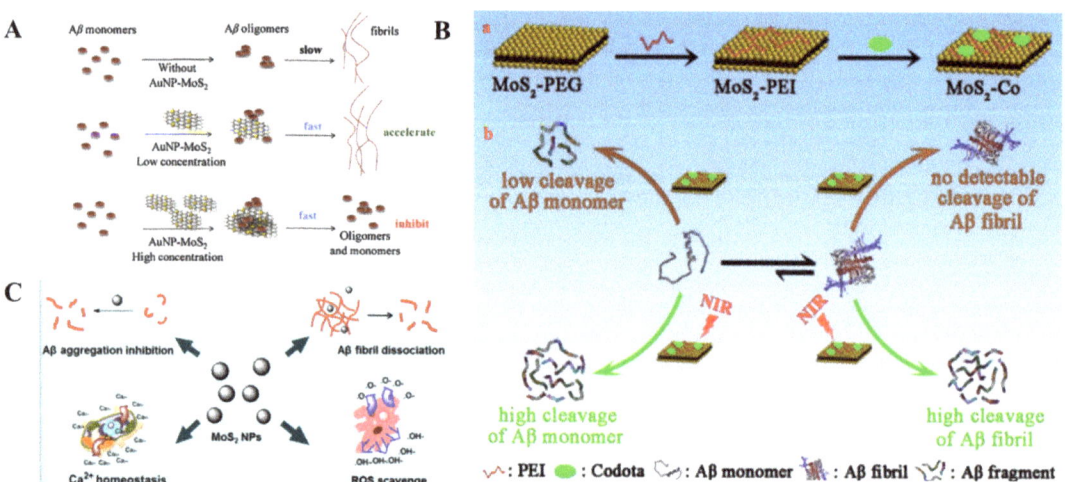

Figure 11. (**A**) Schematic illustration of the mechanism of the concentration-dependent effect of AuNP-MoS$_2$ nanocomposites on Aβ$_{1-40}$ aggregation. Reprinted with permission from reference [146]. Copyright 2019 Elsvier. (**B**) Schematic illustration

of the synthesis route of MoS$_2$-Co and hydrolysis enhanced by MoS$_2$-Co in the presence of an NIR laser. (a) Synthesis route of MoS$_2$-Co. (b) In the presence of NIR laser, MoS$_2$-Co not only improves the hydrolytic activity toward Ab monomers (left side) but also enhances the hydrolytic capacity toward Ab fibrils (rightside). Reprinted with permission from reference [152]. Copyright 2019 Wiley-VCH. (C) Schematic illustration of MoS$_2$ NPs as multifunctional inhibitors against AD. Reprinted with permission from reference [153]. Copyright 2017 American Chemical Society.

MoS$_2$ NPs are also drawing more and more interest as self-lubricating coatings and in biochemical applications. Han et al. prepared spherical polyvinylpyrrolidone-functionalized MoS$_2$ NPs with an average diameter of 100 nm using a pulsed laser ablation method and found that they show multifunctional effects on Aβ_{1-42} aggregation (Figure 11C) [153]. MoS$_2$ NPs could adsorb Aβ_{1-42} monomers or oligomers on the surface based on the interaction between MoS$_2$ NPs and the hydrophobic region of Aβ_{1-42}. This delays the nucleation process, inhibits Aβ_{1-42} aggregation and destabilizes the preformed fibrils. As a result, the calcium channel induced by the incorporation of Aβ_{1-42} oligomers into neuronal cell membranes was blocked to ensure calcium homeostasis and protect neuronal cells. Moreover, MoS$_2$ NPs could reduce the intracellular ROS (·OH) level induced by Aβ_{1-42}.

2.4.3. Graphitic Carbon Nitride

Unlike bulk g-C$_3$N$_4$, the 2D ultrathin g-C$_3$N$_4$ nanosheet is the most stable allotrope of carbon nitride under ambient conditions. It has excellent properties of good biocompatibility, high surface-area-to-volume ratio and nontoxicity and was employed in bioimaging, drug delivery and cancer diagnosis.

A g-C$_3$N$_4$ nanosheet, with a narrow band gap of 2.7 eV, can act as a stable photocatalyst for water splitting and the degradation of organic pollutants. Chung et al. applied photoactive g-C$_3$N$_4$ for the light-induced suppression of Aβ aggregation and toxicity [154]. As shown in Figure 12A, the photosensitized g-C$_3$N$_4$ generated oxidative ROS through photoinduced electron transfer under visible-light illumination, which further oxidized Aβ peptides, preventing the aggregation of Aβ monomers. However, g-C$_3$N$_4$ had no obvious effect on Aβ aggregation under dark conditions. Moreover, doping transition metal ions could promote ROS generation and enhance their inhibition efficiency. To enhance the photodegradation efficiency, Wang et al. used GO/g-C$_3$N$_4$ as the photocatalyst for irreversible disassembly of Aβ_{33-42} aggregate into nontoxic monomers under UV (Figure 12B) [155]. In this nanocomposite, GO acts as an Aβ collector due to its high surface area and abundant functional groups. g-C$_3$N$_4$ was also decorated with AuNPs to separate photoexcited electron-hole pairs [156].

Based on its strong adsorption capacity for metal ions, Li et al. reported that a g-C$_3$N$_4$ nanosheet could act as the chelator to block Cu^{2+}-induced Aβ aggregation, disaggregate the preformed Aβ-Cu^{2+} aggregates, reduce the ROS level induced by Aβ-Cu^{2+} and block Aβ-mediated toxicity [157]. At the same time, they also found that platinum(II)-coordinated g-C$_3$N$_4$ (g-C$_3$N$_4$@Pt) can covalently bind to Aβ monomers and oxygenate Aβ monomers and oligomers upon visible light irradiation, thus inhibiting the aggregation and toxicity of Aβ [158]. Furthermore, they found that the accumulation of oxygenated Aβ can inhibit the aggregation of native Aβ peptides.

For targeted therapy, Gong et al. developed an intelligent Aβ nanocaptor by anchoring C$_3$N$_4$ nanodots to Fe$_3$O$_4$@MSNs and modifying them with benzothiazole aniline (BTA) (B-FeCN), as shown in Figure 12C [159]. In this nanocomposite, C$_3$N$_4$ nanodots could capture Cu^{2+}, subsequently blocking the formation of the Aβ-Cu^{2+} complex and diminishing Aβ aggregation. Fe$_3$O$_4$ could cause local low-temperature hyperthermia to enhance the BBB permeability and dissolute the Aβ plaques. In addition, BTA endowed the nanocaptor with aspecific targeting ability and fluorescent imaging property for monitoring Aβ aggregates.

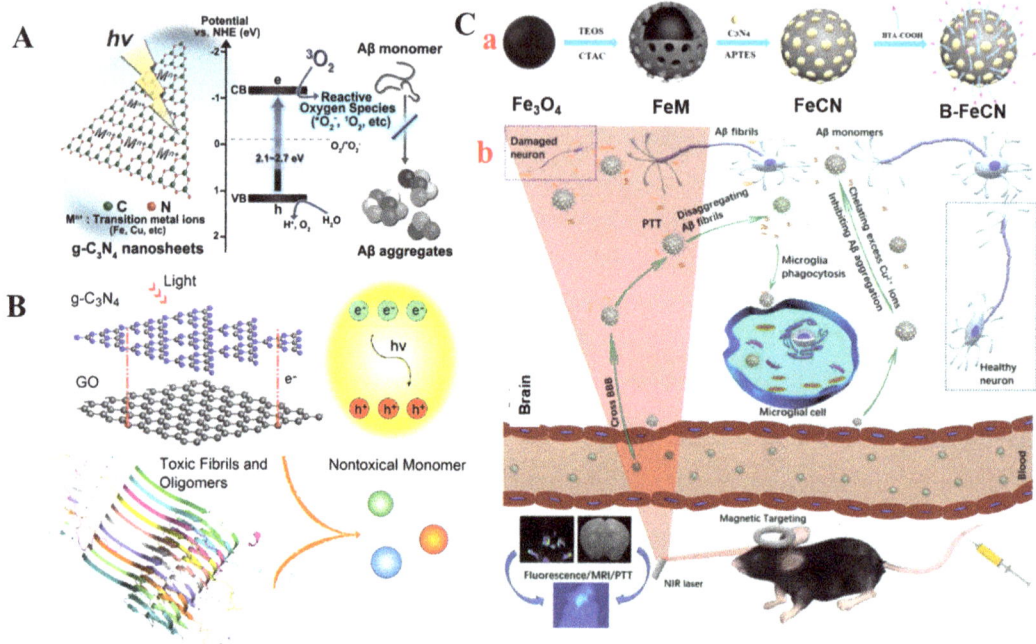

Figure 12. (**A**) Schematic illustration of g-C_3N_4 NSs as an Aβ aggregation inhibitor. Reprinted with permission from reference [154]. Copyright 2016 Wiley-VCH. (**B**) Schematic illustration of the degradation of Aβ aggregates using GO/g-C_3N_4 under light irradiation. Reprinted with permission from reference [155]. Copyright 2019 American Chemical Society. (**C**) (a) Schematic illustration of the preparation of B-FeCN nanocaptors. (b) Schematic illustration of the B-FeCN nanosystem as a multifunctional nanocaptor to inhibit Aβ aggregation for the magnetic targeting phototherapy of AD treatment. Reprinted with permission from reference [159]. Copyright 2021 Elsevier.

2.5. Metal-Organic Frameworks

As increasingly popular crystalline porous materials, metal-organic frameworks (MOFs) are built from metal nodes and organic linkers. Benefitting from the control of chemical functionality, pore size and crystal morphology, they have been used in many fields, including catalysis, gas storage, drug delivery and biosensing. Owing to the exposed metal sites and porphyrin linkers with aromatic rings, porphyrinic MOFs are particularly attractive for biomedical research. Porphyrinic MOF PCN-224 was prepared for the NIR-induced suppression of Aβ peptide aggregation (Figure 13A) [160]. Besides good biocompatibility and excellent stability, PCN-224 showed singlet oxygen generation capability in the NIR window because of the high density of the photosensitizer molecule TCPP in the framework and the easy diffusion of O_2 through the porous structure. The results showed that the photoactivated PCN-224 could effectively inhibit the aggregation of Aβ$_{1-42}$ into a high-order β-sheet-rich structure and rescue the cytotoxicity of Aβ$_{1-42}$. According to the previous report, the nitrogen atoms in porphyrin from porphyrinic MOF possess a high binding affinity to Cu^{2+} ions [161]. Inspired by these findings, Yu et al. utilized porphyrinic MOF as a Cu^{2+}-chelator and photooxidation agent for inhibiting Aβ peptide aggregation (Figure 13B) [162]. To further enhance the selectivity and photooxidation efficiency, MOFs were modified with the Aβ-targeting peptide LPFFD. As one sub-class of the MOF family, Prussian blue (PB) has numerous applications, including electrocatalysis, bioimaging and biosensing. According to the previous reports, it can act as a nanozyme to scavenge ROS and trap metal ions in its lattice cavities. Recently, Kowalczyk et al. studied the dual effects of PB on inhibiting Aβ$_{1-40}$ aggregation and chelating Cu^{2+} [163]. They found that PB-could accelerate the nucleation of Aβ$_{1-40}$ and facilitate the formation of Aβ$_{1-40}$ amorphous aggregates instead of β-sheet fibrils.

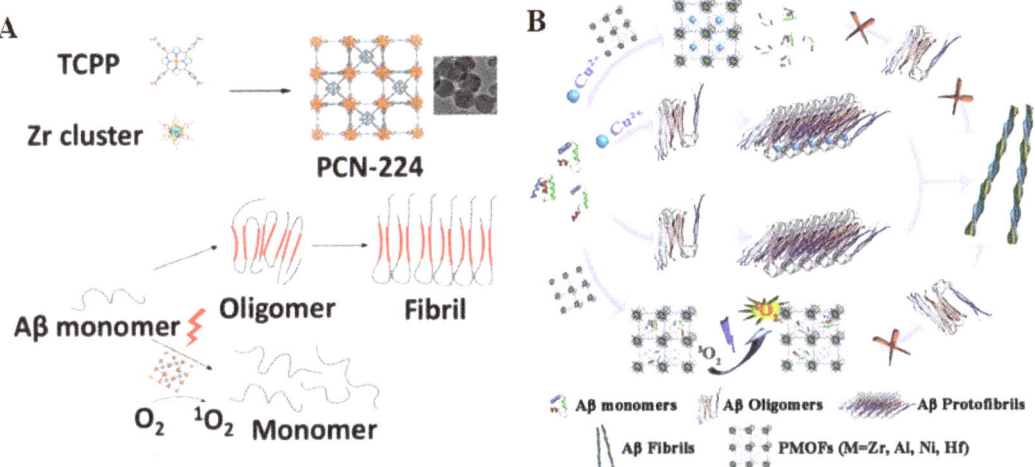

Figure 13. (**A**) Schematic diagram of the photo-inhibition of Aβ$_{1-42}$ aggregation using PCN-224 nanoparticles. Reprinted with permission from reference [160]. Copyright 2018 American Chemical Society. (**B**) Schematic illustration of the possible mechanism of inhibition effect of porphyrinic MOFs on the amyloid fibrillation process. Reprinted with permission from reference [162]. Copyright 2019 Wiley-VCH.

2.6. Semiconductor Quantum Dots

Unlike traditional fluorescent organic dyes, semiconductor quantum dots (QDs) have shown excellent optical properties, including size-dependent emission wavelengths, high resistance to photobleaching and multicolor fluorescence emission with a single excitation. Thus, QDs are widely utilized in various applications, such as drug delivery, fluorescent biosensing and tissue imaging. Furthermore, QDs have been utilized as promising candidates against amyloidosis for monitoring and inhibiting Aβ aggregation [164].

QDs (NAC-QDs) capped with N-acetyl-L-cysteine were reported to quench both the nucleation and elongation processes resulting from the intermolecular attractive interactions, such as hydrogen bonding between NAC-QDs and amyloid fibrils and the blockage of the active elongation sites on the Aβ fibrils [165]. Furthermore, NAC-QDs have a neuro-protective ability against the cytotoxicity induced by Aβ peptides on human neuroblastoma SH-SY5Y cells [166]. Dihydrolipoic acid(DHLA)-capped CdSe/ZnS QDs also reduced the fibrillation process [167].

2.7. Self-Assembled Nanomaterials

2.7.1. Liposomes

Liposomes have been used in drug delivery, because of their non-toxic, high drug-loading capacity and their ease of preparation and modification. In 1999, Maria et al. studied the structure of Aβ$_{25-35}$ and explored its association with different phospholipid membrane vesicles [168]. It was found that three kinds of negatively charged vesicles could accelerate the aggregation of Aβ$_{25-35}$ based on the electrostatic interaction, while vesicles formed by the zwitterionic phospholipid could slow down the aggregation of Aβ$_{25-35}$. Neutral liposomes increase the time of Aβ aggregation in a concentration-dependent manner [169]. The effect of NLs with different sizes on the Aβ aggregation was also investigated by Terakawa and co-workers [170]. Liposomes with smaller sizes (<50 nm) promoted the nucleation and yet those with larger sizes decreased the amount of fibrils and had no influence on the lag time of fibrillation. Shimanouchi et al. reported that Cu^{2+}

affected the fibrillar aggregates formed on the surface of oxidized and negatively charged liposomes, such as the oxidatively damaged neuronal cell membranes [171]. Thus, anionic liposomes can result in the formation of spherulitic Aβ aggregates.

Various methods have been proposed by incorporating or modifying the liposomes with different molecules, peptides or antibodies for targeting the Aβ aggregates and plaques [172–174]. Nanoliposomes containing anionic phosphatidic acid (PA) or cardiolipin (CL) can bind with all formats of Aβ$_{1-42}$ aggregates with high affinity and thus reduce Aβ-induced toxicity [175,176]. Mourtas et al. found that the planarity of curcumin on the liposome has an important influence on the affinity toward Aβ aggregates, which is dependent upon the conjugation method [177]. Moreover, Taylor et al. demonstrated that curcumin-modified liposome synthesized using click chemistry was the most effective in the inhibition of Aβ aggregation [178]. Canovi et al. decorated NLs with an anti-Aβ monoclonal antibody (Aβ–MAb) to achieve a high affinity toward Aβ monomers and fibrils [179]. Moreover, the multifunctional conjugation of NLs containing PA, CL, curcumin with apolipoprotein E or the anti-transferrin receptor antibody can facilitate the crossing of the BBB and enhance the uptake in the brain capillary cells without the sacrifice of Aβ targeting [180–182]. For instance, liposomes bi-functionalized with PA and an ApoE-derived peptide destabilized the preformed Aβ$_{1-42}$ aggregates under the synergic action and could cross the BBB in vitroandin vivo [183,184].

2.7.2. Polymer Nanoparticles

Celia et al. demonstrated that copolymeric NiPAM:BAM nanoparticles increased the nucleation time of Aβ fibrillation, but the elongation step remained largely unaffected, which isdependent uponthe concentrationand hydrophobicity [185]. Through studying the effect of cationic amino-modified PS NPs, they indicated that there is a balance between two different pathways: fibrillation of the free monomer in solution and the nucleation and fibrillation accelerated at the particle surface, which can be determined by the ratio between the peptide and NPs concentration (Figure 14A) [186]. Biopolymeric chitosan-based NPs were also reported to show the ability to inhibit Aβ aggregation and disintegrate the preformed fibrils [187].

The positively charged fluorescent conjugated polymer NPs (CPNPs) were prepared to inhibit Aβ$_{1-40}$ peptide fibrillation (Figure 14B) [188]. Moreover, CPNPs with excellent photophysical properties provided fluorescence signals for probing the interaction with Aβ peptides. They found that CPNPs could not only inhibit the aggregation of Aβ but also bind with the terminal of seed fibrils, preventing further fibrillation. A photosensitive polymer nanodot was designed by modifying it with a photosensitizer for efficient suppression of Aβ aggregation [189]. Dou et al. produced fluorogenic "nanogrenades" based on supermolecular assembly between organic dyes and conjugated polymers [190]. The quenched fluorescence of dyes in the nanogrenades was recovered after binding with hydrophobic Aβ fibril plaques. The conjugated polymers in the nanogrenades could generate ROS to destruct the Aβ plaques usingwhite light irradiation.

NPs assembled using conjugated polymers can also be applied to construct stimuli-responsive drug delivery systems. Recently, to ensure targeting and selectivity, Lai et al. designed versatile NPs with a high Aβ-binding affinity, stimuli-responsive drug release and a photothermal degradation ability for the dissolution of Aβ [191]. As shown in Figure 14C, the NPs were composed of an NIR-absorbing conjugated polymer-formed photothermal core and a thermal-responsive polymer-formed shell as NIR-stimuli gatekeeper. Inhibitor curcumin was loaded into the NPs andthe peptide LPFFDwas modified on the surface of NPs for targeting Aβ. Upon NIR laser irradiation, local heat generated by the core could not only trigger the release of encapsulated curcumin to inhibit the aggregation of Aβ but also effectively dissociate the Aβ deposits. Moreover, the Aβ fibrillation and disassembly could be real-time monitored due to the intrinsic polarity-dependent fluorescence of curcumin.

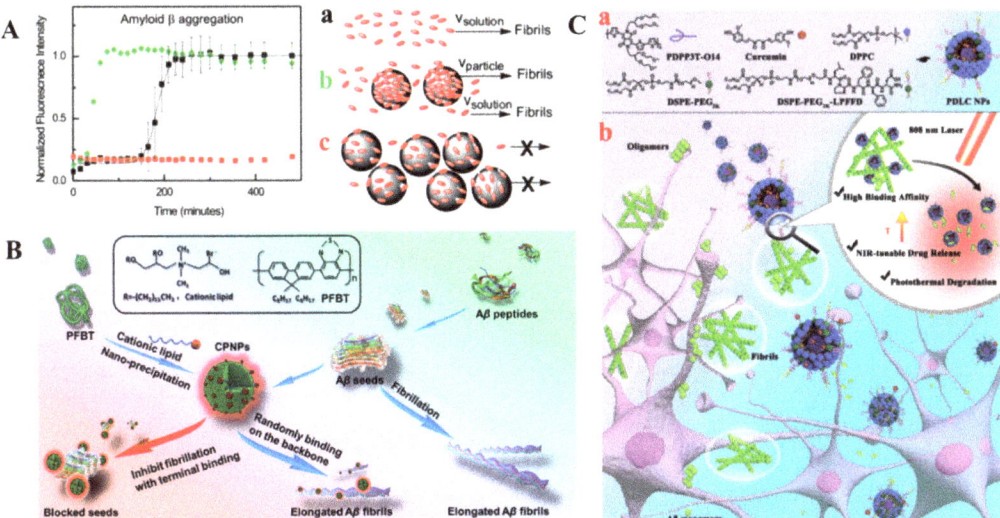

Figure 14. (**A**) Schematic of the dual effect of amino-modified polystyrene nanoparticles on Aβ fibrillation. (a) The fibrillation of Aβ$_{1-40}$ in the absence of nanoparticles shows the typical nucleation-elongation profile. (b) The fibrillation process is accelerated (shorter lag phase) by nanoparticles at low particle concentration (c) At high particle concentration, the fibrillation process is retarded (longer lag phase). Reprinted with permission from reference [186]. Copyright 2010 American Chemical Society. (**B**) Schematic diagram of the procedures for CPNPs fabrication and Aβ$_{1-40}$ fibril inhibition with CPNPs. Reprinted with permission from reference [188]. Copyright 2019 American Chemical Society. (**C**) Schematic illustration of PDLC NPs for chemo-photothermal treatment for Aβ aggregation. (a) Chemical structures and the synthesis of PDLC NPs. (b) Schematic illustration of PDLC NPs-mediated chem-photothermal treatment by combining NIR light-tunable drug release and photodegradation of amyloid β. Reprinted with permission from reference [191]. Copyright 2019 American Chemical Society.

Dopamine can self-assemble into melanin-like poly(dopamine) (PDA) NPs under alkaline conditions with oxygen as the oxidant. PDA NPs with functional groups (i.e., catechol and amine) on the surface can interact with peptides and proteins. Our group was the first to find out that PDA NPs could prevent the formation of Aβ fibrils via the hydrogen bonding and aromatic interactions between Aβ and PDA NPs [192]. Moreover, eumelanin-like particles and pheomelanin-like particles could also perturb the Aβ$_{1-42}$ aggregation and remodel the matured Aβ$_{1-42}$ fibers [192].

Inspired by the self-assembly of biomolecules into complicated functionalized units in cells and nature, researchers put efforts into the self-assembly of different molecules from natural small molecules to peptides, even to proteins. Among those self-assembly blocks, low-molecular-weight peptides have attracted significant attention due to their flexible sequences and biodegradability. Recently, Liu et al. proposed a peptide-based porphyrin supramolecular self-assembly (PKNPs) for target-driving the selective photooxygenation of Aβ [193]. Porphyrin-peptide conjugate (PP-KLVFF) can be self-assembled into PKNPs via hydrophobic interactions and π-π stacking interactions, resulting in the suppression of the intrinsic fluorescence emission, the generation of ROS by free porphyrin and the enhancement of photo-to-thermal conversion ability. The photothermal effect facilitated the crossing of the BBB and then Aβ selectively initiated the disassembly of PKNPs into free porphyrin to produce ROS under light irradiation and thus oxygenated the Aβ.

2.8. Others

In the PDT, visible (or UV) light-activated photosensitizers are always confronted with the problem that the penetration depth of UV–visible light in biological tissues is limited. To solve this problem, the upconversion nanoparticles (UCNPs) with the ability to convert

NIR light into short-wavelength light are attractive for therapeutic applications. As shown in Figure 15A, Kuk et al. proposed a NIR-light-responsive strategy for the suppression of Aβ aggregation [194]. In this work, rattle-structured organosilica-shell-coated, Yb/Er-co-doped NaYF$_4$ NPs were synthesized with an interior cavity to encapsulate numerous rose bengal (RB) molecules with a high loading efficiency and no self-aggregation. Since the absorption of RB partially overlapped with the green emission of UCNPs, visible-light-absorbing RB was activated by UCNPs under 980 nm NIR light, through the highly efficient energy transfer to generate oxidative $^1O_2$, oxidize peptides and preclude the Aβ fibrillogenesis. However, in dark conditions, a delayed elongation rate but an unaltered amount of total Aβ aggregate was recorded, which wasascribed to the intrinsic inhibition ability of the positively charged UCNPs. Moreover, the biocompatible UCNPs also showed effective suppression of the Aβ-induced cytotoxicity under NIR light.

Polyphenol compounds can inhibit Aβ aggregation and decrease the generation of ROS. However, excess metal ions in Aβ plaque can bind with them, resulting in a decreasein efficacy. Ma et al. proposed a NIR-responsive UCNPs-caged system to sequentially release drugs by regulating them using an NIR laser [195]. As shown in Figure 15B, the metal chelator CQ and polyphenol curcumin were conjugated on the surface of UCNPs using two NIR-sensitive linkers. After being irradiated by a low-power laser, CQ was released to remove free metal ions. Then, curcumin was released to clear superfluous ROS by increasing the intensity of the laser, leading to enhanced treatment efficacy.

Chiral amino acids or peptides conjugated on the NPs can endow NPs with chiral properties, which have aroused interest in the applicability of chiral NPs in different fields. Recently, Zhang et al. found that D-type penicillamine (D-Pen)-modified Fe$_x$Cu$_y$Se nanoparticles (NPs) showed higher efficiency in the inhibition of Aβ$_{1-42}$-monomer aggregation and enhancement of the dissociation of Aβ$_{1-42}$ fibrils under NIR light irradiation in 10 min (Figure 15C) [196].

Sulfur nanomaterials have the excellent ability to remove Cu^{2+} ions and radicals. Sun et al. synthesized three RVG-peptide-modified sulfur NPs (SNPs) with different morphologies and study their influence on the aggregation of Aβ-Cu^{2+} complexes and corresponding neurotoxicity [197]. They found that the sphere-like SNPs exhibited the most effective inhibition activity owing to the small size, thus reducing the Aβ-Cu^{2+}-induced ROS and increasingthe cell viability (Figure 15D).

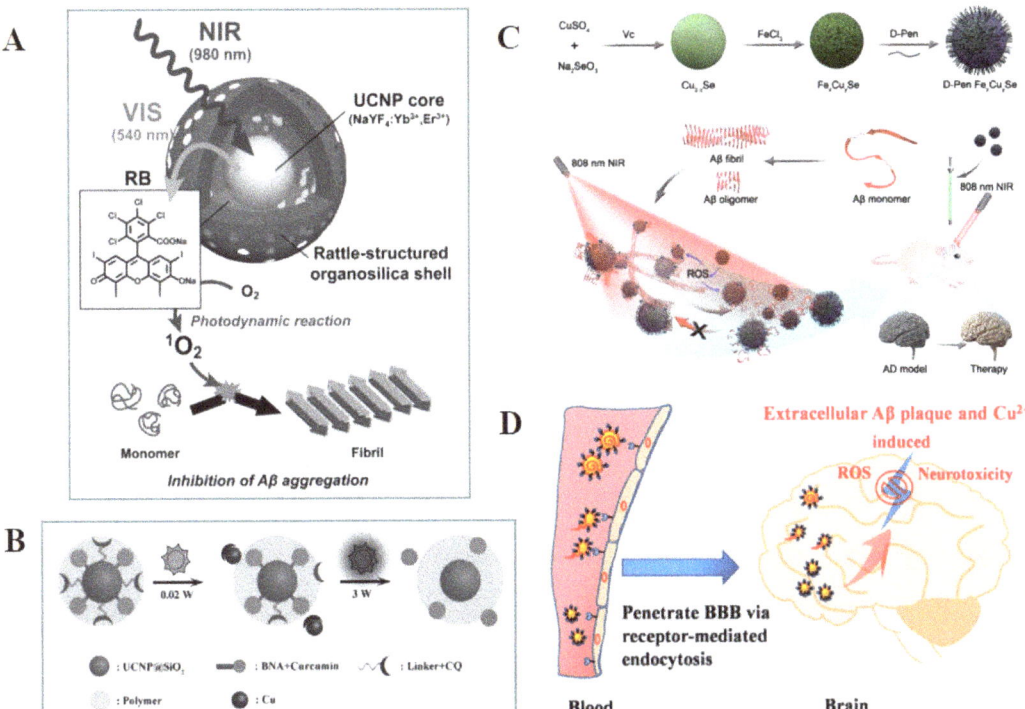

Figure 15. (**A**) Schematic of Aβ aggregation inhibition by NIR-responsive rattle-structured UCNPs. Reprinted with permission from reference [194]. Copyright 2017 Wiley-VCH. (**B**) Illustration of agents that are sequentially released during a process based on 980 nm NIR light-triggered UCNP@SiO$_2$@Cur/CQ. Reprinted with permission from reference [195]. Copyright 2017 Wiley-VCH. (**C**) Schematic of the synthesis of Pen modified Fe$_x$Cu$_y$Se and illustration of the inhibition and disassembly effects of D-Pen-modified Fe$_x$Cu$_y$Se on Aβ$_{1-42}$ aggregation and the mitigation of potential neurotoxicity in an AD mice model. Reprinted with permission from reference [196]. Copyright 2018 Wiley-VCH. (**D**) Schematic of the inhibition Aβ aggregation by sulfur NPs. Reprinted with permission from reference [197]. Copyright 2018 American Chemical Society.

3. Conclusions

In this review, we give a brief overview of recent achievements of nanomaterial-based modulation of Aβ aggregation. Nanomaterials for the treatment of AD play multiple roles. First, most nanomaterials can directly interact with Aβ peptides to accelerate or slow the aggregation. Second, nanomaterials can act as nano-carriers for loading of various drugs to allow them to cross the BBB and improve the local concentration of drugs. Third, nanomaterials with photosensitive properties can influence the format of Aβ through PTT or PDT. Although the development of nanomaterials opens a brand new chapter in the treatment of AD, more efforts are still urgently needed and more novel nanomaterials should be explored and investigated. For example, MXene, which is a novel type of 2D nanosheet that is mainly composed of early transition metal carbides, has attracted a great deal of attention in energy evolution and nanomedicine [198]. Moreover, metal ions on the MXene surface may interact with Aβ peptides or aggregates. Although there are increasing studies focusing on the interactions between nanomaterials and Aβ, a deep and comprehensive understanding of its nature and application is still necessary.

Author Contributions: Conceptualization, Y.H. and L.L.; writing—original draft preparation, Y.H. and Y.C.; writing—review and editing, J.W.; project administration, L.L.; funding acquisition, J.W. All authors have read and agreed to the published version of the manuscript.

Funding: This research was funded by the National Natural Science Foundation of China (22076221) and the Program for Innovative Research Team of Science and Technology in the University of Henan Province (21IRTSTHN005).

Conflicts of Interest: The authors declare no conflict of interest.

References

1. Tao, Y.X.; Conn, P.M. Pharmacoperones as Novel Therapeutics for Diverse Protein Conformational Diseases. *Physiol. Rev.* **2018**, *98*, 697–725. [CrossRef]
2. Jarosz, D.F.; Khurana, V. Specification of Physiologic and Disease States by Distinct Proteins and Protein Conformations. *Cell* **2017**, *171*, 1001–1014. [CrossRef]
3. Klementieva, O.; Willen, K.; Martinsson, I.; Israelsson, B.; Engdahl, A.; Cladera, J.; Uvdal, P.; Gouras, G.K. Pre-Plaque Conformational Changes in Alzheimer's Disease-Linked Aβ and App. *Nat. Commun.* **2017**, *8*, 14726. [CrossRef]
4. Blennow, K.; de Leon, M.J.; Zetterberg, H. Alzheimer's Disease. *Lancet* **2006**, *368*, 387–403. [CrossRef]
5. Kiernan, M.C.; Vucic, S.; Cheah, B.C.; Turner, M.R.; Eisen, A.; Hardiman, O.; Burrell, J.R.; Zoing, M.C. Amyotrophic Lateral Sclerosis. *Lancet* **2011**, *377*, 942–955. [CrossRef]
6. Yepes, M. The Plasminogen Activating System in the Pathogenesis of Alzheimer's Disease. *Neural Regen. Res.* **2021**, *16*, 1973–1977. [CrossRef]
7. Caselli, R.J.; Knopman, D.S.; Bu, G. An Agnostic Reevaluation of the Amyloid Cascade Hypothesis of Alzheimer's Disease Pathogenesis: The Role of App Homeostasis. *Alzheimers Dement.* **2020**, *16*, 1582–1590. [CrossRef] [PubMed]
8. Canevelli, M.; Bruno, G.; Cesari, M. The Sterile Controversy on the Amyloid Cascade Hypothesis. *Neurosci. Biobehav. Rev.* **2017**, *83*, 472–473. [CrossRef]
9. Hu, W.; Zhang, X.; Tung, Y.C.; Xie, S.; Liu, F.; Iqbal, K. Hyperphosphorylation Determines Both the Spread and the Morphology of Tau Pathology. *Alzheimers Dement.* **2016**, *12*, 1066–1077. [CrossRef]
10. Styr, B.; Slutsky, I. Imbalance between Firing Homeostasis and Synaptic Plasticity Drives Early-Phase Alzheimer's Disease. *Nat. Neurosci.* **2018**, *21*, 463–473. [CrossRef]
11. Breijyeh, Z.; Karaman, R. Comprehensive Review on Alzheimer's Disease: Causes and Treatment. *Molecules* **2020**, *25*, 5789. [CrossRef]
12. Flammang, B.; Pardossi-Piquard, R.; Sevalle, J.; Debayle, D.; Dabert-Gay, A.S.; Thevenet, A.; Lauritzen, I.; Checler, F. Evidence That the Amyloid-B Protein Precursor Intracellular Domain, Aicd, Derives from B-Secretase-Generated C-Terminal Fragment. *J. Alzheimers Dis.* **2012**, *30*, 145–153. [CrossRef] [PubMed]
13. Checler, F. Processing of the B-Amyloid Precursor Protein and Its Regulation in Alzheimer's Disease. *J. Neurochem.* **1995**, *65*, 1431–1444. [CrossRef] [PubMed]
14. Iwatsubo, T.; Odaka, A.; Suzuki, N.; Mizusawa, H.; Nukina, N.; Ihara, Y. Visualization of Aβ42(43) and Aβ40 in Senile Plaques with End-Specific Aβ Monoclonals: Evidence That an Initially Deposited Species Is Aβ42(43). *Neuron* **1994**, *13*, 45–53. [CrossRef]
15. Haass, C.; Selkoe, D.J. Soluble Protein Oligomers in Neurodegeneration: Lessons from the Alzheimer's Amyloid B-Peptide. *Nat. Rev. Mol. Cell Biol.* **2007**, *8*, 101–112. [CrossRef]
16. Yang, J.; Zhang, X.; Yuan, P.; Yang, J.; Xu, Y.; Grutzendler, J.; Shao, Y.; Moore, A.; Ran, C. Oxalate-Curcumin-Based Probe for Micro- and Macroimaging of Reactive Oxygen Species in Alzheimer's Disease. *Proc. Natl. Acad. Sci. USA* **2017**, *114*, 12384–12389. [CrossRef] [PubMed]
17. Yan, L.M.; Velkova, A.; Tatarek-Nossol, M.; Andreetto, E.; Kapurniotu, A. Iapp Mimic Blocks Aβ Cytotoxic Self-Assembly: Cross-Suppression of Amyloid Toxicity of Aβ and Iapp Suggests a Molecular Link between Alzheimer's Disease and Type Ii Diabetes. *Angew. Chem. Int. Ed. Engl.* **2007**, *46*, 1246–1252. [CrossRef] [PubMed]
18. Richman, M.; Wilk, S.; Chemerovski, M.; Warmlander, S.K.; Wahlstrom, A.; Graslund, A.; Rahimipour, S. In Vitro and Mechanistic Studies of an Antiamyloidogenic Self-Assembled Cyclic $_{D,L}$-A-Peptide Architecture. *J. Am. Chem. Soc.* **2013**, *135*, 3474–3484. [CrossRef]
19. Liu, W.; Dong, X.; Sun, Y. D-Enantiomeric Rthlvffark-Nh$_2$: A Potent Multifunctional Decapeptide Inhibiting Cu^{2+}-Mediated Amyloid B-Protein Aggregation and Rmodeling Cu^{2+}-Mediated Amyloid B Aggregates. *ACS Chem. Neurosci.* **2019**, *10*, 1390–1401. [CrossRef]
20. Buxbaum, J.N.; Ye, Z.; Reixach, N.; Friske, L.; Levy, C.; Das, P.; Golde, T.; Masliah, E.; Roberts, A.R.; Bartfai, T. Transthyretin Protects Alzheimer's Mice from the Behavioral and Biochemical Effects of Aβ Toxicity. *Proc. Natl. Acad. Sci. USA* **2008**, *105*, 2681–2686. [CrossRef]
21. Luo, J.; Warmlander, S.K.; Graslund, A.; Abrahams, J.P. Human Lysozyme Inhibits the In Vitro Aggregation of Aβ Peptides, Which in Vivo Are Associated with Alzheimer's Disease. *Chem. Commun.* **2013**, *49*, 6507–6509. [CrossRef] [PubMed]
22. Wang, W.; Dong, X.; Sun, Y. Modification of Serum Albumin by High Conversion of Carboxyl to Amino Groups Creates a Potent Inhibitor of Amyloid B-Protein Fbrillogenesis. *Bioconjug. Chem.* **2019**, *30*, 1477–1488. [CrossRef] [PubMed]

23. Gronwall, C.; Jonsson, A.; Lindstrom, S.; Gunneriusson, E.; Stahl, S.; Herne, N. Selection and Characterization of Affibody Ligands Binding to Alzheimer Amyloid B Peptides. *J. Biotechnol.* **2007**, *128*, 162–183. [CrossRef]
24. Fan, Y.; Wu, D.; Yi, X.; Tang, H.; Wu, L.; Xia, Y.; Wang, Z.; Liu, Q.; Zhou, Z.; Wang, J. Tmpyp Inhibits Amyloid-B Aggregation and Alleviates Amyloid-Induced Cytotoxicity. *ACS Omega* **2017**, *2*, 4188–4195. [CrossRef] [PubMed]
25. Taniguchi, A.; Shimizu, Y.; Oisaki, K.; Sohma, Y.; Kanai, M. Switchable Photooxygenation Catalysts That Sense Higher-Order Amyloid Structures. *Nat. Chem.* **2016**, *8*, 974–982. [CrossRef] [PubMed]
26. Taniguchi, A.; Sasaki, D.; Shiohara, A.; Iwatsubo, T.; Tomita, T.; Sohma, Y.; Kanai, M. Attenuation of the Aggregation and Neurotoxicity of Amyloid-B Peptides by Catalytic Photooxygenation. *Angew. Chem. Int. Ed. Engl.* **2014**, *53*, 1382–1385. [CrossRef] [PubMed]
27. Lee, J.S.; Lee, B.I.; Park, C.B. Photo-Induced Inhibition of Alzheimer's B-Amyloid Aggregation In Vitro by Rose Bengal. *Biomaterials* **2015**, *38*, 43–49. [CrossRef]
28. Lee, B.I.; Lee, S.; Suh, Y.S.; Lee, J.S.; Kim, A.-k.; Kwon, O.Y.; Yu, K.; Park, C.B. Photoexcited Porphyrins as a Strong Suppressor of B-Amyloid Aggregation and Synaptic Toxicity. *Angew. Chem.* **2015**, *127*, 11634–11638. [CrossRef]
29. Lee, B.I.; Suh, Y.S.; Chung, Y.J.; Yu, K.; Park, C.B. Shedding Light on Alzheimer's B-Amyloidosis: Photosensitized Methylene Blue Inhibits Self-Assembly of B-Amyloid Peptides and Disintegrates Their Aggregates. *Sci. Rep.* **2017**, *7*, 7523. [CrossRef]
30. Zorkina, Y.; Abramova, O.; Ushakova, V.; Morozova, A.; Zubkov, E.; Valikhov, M.; Melnikov, P.; Majouga, A.; Chekhonin, V. Nano Carrier Drug Delivery Systems for the Treatment of Neuropsychiatric Disorders: Advantages and Limitations. *Molecules* **2020**, *25*, 5294. [CrossRef] [PubMed]
31. Sun, J.; Wei, C.; Liu, Y.; Xie, W.; Xu, M.; Zhou, H.; Liu, J. Progressive Release of Mesoporous Nano-Selenium Delivery System for the Multi-Channel Synergistic Treatment of Alzheimer's Disease. *Biomaterials* **2019**, *197*, 417–431. [CrossRef] [PubMed]
32. Zagorska, A.; Jaromin, A. Perspectives for New and More Efficient Multifunctional Ligands for Alzheimer's Disease Therapy. *Molecules* **2020**, *25*, 3337. [CrossRef]
33. Manek, E.; Darvas, F.; Petroianu, G.A. Use of Biodegradable, Chitosan-Based Nanoparticles in the Treatment of Alzheimer's Disease. *Molecules* **2020**, *25*, 4866. [CrossRef] [PubMed]
34. Wu, W.H.; Sun, X.; Yu, Y.P.; Hu, J.; Zhao, L.; Liu, Q.; Zhao, Y.F.; Li, Y.M. Tio2 Nanoparticles Promote Beta-Amyloid Fibrillation In Vitro. *Biochem. Biophys. Res. Commun.* **2008**, *373*, 315–318. [CrossRef]
35. Daniel, M.-C.; Astruc, D. Gold Nanoparticles: Assembly, Supramolecular Chemistry, Quantum-Size-Related Properties, and Applications toward Biology, Catalysis, and Nanotechnology. *Chem. Rev.* **2004**, *104*, 293–346. [CrossRef] [PubMed]
36. Dykmana, L.; Khlebtsov, N. Gold Nanoparticles in Biomedical Applications: Recent Advances and Perspectives. *Chem. Soc. Rev.* **2012**, *41*, 2256–2282. [CrossRef]
37. Lee, H.; Kim, Y.; Park, A.; Nam, J.M.; Kim, Y.; Park, A.; Nam, J.M. Amyloid-B Aggregation with Gold Nanoparticles on Brain Lipid Bilayer. *Small* **2014**, *10*, 1779–1789. [CrossRef]
38. Mirsadeghi, S.; Dinarvand, R.; Ghahremani, M.H.; Hormozi-Nezhad, M.R.; Mahmoudi, Z.; Hajipour, M.J.; Atyabi, F.; Ghavami, M.; Mahmoudi, M. Protein Corona Composition of Gold Nanoparticles/Nanorods Affects Amyloid Beta Fibrillation Process. *Nanoscale* **2015**, *7*, 5004–5013. [CrossRef]
39. Kim, Y.; Park, J.H.; Lee, H.; Nam, J.M. How Do the Size, Charge and Shape of Nanoparticles Affect Amyloid Beta Aggregation on Brain Lipid Bilayer? *Sci. Rep.* **2016**, *6*, 19548. [CrossRef]
40. Gao, G.; Zhang, M.; Gong, D.; Chen, R.; Hu, X.; Sun, T. The Size-Effect of Gold Nanoparticles and Nanoclusters in the Inhibition of Amyloid-Beta Fibrillation. *Nanoscale* **2017**, *9*, 4107–4113. [CrossRef]
41. Liao, Y.H.; Chang, Y.J.; Yoshiike, Y.; Chang, Y.C.; Chen, Y.R. Negatively Charged Gold Nanoparticles Inhibit Alzheimer's Amyloid-B Fibrillization, Induce Fibril Dissociation, and Mitigate Neurotoxicity. *Small* **2012**, *8*, 3631–3639. [CrossRef]
42. Ma, Q.; Wei, G.; Yang, X. Influence of Au Nanoparticles on the Aggregation of Amyloid-Beta-(25-35) Peptides. *Nanoscale* **2013**, *5*, 10397–10403. [CrossRef]
43. Wang, W.; Han, Y.; Fan, Y.; Wang, Y. Effects of Gold Nanospheres and Nanocubes on Amyloid-Beta Peptide Fibrillation. *Langmuir* **2019**, *35*, 2334–2342. [CrossRef]
44. Liu, Y.; He, G.; Zhang, Z.; Yin, H.; Liu, H.; Chen, J.; Zhang, S.; Yang, B.; Xu, L.-P.; Zhang, X. Size-Effect of Gold Nanorods on Modulating the Kinetic Process of Amyloid-B Aggregation. *Chem. Phys. Lett.* **2019**, *734*, 136702. [CrossRef]
45. Bellucci, L.; Ardevol, A.; Parrinello, M.; Lutz, H.; Lu, H.; Weidner, T.; Corni, S. The Interaction with Gold Suppresses Fiber-Like Conformations of the Amyloid B(16-22) Peptide. *Nanoscale* **2016**, *8*, 8737–8748. [CrossRef]
46. Song, M.; Sun, Y.; Luo, Y.; Zhu, Y.; Liu, Y.; Li, H. Exploring the Mechanism of Inhibition of Au Nanoparticles on the Aggregation of Amyloid-B(16-22) Peptides at the Atom Level by All-Atom Molecular Dynamics. *Int. J. Mol. Sci.* **2018**, *19*, 1815. [CrossRef] [PubMed]
47. Anand, B.G.; Wu, Q.; Karthivashan, G.; Shejale, K.P.; Amidian, S.; Wille, H.; Kar, S. Mimosine Functionalized Gold Nanoparticles (Mimo-Aunps) Suppress B-Amyloid Aggregation and Neuronal Toxicity. *Bioact. Mater.* **2021**, *6*, 4491–4505. [CrossRef] [PubMed]
48. Palmal, S.; Maity, A.R.; Singh, B.K.; Basu, S.; Jana, N.R.; Jana, N.R. Inhibition of Amyloid Fibril Growth and Dissolution of Amyloid Fibrils by Curcumin–Gold Nanoparticles. *Chem. Eur. J.* **2014**, *20*, 6184–6191. [CrossRef] [PubMed]
49. Xiong, N.; Zhao, Y.; Dong, X.; Zheng, J.; Sun, Y. Design of a Molecular Hybrid of Dual Peptide Inhibitors Coupled on Aunps for Enhanced Inhibition of Amyloid B-Protein Aggregation and Cytotoxicity. *Small* **2017**, *13*, 1601666. [CrossRef]

50. Adura, C.; Guerrero, S.; Salas, E.; Medel, L.; Riveros, A.; Mena, J.; Arbiol, J.; Albericio, F.; Giralt, E.; Kogan, M.J. Stable Conjugates of Peptides with Gold Nanorods for Biomedical Applications with Reduced Effects on Cell Viability. *ACS Appl. Mater. Inter.* **2013**, *5*, 4076–4085. [CrossRef]
51. Guerrero, S.; Araya, E.; Fiedler, J.L.; Arias, J.I.; Adura, C.; Albericio, F.; Giralt, E.; Arias, J.L.; Fernandez, M.S.; Kogan, M.J. Improving the Brain Delivery of Gold Nanoparticles by Conjugation with an Amphipathic Peptide. *Nanomedicine* **2010**, *5*, 897–913. [CrossRef] [PubMed]
52. Olmedo, I.; Araya, E.; Sanz, F.; Medina, E.; Arbiol, J.; Toledo, P.; Alvarez-Lueje, A.; Giralt, E.; Kogan, M.J. How Changes in the Sequence of the Peptide Clpffd-Nh$_2$ Can Modify the Conjugation and Stability of Gold Nanoparticles and Their Affinity for Beta-Amyloid Fibrils. *Bioconjug. Chem.* **2008**, *19*, 1154–1163. [CrossRef] [PubMed]
53. Kogan, M.J.; Bastus, N.G.; Amigo, R.; Grillo-Bosch, D.; Araya, E.; Turiel, A.; Labarta, A.; Giralt, E.; Puntes, V.F. Nanoparticle-Mediated Local and Remote Manipulation of Protein Aggregation. *Nano Lett.* **2006**, *6*, 110–115. [CrossRef]
54. Araya, E.; Olmedo, I.; Bastus, N.G.; Guerrero, S.; Puntes, V.F.; Giralt, E.; Kogan, M.J. Gold Nanoparticles and Microwave Irradiation Inhibit Beta-Amyloid Amyloidogenesis. *Nanoscale Res. Lett.* **2008**, *3*, 435–443. [CrossRef]
55. Triulzi, R.C.; Dai, Q.; Zou, J.; Leblanc, R.M.; Gu, Q.; Orbulescu, J.; Huo, Q. Photothermal Ablation of Amyloid Aggregates by Gold Nanoparticles. *Colloids Surf. B* **2008**, *63*, 200–208. [CrossRef]
56. Ruff, J.; Hassan, N.; Morales-Zavala, F.; Steitz, J.; Araya, E.; Kogan, M.J.; Simon, U. Clpffd–Peg Functionalized Nir-Absorbing Hollow Gold Nanospheres and Gold Nanorods Inhibit B-Amyloid Aggregation. *J. Mater. Chem. B* **2018**, *6*, 2432–2443. [CrossRef]
57. Yin, T.; Xie, W.; Sun, J.; Yang, L.; Liu, J. Penetratin Peptide-Functionalized Gold Nanostars: Enhanced Bbb Permeability and Nir Photothermal Treatment of Alzheimer's Disease Using Ultralow Irradiance. *ACS Appl. Mater. Inter.* **2016**, *8*, 19291–19302. [CrossRef]
58. Lin, D.; He, R.; Li, S.; Xu, Y.; Wang, J.; Wei, G.; Ji, M.; Yang, X. Highly Efficient Destruction of Amyloid-B Fibrils by Femtosecond Laser-Induced Nanoexplosion of Gold Nanorods. *ACS Chem. Neurosci.* **2016**, *7*, 1728–1736. [CrossRef]
59. Bush, A.I.; Pettingell, W.H.; Multhaup, G.; d ParadisParadis, M.; Vonsattel, J.P.; Gusella, J.F.; Beyreuther, K.; Masters, C.L.; Tanzi, R.E. Rapid Induction of Alzheimer Aβ Amyloid Formation by Zinc. *Science* **1994**, *265*, 1464–1467. [CrossRef]
60. Geng, J.; Li, M.; Wu, L.; Ren, J.; Qu, X. Liberation of Copper from Amyloid Plaques: Making a Risk Factor Useful for Alzheimer's Disease Treatment. *J. Med. Chem.* **2012**, *55*, 9146–9155. [CrossRef]
61. Kepp, K.P. Bioinorganic Chemistry of Alzheimer's Disease. *Chem. Rev.* **2012**, *112*, 5193–5239. [CrossRef]
62. Cahoon, L. The Curious Case of Clioquinol. *Nat. Med.* **2009**, *15*, 356. [CrossRef] [PubMed]
63. Dedeoglu, A.; Cormier, K.; Payton, S.; Tseitlin, K.A.; Kremsky, J.N.; Lai, L.; Li, X.; Moir, R.D.; Tanzi, R.E.; Bush, A.I.; et al. Preliminary Studies of a Novel Bifunctional Metal Chelator Targeting Alzheimer's Amyloidogenesis. *Exp. Gerontol.* **2004**, *39*, 1641–1649. [CrossRef] [PubMed]
64. Shi, P.; Li, M.; Ren, J.; Qu, X. Gold Nanocage-Based Dual Responsive "Caged Metal Chelator"Release System: Noninvasive Remote Control with near Infrared for Potential Treatment of Alzheimer's Disease. *Adv. Funct. Mater.* **2013**, *23*, 5412–5419. [CrossRef]
65. Hao, S.; Li, X.; Han, A.; Yang, Y.; Fang, G.; Liu, J.; Wang, S. CLVFFA-Functionalized Gold Nanoclusters Inhibit Aβ$_{40}$ Fibrillation, Fibrils' Prolongation, and Mature Fibrils' Disaggregation. *ACS Chem. Neurosci.* **2019**, *10*, 4633–4642. [CrossRef] [PubMed]
66. Sun, T.; He, M.; Luo, Z.; Ma, Z.; Gao, G.; Zhang, W. Au$_{23}$(Cr)$_{14}$ Nanocluster Restores Fibril Aβ's Unfolded State with Abolished Cytotoxicity and Dissolves Endogenous Aβ Plaques. *Natl. Sci. Rev.* **2020**, *7*, 763–774. [CrossRef]
67. Li, Q.; Liu, L.; Zhang, S.; Xu, M.; Wang, X.; Wang, C.; Besenbacher, F.; Dong, M. Modulating Aβ$_{33-42}$ Peptide Assembly by Graphene Oxide. *Chem. Eur. J.* **2014**, *20*, 7236–7240. [CrossRef] [PubMed]
68. Bag, S.; Sett, A.; DasGupta, S.; Dasgupta, S. Hydropathy: The Controlling Factor Behind the Inhibition of Aβ Fibrillation by Graphene Oxide. *RSC Adv.* **2016**, *6*, 103242–103252. [CrossRef]
69. Yu, X.; Wang, Q.; Lin, Y.; Zhao, J.; Zhao, C.; Zheng, J. Structure, Orientation, and Surface Interaction of Alzheimer Amyloid-Beta Peptides on the Graphite. *Langmuir* **2012**, *28*, 6595–6605. [CrossRef]
70. Yang, Z.; Ge, C.; Liu, J.; Chong, Y.; Gu, Z.; Jimenez-Cruz, C.A.; Chai, Z.; Zhou, R. Destruction of Amyloid Fibrils by Graphene through Penetration and Extraction of Peptides. *Nanoscale* **2015**, *7*, 18725–18737. [CrossRef]
71. Mahmoudi, M.; Akhavan, O.; Ghavami, M.; Rezaee, F.; Ghiasi, S.M. Graphene Oxide Strongly Inhibits Amyloid Beta Fibrillation. *Nanoscale* **2012**, *4*, 7322–7325. [CrossRef] [PubMed]
72. Wang, J.; Cao, Y.; Li, Q.; Liu, L.; Dong, M. Size Effect of Graphene Oxide on Modulating Amyloid Peptide Assembly. *Chem. Eur. J.* **2015**, *21*, 9632–9637. [CrossRef]
73. Qing, G.; Zhao, S.; Xiong, Y.; Lv, Z.; Jiang, F.; Liu, Y.; Chen, H.; Zhang, M.; Sun, T. Chiral Effect at Protein/Graphene Interface: A Bioinspired Perspective to Understand Amyloid Formation. *J. Am. Chem. Soc.* **2014**, *136*, 10736–10742. [CrossRef] [PubMed]
74. Li, M.; Yang, X.; Ren, J.; Qu, K.; Qu, X. Using Graphene Oxide High near-Infrared Absorbance for Photothermal Treatment of Alzheimer's Disease. *Adv. Mater.* **2012**, *24*, 1722–1728. [CrossRef]
75. Xu, C.; Shi, P.; Li, M.; Ren, J.; Qu, X. A Cytotoxic Amyloid Oligomer Self-Triggered and Nir-Enhanced Amyloidosis Therapeutic System. *Nano Res.* **2015**, *8*, 2431–2444. [CrossRef]
76. Li, J.; Han, Q.; Wang, X.; Yu, N.; Yang, L.; Yang, R.; Wang, C. Reduced Aggregation and Cytotoxicity of Amyloid Peptides by Graphene Oxide/Gold Nanocomposites Prepared by Pulsed Laser Ablation in Water. *Small* **2014**, *10*, 4386–4394. [CrossRef]

77. Ahmad, I.; Mozhi, A.; Yang, L.; Han, Q.; Liang, X.; Li, C.; Yang, R.; Wang, C. Graphene Oxide-Iron Oxide Nanocomposite as an Inhibitor of Aβ42 Amyloid Peptide Aggregation. *Colloids Surf. B* **2017**, *159*, 540–545. [CrossRef] [PubMed]
78. Liu, F.; Wang, W.; Sang, J.; Jia, L.; Lu, F. Hydroxylated Single-Walled Carbon Nanotubes Inhibit Aβ42 Fibrillogenesis, Disaggregate Mature Fibrils, and Protect against Aβ42-Induced Cytotoxicity. *ACS Chem. Neurosci.* **2019**, *10*, 588–598. [CrossRef]
79. Kam, N.W.; O'Connell, M.; Wisdom, J.A.; Dai, H. Carbon Nanotubes as Multifunctional Biological Transporters and near-Infrared Agents for Selective Cancer Cell Destruction. *Proc. Natl. Acad. Sci. USA* **2005**, *102*, 11600–11605. [CrossRef]
80. Luo, J.; Warmlander, S.K.; Yu, C.H.; Muhammad, K.; Graslund, A.; Pieter Abrahams, J. The Abeta Peptide Forms Non-Amyloid Fibrils in the Presence of Carbon Nanotubes. *Nanoscale* **2014**, *6*, 6720–6726. [CrossRef] [PubMed]
81. Xie, L.; Lin, D.; Luo, Y.; Li, H.; Yang, X.; Wei, G. Effects of Hydroxylated Carbon Nanotubes on the Aggregation of Aβ16-22 Peptides: A Combined Simulation and Experimental Study. *Biophys. J.* **2014**, *107*, 1930–1938. [CrossRef] [PubMed]
82. Ma, M.; Gao, N.; Li, X.; Liu, Z.; Pi, Z.; Du, X.; Ren, J.; Qu, X. A Biocompatible Second near-Infrared Nanozyme for Spatiotemporal and Non-Invasive Attenuation of Amyloid Deposition through Scalp and Skull. *ACS Nano* **2020**, *14*, 9894–9903. [CrossRef] [PubMed]
83. Sun, Y.; Qian, Z.; Wei, G. The Inhibitory Mechanism of a Fullerene Derivative against Amyloid-Beta Peptide Aggregation: An Atomistic Simulation Study. *Phys. Chem. Chem. Phys.* **2016**, *18*, 12582–12591. [CrossRef] [PubMed]
84. Xie, L.; Luo, Y.; Lin, D.; Xi, W.; Yang, X.; Wei, G. The Molecular Mechanism of Fullerene-Inhibited Aggregation of Alzheimer's Β-Amyloid Peptide Fragment. *Nanoscale* **2014**, *6*, 9752–9762. [CrossRef] [PubMed]
85. Kim, J.E.; Lee, M. Fullerene Inhibits Β-Amyloid Peptide Aggregation. *Biochem. Biophys. Res. Commun.* **2003**, *303*, 576–579. [CrossRef]
86. Podolski, I.Y.; Podlubnaya, Z.A.; Kosenko, E.A.; Mugantseva, E.A.; Makarova, E.G.; Marsagishvili, L.G.; Shpagina, M.D.; Kaminsky, Y.G.; Andrievsky, G.V.; Klochkov, V.K. Effects of Hydrated Forms of C_{60} Fullerene on Amyloid Β-Peptide Fibrillization In Vitro and Performance of the Cognitive Task. *J. Nanosci. Nanotechnol.* **2007**, *7*, 1479–1485. [CrossRef]
87. Bobylev, A.G.; Kornev, A.B.; Bobyleva, L.G.; Shpagina, M.D.; Fadeeva, I.S.; Fadeev, R.S.; Deryabin, D.G.; Balzarini, J.; Troshin, P.A.; Podlubnaya, Z.A. Fullerenolates: Metallated Polyhydroxylated Fullerenes with Potent Anti-Amyloid Activity. *Org. Biomol. Chem.* **2011**, *9*, 5714–5719. [CrossRef]
88. Bednarikova, Z.; Huy, P.D.; Mocanu, M.M.; Fedunova, D.; Li, M.S.; Gazova, Z. Fullerenol $C_{60}(Oh)_{16}$ Prevents Amyloid Fibrillization of Aβ40-In Vitro and in Silico Approach. *Phys. Chem. Chem. Phys.* **2016**, *18*, 18855–18867. [CrossRef]
89. Melchor, M.-H.; Susana, F.-G.; Francisco, G.-S.; Hiram I, B.; Norma, R.-F.; Jorge A, L.-R.; Perla Y, L.-C.; Gustavo, B.-I. Fullerene-malonates Inhibit Amyloid Beta Aggregation, In Vitro and in Silico Evaluation. *RSC Adv.* **2018**, *8*, 39667–39677. [CrossRef]
90. Bobylev, A.G.; Kraevaya, O.A.; Bobyleva, L.G.; Khakina, E.A.; Fadeev, R.S.; Zhilenkov, A.V.; Mishchenko, D.V.; Penkov, N.V.; Teplov, I.Y.; Yakupova, E.I.; et al. Anti-amyloid Activities of Three Different Types of Water-Soluble Fullerene Derivatives. *Colloids Surf. B* **2019**, *183*, 110426. [CrossRef]
91. Prat, F.; Hou, C.-C.; Foote, C.S. Determination of the Quenching Rate Constants of Singlet Oxygen by Derivatized Nucleosides in Nonaqueous Solution. *J. Am. Chem. Soc.* **1997**, *119*, 5051–5052. [CrossRef]
92. Tanimoto, S.; Sakai, S.; Matsumura, S.; Takahashi, D.; Toshima, K. Target-Selective Photo-Degradation of Hiv-1 Protease by a Fullerene-Sugar Hybrid. *Chem. Commun.* **2008**, 5767–5769. [CrossRef] [PubMed]
93. Ishida, Y.; Tanimoto, S.; Takahashi, D.; Toshima, K. Photo-Degradation of Amyloid Β by a Designed Fullerene-Sugar Hybrid. *MedChemComm* **2010**, *1*, 212. [CrossRef]
94. Ishida, Y.; Fujii, T.; Oka, K.; Takahashi, D.; Toshima, K. Inhibition of Amyloi Β Aggregation and Cytotoxicity by Photodegradation Using a Designed Fullerene Derivative. *Chem. Asian J.* **2011**, *6*, 2312–2315. [CrossRef]
95. Du, Z.; Gao, N.; Wang, X.; Ren, J.; Qu, X. Near-Infrared Switchable Fullerene-Based Synergy Therapy for Alzheimer's Disease. *Small* **2018**, *14*, 1801852. [CrossRef]
96. Xu, X.; Ray, R.; Gu, Y.; Ploehn, H.J.; Gearheart, L.; Raker, K.; Scrivens, W.A. Electrophoretic Analysis and Purification of Fluorescent Single-Walled Carbon Nanotube Fragments. *J. Am. Chem. Soc.* **2004**, *126*, 12736–12737. [CrossRef]
97. Liu, Y.; Xu, L.P.; Dai, W.; Dong, H.; Wen, Y.; Zhang, X. Graphene Quantum Dots for the Inhibition of Β Amyloid Aggregation. *Nanoscale* **2015**, *7*, 19060–19065. [CrossRef]
98. Sun, D.; Zhang, W.; Yu, Q.; Chen, X.; Xu, M.; Zhou, Y.; Liu, J. Chiral Penicillamine-Modified Selenium Nanoparticles Enantioselectively Inhibit Metal-Induced Amyloid Beta Aggregation for Treating Alzheimer's Disease. *J. Colloid Interface Sci.* **2017**, *505*, 1001–1010. [CrossRef]
99. Malishev, R.; Arad, E.; Bhunia, S.K.; Shaham-Niv, S.; Kolusheva, S.; Gazit, E.; Jelinek, R. Chiral Modulation of Amyloid Beta Fibrillation and Cytotoxicity by Enantiomeric Carbon Dots. *Chem. Commun.* **2018**, *54*, 7762–7765. [CrossRef] [PubMed]
100. Xiao, S.; Zhou, D.; Luan, P.; Gu, B.; Feng, L.; Fan, S.; Liao, W.; Fang, W.; Yang, L.; Tao, E.; et al. Graphene Quantum Dots Conjugated Neuroprotective Peptide Improve Learning and Memory Capability. *Biomaterials* **2016**, *106*, 98–110. [CrossRef] [PubMed]
101. Gao, W.; Wang, W.; Dong, X.; Sun, Y. Nitrogen-Doped Carbonized Polymer Dots: A Potent Scavenger and Detector Targeting Alzheimer's Β-Amyloid Plaques. *Small* **2020**, *16*, e2002804. [CrossRef] [PubMed]
102. Chung, Y.J.; Kim, K.; Lee, B.I.; Park, C.B. Carbon Nanodot-Sensitized Modulation of Alzheimer's Β-Amyloid Self-Assembly, Disassembly, and Toxicity. *Small* **2017**, *13*, 1700983. [CrossRef] [PubMed]

103. Chung, Y.J.; Lee, C.H.; Lim, J.; Jang, J.; Kang, H.; Park, C.B. Photomodulating Carbon Dots for Spatiotemporal Suppression of Alzheimer's B-Amyloid Aggregation. *ACS Nano* **2020**, *14*, 16973–16983. [CrossRef]
104. Mahmoudi, M.; Quinlan-Pluck, F.; Monopoli, M.P.; Sheibani, S.; Vali, H.; Dawson, K.A.; Lynch, I. Influence of the Physiochemical Properties of Superparamagnetic Iron Oxide Nanoparticles on Amyloid Beta Protein Fibrillation in Solution. *ACS Chem. Neurosci.* **2013**, *4*, 475–485. [CrossRef] [PubMed]
105. Margel, S.; Skaat, H.; Corem-Salkmon, E.; Grinberg, I.; Last, D.; Goez, D.; Mardor, Y. Antibody-Conjugated, Dual-Modal, near-Infrared Fluorescent Iron Oxide Nanoparticles for Antiamyloidgenic Activity and Specific Detection of Amyloid-B Fibrils. *Int. J. Nanomed.* **2013**, *8*, 4063–4076. [CrossRef] [PubMed]
106. Skaat, H.; Shafir, G.; Margel, S. Acceleration and Inhibition of Amyloid-B Fibril Formation by Peptide-Conjugated Fluorescent-Maghemite Nanoparticles. *J. Nanopart. Res.* **2011**, *13*, 3521–3534. [CrossRef]
107. Halevas, E.; Mavroidi, B.; Nday, C.M.; Tang, J.; Smith, G.C.; Boukos, N.; Litsardakis, G.; Pelecanou, M.; Salifoglou, A. Modified Magnetic Core-Shell Mesoporous Silica Nano-Formulations with Encapsulated Quercetin Exhibit Anti-Amyloid and Antioxidant Activity. *J. Inorg. Biochem.* **2020**, *213*, 111271. [CrossRef]
108. Hirohata, M.; Hasegawa, K.; Tsutsumi-Yasuhara, S.; Ohhashi, Y.; Ookoshi, T.; Ono, K.; Yamada, M.; Naiki, H. The Anti-Amyloidogenic Effect Is Exerted against Alzheimer's Beta-Amyloid Fibrils In Vitro by Preferential and Reversible Binding of Flavonoids to the Amyloid Fibril Structure. *Biochemistry* **2007**, *46*, 1888–1899. [CrossRef]
109. Li, M.; Liu, Z.; Ren, J.; Qu, X. Inhibition of Metal-Induced Amyloid Aggregation Using Light-Responsive Magnetic Nanoparticle Prochelator Conjugates. *Chem. Sci.* **2012**, *3*, 868–873. [CrossRef]
110. Loynachan, C.N.; Romero, G.; Christiansen, M.G.; Chen, R.; Ellison, R.; O'Malley, T.T.; Froriep, U.P.; Walsh, D.M.; Anikeeva, P. Targeted Magnetic Nanoparticles for Remote Magnetothermal Disruption of Amyloid-B Aggregates. *Adv. Healthc. Mater.* **2015**, *4*, 2100–2109. [CrossRef]
111. Chen, R.; Romero, G.; Christiansen, M.G.; Mohr, A.; Anikeeva, P. Wireless Magnetothermal Deep Brain Stimulation. *Science* **2015**, *347*, 1477–1480. [CrossRef]
112. Riedinger, A.; Guardia, P.; Curcio, A.; Garcia, M.A.; Cingolani, R.; Manna, L.; Pellegrino, T. Subnanometer Local Temperature Probing and Remotely Controlled Drug Release Based on Azo-Functionalized Iron Oxide Nanoparticles. *Nano Lett.* **2013**, *13*, 2399–2406. [CrossRef]
113. Dyne, E.; Prakash, P.S.; Li, J.; Yu, B.; Schmidt, T.L.; Huang, S.; Kim, M.H. Mild Magnetic Nanoparticle Hyperthermia Promotes the Disaggregation and Microglia-Mediated Clearance of Beta-Amyloid Plaques. *Nanomedicine* **2021**, *34*, 102397. [CrossRef]
114. Du, Z.; Gao, N.; Guan, Y.; Ding, C.; Sun, Y.; Ren, J.; Qu, X. Rational Design of a "Sense and Treat" System to Target Amyloid Aggregates Related to Alzheimer's Disease. *Nano Res.* **2018**, *11*, 1987–1997. [CrossRef]
115. Rhule, J.T.; Hill, C.L.; Judd, D.A.; Schinazi, R.F. Polyoxometalates in Medicine. *Chem. Rev.* **1998**, *98*, 327–358. [CrossRef] [PubMed]
116. Judd, D.A.; Nettles, J.H.; Nevins, N.; Snyder, J.P.; Liotta, D.C.; Tang, J.; Ermolieff, J.; Schinazi, R.F.; Hill, C.L. Polyoxometalate Hiv-1 Protease Inhibitors. A New Mode of Protease Inhibition. *J. Am. Chem. Soc.* **2001**, *123*, 886–897. [CrossRef]
117. Geng, J.; Li, M.; Ren, J.; Wang, E.; Qu, X. Polyoxometalates as Inhibitors of the Aggregation of Amyloid Beta Peptides Associated with Alzheimer's Disease. *Angew. Chem. Int. Ed. Engl.* **2011**, *50*, 4184–4188. [CrossRef]
118. Zhou, Y.; Zheng, L.; Han, F.; Zhang, G.; Ma, Y.; Yao, J.; Keita, B.; de Oliveira, P.; Nadjo, L. Inhibition of Amyloid-B Protein Fibrillization Upon Interaction with Polyoxometalates Nanoclusters. *Colloids Surface A* **2011**, *375*, 97–101. [CrossRef]
119. Gao, N.; Sun, H.; Dong, K.; Ren, J.; Duan, T.; Xu, C.; Qu, X. Transition-Metal-Substituted Polyoxometalate Derivatives as Functional Anti-Amyloid Agents for Alzheimer's Disease. *Nat. Commun.* **2014**, *5*, 3422. [CrossRef]
120. Zhao, J.; Li, K.; Wan, K.; Sun, T.; Zheng, N.; Zhu, F.; Ma, J.; Jiao, J.; Li, T.; Ni, J.; et al. Organoplatinum-substituted polyoxometalate inhibits B-amyloid aggregation for Alzheimer's therapy. *Angew. Chem.* **2019**, *131*, 18200–18207. [CrossRef]
121. Chen, Q.; Yang, L.; Zheng, C.; Zheng, W.; Zhang, J.; Zhou, Y.; Liu, J. Mo Polyoxometalate Nanoclusters Capable of Inhibiting the Aggregation of Aβ-Peptide Associated with Alzheimer's Disease. *Nanoscale* **2014**, *6*, 6886–6897. [CrossRef]
122. Bernardini, G.; Wedd, A.G.; Zhao, C.; Bond, A.M. Photochemical Oxidation of Water and Reduction of Polyoxometalate Anions at Interfaces of Water with Ionic Liquids or Diethylether. *Proc. Natl. Acad. Sci. USA* **2012**, *109*, 11552–11557. [CrossRef]
123. Bonchio, M.; Carraro, M.; Conte, V.; Scorrano, G. Aerobic Photooxidation in Water by Polyoxotungstates: The Case of Uracil. *Eur. J. Org. Chem.* **2005**, *2005*, 4897–4903. [CrossRef]
124. Li, M.; Xu, C.; Ren, J.; Wang, E.; Qu, X. Photodegradation of Beta-Sheet Amyloid Fibrils Associated with Alzheimer's Disease by Using Polyoxometalates as Photocatalysts. *Chem. Commun.* **2013**, *49*, 11394–11396. [CrossRef]
125. Ma, M.; Gao, N.; Sun, Y.; Du, X.; Ren, J.; Qu, X. Redox-Activated near-Infrared-Responsive Polyoxometalates Used for Photothermal Treatment of Alzheimer's Disease. *Adv. Healthc. Mater.* **2018**, *7*, e1800320. [CrossRef] [PubMed]
126. Li, M.; Xu, C.; Wu, L.; Ren, J.; Wang, E.; Qu, X. Self-Assembled Peptide-Polyoxometalate Hybrid Nanospheres: Two in One Enhances Targeted Inhibition of Amyloid Beta-Peptide Aggregation Associated with Alzheimer's Disease. *Small* **2013**, *9*, 3455–3461. [CrossRef]
127. Gao, N.; Sun, H.; Dong, K.; Ren, J.; Qu, X. Gold-Nanoparticle-Based Multifunctional Amyloid-B Inhibitor against Alzheimer's Disease. *Chem. Eur. J.* **2015**, *21*, 829–835. [CrossRef]
128. Li, M.; Guan, Y.; Zhao, A.; Ren, J.; Qu, X. Using Multifunctional Peptide Conjugated Au Nanorods for Monitoring Beta-Amyloid Aggregation and Chemo-Photothermal Treatment of Alzheimer's Disease. *Theranostics* **2017**, *7*, 2996–3006. [CrossRef]

129. Xu, C.; Qu, X. Cerium Oxide Nanoparticle: A Remarkably Versatile Rare Earth Nanomaterial for Biological Applications. *NPG Asia Mater.* **2014**, *6*, e90. [CrossRef]
130. D'Angelo, B.; Santucci, S.; Benedetti, E.; Di Loreto, S.; Phani, R.; Falone, S.; Amicarelli, F.; Ceru, M.; Cimini, A. Cerium Oxide Nanoparticles Trigger Neuronal Survival in Ahuman Alzheimer Disease Model by Modulating Bdnf Pathway. *Curr. Nanosci.* **2009**, *5*, 167–176. [CrossRef]
131. Dowding, J.M.; Song, W.; Bossy, K.; Karakoti, A.; Kumar, A.; Kim, A.; Bossy, B.; Seal, S.; Ellisman, M.H.; Perkins, G.; et al. Cerium Oxide Nanoparticles Protect against Aβ-Induced Mitochondrial Fragmentation and Neuronal Cell Death. *Cell Death Differ.* **2014**, *21*, 1622–1632. [CrossRef]
132. Li, M.; Shi, P.; Xu, C.; Ren, J.; Qu, X. Cerium Oxide Caged Metal Chelator: Anti-Aggregation and Anti-Oxidation Integrated H_2O_2-Responsive Controlled Drug Release for Potential Alzheimer's Disease Treatment. *Chem. Sci.* **2013**, *4*, 2536–2542. [CrossRef]
133. Guan, Y.; Gao, N.; Ren, J.; Qu, X. Rationally Designed Cenp@Mnmos4 Core-Shell Nanoparticles for Modulating Multiple Facets of Alzheimer's Disease. *Chem. Eur. J.* **2016**, *22*, 14523–14526. [CrossRef]
134. Absillis, G.; Parac-Vogt, T.N. Peptide Bond Hydrolysis Catalyzed by the Wells-Dawson $Zr(A_2-P_2W_{17}O_{61})_2$ Polyoxometalate. *Inorg. Chem.* **2012**, *51*, 9902–9910. [CrossRef]
135. Guan, Y.; Li, M.; Dong, K.; Gao, N.; Ren, J.; Zheng, Y.; Qu, X. Ceria/Poms Hybrid Nanoparticles as a Mimicking Metallopeptidase for Treatment of Neurotoxicity of Amyloid-B Peptide. *Biomaterials* **2016**, *98*, 92–102. [CrossRef] [PubMed]
136. Kim, D.; Kwon, H.J.; Hyeon, T. Magnetite/Ceria Nanoparticle Assemblies for Extracorporeal Cleansing of Amyloid-B in Alzheimer's Disease. *Adv. Mater.* **2019**, *31*, e1807965. [CrossRef] [PubMed]
137. Lim, Y.J.; Zhou, W.H.; Li, G.; Hu, Z.W.; Hong, L.; Yu, X.F.; Li, Y.M. Black Phosphorus Nanomaterials Regulate the Aggregation of Amyloid-B. *ChemNanoMat* **2019**, *5*, 606–611. [CrossRef]
138. Yang, J.; Liu, W.; Sun, Y.; Dong, X. Lvffark-Peg-Stabilized Black Phosphorus Nanosheets Potently Inhibit Amyloid-B Fibrillogenesis. *Langmuir* **2020**, *36*, 1804–1812. [CrossRef]
139. Wang, H.; Yang, X.; Shao, W.; Chen, S.; Xie, J.; Zhang, X.; Wang, J.; Xie, Y. Ultrathin Black Phosphorus Nanosheets for Efficient Singlet Oxygen Generation. *J. Am. Chem. Soc.* **2015**, *137*, 11376–11382. [CrossRef]
140. Sun, Z.; Xie, H.; Tang, S.; Yu, X.-F.; Guo, Z.; Shao, J.; Zhang, H.; Huang, H.; Wang, H.; Chu, P.K. Ultrasmall Black Phosphorus Quantum Dots: Synthesis and Use as Photothermal Agents. *Angew. Chem.* **2015**, *127*, 11688–11692. [CrossRef]
141. Sun, C.; Wen, L.; Zeng, J.; Wang, Y.; Sun, Q.; Deng, L.; Zhao, C.; Li, Z. One-Pot Solventless Preparation of Pegylated Black Phosphorus Nanoparticles for Photoacoustic Imaging and Photothermal Therapy of Cancer. *Biomaterials* **2016**, *91*, 81–89. [CrossRef]
142. Chen, W.; Ouyang, J.; Liu, H.; Chen, M.; Zeng, K.; Sheng, J.; Liu, Z.; Han, Y.; Wang, L.; Li, J.; et al. Black Phosphorus Nanosheet-Based Drug Delivery System for Synergistic Photodynamic/Photothermal/Chemotherapy of Cancer. *Adv. Mater.* **2017**, *29*, 1603864. [CrossRef]
143. Li, Y.; Du, Z.; Liu, X.; Ma, M.; Yu, D.; Lu, Y.; Ren, J.; Qu, X. Near-Infrared Activated Black Phosphorus as a Nontoxic Photo-Oxidant for Alzheimer's Amyloid-B Peptide. *Small* **2019**, *15*, 1901116. [CrossRef]
144. Mudedla, S.K.; Murugan, N.A.; Subramanian, V.; Agren, H. Destabilization of Amyloid Fibrils on Interaction with Mos2-Based Nanomaterials. *RSC Adv.* **2019**, *9*, 1613–1624. [CrossRef]
145. Wang, J.; Liu, L.; Ge, D.; Zhang, H.; Feng, Y.; Zhang, Y.; Chen, M.; Dong, M. Differential Modulating Effect of Mos2 on Amyloid Peptide Assemblies. *Chem. Eur. J.* **2018**, *24*, 3397–3402. [CrossRef]
146. Liu, Y.; Zheng, Y.; Li, S.; Li, J.; Du, X.; Ma, Y.; Liao, G.; Wang, Q.; Yang, X.; Wang, K. Contradictory Effect of Gold Nanoparticle-Decorated Molybdenum Sulfide Nanocomposites on Amyloid-B-40 Aggregation. *Chin. Chem. Lett.* **2020**, *31*, 3113–3116. [CrossRef]
147. Chou, S.S.; Kaehr, B.; Kim, J.; Foley, B.M.; De, M.; Hopkins, P.E.; Huang, J.; Brinker, C.J.; Dravid, V.P. Chemically Exfoliated Mos2 as near-Infrared Photothermal Agents. *Angew. Chem. Int. Ed. Engl.* **2013**, *52*, 4160–4164. [CrossRef]
148. Li, M.; Zhao, A.; Dong, K.; Li, W.; Ren, J.; Qu, X. Chemically Exfoliated Ws2 Nanosheets Efficiently Inhibit Amyloid B-Peptide Aggregation and Can Be Used for Photothermal Treatment of Alzheimer's Disease. *Nano Res.* **2015**, *8*, 3216–3227. [CrossRef]
149. Wang, X.; Han, Q.; Liu, X.; Wang, C.; Yang, R. Multifunctional Inhibitors of B-Amyloid Aggregation Based on Mos2/Aunr Nanocomposites with High near-Infrared Absorption. *Nanoscale* **2019**, *11*, 9185–9193. [CrossRef]
150. Suh, J.; Yoo, S.H.; Kim, M.G.; Jeong, K.; Ahn, J.Y.; Kim, M.-s.; Chae, P.S.; Lee, T.Y.; Lee, J.; Lee, J.; et al. Cleavage Agents for Soluble Oligomers of Amyloid B Peptides. *Angew. Chem.* **2007**, *119*, 7194–7197. [CrossRef]
151. Derrick, J.S.; Lee, J.; Lee, S.J.; Kim, Y.; Nam, E.; Tak, H.; Kang, J.; Lee, M.; Kim, S.H.; Park, K.; et al. Mechanistic Insights into Tunable Metal-Mediated Hydrolysis of Amyloid-B Peptides. *J. Am. Chem. Soc.* **2017**, *139*, 2234–2244. [CrossRef]
152. Ma, M.; Wang, Y.; Gao, N.; Liu, X.; Sun, Y.; Ren, J.; Qu, X. A near-Infrared-Controllable Artificial Metalloprotease Used for Degrading Amyloid-B Monomers and Aggregates. *Chem. Eur. J.* **2019**, *25*, 11852–11858. [CrossRef] [PubMed]
153. Han, Q.; Cai, S.; Yang, L.; Wang, X.; Qi, C.; Yang, R.; Wang, C. Molybdenum Disulfide Nanoparticles as Multifunctional Inhibitors against Alzheimer's Disease. *ACS Appl. Mater. Inter.* **2017**, *9*, 21116–21123. [CrossRef]
154. Chung, Y.J.; Lee, B.I.; Ko, J.W.; Park, C.B. Photoactive G-C_3N_4 Nanosheets for Light-Induced Suppression of Alzheimer's B-Amyloid Aggregation and Toxicity. *Adv. Healthc. Mater.* **2016**, *5*, 1560–1565. [CrossRef]
155. Wang, J.; Zhang, Z.; Zhang, H.; Li, C.; Chen, M.; Liu, L.; Dong, M. Enhanced Photoresponsive Graphene Oxide-Modified G-C_3N_4 for Disassembly of Amyloid B Fibrils. *ACS Appl. Mater. Inter.* **2019**, *11*, 96–103. [CrossRef]

156. Wang, J.; Feng, Y.; Tian, X.; Li, C.; Liu, L. Disassembling and Degradation of Amyloid Protein Aggregates Based on Gold Nanoparticle-Modified G-C$_3$n$_4$. *Colloids Surf. B* **2020**, *192*, 111051. [CrossRef]
157. Li, M.; Guan, Y.; Ding, C.; Chen, Z.; Ren, J.; Qu, X. An Ultrathin Graphitic Carbon Nitride Nanosheet: A Novel Inhibitor of Metal-Induced Amyloid Aggregation Associated with Alzheimer's Disease. *J. Mater. Chem. B* **2016**, *4*, 4072–4075. [CrossRef]
158. Li, M.; Guan, Y.; Chen, Z.; Gao, N.; Ren, J.; Dong, K.; Qu, X. Platinum-Coordinated Graphitic Carbon Nitride Nanosheet Used for Targeted Inhibition of Amyloid B-Peptide Aggregation. *Nano Res.* **2016**, *9*, 2411–2423. [CrossRef]
159. Gong, L.; Zhang, X.; Ge, K.; Yin, Y.; Machuki, J.O.; Yang, Y.; Shi, H.; Geng, D.; Gao, F. Carbon Nitride-Based Nanocaptor: An Intelligent Nanosystem with Metal Ions Chelating Effect for Enhanced Magnetic Targeting Phototherapy of Alzheimer's Disease. *Biomaterials* **2021**, *267*, 120483. [CrossRef] [PubMed]
160. Wang, J.; Fan, Y.; Tan, Y.; Zhao, X.; Zhang, Y.; Cheng, C.; Yang, M. Porphyrinic Metal-Organic Framework Pcn-224 Nanoparticles for near-Infrared-Induced Attenuation of Aggregation and Neurotoxicity of Alzheimer's Amyloid-Beta Peptide. *ACS Appl. Mater. Inter.* **2018**, *10*, 36615–36621. [CrossRef] [PubMed]
161. Chen, Y.-Z.; Jiang, H.-L. Porphyrinic Metal-Organic Framework Catalyzed Heck-Reaction: Fluorescence "Turn-on" Sensing of Cu(Ii) Ion. *Chem. Mater.* **2016**, *28*, 6698–6704. [CrossRef]
162. Yu, D.; Guan, Y.; Bai, F.; Du, Z.; Gao, N.; Ren, J.; Qu, X. Metal-Organic Frameworks Harness Cu Chelating and Photooxidation against Amyloid B Aggregation in Vivo. *Chem. Eur. J.* **2019**, *25*, 3489–3495. [CrossRef] [PubMed]
163. Kowalczyk, J.; Grapsi, E.; Espargaro, A.; Caballero, A.B.; Juarez-Jimenez, J.; Busquets, M.A.; Gamez, P.; Sabate, R.; Estelrich, J. Dual Effect of Prussian Blue Nanoparticles on Aβ$_{40}$ Aggregation: B-Sheet Fibril Reduction and Copper Dyshomeostasis Regulation. *Biomacromolecules* **2021**, *22*, 430–440. [CrossRef] [PubMed]
164. Prabhu, M.P.T.; Sarkar, N. Quantum Dots as Promising Theranostic Tools Againstamyloidosis:A Review. *Protein Pept. Lett.* **2019**, *26*, 555–563. [CrossRef] [PubMed]
165. Xiao, L.; Zhao, D.; Chan, W.H.; Choi, M.M.; Li, H.W. Inhibition of Beta 1-40 Amyloid Fibrillation with N-Acetyl-L-Cysteine Capped Quantum Dots. *Biomaterials* **2010**, *31*, 91–98. [CrossRef] [PubMed]
166. Ng, O.T.W.; Wong, Y.; Chan, H.M.; Cheng, J.; Qi, X.; Chan, W.H.; Yung, K.K.L.; Li, H.W. N-Acetyl-L-Cysteine Capped Quantum Dots Offer Neuronal Cell Protection by Inhibiting Beta(1-40) Amyloid Fibrillation. *Biomater. Sci.* **2013**, *1*, 577–580. [CrossRef]
167. Thakur, G.; Micic, M.; Yang, Y.; Li, W.; Movia, D.; Giordani, S.; Zhang, H.; Leblanc, R.M. Conjugated Quantum Dots Inhibit the Amyloid B (1-42) Fibrillation Process. *Int. J. Alzheimers Dis.* **2011**, *2011*, 502386. [CrossRef] [PubMed]
168. Del Mar Martinez-Senac, M.; Villalain, J.; Gomez-Fernandez, J.C. Structure of the Alzheimer B-Amyloid Peptide (25-35) and Its Interaction with Negatively Charged Phospholipid Vesicles. *Eur. J. Biochem.* **1999**, *265*, 744–753. [CrossRef]
169. Sabaté, R.; Gallardo, M.; Estelrich, J. Spontaneous Incorporation of B-Amyloid Peptide into Neutral Liposomes. *Colloids Surface A* **2005**, *270-271*, 13–17. [CrossRef]
170. Terakawa, M.S.; Yagi, H.; Adachi, M.; Lee, Y.H.; Goto, Y. Small Liposomes Accelerate the Fibrillation of Amyloid B(1-40). *J. Biol. Chem.* **2015**, *290*, 815–826. [CrossRef]
171. Shimanouchi, T.; Onishi, R.; Kitaura, N.; Umakoshi, H.; Kuboi, R. Copper-Mediated Growth of Amyloid Beta Fibrils in the Presence of Oxidized and Negatively Charged Liposomes. *J. Biosci. Bioeng.* **2011**, *112*, 611–615. [CrossRef]
172. Tanifum, E.A.; Dasgupta, I.; Srivastava, M.; Bhavane, R.C.; Sun, L.; Berridge, J.; Pourgarzham, H.; Kamath, R.; Espinosa, G.; Cook, S.C.; et al. Intravenous Delivery of Targeted Liposomes to Amyloid-Beta Pathology in App/Psen1 Transgenic Mice. *PLoS ONE* **2012**, *7*, e48515. [CrossRef]
173. Airoldi, C.; Mourtas, S.; Cardona, F.; Zona, C.; Sironi, E.; D'Orazio, G.; Markoutsa, E.; Nicotra, F.; Antimisiaris, S.G.; La Ferla, B. Nanoliposomes Presenting on Surface a Cis-Glycofused Benzopyran Compound Display Binding Affinity and Aggregation Inhibition Ability Towards Amyloid B1-42 Peptide. *Eur. J. Med. Chem.* **2014**, *85*, 43–50. [CrossRef]
174. Carlred, L.; Gunnarsson, A.; Sole-Domenech, S.; Johansson, B.; Vukojevic, V.; Terenius, L.; Codita, A.; Winblad, B.; Schalling, M.; Hook, F.; et al. Simultaneous Imaging of Amyloid-Beta and Lipids in Brain Tissue Using Antibody-Coupled Liposomes and Time-of-Flight Secondary Ion Mass Spectrometry. *J. Am. Chem. Soc.* **2014**, *136*, 9973–9981. [CrossRef]
175. Gobbi, M.; Re, F.; Canovi, M.; Beeg, M.; Gregori, M.; Sesana, S.; Sonnino, S.; Brogioli, D.; Musicanti, C.; Gasco, P.; et al. Lipid-Based Nanoparticles with High Binding Affinity for Amyloid-B$_{1-42}$ Peptide. *Biomaterials* **2010**, *31*, 6519–6529. [CrossRef]
176. Bereczki, E.; Re, F.; Masserini, M.E.; Winblad, B.; Pei, J.J. Liposomes Functionalized with Acidic Lipids Rescue Aβ-Induced Toxicity in Murine Neuroblastoma Cells. *Nanomedicine* **2011**, *7*, 560–571. [CrossRef]
177. Mourtas, S.; Canovi, M.; Zona, C.; Aurilia, D.; Niarakis, A.; La Ferla, B.; Salmona, M.; Nicotra, F.; Gobbi, M.; Antimisiaris, S.G. Curcumin-Decorated Nanoliposomes with Very High Affinity for Amyloid-B1-42 Peptide. *Biomaterials* **2011**, *32*, 1635–1645. [CrossRef] [PubMed]
178. Taylor, M.; Moore, S.; Mourtas, S.; Niarakis, A.; Re, F.; Zona, C.; La Ferla, B.; Nicotra, F.; Masserini, M.; Antimisiaris, S.G.; et al. Effect of Curcumin-Associated and Lipid Ligand-Functionalized Nanoliposomes on Aggregation of the Alzheimer's Aβ Peptide. *Nanomedicine* **2011**, *7*, 541–550. [CrossRef] [PubMed]
179. Canovi, M.; Markoutsa, E.; Lazar, A.N.; Pampalakis, G.; Clemente, C.; Re, F.; Sesana, S.; Masserini, M.; Salmona, M.; Duyckaerts, C.; et al. The Binding Affinity of Anti-Aβ$_{1-42}$ Mab-Decorated Nanoliposomes to Aβ$_{1-42}$ Peptides In Vitro and to Amyloid Deposits in Post-Mortem Tissue. *Biomaterials* **2011**, *32*, 5489–5497. [CrossRef] [PubMed]

180. Re, F.; Cambianica, I.; Sesana, S.; Salvati, E.; Cagnotto, A.; Salmona, M.; Couraud, P.O.; Moghimi, S.M.; Masserini, M.; Sancini, G. Functionalization with Apoe-Derived Peptides Enhances the Interaction with Brain Capillary Endothelial Cells of Nanoliposomes Binding Amyloid-Beta Peptide. *J. Biotechnol.* **2011**, *156*, 341–346. [CrossRef]
181. Salvati, E.; Re, F.; Sesana, S.; Cambianica, I.; Sancini, G.; Masserini, M.; Gregori, M. Liposomes Functionalized to Overcome the Blood-Brain Barrier and to Target Amyloid-Beta Peptide: The Chemical Design Affects the Permeability across an In Vitro Model. *Int. J. Nanomed.* **2013**, *8*, 1749–1758. [CrossRef]
182. Mourtas, S.; Lazar, A.N.; Markoutsa, E.; Duyckaerts, C.; Antimisiaris, S.G. Multifunctional Nanoliposomes with Curcumin-Lipid Derivative and Brain Targeting Functionality with Potential Applications for Alzheimer Disease. *Eur. J. Med. Chem.* **2014**, *80*, 175–183. [CrossRef]
183. Bana, L.; Minniti, S.; Salvati, E.; Sesana, S.; Zambelli, V.; Cagnotto, A.; Orlando, A.; Cazzaniga, E.; Zwart, R.; Scheper, W.; et al. Liposomes Bi-Functionalized with Phosphatidic Acid and an Apoe-Derived Peptide Affect Abeta Aggregation Features and Cross the Blood-Brain-Barrier: Implications for Therapy of Alzheimer Disease. *Nanomedicine* **2014**, *10*, 1583–1590. [CrossRef]
184. Balducci, C.; Mancini, S.; Minniti, S.; La Vitola, P.; Zotti, M.; Sancini, G.; Mauri, M.; Cagnotto, A.; Colombo, L.; Fiordaliso, F.; et al. Multifunctional Liposomes Reduce Brain B-Amyloid Burden and Ameliorate Memory Impairment in Alzheimer's Disease Mouse Models. *J. Neurosci.* **2014**, *34*, 14022–14031. [CrossRef]
185. Cabaleiro-Lago, C.; Quinlan-Pluck, F.; Lynch, I.; Lindman, S.; Minogue, A.M.; Thulin, E.; Walsh, D.M.; Dawson, K.A.; Linse, S. Inhibition of Amyloid Beta Protein Fibrillation by Polymeric Nanoparticles. *J. Am. Chem. Soc.* **2008**, *130*, 15437–15443. [CrossRef]
186. Cabaleiro-Lago, C.; Quinlan-Pluck, F.; Lynch, I.; Dawson, K.A.; Linse, S. Dual Effect of Amino Modified Polystyrene Nanoparticles on Amyloid Beta Protein Fibrillation. *ACS Chem. Neurosci.* **2010**, *1*, 279–287. [CrossRef]
187. Jha, A.; Ghormade, V.; Kolge, H.; Paknikar, K.M. Dual Effect of Chitosan-Based Nanoparticles on the Inhibition of B-Amyloid Peptide Aggregation and Disintegration of the Preformed Fibrils. *J. Mater. Chem. B* **2019**, *7*, 3362–3373. [CrossRef]
188. Ye, Z.; Wei, L.; Li, Y.; Xiao, L. Efficient Modulation of B-Amyloid Peptide Fibrillation with Polymer Nanoparticles Revealed by Super-Resolution Optical Microscopy. *Anal. Chem.* **2019**, *91*, 8582–8590. [CrossRef]
189. Xu, Y.; Xiao, L. Efficient Suppression of Amyloid-Beta Peptide Aggregation and Cytotoxicity with Photosensitive Polymer Nanodots. *J. Mater. Chem. B* **2020**, *8*, 5776–5782. [CrossRef]
190. Dou, W.T.; Lv, Y.; Tan, C.; Chen, G.R.; He, X.P. Irreversible Destruction of Amyloid Fibril Plaques by Conjugated Polymer Based Fluorogenic Nanogrenades. *J. Mater. Chem. B* **2016**, *4*, 4502–4506. [CrossRef]
191. Lai, Y.; Zhu, Y.; Xu, Z.; Hu, X.; Saeed, M.; Yu, H.; Chen, X.; Liu, J.; Zhang, W. Engineering Versatile Nanoparticles for near-Infrared Light-Tunable Drug Release and Photothermal Degradation of Amyloid B. *Adv. Funct. Mater.* **2020**, *30*, 1908473. [CrossRef]
192. Liu, L.; Chang, Y.; Yu, J.; Jiang, M.; Xia, N. Two-in-One Polydopamine Nanospheres for Fluorescent Determination of Beta-Amyloid Oligomers and Inhibition of Beta-Amyloid Aggregation. *Sensor. Actuat. B-Chem.* **2017**, *251*, 359–365. [CrossRef]
193. Liu, Z.; Ma, M.; Yu, D.; Ren, J.; Qu, X. Target-Driven Supramolecular Self-Assembly for Selective Amyloid-B Photooxygenation against Alzheimer's Disease. *Chem. Sci.* **2020**, *11*, 11003–11008. [CrossRef]
194. Kuk, S.; Lee, B.I.; Lee, J.S.; Park, C.B. Rattle-Structured Upconversion Nanoparticles for near-Ir-Induced Suppression of Alzheimer's B-Amyloid Aggregation. *Small* **2017**, *13*, 1603139. [CrossRef]
195. Ma, M.; Gao, N.; Sun, Y.; Ren, J.; Qu, X. A near-Infrared Responsive Drug Sequential Release System for Better Eradicating Amyloid Aggregates. *Small* **2017**, *13*, 1701817. [CrossRef]
196. Zhang, H.; Hao, C.; Qu, A.; Sun, M.; Xu, L.; Xu, C.; Kuang, H. Light-Induced Chiral Iron Copper Selenide Nanoparticles Prevent B-Amyloidopathy in Vivo. *Angew. Chem. Int. Ed. Engl.* **2020**, *59*, 7131–7138. [CrossRef]
197. Sun, J.; Xie, W.; Zhu, X.; Xu, M.; Liu, J. Sulfur Nanoparticles with Novel Morphologies Coupled with Brain-Targeting Peptides Rvg as a New Type of Inhibitor against Metal-Induced Aβ Aggregation. *ACS Chem. Neurosci.* **2018**, *9*, 749–761. [CrossRef]
198. Huang, K.; Li, Z.; Lin, J.; Han, G.; Huang, P. Two-Dimensional Transition Metal Carbides and Nitrides (Mxenes) for Biomedical Applications. *Chem. Soc. Rev.* **2018**, *47*, 5109–5124. [CrossRef]

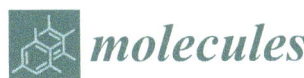

Article

Endosomal pH-Responsive Fe-Based Hyaluronate Nanoparticles for Doxorubicin Delivery

Yangmun Bae [1,†], Yoonyoung Kim [1,†] and Eun Seong Lee [1,2,*]

1. Department of Biotechnology, The Catholic University of Korea, 43 Jibong-ro, Bucheon-si 14662, Gyeonggi-do, Korea; beebe1@naver.com (Y.B.); rladbsdud727@naver.com (Y.K.)
2. Department of Biomedical-Chemical Engineering, The Catholic University of Korea, 43 Jibong-ro, Bucheon-si 14662, Gyeonggi-do, Korea
* Correspondence: eslee@catholic.ac.kr; Tel.: +82-2-2164-4921
† These authors contributed equally to this paper.

Abstract: In this study, we report pH-responsive metal-based biopolymer nanoparticles (NPs) for tumor-specific chemotherapy. Here, aminated hyaluronic acid (aHA) coupled with 2,3-dimethylmaleic anhydride (DMA, as a pH-responsive moiety) (aHA-DMA) was electrostatically complexed with ferrous chloride tetrahydrate ($FeCl_2/4H_2O$, as a chelating metal) and doxorubicin (DOX, as an antitumor drug model), producing DOX-loaded Fe-based hyaluronate nanoparticles (DOX@aHA-DMA/Fe NPs). Importantly, the DOX@aHA-DMA/Fe NPs improved tumor cellular uptake due to HA-mediated endocytosis for tumor cells overexpressing CD44 receptors. As a result, the average fluorescent DOX intensity observed in MDA-MB-231 cells (with CD44 receptors) was ~7.9 × 10^2 (DOX@HA/Fe NPs, without DMA), ~8.1 × 10^2 (DOX@aHA-$DMA_{0.36}$/Fe NPs), and ~9.3 × 10^2 (DOX@aHA-$DMA_{0.60}$/Fe NPs). Furthermore, the DOX@aHA-DMA/Fe NPs were destabilized due to ionic repulsion between Fe^{2+} and DMA-detached aHA (i.e., positively charged free aHA) in the acidic environment of tumor cells. This event accelerated the release of DOX from the destabilized NPs. Our results suggest that these NPs can be promising tumor-targeting drug carriers responding to acidic endosomal pH.

Keywords: Fe-based nanoparticles; endosomal pH-responsive hyaluronate; CD44 receptor-mediated endocytosis; tumor therapy

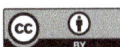

1. Introduction

Recently, the biological or physical properties of metal molecules have inspired the development of various bioactive nanoparticles (e.g., bacteria-killing nanoparticles and tumor-targeting nanoparticles) [1,2] and the development of simple biomimetic particles. In particular, metal-containing biopolymer nanocomposites have been actively designed for engineering multifunctional drug carriers with specific biological functions and tunable hyperstructures [1–3]. For example, the complexation of Fe and biopolymers is an effective and simple approach to fabricate biocompatible nanosized drug carriers in that Fe is an element present in living organisms and can be used as a chelating agent for negatively charged biopolymers [4–7]. Moreover, Fe-based nanocomposites are easy to control in terms of their composition, shape, size, and surface characteristics as a result of different mixing ratios and biopolymer types [4–7]. It is also interesting to note that the combination of biopolymers reactive to specific stimuli (light, temperature, pH, etc.) and Fe can contribute to the development of stimuli-responsive drug delivery systems [4–9].

In this study, we synthesized the aminated hyaluronic acid (aHA) coupled with 2,3-dimethylmaleic anhydride (aHA-DMA), which can target tumor cells with CD44 receptors and is responsive to acidic endosomal pH [10–13]. Furthermore, we could prepare acidic pH-responsive Fe-based hyaluronate nanoparticles using aHA-DMA, ferrous chloride tetrahydrate ($FeCl_2/4H_2O$) [5,9,12], and doxorubicin (DOX, as an antitumor drug model).

It is important that the DMA moiety present in aHA-DMA can be detached from aHA resulting from hydrolysis of DMA at a weakly acidic pH [10,12,14], resulting in the production of positively charged aHA. We expect that our NPs have low cytotoxicity because of the use of biodegradable/biocompatible components (HA and Fe) [12,13,15,16] and exhibit fascinating biological/physicochemical functionality in tumor environments as a result of HA-mediated specific binding to the CD44 receptors of tumor cells and DMA-mediated reactivity to acidic endosomal pH [11,14,15,17–21], resulting in improved antitumor activity (Figure 1a). In this study, we focused not only on the development of Fe-based NPs that have a specific binding ability [11,15] to tumor cells and reactivity to acidic endosomal pH but also on the analysis of the physicochemical properties of NPs.

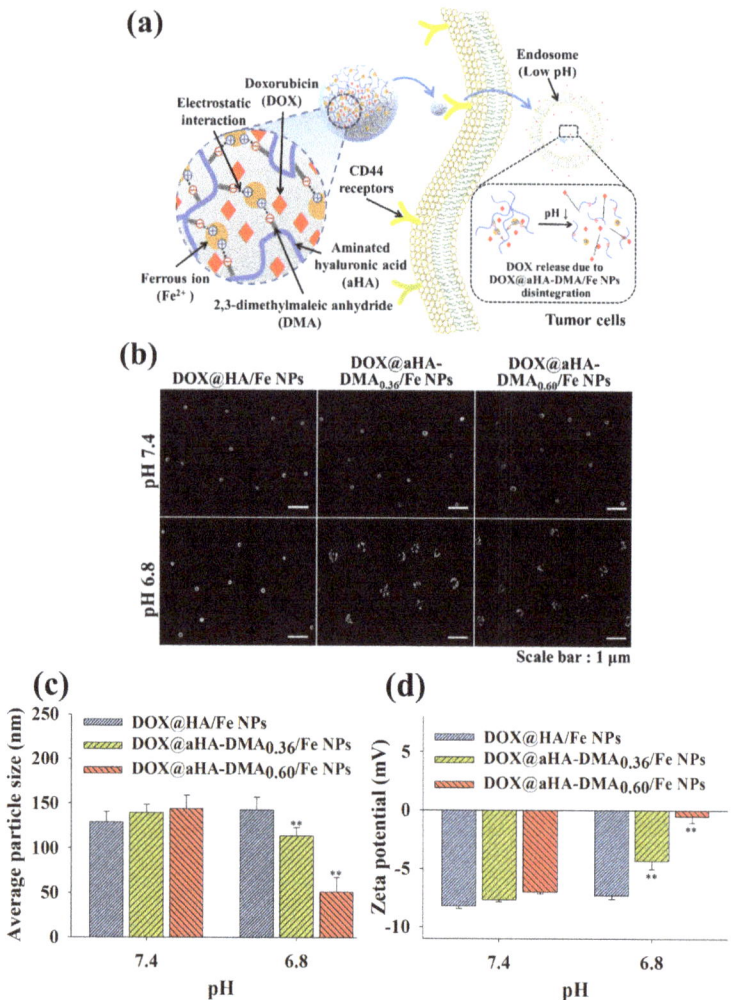

Figure 1. (a) Schematic illustration of DOX@aHA-DMA/Fe NPs. (b) FE-SEM images of DOX@HA/Fe NPs, DOX@aHA-DMA$_{0.36}$/Fe NPs, and DOX@aHA-DMA$_{0.60}$/Fe NPs at pH 7.4 or 6.8. (c) Average particle size and (d) zeta potential values of DOX@HA/Fe NPs, DOX@aHA-DMA$_{0.36}$/Fe NPs, and DOX@aHA-DMA$_{0.60}$/Fe NPs at pH 7.4 or 6.8 (n = 3, as multiple experiments; ** p < 0.01 compared to DOX@HA/Fe NPs).

2. Materials and Methods

2.1. Materials

Hyaluronic acid (HA, M_w = 4.8 kDa), adipic acid dihydrazide (ADH), N,N'-dicyclohexylcarbodiimide (DCC), N-hydroxysuccinimide (NHS), dimethyl sulfoxide (DMSO), triethylamine (TEA), 2,3-dimethylmaleic anhydride (DMA), sodium hydroxide (NaOH), ferrous chloride tetrahydrate ($FeCl_2 \cdot 4H_2O$), doxorubicin hydrochloride (DOX), formaldehyde, and triton X-100 were purchased from Sigma-Aldrich (St. Louis, MO, USA). Phosphate buffered saline (PBS), Roswell Park Memorial Institute-1640 (RPMI-1640), fetal bovine serum (FBS), penicillin, streptomycin, trypsin, and ethylene diaminetetraacetic acid (EDTA) were purchased from Welgene Inc. (Seoul, Korea). Cell Counting Kit-8 (CCK-8) was purchased from Dojindo Molecular Technologies Inc. (Rockville, MD, USA).

2.2. Synthesis of DOX-Loaded Fe-Based HA NPs

HA (300 mg) was preactivated (i.e., aminated) with ADH (644 mg), DCC (770 mg), and NHS (434 mg) in DMSO (15 mL) containing TEA (1 mL) at 25 °C for 4 days. The resulting solution was dialyzed (Spectra/Por® MWCO 3.5 kDa) against fresh DMSO at 25 °C for 3 days and deionized water for 3 days to remove the unreacted chemicals [22]. The aminated HA powder (aHA, 100 mg) obtained through freeze-drying for 2 days was reacted with DMA (174 mg or 87 mg) in 0.1 M NaOH aqueous solution (10 mL, adjusted to pH 9.0 using 0.1 M HCl) for 3 days [10]. This solution was dialyzed using a preswollen dialysis membrane (Spectra/Por® MWCO 3.5 kDa; Spectrum Lab., Rancho Dominguez, CA, USA) against PBS (150 mM, pH 7.4) at 25 °C for 3 days and then lyophilized, producing aHA-$DMA_{0.60}$ or aHA-$DMA_{0.36}$; the numerals indicate the number of moles of DMA conjugated to 1 repeating unit of aHA (Figure S1).

Next, aHA-$DMA_{0.60}$ (200 mg) or aHA-$DMA_{0.36}$ (200 mg) was mixed with $FeCl_2 \cdot 4H_2O$ (47 mg) and DOX (40 mg) in 0.1 M NaOH aqueous solution (10 mL). The resulting solution was dialyzed using a preswollen dialysis membrane (Spectra/Por® MWCO 3.5 kDa) against PBS (150 mM, pH 7.4) for 3 days and then lyophilized [23–25], producing DOX-loaded Fe-based aHA-DMA NPs (DOX@aHA-$DMA_{0.60}$/Fe NPs and DOX@aHA-$DMA_{0.36}$/Fe NPs). In addition, HA (200 mg) was mixed with $FeCl_2 \cdot 4H_2O$ (47 mg) and DOX (40 mg) in 0.1 M NaOH aqueous solution (10 mL) for 3 days to prepare a pH-nonresponsive control group (DOX@HA/Fe NPs). The amount of DOX encapsulated in the NPs was calculated after measuring the fluorescence intensity (λ_{ex} of 470 nm and λ_{em} of 592 nm) of DOX remaining in the supernatant (obtained after the centrifugation of solution at 100,000 rpm for 15 min at 4 °C) using a fluorescence spectrophotometer (RF-5301PC, Shimadzu, Kyoto, Japan) [17,18]. The loading efficiency (%) of DOX in the NPs was calculated as the weight percentage of DOX in the NPs relative to the initial feeding amount of DOX. The loading content (%) of DOX in the NPs was calculated as the weight percentage of DOX encapsulated in the NPs [17,18].

2.3. Characterization of Fe-Based HA NPs

The surface morphology and particle size of the NPs were monitored using field emission scanning electron microscopy (FE-SEM, Hitach S-400, Nagano, Japan) [12,26]. Before testing, the NPs were stabilized in PBS (150 mM, pH 7.4 or 6.8) at 25 °C for 4 h and then lyophilized. The average particle size and zeta potentials of the NPs (0.1 mg/mL) in PBS (150 mM, pH 7.4 or 6.8) were measured using a Zetasizer 3000 instrument (Malvern Instruments, Malvern, UK) [27,28]. Prior to the experiments, the NPs were stabilized in PBS (150 mM, pH 7.4 or 6.8) at 25 °C for 24 h. In addition, the concentration of Fe in the NPs was measured using an inductively coupled plasma mass spectrometer (ICP-MS, Thermo Scientific Inc., Waltham, MA, USA) [29].

2.4. In Vitro DOX Release Behavior

To confirm the pH-dependent DOX release profiles of the NPs at pH 7.4 (i.e., normal body pH) or 6.8 (i.e., acidic endosomal pH), each NP (equivalent to DOX 10 µg/mL) in

1 mL of PBS (150 mM, pH 7.4 or 6.8) was added to a dialysis membrane tube (Spectra/Por® MWCO 50 kDa) and immersed in 15 mL of fresh PBS (150 mM, pH 7.4 or 6.8) [17,18,20,30]. The preswollen membrane tubes were placed in a water bath shaking incubator (100 rpm) at 37 °C. The aqueous solution outside of the dialysis tubes was extracted and changed to a fresh PBS at each time point [17,18,20,30]. The amount of DOX present in the extracted solution was determined by measuring the DOX fluorescence intensity (λ_{ex} of 470 nm, λ_{em} of 592 nm) using a fluorescence spectrophotometer (RF-5301, Shimadzu, Kyoto, Japan) [17,18].

2.5. Cell Culture

Human breast carcinoma MDA-MB-231 cells and human liver carcinoma Huh7 cells were purchased from the Korea Cell Line Bank (Seoul, Korea) and cultured in RPMI-1640 medium supplemented with 10% FBS and 1% penicillin-streptomycin. The cells were maintained in a humidified incubator with a 5% CO_2 atmosphere at 37 °C and then harvested via trypsinization using a trypsin/EDTA solution (0.25% (wt./vol.)/0.03% (wt./vol.)). The collected cells (1×10^6 cells/mL) were seeded into a 96-well culture plate and cultured in RPMI-1640 medium for 24 h [11,18–20,31,32].

2.6. In Vitro Cellular Uptake Experiments

The NPs (equivalent to DOX 10 µg/mL) or free DOX (10 µg/mL) suspended in an RPMI-1640 medium (pH 7.4 or 6.8) were incubated with MDA-MB-231 cells (CD44 receptor-positive cells) and Huh7 cells (CD44 receptor-negative cells) at 37 °C for 4 h. The treated cells were washed three times with fresh PBS (pH 7.4). The DOX fluorescence intensity (λ_{ex} of 470 nm and λ_{em} of 592 nm) of the treated cells was analyzed using a flow cytometer (FACS Calibur, Becton Dickinson, Franklin Lakes, NJ, USA) [11,17,31].

To visualize the cellular uptake of DOX, MDA-MB-231 cells and Huh7 cells treated with NPs (equivalent to DOX 10 µg/mL) at pH 7.4 or 6.8 for 4 h were fixed using a 3.7% (wt./vol.) formaldehyde solution and monitored using a visible and near-infrared (VNIR) hyperspectral camera (CytoViva, Auburn, AL, USA). The scanned area of the treated cells was merged with the collected spectral data to visualize the cellular uptake of fluorescent DOX in the cells [11,17].

2.7. In Vitro Cytotoxicity

The cells were incubated with NPs (equivalent to DOX 10 µg/mL) or free DOX (10 µg/mL) suspended in an RPMI-1640 medium (pH 7.4 or 6.8) at 37 °C for 4 h and then washed three times with fresh PBS (pH 7.4). The CCK-8 assay was used to evaluate the cell viability of cells treated with the NPs. In addition, the cells were incubated at 37 °C for 24 h with the NPs (1–200 µg/mL, without DOX) at pH 7.4 to evaluate the original toxicity of NPs [11,17].

2.8. Hemolysis Test

A hemolysis test was conducted using red blood cells (RBCs) collected from BALB/c mice (7-week-old female) to determine the endosomolytic activity of the NPs. The RBC solution (10^6 cells/mL, pH 7.4–6.0) was incubated with the NPs (30 µg/mL, without DOX) at 37 °C for 1 h. The solutions were centrifuged at 1500 rpm for 10 min at 4 °C, and the supernatant was collected. The light absorbance (LA) value of the supernatant was measured using a spectrophotometer at a wavelength of 541 nm. The 0% LA value (as a negative control) was acquired from a PBS-treated intact RBC solution and the 100% LA value (as a positive control) was obtained from a completely-lysed RBC solution using 2 wt.% Triton X-100. The hemolysis (%) of NPs was determined as the LA of the RBC solution treated with NPs against the control LA value [11,12,17,18].

2.9. Local Healing Assay

The culture dish containing MDA-MB-231 cells treated with NPs (equivalent to DOX 10 µg/mL) or free DOX (10 µg/mL) suspended in RPMI-1640 medium at 37 °C for 4 h was scraped with a 200 μL pipette tip and observed with a light microscope after 24 h to evaluate the cell migration (proliferation) activity of tumor cells [33].

2.10. Statistical Evaluation

All data were evaluated using Student's *t*-test or analysis of variance (ANOVA) at a significance level of $p < 0.01$ (**) [18–22,27–32].

3. Results and Discussion

3.1. Synthesis of DOX-Loaded Fe-Based HA NPs

To fabricate biofunctional DOX@aHA-DMA/Fe NPs, we first synthesized aHA-DMA using a biocompatible HA and a pH-responsive DMA. Briefly, aHA-DMA was synthesized by coupling DMA to aHA (obtained after the amination process of HA using ADH, DCC, NHS, and TEA) [10,22], as shown in Figure S1. As a result, we prepared two types of aHA-DMA with different DMA conjugation ratios (aHA-DMA$_{0.36}$ and aHA-DMA$_{0.60}$). Here, the molar conjugation ratio of DMA to aHA was defined as the number of conjugated DMA molecules per repeating unit of aHA and calculated after analyzing the ^{1}H-NMR peaks at δ 2.4 ppm (-CH$_3$, HA part) and δ 1.9 ppm (-CH$_3$, DMA part) (Figures S2 and S3) [10,14,22]. Additionally, to determine the acidic pH-induced degradation of DMA moieties, we incubated aHA-DMA in an acidic PBS (150 mM, pH 6.8) environment for 24 h at 37 °C. We observed the disappearance of the ^{1}H-NMR peaks at δ 1.9 ppm (-CH$_3$, DMA part) (Figure S4) as a result of DMA degradation at pH 6.8 [14].

Next, we prepared three types of DOX-loaded Fe-based HA NPs (DOX@HA/Fe NPs, DOX@aHA-DMA$_{0.36}$/Fe NPs, and DOX@aHA-DMA$_{0.60}$/Fe NPs) after electrostatic interactions [4,5,12] between polymers (HA, aHA-DMA$_{0.36}$, and aHA-DMA$_{0.60}$), Fe^{2+}, and DOX. The weight percentages (wt.%) of Fe^{2+} in DOX@HA/Fe NPs, DOX@aHA-DMA$_{0.36}$/Fe NPs, and DOX@aHA-DMA$_{0.60}$/Fe NPs were 0.63 ± 0.02 wt.%, 0.84 ± 0.03 wt.%, and 0.93 ± 0.02 wt.%, respectively. The loading efficiencies of DOX in DOX@HA/Fe NPs, DOX@aHA-DMA$_{0.36}$/Fe NPs, and DOX@aHA-DMA$_{0.60}$/Fe NPs were 65 wt.%, 63 wt.%, and 63 wt.%, respectively. The loading contents of DOX in DOX@HA/Fe NPs, DOX@aHA-DMA$_{0.36}$/Fe NPs, and DOX@aHA-DMA$_{0.60}$/Fe NPs were 20 wt.%, 20 wt.%, and 21 wt.%, respectively (Figure S5).

3.2. Characterization of DOX-Loaded Fe-Based HA NPs

We anticipated that the electrostatically complexed DOX@aHA-DMA/Fe NPs could have improved tumor uptake through binding CD44 receptors [11,15,17,18] of tumor cells due to the presence of HA and the accelerated DOX release rate by removal of DMA (i.e., pH-responsive property) at weakly acidic endosomal pH (i.e., pH 6.8) [11,12,14] (Figure 1a). First, we analyzed the pH-responsive property of DOX@aHA-DMA/Fe NPs using an FE-SEM instrument. Figure 1b shows that DOX@aHA-DMA$_{0.36}$/Fe NPs and DOX@aHA-DMA$_{0.60}$/Fe NPs became unstable at pH 6.8, and their nanostructures were collapsed probably due to ionic repulsion between Fe^{2+} and DMA-detached aHA (Figure S4). However, DOX@HA/Fe NPs (used as the control group) maintained no difference in nanostructured morphology regardless of the pH change. Similarly, Figure 1c shows that the average particle sizes of DOX@HA/Fe NPs, DOX@aHA-DMA$_{0.36}$/Fe NPs, and DOX@aHA-DMA$_{0.60}$/Fe NPs at pH 7.4 were 128 nm, 140 nm, and 144 nm, respectively. However, the average particle sizes of DOX@HA/Fe NPs, DOX@aHA-DMA$_{0.36}$/Fe NPs, and DOX@aHA-DMA$_{0.60}$/Fe NPs at pH 6.8 were shifted to 142 nm, 113 nm, and 52 nm, respectively. As expected, it was apparent that DOX@aHA-DMA$_{0.60}$/Fe NPs with a high DMA conjugation ratio appears to have more reactivity to pH 6.8. In addition, the zeta potential values of DOX@HA/Fe NPs, DOX@aHA-DMA$_{0.36}$/Fe NPs, and DOX@aHA-DMA$_{0.60}$/Fe NPs at pH 7.4 were -8.2 mV, -7.6 mV, and -7.0 mV, respectively (Figure 1d). However, the zeta potential values of DOX@HA/Fe NPs, DOX@aHA-DMA$_{0.36}$/Fe NPs, and DOX@aHA-DMA$_{0.60}$/Fe NPs at pH 6.8 were shifted to -7.2 mV, -4.3 mV, and -0.5 mV, respectively. These results reveal that the degradation of DMA moieties in DOX@aHA-DMA$_{0.36}$/Fe NPs and DOX@aHA-DMA$_{0.60}$/Fe NPs at pH 6.8 promoted the electrostatic repulsion between aHA and Fe^{2+}, resulting in mediating the destabilization of NPs.

In addition, all NPs showed no significant particle size change in PBS (150 mM, pH 7.4) containing 10% FBS for 7 days (data not shown).

3.3. In Vitro DOX Release

We also monitored the DOX release behaviors of the DOX-loaded Fe-based HA NPs at pH 7.4 and 6.8. As shown in Figure 2, DOX-loaded Fe-based HA NPs showed a maximum 30 wt.% DOX release at pH 7.4, but it was confirmed that the cumulative DOX release of DOX@aHA-DMA$_{0.36}$/Fe NPs and DOX@aHA-DMA$_{0.60}$/Fe NPs increased at pH 6.8. In particular, DOX@aHA-DMA$_{0.36}$/Fe NPs and DOX@aHA-DMA$_{0.60}$/Fe NPs showed approximately 68 wt.% and 72 wt.% DOX release at pH 6.8, respectively. Here, the DOX release of DOX@aHA-DMA$_{0.36}$/Fe NPs and DOX@aHA-DMA$_{0.60}$/Fe NPs was rapid, reaching a plateau between 4 h and 12 h. These results indicate that DOX@aHA-DMA$_{0.36}$/Fe NPs and DOX@aHA-DMA$_{0.60}$/Fe NPs destabilized at pH 6.8 promote DOX release.

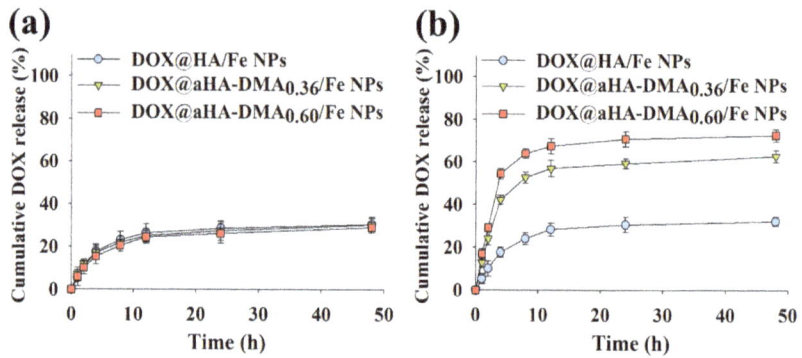

Figure 2. Cumulative DOX release profiles of DOX@HA/Fe NPs, DOX@aHA-DMA$_{0.36}$/Fe NPs, and DOX@aHA-DMA$_{0.60}$/Fe NPs at (**a**) pH 7.4 or (**b**) 6.8 for 48 h ($n = 3$, as multiple experiments).

3.4. In Vitro Cellular Uptake of DOX-Loaded Fe-Based HA NPs

To study the cellular internalization behaviors of the DOX-loaded Fe-based HA NPs, we performed in vitro cell tests using two types of tumor cells with or without CD44 receptors [11]. The quantitative cellular uptake of the DOX-loaded Fe-based HA NPs was measured using a flow cytometer. As shown in Figure 3a, the average fluorescent DOX intensity observed in MDA-MB-231 cells (with CD44 receptors) [11,31] was ~8.3 × 10^3 (free DOX), ~7.9 × 10^2 (DOX@HA/Fe NPs), ~8.1 × 10^2 (DOX@aHA-DMA$_{0.36}$/Fe NPs), and ~9.3 × 10^2 (DOX@aHA-DMA$_{0.60}$/Fe NPs). However, the DOX@HA/Fe NPs, DOX@aHA-DMA$_{0.36}$/Fe NPs, and DOX@aHA-DMA$_{0.60}$/Fe NPs showed low cellular internalization in Huh7 cells (without CD44 receptors) (Figure 3b) [11]. These results indicate that the DOX-loaded Fe-based HA NPs with HA moieties (DOX@HA/Fe NPs, DOX@aHA-DMA$_{0.36}$/Fe NPs, and DOX@aHA-DMA$_{0.60}$/Fe NPs) had excellent cellular uptake in MDA-MB-231 tumor cells with CD44 receptors due to HA-mediated binding to CD44 receptors. We further performed hyperspectral image analysis [11,17] to visualize the tumoral uptake of DOX-loaded Fe-based HA NPs by mapping the DOX signal spectrum in the cells. Figure 3c shows that MDA-MB-231 cells treated with DOX-loaded Fe-based HA NPs (DOX@HA/Fe NPs, DOX@aHA-DMA$_{0.36}$/Fe NPs, and DOX@aHA-DMA$_{0.60}$/Fe NPs) exhibited high cellular localization of DOX, unlike Huh7 cells (Figure 3d) treated with DOX-loaded Fe-based HA NPs. In addition, free DOX treatment showed high cellular localization regardless of the cell type [11].

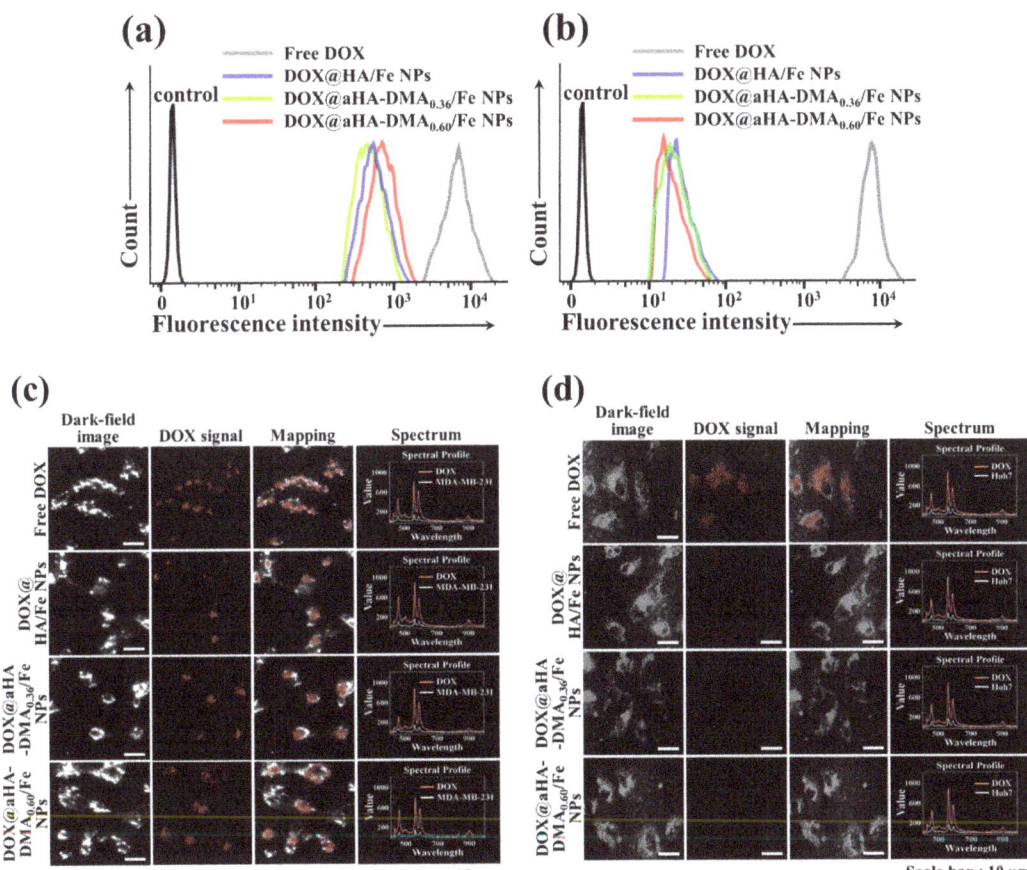

Figure 3. Flow cytometry analysis of (**a**) MDA-MB-231 cells and (**b**) Huh7 cells treated with free DOX (10 µg/mL) or NPs (equivalent to DOX 10 µg/mL) for 4 h of incubation at 37 °C. Here, control refers to cells that were not treated with drugs. Hyperspectral images of (**c**) MDA-MB-231 cells and (**d**) Huh7 cells treated with free DOX (10 µg/mL) or NPs (equivalent to DOX 10 µg/mL) for 4 h incubation at 37 °C.

3.5. In Vitro Tumor Inhibition of DOX-Loaded Fe-Based HA NPs

To evaluate the in vitro tumor cytotoxicity of the DOX-loaded Fe-based HA NPs, we measured the cell viability of tumor cells treated with each sample [11,17,31]. Figure 4a shows that the DOX@aHA-DMA$_{0.60}$/Fe NPs exhibited an excellent tumor cell death rate for MDA-MB-231 tumor cells compared with Huh7 cells. Interestingly, DOX@aHA-DMA$_{0.60}$/Fe NPs resulted in an ~70% cell death rate for MDA-MB-231 tumor cells, unlike other HA-based NPs (DOX@HA/Fe NPs and DOX@aHA-DMA$_{0.36}$/Fe NPs). This is thought to be due to the other properties (probably due to pH-dependent changes in NPs, Figure 2) in addition to the ability to bind CD44 receptors expressed in MDA-MB-231 tumor cells [11,17,31]. In addition, free DOX treatment resulted in high cytotoxicity to both cell lines. However, the NPs without DOX showed negligible cell cytotoxicity, indicating the non-toxic properties of NPs [11,17,31] (Figure 4b).

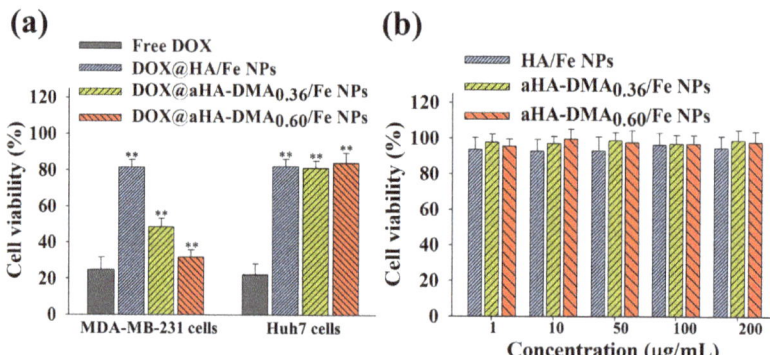

Figure 4. (a) Cell viability was determined by CCK-8 assay of MDA-MB-231 cells and Huh7 cells treated with free DOX (10 µg/mL) or NPs (equivalent to DOX of 10 µg/mL) for 24 h of incubation at 37 °C (n = 7, as multiple experiments, ** $p < 0.01$ compared to free DOX). (b) Cell viability was determined by CCK-8 assay of MDA-MB-231 cells treated with NPs (1–200 µg/mL, without DOX) for 24 h (n = 7, as multiple experiments).

Figure 5 shows the pH-dependent functionality of DOX@aHA-DMA$_{0.60}$/Fe NPs in the cells. Here, we performed a hemolysis test [11,12,17,18] at pH 7.4, 6.8, or 6.0 using RBCs (as a model substance similar to the endosomal membrane) [11,12,17,18] to estimate the pH-dependent endosomolytic activity of NPs. First, negligible hemolytic activity of all NP samples at pH 7.4 was observed. However, the DOX@aHA-DMA$_{0.60}$/Fe NPs resulted in remarkable hemolysis activity at pH 6.8 and 6.0, probably due to the proton sponge effect by the hydrolysis of DMA in aHA-DMA and the protonation of aHA at pH 6.8 and 6.0. In particular, the DOX@aHA-DMA$_{0.60}$/Fe NPs with more DMA showed slightly better hemolysis activity than the DOX@aHA-DMA$_{0.36}$/Fe NPs. This hemolysis activity of DOX@aHA-DMA$_{0.60}$/Fe NPs is thought to mediate the endosomal escape of DOX released from NPs, resulting in improved cell cytotoxicity.

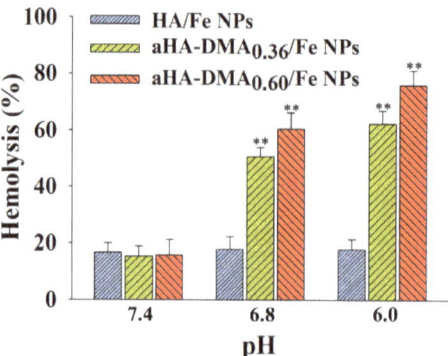

Figure 5. Hemolysis activity of the NPs (100 µg/mL, without DOX) at pH 7.4, 6.8, or 6.0 (n = 3, as multiple experiments, ** $p < 0.01$ compared to HA/Fe NPs).

We also investigated the therapeutic efficacy of DOX-loaded Fe-based HA NPs using a local healing test in MDA-MB-231 cells. As shown in Figure 6, MDA-MB-231 cells treated with DOX@aHA-DMA$_{0.60}$/Fe NPs exhibited reduced tumor cell migration events [33] after 24 h of incubation, which is similar to the results of cells treated with free DOX. However,

MDA-MB-231 cells treated with DOX@HA/Fe NPs presented some cell migration events, revealing their poor therapeutic efficacy [11,17,31,33].

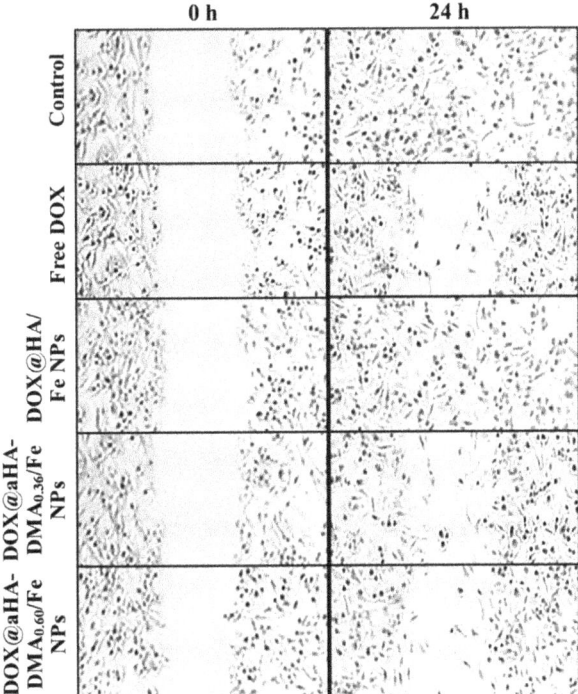

Figure 6. Local healing assays of MDA-MB-231 cells treated with free DOX (10 µg/mL) or NPs (equivalent to DOX 10 µg/mL) for 24 h of incubation at 37 °C.

Overall, our results suggest that the DOX released from DOX@aHA-DMA$_{0.60}$/Fe NPs in an acidic endosomal environment (pH 6.0) is effective in inhibiting tumor cell proliferation and increasing tumor cell death.

4. Conclusions

In this study, we successfully engineered a metal-based multifunctional DOX@aHA-DMA$_{0.60}$/Fe NPs to inhibit tumor cell proliferation. The electrostatically complexed DOX@aHA-DMA$_{0.60}$/Fe NPs were selectively internalized to MDA-MB-231 tumor cells via CD44-mediated endocytosis. Importantly, DMA-detached aHA at acidic pH mediated ionic repulsion against Fe^{2+} ions in NPs and accelerated DOX release. The comprehensive results from in vitro studies indicate that DOX@aHA-DMA$_{0.60}$/Fe NPs were effective in enhancing tumor cell suppression. Of course, further investigation is needed to confirm the antitumor activity of this formulation in vivo.

Supplementary Materials: The following are available online, Figure S1: Synthesis procedure of aHA-DMA; Figure S2: ^{1}H-NMR peaks of aHA; Figure S3: ^{1}H-NMR peaks of aHA-DMA$_{0.60}$; Figure S4: ^{1}H-NMR peaks of DMA-detached aHA; Figure S5: DOX loading efficiency and loading content of DOX@HA/Fe NPs, DOX@aHA-DMA$_{0.36}$/Fe NPs, and DOX@aHA-DMA$_{0.60}$/Fe NPs (n = 3, as multiple experiments).

Author Contributions: Y.B. and Y.K. contributed equally to this work as first authors. Conceptualization, E.S.L.; methodology, Y.B.; investigation, Y.B.; data curation, Y.B., Y.K., and E.S.L.; writing—

original draft preparation, E.S.L., Y.B., and Y.K.; writing—review and editing, E.S.L.; supervision, E.S.L.; project administration, E.S.L.; funding acquisition, E.S.L. All authors have read and agreed to the published version of the manuscript.

Funding: This work was financially supported by the 2021 Research Fund of the Catholic University of Korea, by the National Research Foundation of Korea (NRF) grant funded by the Korean government (MSIT) (grant number: NRF-2021R1A2B5B01001932).

Informed Consent Statement: Not applicable.

Conflicts of Interest: The authors declare no conflict of interest.

Sample Availability: Samples of aHA-DMA and NPs are available from the authors.

References

1. Akhtar, M.J.; Alhadlaq, H.A.; Kumar, S.; Alrokayan, S.A.; Ahamed, M. Selective cancer-killing ability of metal-based nanoparticles: Implications for cancer therapy. *Arch. Toxicol.* **2015**, *89*, 1895–1907. [CrossRef] [PubMed]
2. Dzhardimalieva, G.I.; Uflyand, I.E. Preparation of metal-polymer nanocomposites by chemical reduction of metal ions: Functions of polymer matrices. *J. Polym. Res.* **2018**, *25*, 255. [CrossRef]
3. Malola, S.; Nieminen, P.; Pihlajamaki, A.; Hamalainen, J.; Karkkainen, T.; Hakkinen, H. A method for structure prediction of metal-ligand interfaces of hybrid nanoparticles. *Nat. Commun.* **2019**, *10*, 3973. [CrossRef]
4. Kang, S.; He, Y.; Yu, D.G.; Li, W.; Wang, K. Drug-zein@lipid hybrid nanoparticles: Electrospraying preparation and drug extended release application. *Colloids Surf. B* **2021**, *201*, 111629. [CrossRef] [PubMed]
5. Wang, M.; Hou, J.; Yu, D.; Li, S.; Zhu, J.; Chen, Z. Electrospun tri-layer nanodepots for sustained release of acyclovir. *J. Alloys Compd.* **2020**, *846*, 156471. [CrossRef]
6. Herrera, S.E.; Agazzi, M.L.; Cortez, M.L.; Marmisolle, W.A.; Tagliazucchi, M.; Azzaroni, O. Multitasking polyamine/ferrioxalate nano-sized assemblies: Thermo-, photo-, and redox-responsive soft materials made easy. *Chem. Commun.* **2019**, *55*, 14653–14656. [CrossRef]
7. Neumann, L.N.; Urban, D.A.; Lemal, P.; Ramani, S.; Petri-Fink, A.; Balog, S.; Weder, C.; Schrettl, S. Preparation of metallo-supramolecular single-chain polymeric nanoparticles and their characterization by Taylor dispersion. *Polym. Chem.* **2020**, *11*, 586–592. [CrossRef]
8. Gao, W.; Chan, J.M.; Farokhzad, O.C. pH-responsive nanoparticles for drug delivery. *Mol. Pharm.* **2010**, *7*, 1913–1920. [CrossRef]
9. Kanamala, M.; Wilson, W.R.; Yang, M.; Palmer, B.D.; Wu, Z. Mechanisms and biomaterials in pH-responsive tumour targeted drug delivery: A review. *Biomaterials* **2016**, *85*, 152–167. [CrossRef]
10. Huo, Q.; Zhu, J.; Niu, Y.; Shi, H.; Gong, Y.; Li, Y.; Song, H.; Liu, Y. pH-triggered surface charge-switchable polymer micelles for the co-delivery of paclitaxel/disulfiram and overcoming multidrug resistance in cancer. *Int. J. Nanomed.* **2017**, *12*, 8631–8647. [CrossRef]
11. Noh, G.J.; Oh, K.T.; Youn, Y.S.; Lee, E.S. Cyclic RGD-conjugated hyaluronate dot bearing cleavable doxorubicin for multivalent tumor targeting. *Biomacromolecules* **2020**, *21*, 2525–2535. [CrossRef] [PubMed]
12. Yoon, S.; Kim, Y.; Youn, Y.S.; Oh, K.T.; Kim, D.; Lee, E.S. Transferrin-conjugated pH-responsive gamma-cyclodextrin nanoparticles for antitumoral topotecan delivery. *Pharmaceutics* **2020**, *12*, 1109. [CrossRef] [PubMed]
13. Kim, K.; Choi, H.; Choi, E.S.; Park, M.H.; Ryu, J.H. Hyaluronic acid-coated nanomedicine for targeted cancer therapy. *Pharmaceutics* **2019**, *11*, 301. [CrossRef] [PubMed]
14. Oh, N.M.; Kwag, D.S.; Oh, K.T.; Youn, Y.S.; Lee, E.S. Electrostatic charge conversion processes in engineered tumor-identifying polypeptides for targeted chemotherapy. *Biomaterials* **2012**, *33*, 1884–1893. [CrossRef] [PubMed]
15. Yang, Y.; Zhao, Y.; Lan, J.; Kang, Y.; Zhang, T.; Ding, Y.; Zhang, X.; Lu, L. Reduction-sensitive CD44 receptor-targeted hyaluronic acid derivative micelles for doxorubicin delivery. *Int. J. Nanomed.* **2018**, *13*, 4361–4378. [CrossRef]
16. Sarkar, S.; Ponce, N.T.; Banerjee, A.; Bandopadhyay, R.; Rajendran, S.; Lichtfouse, E. Green polymeric nanomaterials for the photocatalytic degradation of dyes: A review. *Environ. Chem. Lett.* **2020**, *18*, 1569–1580. [CrossRef]
17. Park, J.; Lee, H.; Youn, Y.S.; Oh, K.T.; Lee, E.S. Tumor-homing pH-sensitive extracellular vesicles for targeting heterogeneous tumors. *Pharmaceutic* **2020**, *12*, 372. [CrossRef]
18. Lee, H.; Park, H.; Noh, G.J.; Lee, E.S. pH-responsive hyaluronate-anchored extracellular vesicles to promote tumor-targeted drug delivery. *Carbohydr. Polym.* **2018**, *202*, 323–333. [CrossRef]
19. Kim, Y.; Youn, Y.S.; Oh, K.T.; Kim, D.; Lee, E.S. Tumor-targeting liposomes with transient holes allowing intact rituximab internally. *Biomacromolecules* **2021**, *22*, 723–731. [CrossRef]
20. Lee, J.M.; Park, H.; Oh, K.T.; Lee, E.S. pH-responsive hyaluronated liposomes for docetaxel delivery. *Int. J. Pharm.* **2018**, *547*, 377–384. [CrossRef]
21. Choi, E.J.; Lee, J.M.; Youn, Y.S.; Na, K.; Lee, E.S. Hyaluronate dots for highly efficient photodynamic therapy. *Carbohydr. Polym.* **2018**, *181*, 10–18. [CrossRef] [PubMed]
22. Luo, Y.; Kirker, K.R.; Prestwich, G.D. Cross-linked hyaluronic acid hydrogel films: New biomaterials for drug delivery. *J. Control. Release* **2000**, *69*, 169–184. [CrossRef]

23. Koo, M.; Oh, K.T.; Noh, G.; Lee, E.S. Gold nanoparticles bearing a tumor pH-sensitive cyclodextrin cap. *ACS Appl. Mater. Interfaces* **2018**, *10*, 24450–24458. [CrossRef] [PubMed]
24. Yu, H.S.; Lee, J.M.; Youn, Y.S.; Oh, K.T.; Na, K.; Lee, E.S. Gamma-cyclodextrin-phenylacetic acid mesh as a drug trap. *Carbohydr. Polym.* **2018**, *184*, 390–400. [CrossRef]
25. Lee, U.Y.; Oh, Y.T.; Kim, D.; Lee, E.S. Multimeric grain-marked micelles for highly efficient photodynamic therapy and magnetic resonance imaging of tumors. *Int. J. Pharm.* **2014**, *471*, 166–172. [CrossRef] [PubMed]
26. Lee, U.Y.; Oh, N.M.; Kwag, D.S.; Oh, K.T.; Oh, Y.T.; Youn, Y.S.; Lee, E.S. Facile synthesis of multimeric micelles. *Angew. Chem. Int. Ed. Engl.* **2012**, *51*, 7287–7291. [CrossRef] [PubMed]
27. Kwag, D.S.; Oh, K.T.; Lee, E.S. Facile synthesis of multilayered polysaccharidic vesicles. *J. Control Release* **2014**, *187*, 83–90. [CrossRef] [PubMed]
28. Yu, H.S.; Park, H.; Tran, T.H.; Hwang, S.Y.; Na, K.; Lee, E.S.; Oh, K.T.; Oh, D.X.; Park, A.J. Poisonous caterpillar-inspired chitosan nanofiber enabling dual photothermal and photodynamic tumor ablation. *Pharmaceutics* **2019**, *11*, 258. [CrossRef]
29. Lee, U.Y.; Youn, Y.S.; Park, J.; Lee, E.S. Y-shaped ligand-driven gold nanoparticles for highly efficient tumoral uptake and photothermal ablation. *ACS Nano* **2014**, *8*, 12858–12865. [CrossRef]
30. Noh, G.; Youn, Y.S.; Lee, E.S. Preparation of iron oxide nanoparticles functionalized with Y-shaped ligands for brain tumor targeting. *J. Mater. Chem. B* **2016**, *4*, 6074–6080. [CrossRef]
31. Lee, E.; Park, J.; Youn, Y.S.; Oh, K.T.; Kim, D.; Lee, E.S. Alendronate/cRGD-decorated ultrafine hyaluronate dot targeting bone metastasis. *Biomedicines* **2020**, *8*, 492. [CrossRef] [PubMed]
32. Yu, H.S.; Lee, E.S. Honeycomb-like pH-responsive gamma-cyclodextrin electrospun particles for highly efficient tumor therapy. *Carbohydr. Polym.* **2020**, *230*, 115563. [CrossRef] [PubMed]
33. Wang, X.; Decker, C.C.; Zechner, L.; Krstin, S.; Wink, M. In vitro wound healing of tumor cells: Inhibition of cell migration by selected cytotoxic alkaloids. *BMC Pharmacol. Toxicol.* **2019**, *20*, 4. [CrossRef] [PubMed]

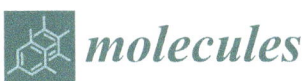

Review

Recent Advances of Cell Membrane Coated Nanoparticles in Treating Cardiovascular Disorders

Chaojie Zhu [1,2,3,†], Junkai Ma [2,3,†], Zhiheng Ji [2,3], Jie Shen [4,*] and Qiwen Wang [1,*]

1. Department of Cardiology, The First Affiliated Hospital, Zhejiang University School of Medicine, Hangzhou 310003, China; 3180101530@zju.edu.cn
2. Chu Kochen Honors College, Zhejiang University, Hangzhou 310058, China; 3180101531@zju.edu.cn (J.M.); 3180103158@zju.edu.cn (Z.J.)
3. Institute of Pharmaceutics, College of Pharmaceutical Sciences, Zhejiang University, Hangzhou 310058, China
4. Department of Pharmacy, School of Medicine, Zhejiang University City College, Hangzhou 310015, China
* Correspondence: shenj@zucc.edu.cn (J.S.); wangqiwen@zju.edu.cn (Q.W.)
† These authors contribute equally.

Abstract: Cardiovascular diseases (CVDs) are the leading cause of death worldwide, causing approximately 17.9 million deaths annually, an estimated 31% of all deaths, according to the WHO. CVDs are essentially rooted in atherosclerosis and are clinically classified into coronary heart disease, stroke and peripheral vascular disorders. Current clinical interventions include early diagnosis, the insertion of stents, and long-term preventive therapy. However, clinical diagnostic and therapeutic tools are subject to a number of limitations including, but not limited to, potential toxicity induced by contrast agents and unexpected bleeding caused by anti-platelet drugs. Nanomedicine has achieved great advancements in biomedical area. Among them, cell membrane coated nanoparticles, denoted as CMCNPs, have acquired enormous expectations due to their biomimetic properties. Such membrane coating technology not only helps avoid immune clearance, but also endows nanoparticles with diverse cellular and functional mimicry. In this review, we will describe the superiorities of CMCNPs in treating cardiovascular diseases and their potentials in optimizing current clinical managements.

Keywords: cell membrane coated nanoparticle; atherosclerosis; thrombosis; diagnosis and therapy; cardiovascular disease

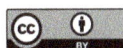

1. Introduction

Cardiovascular disease (CVD) surpasses cancer as the most common cause of mortality [1], contributing to almost 40% total deaths in China [2]. Conventional therapeutic options include medications embodying anticoagulants [3], antiplatelet [4], thrombolytic [5] and antilipemic agents [6], and surgery including vessel bypass grafting [7] and stent insertion [8,9]. Nonetheless, disease reoccurrences, which have been reported to be 50% for any CVD event or subsequent revascularization in the year after myocardial infarction [10], side effects, for example bleeding events (occurring in around 1-8%) induced by dual antiplatelet therapy in treating acute coronary heart syndrome [11], and a high frequency of adverse drug reactions (~20%) [12], remain challenging. This is especially true for small-molecule based agents, which are organic compounds influencing molecule pathways by targeting vital functional proteins displayed on blood vessels and the heart; off-target toxicities, systemic degradation, short half-life and low bioavailability hinder clinical treatment [13–15].

Nanotechnology has achieved great advancements in the biomedical field. Nanomaterials facilitate targeted small-molecule drug delivery to the specific lesion site, or they may sometimes perform as a pharmacological active compound per se due to their unique physical and chemical properties [16]. Nevertheless, without any surface modifications, these nanoplatforms are rapidly removed from circulation into the liver and spleen by the body's reticuloendothelial system (RES), which severely hampers their therapeutic efficacy [17]. Nanomaterials surface PEGylation is the most extensive measurement taken to improve their biocompatibility and prolong the circulation time [18]. However, such a method has been associated with the potential toxicity effect of inducing hypersensitivity reactions which can provoke an anaphylactic shock [19]. Alternatively, cell membrane coating technology has been reported to elicit immune evasion and prolong nanocarriers' circulation time. Furthermore, the functional proteins on the cloaked cell membranes render additional biological properties for nanoparticles, such as selective adherence, inflammatory site targeting and endothelium penetration [20]. In this review, we briefly introduce the pathogenesis, therapeutic targets and current clinical medications of several main cardiovascular diseases. Then, we will explain fundamental information about cell membrane coated nanoparticles, including their history, characteristics and synthetic routes. To elucidate the significance of CMCNPs, we describe the evolution of CVD treatments. Through highlighting the bottlenecks of clinical medications and conventional nanomedicine in chronological sequence, we demonstrate the superiority of CMCNPs in treating CVDs. In particular, we show that CMCNPs boast a number of unique therapeutic characteristics, such as their intrinsic capacity to target lesions. As far as we know, it is the first work that describes the evolution of CVDs treatments—from clinical medications, to conventional nanomedicine, and finally to CMCNPs, with a special focus on CMCNPs.

2. Cardiovascular Diseases

The cardiovascular system, or circulatory system, consisting of the heart and numerous vessels, is responsible for blood circulation in the body and crucial for oxygen, nutrition and cellular traffic. Behavioral risk factors such as smoking [21], hypertension [22], and diabetes [23] and biological risk factors such as age, gender [24], and family history [25], increase the prevalence of cardiovascular disease worldwide [26]. The main categories of CVDs include coronary heart disease, stroke and peripheral vascular disorders. These aforementioned CVDs are triggered by abnormal blood flow, either due to blood blockage or bleeding, the occurrence of which is essentially on account of atherosclerosis or thrombosis (Figure 1) [27]. Clinical measurements include early diagnosis, preventive care or surgical intervention. Despite these efforts to prevent and treat CVDs, progress has been moderate, and the annual total of CVD cases has seen a continuous increase in the last 30 years [28].

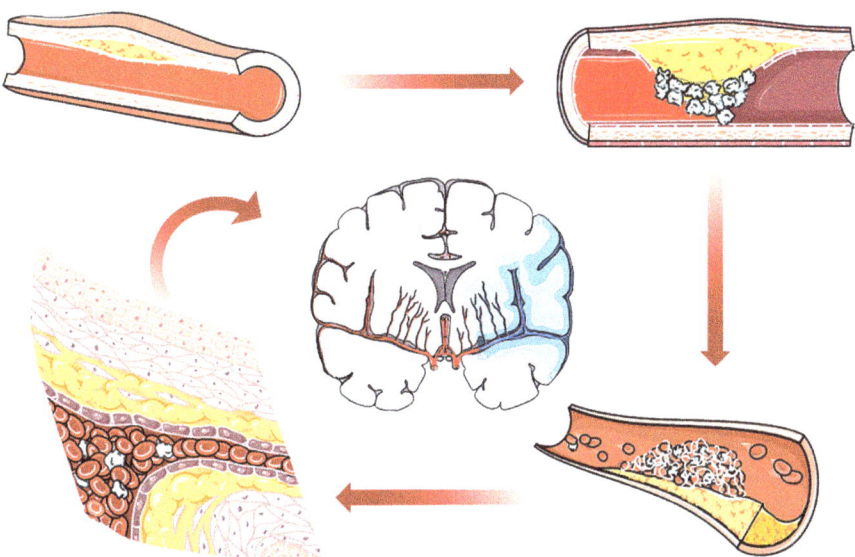

Figure 1. Schematic diagram showing the process of atherosclerosis. Under pathologic conditions, atherosclerosis develops with plaque formation. Atherosclerotic plaque will rupture with thrombus formation. Both thrombosis and atherosclerosis will cause local ischemia, resulting in coronary disease or peripheral arterial disease. In addition, thrombus may travel to the brain arteries, which induces ischemic stroke.

2.1. Mechanisms of Atherosclerosis and Thrombosis

2.1.1. Atherosclerosis

Atherosclerosis (AS) is the most common cause of myocardial infarction and ischemia, which is featured by chronic inflammation. An intimate correlation has been reported between low-density lipoprotein (LDL), one of the five major groups of lipoprotein responsible for fat molecules transporting throughout the body in the extracellular water, and atherosclerosis [29]. Elevated levels of LDL upregulate the expression of endothelial cell adhesion molecules which can drive the infiltration of leukocytes into vessels through classical recruitment cascades [30]. Furthermore, the chemokines released from endothelial cells and activated macrophages recruit peripheral neutrophils and monocytes. In the late stage of the disease, monocytes recruited to the lesion continuously digest modified lipoprotein, differentiating into foam cells [31]. Proteases released by the apoptotic foam cells further destroy the thin endothelial cell layer which covers and protects the atherosclerotic plaque, eventually leading to plaque rupture and thrombus formation [32].

2.1.2. Thrombosis

Thrombosis is defined as the formation of a blood clot within the vascular system, which severely obstructs normal blood circulation and may eventually lead to myocardial infarction and ischemic stroke. Under normal conditions, endothelial cells will actively prevent the formation of thrombus through various factors which block platelet adhesion and aggregation, inhibit coagulation and lyse the clots. Three main abnormalities of circulation facilitate thrombus formation; endothelial injury, alterations in blood flow and hypercoagulation, collectively named "Virchow's Triad" [33]. The clot formed during this process promotes hypoxia and inflammation at the lesion site, subsequently promoting the infiltration of activated immune cells. Lesional monocytes and macrophages express metalloproteinase (MMP), which can facilitate thrombus resolution. When unresolved, clots will induce ischemia-related cardiovascular diseases, such as lower limb ischemia and ischemic stroke [34].

2.2. Classifications of CVDs

Cardiovascular diseases can be mainly classified into three categories—including coronary heart disease, stroke and peripheral vascular disorders—based on the location of the injury. In the next section, the main risks, manifestations, and disease mechanisms will be discussed.

2.2.1. Coronary Heart Disease

Coronary heart disease, otherwise called ischemic heart disease, occurs due to insufficient blood flow to the heart and the necrosis of myocardial tissues induced by a lack of oxygen. In the early stages of the disease, a shortage of blood flow is mainly caused by atherosclerotic plaque obstruction. When the atherosclerotic plaque suddenly breaks off, it exposes its highly thrombotic components, consequently leading to thrombus formation. Thrombus formed during this process may completely obstruct the blood vessel through thrombo-embolism, which potentiates myocardial infarction [35,36].

2.2.2. Stroke

Stroke will occur when the supply of blood to the brain tissue is impacted. Strokes can be divided into two subtypes—ischemic stroke and hemorrhagic stroke—based on their mechanism of formation. Hemorrhagic stroke, which makes up almost 13% of total clinical cases, is usually caused by hypertension, which results in intracranial hypertension and oxygen and nutrition depletion in the downstream tissues, rapidly inducing damage to the brain tissues [37]. On the other hand, atherosclerosis is the major cause of ischemic stroke. As a result, thrombus forms due to the local inflammation and ulceration of the fibrous plaques. The clot occludes the atherosclerotic vessel or travels further to block the brain's arteries, causing ischemic stroke [38]. The resulting oxygen- and glucose-depleted environment downregulates junctional protein expression, which in turn facilitates the extravasation of proteins and leukocytes infiltration. Leukocytes, e.g., neutrophils, recruited to the brain lesion site during the acute inflammatory phase exacerbate inflammation through the generation of reactive oxygen species, worsening the disease condition [39,40].

2.2.3. Peripheral Vascular Disorders

Peripheral vascular disorder, or peripheral arterial disease, occurs in parts of the body other than the brain and heart, such as legs and arms, the major causes of which include atherosclerosis and thrombo-embolism. Narrowing lumens induce insufficient blood flow into the lesion site, leading to local ischemia, and eventually developing into intermittent claudication. Aggravating intermittent claudication may cause critical limb ischemia, and ultimately progress into acute limb ischemia when the blood flow is completely obstructed [41].

2.3. Clinical Management and Its Bottleneck

Before therapeutic intervention, appropriate diagnosis should be implemented. Current clinic diagnostic tools mainly include X-ray, doppler ultrasound, CT angiography and magnetic resonance imaging angiography. However, early stage diagnosis of atherosclerosis remains a major issue due to inadequate diagnostic clarity and clinical acumen. To facilitate early diagnosis of atherosclerosis, iodinated compounds and gadolinium are two representative contrast dyes applied for CT angiography and magnetic resonance imaging angiograph, respectively. Although these measurements have achieved success to a certain degree, the biosafety of contrast agents has aroused concerns. For example, iodinated compounds are limiting in those with hypersensitivity or significant renal dysfunction. Gadolinium can also be limiting due to its potential toxicity in inducing nephrogenic systemic fibrosis, which is a rare but unmanageable scleroderma like disease [42].

Apart from diagnosis, there are also hurdles for the management and prevention of cardiovascular diseases. For high-risk patients who have not yet experienced CVDs, long-term preventive medications, such as statins, are recommended. However, a lack of patient compliance hinders our fight against CVDs [43]. In addition, anticoagulant, thrombolysis and antiplatelet agents are clinically used to treat thrombo-embolism-related CVDs. Despite the efficacy of these drugs at impeding the process of plaque development and thrombus formation, they come with a significant risk of unexpected bleeding, for example coumarin, a vitamin K antagonist, is related to a risk of major bleeding that ranges from 2% to 13% during the mean duration of follow-up of 6 to 30 months [44]. Furthermore, the therapeutic dosage varies between patients and with disease stage. Last but not least, clinical strategies against acute ischemic stroke are mainly divided into intravenous thrombolysis and endovascular thrombectomy, both of which are time-critical and have extremely limited therapeutic time windows [45]. The performance of stents also encounters bottlenecks. Bare metal stents (BMS) and drug-eluting stents (DES) are two conventional classes applied in clinical settings. DES are platforms for delivering therapeutic molecules locally, which were developed to overcome several side effects associated with BMS, such as thrombosis and neointimal hyperplasia. Although DES exhibit efficacies in preventing restenosis and scar tissue formation to some extent, in-stent thrombosis due to inflammation or certain gradient on stents, for example polymers, is the main challenge [46]. Therefore, there remains an urgent need for better alternatives with improved diagnostic and therapeutic efficacy.

3. Nanomedicine against CVDs

Recent advancements achieved in nanomedicine exhibit great potential to improve off-target side effects, long-term toxicity and limited diagnostic or therapeutic efficacy [47]. For example, conventional use of stents are accompanied with risks of thrombosis and restenosis. Especially for DES, late stent thrombosis (>30 days) is a main challenge. Nanoparticles have been incorporated into stents' formulations to modulate their drug releasing properties and achieve robust endothelial healing. Liu et al. developed advanced DES, which were composed of collagen and nitric oxide (NO) donor-loaded PLGA nanoparticles [48]. As a result, such platform alleviated intima formation and exhibited a sustained release capability of NO, which significantly reduced platelet aggregation in rabbit blood, thus mitigating thrombosis.

Conventional diagnostic contrast agents, such as gadopentetic, take effect through revealing the narrowing of the vessels, termed stenosis. In contrast, nano-based molecular contrast agent could directly disclose the location of atherosclerotic plaques through active targeting [49]. For example, Qiao et al. developed an osteopontin antibody conjugated upconversion nanoplatform to achieve noninvasive targeting and imaging of vulnerable plaques [50]. Morishige et al. reported dextran coated superparamagnetic nanoparticles, which exhibited affinity towards macrophages and could be utilized to assess macrophage burden in atherosclerosis, providing a useful tool for identifying inflamed plaques and monitoring disease conditions [51].

Nanoparticles have also achieved breathtaking therapeutic improvements. The current clinical prevention of atherosclerosis mainly relies on the long term oral administration of statins, with insignificant effects unless taking an extremely high dosage [52]. However, such high dosage will inevitably induce hepatotoxicity and myopathy [53]. To address this predicament, Kim et al. reported a cargo-switching nanoparticles composed of a cyclodextrin shell component and simvastatin as a loaded drug to achieve higher affinity towards atherosclerotic lesion and plaque regression [54]. In another way, Flores et al. developed single walled carbon nanotubes loaded with a chemical inhibitor of the antiphagocytic CD47-SIRPα signaling axis. Such nanoplatforms exhibited macrophage-specific targeting ability and could reactivate lesional phagocytosis to effectively reduce plaque burden [55]. Reperfusion is vital for better prognosis in acute stroke. Marsh et al. reported fibrin-targeted perfluorocarbon nanoparticles, the surface of which is modified to deliver the plasminogen activator streptokinase, a thrombolytic agent. Such a nanoplatform exhibited an improved clot-targeting ability with a lower risk of adverse hemorrhagic events [56].

However, these strategies still face the problem of fast clearance by RES. Better therapeutic or diagnostic capabilities can be obtained via prolonging their circulation. In addition, the targeting abilities of these platforms usually rely on peptide or protein (antibody) conjugation. Many factors limit their biofunctions and targeting abilities, for example, proteases in circulation in the body may interact with them, thus depriving them of their functions [57]. Alternative solutions are needed to address these drawbacks.

4. Cell Membrane Coated Nanoparticle and Its Applications in CVDs

Cell membrane coating technology, an alternative surface passivation method substituting for PEGylation, generally exploits innate cell membranes to coat synthetic nanoparticles. Such a coating measurement helps to disguise nanoparticles as some of the body's intrinsic cells, which not only assists them in avoiding the body's immune clearance, thus prolonging their circulation (higher biocompatibility), but also endows them with various cell-like biofunctions via the diverse functional membrane proteins on CMCNPs' surface (cell-mimicking properties).

4.1. Cell Membrane Coated Nanoparticles

Cell membrane cloaking technology was first achieved by Hu et al. who applied red blood cells' membranes to coat poly-(D,L-lactic-co-glycolic) acid (PLGA) nanoparticles, successfully prolonging their circulation by up to 72 h [58]. Considerable research has been conducted to expand cell membranes sources, inner nanoparticles and synthetic routes. Generally, this technique is divided into three procedures to synthesize cell membrane coated nanoparticles: cell membrane extraction, inner core nanoparticle preparation and the fusion process (Figure 2) [59].

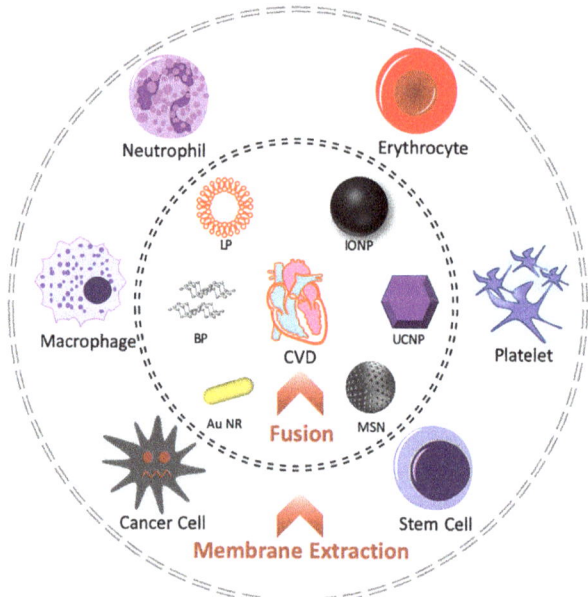

Figure 2. Schematic diagram showing the synthetic process of cell membrane coated nanoparticles. Basically, interested membranes are first extracted from the cell sources, e.g., macrophages, neutrophils, erythrocytes, platelets, cancer cells and stem cells. The membranes are further coated on selected nanoparticles, e.g., black phosphorous, liposome, iron oxide nanoparticle, upconversion nanoparticle, gold nanorod and mesoporous silica nanoparticle. The membrane–core hybrid system can be applied to treat cardiovascular diseases. Abbreviations: BP: black phosphorous; LP: liposome; IONP: iron oxide nanoparticle; UCNP: upconversion nanoparticle; Au NR: gold nanorod; MSN: mesoporous silica nanoparticle.

4.1.1. Cell Membrane Extraction

Cell membranes are mainly composed of phospholipids and diverse functional proteins [60]. The membrane plays a vital role in dividing cell types, cells' intercommunications, signal transduction and cargo selective permeability. Current procedures of cell membrane extraction include membrane lysis and purification [61]. Generally, interested cells are first isolated from whole blood. Following hypotonic treatment for cell lysis, discontinuous sucrose gradient centrifugations are implemented to remove the nucleic and cytoplasmic contents. Further purifications are carried out through washing with specific buffers and extrusion through porous polycarbonate membrane to obtain the purified extracted cell membranes [62].

4.1.2. Core Preparation

A number of novel nanocarriers have emerged (Table 1), e.g., liposomes [62,63], gold nanoparticles [64], mesoporous silica nanoparticles [65,66], iron oxide nanoparticles [67,68], black phosphorous [69–71], PLGA nanoparticles [58,72], and layered double hydroxide [73]. These nanocarriers can either act as drug delivery platforms or as active components in themselves due to their intrinsic physical and chemical properties. For example, black phosphorous 2D nanosheets can be used in photothermal therapy due to its efficient photothermal conversion property [71]. Layered double hydroxide can not only perform as lipid regulator to treat CVDs [74], but can also serve as an immune adjuvant and antigen carrier bi-functional nanoplatform in cancer immunotherapy [75]. To achieve various biological functions, e.g., magnetic resonance imaging, drug carrying or reactive oxygen species scavenging, appropriate inner nanoparticle selection is essential to fulfill the therapeutic potential of cell membrane coated nanoparticles.

Table 1. Common inner particles applied in core–membrane strategy.

Core Particle	Properties	Application	Ref.
PLGA	Biocompatibility and biodegradability Easy manipulation	Drug carrier	[58]
Liposome	Hydrophobic and hydrophilic drug delivery Sustained drug release	Drug carrier	[62,63]
MSN	Tunable pore size High pore volume	Drug carrier	[65,66]
UCNP	Convert NIR into visible light	Deep tissue imaging	[76]
Gold NPs	Photothermal effect	Photothermal therapy	[64]
IONP	Magnetic property	MRI Magnetic targeting	[67,68]
BP Nanosheet	Photothermal conversion	Photothermal therapy	[69–71]

4.1.3. Fusion Process

The fusion process covers the inner core nanoparticles with the extracted and purified cell membranes. Generally, this process is divided into two main approaches: membrane extrusion or sonication bath. The membrane extrusion process is achieved through mixing the cell membrane vesicles and inner nanoparticles and extruding them through porous polycarbonate membranes for several repeated cycles. This method is mainly applied for small-scale production, which is suitable for laboratory use [77]. A sonication bath is a route providing higher yields but requires strictly controlled sonication power. Excessively high temperatures will denature the functional proteins on the obtained cell membrane vesicles, which severely impacts their biological performance. In addition, core–membrane nanoparticles produced through sonication methods exhibit poor size uniformity [78].

Therefore, new strategies are urgently needed with higher production efficiency, improved particle uniformity and valid membrane protein functions.

4.2. Cell Membrane Coated Nanoparticles in Treating Cardiovascular Disease

Cell membrane coated nanoparticles are expected to exhibit some intrinsic cell properties, e.g., specific targeting to inflammatory site, immune evasion, binding affinity to targeted receptors or cells (Table 2). In dealing with cardiovascular diseases, CMCNPs are exploited to mimic peripheral cells, such as erythrocytes [79], platelets [80], or immune cells [81], which have been reported to exhibit a crucial role in disease progression. In the following section, cell membrane coated nanoparticles will be discussed based on the context of their sources and their potential for treating CVDs.

Table 2. Main usage of several common cell membranes.

Membrane Source	Properties	Application	Ref.
Red blood cell	Immune evasion	Prolong circulation	[82]
Platelet	Selective targeting to injured tissue Adherence to inflammatory neutrophil	Targeting cancer metastasis Targeting vascular injury	[83]
Macrophage	Immune evasion Cytokine sequestration	Inflammatory site targeting Anti-inflammation	[84,85]
Neutrophil	Selective targeting to inflammatory tissue	Inflammatory site targeting	[86]
Cancer cell	Tumor targeting Antigen delivery	Homotypic targeting Cancer vaccine	[87]
Stem cell	Penetration across the endothelium	Tumor targeting Inflammatory migratory	[88]
Bacterium	Elicit immune response Anti-adhesion	Cancer immune therapy Bacterial infection	[89,90]

4.2.1. Erythrocytes Cell Membranes

Erythrocytes (or red-blood cells, RBC) are the most abundant cells in the human body, taking the responsibility of oxygen and carbon dioxide transport. Mechanistically, healthy erythrocytes can evade the mononuclear phagocyte system (MPS) through surface membrane protein CD47, which act as "do not eat me" signals to immune cells [91]. Therefore, erythrocytes membranes are intrinsically biocompatible and nonimmunogenic, so they can be utilized to prolong the circulation time of nanoparticles. Apart from this, RBC membrane coated nanoparticles are also explored to act as biomimetic nanosponges for detoxification [92], or serve as nanotoxoids for safe and effective toxin nanovaccination [93].

As mentioned above, Zhang et al. were the first to apply erythrocyte membrane coating on PLGA nanoparticles [58]. In their study, the RBC membrane was extracted through hypotonic medium hemolysis and fused with PLGA nanoparticles to obtain RBC membrane camouflaged NPs (RBC-NPs), with an 80 nm average diameter (Figure 3A). They further proved that the RBC membrane proteins were successfully transferred onto PLGA nanoparticles (Figure 3B). Additionally, RBC membrane coated nanoparticles exhibited outstanding stability in vitro, maintaining its core-shell structure even after 6 h co-incubation with HeLa (Figure 3C). As a result, such a nanoplatform exhibits an outstanding ability to avoid immune clearance, greatly prolonging its circulation time (Figure 3D). Due to its long circulation time, this nanostructure could serve as a universally effective drug delivery platform against CVDs when suitable small-molecule agents are loaded in the inner PLGA core. For example, Wang et al. reported rapamycin-loaded PLGA nanoparticles, which were cloaked with RBC membranes (RBC/RAP@PLGA). As a result, this nanoplatform effectively attenuated the progression of atherosclerosis, in which the average area ration of plaque to vascular lumen decreased from 47.95% to 31.34% after treatment, superior to the free drug group (from 47.95% to 42.42%) [94].

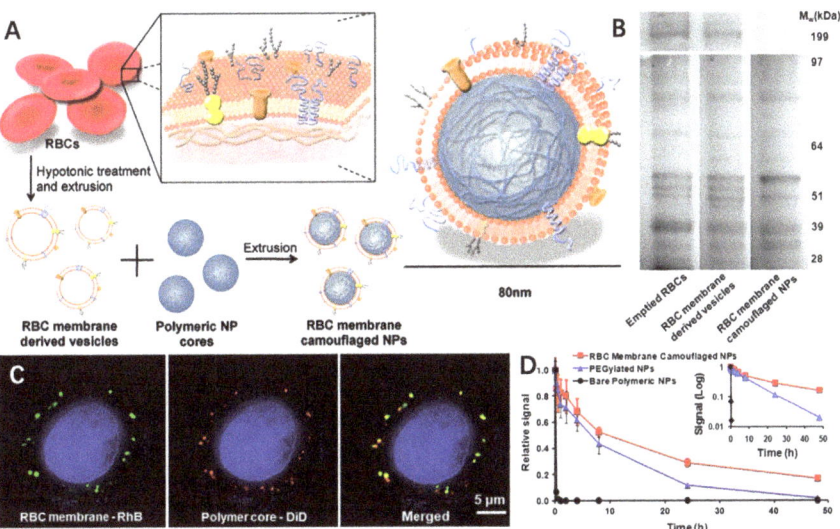

Figure 3. (**A**) Synthetic route of RBC-NPs; (**B**) SDS-PAGE result of emptied RBCs, RBC membrane-derived vesicles and RBC membrane camouflaged NPs; (**C**) Scanning fluorescence microscopy images of colocalization of RBC membranes (marked with green rhodamine-DMPE dyes) and polymeric cores (marked with red DiD dyes) after being internalized by HeLa cells; (**D**) Comparison of systemic circulation time between RBC-NPs, PEGylated NPs and PLGA nanoparticles. Reproduced with permission [41]. Copyright 2011, National Academy of Sciences.

Alternatively, Shao et al. prepared a Janus-type polymeric micromotors (JPMs), composed of heparin (Hep) and chitosan (CHI), coated with RBC membrane [95]. This functional nanoparticle achieved efficient motion toward the thrombus in response to near-infrared (NIR) irradiation via thermal effects and could synergize with photothermal therapy for thrombus alleviation.

The nanoplatforms discussed above mainly utilize the biggest advantage of red blood cell membrane: biocompatibility and immune evasion. Commonly, RBC membranes are coated on drug-loaded PLGA nanoparticles to achieve better drug on-target delivery against cardiovascular diseases.

4.2.2. Platelet Membrane

Platelets are small anucleated blood cells engaged in the blood clotting process. Upon hemorrhage, platelets rapidly migrate to the damaged lesion to form a clot and prevent excessive bleeding. Platelets are the connectors between thrombosis, inflammation and atherosclerosis. When atherosclerotic plaque rupture, vascular injury and decelerated blood flow facilitate platelet activation and binding to the injured vascular wall, eventually leading to thrombus formation [96]. Nanoparticles coated with platelet membrane can exhibit many similar characteristics to platelets, for example, adherence to injured vasculature.

Inspired by this, Zhang et al. firstly developed platelet membrane coated PLGA nanoparticles, which exhibited selective adhesion to damaged human and rodent vasculature and MRSA252 [78]. These platelet membrane coated nanoformulations could be utilized to treat thrombus, arterial injuries and sepsis with appropriate loading agents in the inner PLGA core. For example, when dealing with thrombus, Wang et al. synthesized platelet membrane coated PLGA nanoparticles, loaded with lumbrokinase, a conventional anticoagulant agent (PNPs/LBK) [97]. As a result, PNP/LBK exhibits better thrombus targeting ability with lower hemorrhagic risks.

When thrombus occurs, insufficient blood flow lead to a hypoxic environment that promotes reactive oxygen species (ROS) generation and tissue damage in the lesion site. Inspired by this, Zhao et al. recently developed H_2O_2-responsive platelet membrane cloaked argatroban-loaded polymeric nanoparticles (PNPArg) to treat thrombus [98]. In their strategy, the inner core, Poly(vanillyl alcohol-co-oxalate) (PVAX), is a H_2O_2 degradable polymer that can scavenge excessive ROS and could synergize with argatroban, an anticoagulant agent, showing great therapeutic effects toward various thrombotic diseases.

CMCNPs can also serve as novel diagnostic tools. Ma et al. prepared a platelet membrane coated nanoconstruct (PM-PAAO-UCNPs), which consists of upconversion nanoparticles and Ce6 photosensitizer for accurate localization and non-invasive photodynamic therapy of atherosclerosis [99]. In their study, the platelet membrane coating strategy effectively increased the binding affinity of nanoparticles to foam cells, the features of which include unregulated lipid metabolism, and play a central role throughout the disease stages. Near-infrared light was then applied to induce ROS-mediated apoptosis and regulated metabolism of foam cells to treat atherosclerosis.

Apart from targeting vascular endothelial cells and foam cells, platelets also exhibit binding affinity towards activated neutrophils. During acute ischemic stroke (AIS), neutrophils migrate into cerebral ischemic regions with the aid of platelets. Recruited neutrophils release reactive oxygen species, which are the prime cause of reperfusion injury following AIS [100,101]. Studies have shown potential curative benefits through alleviating the infiltration of neutrophils [102]. Inspired by these findings, Tang et al. innovatively constructed a platelet membrane coated PLGA nanoplatform with superparamagnetic iron oxide nanoparticles and piceatannol loaded (PTNPs) (Figure 4A) [103]. In their study, the coated platelet membranes facilitated binding between nanoparticles and neutrophils through the recognition of P-selectin (platelet) and PSGL-1 (neutrophil). The internalized nanoconstructs then released piceatannol, which alleviated neutrophils' infiltrations in the cerebral ischemic regions (Figure 4B). As a result, PTNPs significantly decreased the infarct volume of mice by approximately 26.2% compared with the group treated with PLGA nanoparticles containing piceatannol and superparamagnetic iron oxide.

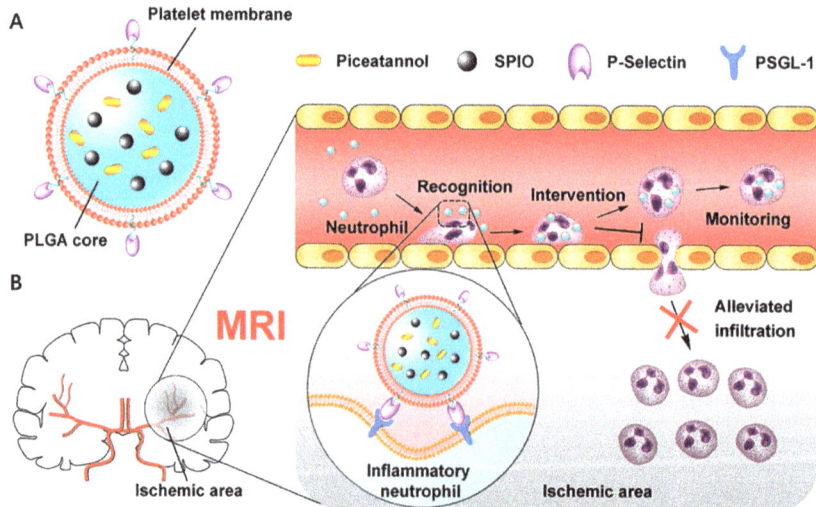

Figure 4. (**A**) Structure of platelet membrane coated PLGA nanoparticle; (**B**) Schematic diagram of therapeutic mechanism. Platelet membrane coated nanoparticles can straightly target the inflammatory neutrophils and take effect through releasing piceatannol to block neutrophils' infiltration. Reproduced with permission [85]. Copyright 2019, American Chemical Society.

Overall, platelet membrane coated nanoparticles have been extensively researched for thrombus, injured vessels and immune cell targeting to achieve higher on-target payload delivery and lower off-target side effects.

4.2.3. Macrophage Membrane

Macrophages are specialized cells responsible for the detection, phagocytosis and destruction of "invaders". Recent reviews have discovered the central role of macrophages in various cardiovascular-related processes including atherosclerotic coronary artery, post myocardial infarction remodeling and cardiac regeneration [104,105]. The macrophage membrane coating strategy is extensively applied to elevate tumor targeting ability through the driving force of CCR2-CCL2 axis, which could also be used to target inflammatory lesion sites [106,107].

Inspired by this, Gao et al. successfully utilized macrophage-derived membranes to coat nanoparticles and achieved enhanced therapeutic efficacy in atherosclerosis treatment [108]. In their study, they produced a ROS-responsive inner core to achieve burst release of the drug. The macrophage membrane coating strategy not only facilitates nanoparticles' evasion of the monocyte phagocyte system (MPS) but also helps targeted delivery to the lesion, where the inner drug is rapidly released due to the oxidative environment of atherosclerosis. In addition, macrophage membranes can sequester proinflammatory cytokines, which could restrict local inflammation. A combination of pharmacotherapy and inflammatory cytokine clearance can significantly improve the therapeutic efficacy against atherosclerosis. Utilizing macrophage membranes' intrinsic tendency toward atherosclerotic plaque, Wang et al. similarly constructed a macrophage membrane coated PLGA nanoplatform with anti-inflammation agent Rapamycin (RAP) loaded [109]. As a result, such nanoplatform exhibited outstanding therapeutic efficacy, in which lipid deposition in plaques were reduced from 36.45% to 17.41%, which was superior to free RAP group (from 36.45% to 31.54%).

Additionally, applying cytokine neutralization strategy, Xue et al. innovatively constructed a macrophage membrane enveloped NPs encapsulating anti-myocardial infarction (MI) agent miR-199a-3 ($MMNP_{miR199a-3p}$) to manage MI [110]. In the study, they bioengineered macrophages to achieve enhanced expression of IL-1βR, IL-6R and TNF-αR. As a result, $MMNP_{miR199a-3p}$ exhibits efficient uptake by myocardial cells and effective inhibition of inflammatory response through inflammatory cytokines neutralization.

Conclusively, inflammatory lesion site targeting ability and cytokine neutralization capacity are the most common usage of macrophage membrane in treating CVDs.

4.2.4. Neutrophil Membrane

As mentioned above, neutrophils can sense and move to the inflammatory body site. Such inflammatory chemotaxis capability has been exploited to enhance drug on-target delivery. For example, Xue et al. achieved effective delivery of paclitaxel (PTX)-contained liposomes to the inflamed post-resection lesion sites mediated by neutrophils, resulting in suppressed glioma reoccurrence [111]. In addition, the feasibility of utilizing neutrophil-derived membranes to target the inflamed lesion has also been proven in rheumatoid arthritis [112].

At the inflamed lesion site, neutrophils are activated and subsequently release reactive oxygen species, bioactive lipid mediators and neutrophils extracellular traps (NETs), which induce inflammatory damage. Many cardiovascular therapies are based on targeting neutrophils, either through blocking neutrophils' infiltration or preventing NET-driven inflammation [39].

Inspired by this, Dong et al. developed neutrophil membrane-derived nanovesicles containing Resolvin D2 (RvD2), an anti-inflammation agent, to treat postischemic stroke brain injury through inhibiting endothelial activation, cytokine release and the infiltration of neutrophils into the cerebral ischemic lesion [113].

In addition, Feng et al. also successfully constructed a neutrophil-mimic membrane coated mesoporous Prussian blue nanozyme (MPBzyme@NCM) (Figure 5A) [114]. In their study, MPBzyme@NCM exhibits active targeting ability to the inflamed brain microvascular endothelial cells, where nanoparticles are then phagocytosed by microglia and subsequently scavenge ROS through MPBzyme. As a result, this nanoplatform can promote microglia polarizing to M2 and reduce the neutrophils recruitment (Figure 5B), exhibiting prospective therapeutic efficacy against ischemic stroke.

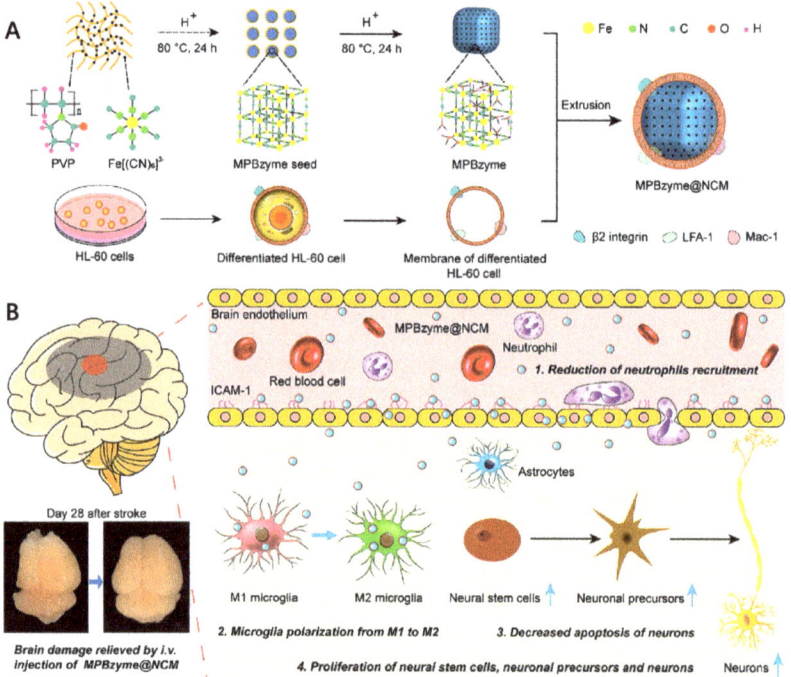

Figure 5. (**A**) Schematic structure of neutrophil-mimic membrane coated mesoporous Prussian blue nanozyme (MPBzyme@NCM); (**B**) Schematic diagram of the therapeutic mechanism. Combination of reduction of neutrophils' recruitment, microglia polarization from M1 to M2, decreased apoptosis of neurons and proliferation of neural stem cells, neuronal precursors and neurons explain the therapeutic efficacy of MPBzyme@NCM. Reproduced with permission [114]. Copyright 2021, American Chemical Society.

In conclusion, the mainstream usage of neutrophil membrane against CVDs still focused on its inflammatory-lesion targeting ability. Further research is needed to explore other biomedical applications of neutrophil-derived membranes, such as cytokine neutralization.

4.2.5. Stem Cell Membrane

The ischemic tissue-directed homing ability of mesenchymal stem cells has been reported. This process is mediated by the interaction of chemokine receptors on the surface of neural stem cells (NSCs) and their ligands enriched in the ischemic microenvironment such as SDF-1/CXCR4 axis [115,116]. Bose et al. first bioengineered human adipose-derived stem cells (hASCs) through mRNA vector transduction to overexpress CXCR4 [117]. This engineered stem cell membranes were then coated on the PLGA nanoparticles with vascular endothelial growth factor (VEGF) loaded to achieve better endothelial cell barrier penetration and increase retention time in ischemic tissues. As a result, this nanoplatform significantly improved therapeutic outcomes, achieving a lower risk of limb loss (17%) compared with the untreated group (83%).

To further improve the targeting ability, Kim et al. recently developed mesenchymal stem cell (MSC)-derived magnetic extracellular nanovesicles to treat ischemic stroke [118]. In their study, iron oxide nanoparticles were first co-incubated with MSC to elevate its expression of therapeutic growth factor. The whole MSCs were then extruded through serial membrane filters and purified to obtain magnetic nanovesicles (MNV). Overall, MNV enhanced lesion targeting ability through magnetic attraction and improved therapeutic efficacy against ischemic stroke.

5. Conclusions and Prospects

Ever since RBC membrane coating technology was first reported, countless investigations have been implemented to explore its therapeutic and diagnostic potential, for example in cancer therapy [119,120]. As mentioned in this review, various cell membranes are applied to prolong circulation time and endow nanoparticles with active targeting properties and inflammatory cytokines neutralization activity to treat CVDs (related studies have been integrated in Table 3).

However, we still lack a basic understanding of complex cell membrane properties. An inappropriate selection of blood type induces hemolysis during blood transfusion, which is attributed to the activation of the host immune system [121]. Therefore, autologous cells should be taken into prior consideration. Current studies on CMCNPs' biomedical applications remain at the laboratory research stage, as most studies have been carried out in mice. With no current clinical usage of CMCNPs, investigations on their biosafety need to be implemented to accelerate their clinical translation.

Apart from biosafety issues, comprehensive studies on pharmacokinetics and cellular uptake of small molecule loaded CMCNPs need to be implemented. As various cell membranes and inner nanoparticles are involved in the synthetic procedure of CMCNPs, the impacts of membrane types and inner nanoparticles' physical and chemical properties on the drug release ability of small molecules and cellular uptake of CMCNPs should be investigated extensively to facilitate their clinical translation.

The feasibility of large-scale production of CMCNPs is another barrier hindering their clinical translation. As aforementioned, membrane extrusion and sonication baths are two major routes to synthesize CMCNPs. However, these two approaches have distinctive strengths and weakness. For example, membrane extrusion is characterized with high uniformity but low-production efficiency, while the sonication method has contrary results. A better synthetic route is needed to overcome this obstacle.

Table 3. Cell membrane coated nanomedicine applied in treating cardiovascular diseases.

Target Disease	Structure (Membrane/Inner Core)	Membrane Source	Efficacy	Ref.
Atherosclerosis	RBC/PLGA	C57BL/6 Mice	(1) Enhanced accumulation in atherosclerotic plaques (2) Higher drug on-target release	[94]
	Platelet/UCNP	Healthy ApoE$^{-/-}$ Mice	(1) Specific targeting to foam cells (2) Photodynamic therapy induced apoptosis and regulated lipid metabolism	[99]
	Platelet/PLGA	Human Type O$^-$ Blood	(1) Avoid severe systematic toxicity of rapamycin (2) Enhanced 4.98-fold greater radiant efficiency than control nanoparticle group	[122]
	Macrophage/ROS-responsive core	RAW264.7 Cells	(1) Avoid immune clearance (2) ROS-responsive drug release (3) Inflammatory cytokine sequestration	[108]
	Macrophage/PLGA	RAW264.7 Cells	(1) Effectively inhibit phagocytosis by macrophages (2) Target and accumulate in atherosclerotic lesion	[109]

Table 3. Cont.

Target Disease	Structure (Membrane/Inner Core)	Membrane Source	Efficacy	Ref.
Thrombus	RBC/Janus-type NPs	Balb/c, Male	(1) Achieve movement through self-thermophoresis effect (2) RBC Membrane facilitate efficient movement in relevant biological environment	[95]
	Platelet/PLGA	ICR Mice	(1) Affinity between platelet membrane and thrombus (2) Lower the risks of adverse effect on the function of coagulation system	[97]
	Platelet/H_2O_2-degradable NPs	Human Type O$^-$ Blood	(1) Thrombus homing ability of platelet membrane (2) H_2O_2 scavenging ability of inner polymer core (3) H_2O_2 responsive drug release ability	[98]
Ischemic myocardium	RBC/Mesoporous iron NPs	Male Sprague Dawley Rats	(1) Excellent biocompatibility (2) Extended circulatory time (3) Controlled-release of H_2S	[123]
	Macrophage/miR$_{199a-3p}$	RAW264.7 Cells	(1) Inflammatory cytokine sequestration (2) Gene delivery	[110]
	Platelet/IONP	C57BL/6 Mice	(1) Specific targeting to inflammatory neutrophils (2) Alleviate infiltrations of neutrophils into hypoxic lesion (3) Disease stage monitoring and nanoparticles localization through MRI	[103]
Ischemic stroke	Platelet/γ-Fe_2O_3 magnetic NPs	Blood Center	(1) Combination targeting ability of platelet membrane and magnetic forces (2) Disease stage monitoring and nanoparticles localization through MRI	[124]
	Neutrophil/MPBzyme	HL-60 Cells	(1) Reduction of neutrophils' recruitment (2) Microglia polarization from M1 to M2 (3) Decreased apoptosis of neurons (4) Facilitate neuronal cells proliferation	[114]
	Stem cell/PLGA	C57BL/6 Mice	(1) Specific targeting ability toward ischemic microenvironment via stem cell membrane coating (2) Significantly augmented the efficacy of glyburide, an antiedema agent, for stroke treatment	[125]
Hindlimb ischemia	Stem cell/PLGA	Patients	(1) Bioengineered stem cell membrane coating for improved ischemic lesion targeting ability (2) Avoid macrophages phagocytosis	[117]
	Stem cell/IONP	Human Bone Marrow	(1) Stem cell preincubated with IONPs to elevate expression of therapeutic factors (2) Magnetic navigation improved the ischemic-lesion targeting	[118]

On the other hand, challenges and opportunities coexist in this field. Many alternative membrane options are under investigation, such as cancer cells [66,87], bacteria [89,90] and even hybrid cell membrane vesicles [89,126]. For example, Gu et al. successfully fabricated "Nano-Ag@erythrosome" nanocomplexes by fusing red blood cell membranes and cancer cell membranes [127]. Such nanocomplexes can effectively target the spleen due to the property of senescent red blood cell membrane, and induce antigen presentation on antigen presenting cells (APCs) to activate an antitumor immune response. Further research may well grasp this strategy and further modify this method by adjusting the adding ratio of different membrane sources to achieve elevated targeting efficiency and improved therapeutic efficacy against cardiovascular diseases [128].

Furthermore, recent research has reported a selective organ targeting (SORT) system for specific tissue mRNA delivery by introducing different SORT lipid into lipid nanoparticles through a bottom-up chemical synthesis method [129]. A combination of bottom-up and top-down CMCNPs synthesizing strategies exhibits great promise in extending their biofunctions and broadening their biomedical applications. Apart from this, lipid insertion, metabolic substrates engineering and genetic modification are other conventional membrane engineering methods, which also exhibit promise to extend the biofunctions of the derived cell membranes and have already been summarized extensively elsewhere [130–133]. In general, these abovementioned measurements, which aim to expand the biomedical application of CMCNPs, are all based on membrane engineering. The appropriate combination of inner functional nanoparticles with selected and modified outer-membranes will significantly enhance the therapeutic efficacies of CMCNPs. Overall, more innovative strategies will be explored in the future to unlock a new stage for cell membrane coated nanoparticles to treat cardiovascular diseases.

Author Contributions: Conceptualization, C.Z., J.S. and Q.W.; methodology, C.Z. and Z.J.; validation, C.Z. and Q.W.; investigation, C.Z. and J.M.; writing—original draft preparation, C.Z. and J.M.; writing—review and editing, C.Z. and J.M.; supervision, C.Z., J.S. and Q.W.; funding acquisition, Q.W. All authors have read and agreed to the published version of the manuscript.

Funding: This research was funded by National Natural Science Foundation of China (81800442).

Institutional Review Board Statement: Not applicable.

Informed Consent Statement: Not applicable.

Data Availability Statement: Not applicable.

Acknowledgments: The authors are grateful for grants received from the National Natural Science Foundation.

Conflicts of Interest: The authors declare that they have no known competing financial interests or personal relationships that could have appeared to influence the work reported in this paper.

Sample Availability: Samples of the compounds are not available from the authors.

References

1. Wang, H.; Naghavi, M.; Allen, C.; Barber, R.M.; Bhutta, Z.A.; Carter, A.; Casey, D.C.; Charlson, F.J.; Chen, A.Z.; Coates, M.M.; et al. Global, regional, and national life expectancy, all-cause mortality, and cause-specific mortality for 249 causes of death, 1980–2015: A systematic analysis for the global burden of disease study 2015. *Lancet* **2016**, *388*, 1459–1544. [CrossRef]
2. Zhou, M.; Wang, H.; Zhu, J.; Chen, W.; Wang, L.; Liu, S.; Li, Y.; Wang, L.; Liu, Y.; Yin, P.; et al. Cause-specific mortality for 240 causes in china during 1990–2013: A systematic subnational analysis for the global burden of disease study 2013. *Lancet* **2016**, *387*, 251–272. [CrossRef]
3. Makaryus, J.; Halperin, J.; Lau, J. Oral anticoagulants in the management of venous thromboembolism. *Nat. Rev. Cardiol.* **2013**, *10*, 397–409. [CrossRef] [PubMed]
4. Michelson, A.D. Antiplatelet therapies for the treatment of cardiovascular disease. *Nat. Rev. Drug Discov.* **2010**, *9*, 154–169. [CrossRef]
5. Lansberg, M.G.; O'Donnell, M.J.; Khatri, P.; Lang, E.S.; Nguyen-Huynh, M.N.; Schwartz, N.E.; Sonnenberg, F.A.; Schulman, S.; Vandvik, P.O.; Spencer, F.A.; et al. Antithrombotic and thrombolytic therapy for ischemic stroke: Antithrombotic therapy and prevention of thrombosis, 9th ed: American College of Chest Physicians Evidence-Based Clinical Practice Guidelines. *Chest* **2012**, *141* (Suppl. S2), e601S–e636S. [CrossRef]
6. Adhyaru, B.B.; Jacobson, T.A. Safety and efficacy of statin therapy. *Nat. Rev. Cardiol.* **2018**, *15*, 757–769. [CrossRef] [PubMed]
7. Cappelletto, A.; Zacchigna, S. Cardiac revascularization: State of the art and perspectives. *Vasc. Biol.* **2019**, *1*, H47–H51. [CrossRef]
8. Byrne, R.A.; Joner, M.; Alfonso, F.; Kastrati, A. Drug-coated balloon therapy in coronary and peripheral artery disease. *Nat. Rev. Cardiol.* **2014**, *11*, 13–23. [CrossRef]
9. McKavanagh, P.; Zawadowski, G.; Ahmed, N.; Kutryk, M. The evolution of coronary stents. *Expert Rev. Cardiovasc. Ther.* **2018**, *16*, 219–228. [CrossRef] [PubMed]

10. Bansilal, S.; Castellano, J.M.; Fuster, V. Global burden of CVD: Focus on secondary prevention of cardiovascular disease. *Int. J. Cardiol.* **2015**, *201*, S1–S7. [CrossRef]
11. Tersalvi, G.; Biasco, L.; Cioffi, G.M.; Pedrazzini, G. Acute coronary syndrome, antiplatelet therapy, and bleeding: A clinical perspective. *JCM* **2020**, *9*, 2064. [CrossRef] [PubMed]
12. Mohebbi, N.; Shalviri, G.; Salarifar, M.; Salamzadeh, J.; Gholami, K. Adverse drug reactions induced by cardiovascular drugs in cardiovascular care unit patients: Adverse drug reactions induced by cardiovascular drugs. *Pharmacoepidemiol. Drug Saf.* **2010**, *19*, 889–894. [CrossRef] [PubMed]
13. Oza, R.; Rundell, K.; Garcellano, M. Recurrent ischemic stroke: Strategies for prevention. *Am. Fam. Physician* **2017**, *96*, 436–440.
14. Dai, Y.; Ge, J. Clinical use of aspirin in treatment and prevention of cardiovascular disease. *Thrombosis* **2012**, *2012*, 245037. [CrossRef] [PubMed]
15. Guthrie, R. Review and management of side effects associated with antiplatelet therapy for prevention of recurrent cerebrovascular events. *Adv. Ther.* **2011**, *28*, 473–482. [CrossRef] [PubMed]
16. Mitchell, M.J.; Billingsley, M.M.; Haley, R.M.; Wechsler, M.E.; Peppas, N.A.; Langer, R. Engineering precision nanoparticles for drug delivery. *Nat. Rev. Drug Discov.* **2021**, *20*, 101–124. [CrossRef]
17. Gustafson, H.H.; Holt-Casper, D.; Grainger, D.W.; Ghandehari, H. Nanoparticle uptake: The phagocyte problem. *Nano Today* **2015**, *10*, 487–510. [CrossRef]
18. Fam, S.Y.; Chee, C.F.; Yong, C.Y.; Ho, K.L.; Mariatulqabtiah, A.R.; Tan, W.S. Stealth coating of nanoparticles in drug-delivery systems. *Nanomaterials* **2020**, *10*, 787. [CrossRef]
19. Knop, K.; Hoogenboom, R.; Fischer, D.; Schubert, U.S. Poly (Ethylene Glycol) in drug delivery: Pros and cons as well as potential alternatives. *Angew. Chem. Int. Ed.* **2010**, *49*, 6288–6308. [CrossRef]
20. Chen, Z.; Wang, Z.; Gu, Z. Bioinspired and biomimetic nanomedicines. *Acc. Chem. Res.* **2019**. [CrossRef]
21. Keto, J.; Ventola, H.; Jokelainen, J.; Linden, K.; Keinänen-Kiukaanniemi, S.; Timonen, M.; Ylisaukko-oja, T.; Auvinen, J. Cardiovascular disease risk factors in relation to smoking behaviour and history: A population-based cohort study. *Open Heart* **2016**, *3*, e000358. [CrossRef] [PubMed]
22. Fuchs, F.D.; Whelton, P.K. High blood pressure and cardiovascular disease. *Hypertension* **2020**, *75*, 285–292. [CrossRef]
23. Leon, B.M. Diabetes and cardiovascular disease: Epidemiology, biological mechanisms, treatment recommendations and future research. *WJD* **2015**, *6*, 1246. [CrossRef] [PubMed]
24. Rodgers, J.L.; Jones, J.; Bolleddu, S.I.; Vanthenapalli, S.; Rodgers, L.E.; Shah, K.; Karia, K.; Panguluri, S.K. cardiovascular risks associated with gender and aging. *JCDD* **2019**, *6*, 19. [CrossRef]
25. Valerio, L.; Peters, R.J.; Zwinderman, A.H.; Pinto-Sietsma, S. Association of family history with cardiovascular disease in hypertensive individuals in a multiethnic population. *JAHA* **2016**, *5*. [CrossRef]
26. Van Camp, G. Cardiovascular disease prevention. *Acta Clin. Belg.* **2014**, *69*, 407–411. [CrossRef]
27. Bentzon, J.F.; Otsuka, F.; Virmani, R.; Falk, E. Mechanisms of plaque formation and rupture. *Circ. Res.* **2014**, *114*, 1852–1866. [CrossRef]
28. Zhao, D.; Liu, J.; Wang, M.; Zhang, X.; Zhou, M. Epidemiology of cardiovascular disease in China: Current features and implications. *Nat. Rev. Cardiol.* **2019**, *16*, 203–212. [CrossRef]
29. Falk, E. Pathogenesis of atherosclerosis. *J. Am. Coll. Cardiol.* **2006**, *47*, C7–C12. [CrossRef]
30. Verna, L.; Ganda, C.; Stemerman, M.B. In vivo low-density lipoprotein exposure induces intercellular adhesion molecule-1 and vascular cell adhesion molecule-1 correlated with activator protein-1 expression. *ATVB* **2006**, *26*, 1344–1349. [CrossRef]
31. Moore, K.J.; Sheedy, F.J.; Fisher, E.A. Macrophages in atherosclerosis: A dynamic balance. *Nat. Rev. Immunol.* **2013**, *13*, 709–721. [CrossRef] [PubMed]
32. Shah, P.K. Mechanisms of plaque vulnerability and rupture. *J. Am. Coll. Cardiol.* **2003**, *41* (Suppl. S4), 15S–22S. [CrossRef]
33. Esmon, C.T. Basic mechanisms and pathogenesis of venous thrombosis. *Blood Rev.* **2009**, *23*, 225–229. [CrossRef]
34. Mackman, N. Triggers, targets and treatments for thrombosis. *Nature* **2008**, *451*, 914–918. [CrossRef]
35. Badimon, L.; Padró, T.; Vilahur, G. Atherosclerosis, platelets and thrombosis in acute ischaemic heart disease. *Eur. Heart J. Acute Cardiovasc. Care* **2012**, *1*, 60–74. [CrossRef] [PubMed]
36. Asada, Y.; Yamashita, A.; Sato, Y.; Hatakeyama, K. Thrombus formation and propagation in the onset of cardiovascular events. *J Atheroscler. Thromb.* **2018**, *25*, 653–664. [CrossRef] [PubMed]
37. Writing Group Members; Rosamond, W.; Flegal, K.; Furie, K.; Go, A.; Greenlund, K.; Haase, N.; Hailpern, S.M.; Ho, M.; Howard, V.; et al. Heart disease and stroke statistics—2008 update: A report from the american heart association statistics committee and stroke statistics subcommittee. *Circulation* **2008**, *117*. [CrossRef]
38. Lyaker, M.; Tulman, D.; Dimitrova, G.; Pin, R.; Papadimos, T. Arterial embolism. *Int. J. Crit. Illn. Inj. Sci.* **2013**, *3*, 77. [CrossRef]
39. Németh, T.; Sperandio, M.; Mócsai, A. Neutrophils as emerging therapeutic targets. *Nat. Rev. Drug Discov.* **2020**, *19*, 253–275. [CrossRef]
40. Chen, Q.; Wang, Q.; Zhu, J.; Xiao, Q.; Zhang, L. Reactive oxygen species: Key regulators in vascular health and diseases: ROS in vascular diseases. *Br. J. Pharmacol.* **2018**, *175*, 1279–1292. [CrossRef]
41. Bloom, B.S.; Banta, H.D.; Gross, P.F.; Peña-Mohr, J.; Sisk, J.E.; Stocking, B. The Swedish council on technology assessment in health care. *Int. J. Technol. Assess. Health Care* **1989**, *5*, 154–158. [CrossRef]

42. Nelson, A.J.; Ardissino, M.; Psaltis, P.J. Current approach to the diagnosis of atherosclerotic coronary artery disease: More questions than answers. *Ther. Adv. Chronic Dis.* **2019**, *10*, 204062231988481. [CrossRef] [PubMed]
43. Fung, V.; Graetz, I.; Reed, M.; Jaffe, M.G. Patient-reported adherence to statin therapy, barriers to adherence, and perceptions of cardiovascular risk. *PLoS ONE* **2018**, *13*, e0191817. [CrossRef]
44. Crowther, M.A.; Warkentin, T.E. Bleeding risk and the management of bleeding complications in patients undergoing anticoagulant therapy: Focus on new anticoagulant agents. *Blood* **2008**, *111*, 4871–4879. [CrossRef]
45. Wolberg, A.S.; Rosendaal, F.R.; Weitz, J.I.; Jaffer, I.H.; Agnelli, G.; Baglin, T.; Mackman, N. Venous thrombosis. *Nat. Rev. Dis. Primers* **2015**, *1*, 15006. [CrossRef]
46. Bagheri, M.; Mohammadi, M.; Steele, T.W.; Ramezani, M. Nanomaterial coatings applied on stent surfaces. *Nanomedicine* **2016**, *11*, 1309–1326. [CrossRef]
47. Patra, J.K.; Das, G.; Fraceto, L.F.; Campos, E.V.R.; del Pilar Rodriguez-Torres, M.; Acosta-Torres, L.S.; Diaz-Torres, L.A.; Grillo, R.; Swamy, M.K.; Sharma, S.; et al. Nano based drug delivery systems: Recent developments and future prospects. *J. Nanobiotechnol.* **2018**, *16*, 71. [CrossRef]
48. Liu, Y.; Wang, W.; Acharya, G.; Shim, Y.-B.; Choe, E.S.; Lee, C.H. Advanced stent coating for drug delivery and in vivo biocompatibility. *J. Nanopart. Res.* **2013**, *15*, 1962. [CrossRef]
49. Palekar, R.U.; Jallouk, A.P.; Lanza, G.M.; Pan, H.; Wickline, S.A. Molecular imaging of atherosclerosis with nanoparticle-based fluorinated MRI contrast agents. *Nanomedicine* **2015**, *10*, 1817–1832. [CrossRef]
50. Qiao, R.; Qiao, H.; Zhang, Y.; Wang, Y.; Chi, C.; Tian, J.; Zhang, L.; Cao, F.; Gao, M. Molecular imaging of vulnerable atherosclerotic plaques in vivo with osteopontin-specific upconversion nanoprobes. *ACS Nano* **2017**, *11*, 1816–1825. [CrossRef]
51. Morishige, K.; Kacher, D.F.; Libby, P.; Josephson, L.; Ganz, P.; Weissleder, R.; Aikawa, M. High-resolution magnetic resonance imaging enhanced with superparamagnetic nanoparticles measures macrophage burden in atherosclerosis. *Circulation* **2010**, *122*, 1707–1715. [CrossRef] [PubMed]
52. Sparrow, C.P.; Burton, C.A.; Hernandez, M.; Mundt, S.; Hassing, H.; Patel, S.; Rosa, R.; Hermanowski-Vosatka, A.; Wang, P.R.; Zhang, D.; et al. Simvastatin has anti-inflammatory and antiatherosclerotic activities independent of plasma cholesterol lowering. *Arterioscler. Thromb. Vasc. Biol.* **2001**, *21*, 115–121. [CrossRef] [PubMed]
53. Armitage, J. The safety of statins in clinical practice. *Lancet* **2007**, *370*, 1781–1790. [CrossRef]
54. Kim, H.; Kumar, S.; Kang, D.-W.; Jo, H.; Park, J.-H. Affinity-driven design of cargo-switching nanoparticles to leverage a cholesterol-rich microenvironment for atherosclerosis therapy. *ACS Nano* **2020**, *14*, 6519–6531. [CrossRef] [PubMed]
55. Flores, A.M.; Hosseini-Nassab, N.; Jarr, K.-U.; Ye, J.; Zhu, X.; Wirka, R.; Koh, A.L.; Tsantilas, P.; Wang, Y.; Nanda, V.; et al. Pro-efferocytic nanoparticles are specifically taken up by lesional macrophages and prevent atherosclerosis. *Nat. Nanotechnol.* **2020**, *15*, 154–161. [CrossRef]
56. Marsh, J.; Senpan, A.; Hu, G.; Scott, M.; Gaffney, P.; Wickline, S.; Lanza, G. Fibrin-targeted perfluorocarbon nanoparticles for targeted thrombolysis. *Nanomedicine* **2007**, *2*, 533–543. [CrossRef]
57. Spicer, C.D.; Jumeaux, C.; Gupta, B.; Stevens, M.M. Peptide and protein nanoparticle conjugates: Versatile platforms for biomedical applications. *Chem. Soc. Rev.* **2018**, *47*, 3574–3620. [CrossRef]
58. Hu, C.-M.J.; Zhang, L.; Aryal, S.; Cheung, C.; Fang, R.H.; Zhang, L. Erythrocyte membrane-camouflaged polymeric nanoparticles as a biomimetic delivery platform. *Proc. Natl. Acad. Sci. USA* **2011**, *108*, 10980–10985. [CrossRef]
59. Zou, S.; Wang, B.; Wang, C.; Wang, Q.; Zhang, L. Cell membrane-coated nanoparticles: Research advances. *Nanomedicine* **2020**, *15*, 625–641. [CrossRef]
60. Simons, K.; Ikonen, E. Functional rafts in cell membranes. *Nature* **1997**, *387*, 569–572. [CrossRef] [PubMed]
61. Zhai, Y.; Su, J.; Ran, W.; Zhang, P.; Yin, Q.; Zhang, Z.; Yu, H.; Li, Y. Preparation and application of cell membrane-camouflaged nanoparticles for cancer therapy. *Theranostics* **2017**, *7*, 2575–2592. [CrossRef]
62. Cao, H.; Dan, Z.; He, X.; Zhang, Z.; Yu, H.; Yin, Q.; Li, Y. Liposomes coated with isolated macrophage membrane can target lung metastasis of breast cancer. *ACS Nano* **2016**, *10*, 7738–7748. [CrossRef] [PubMed]
63. Liu, X.; Zhang, L.; Jiang, W.; Yang, Z.; Gan, Z.; Yu, C.; Tao, R.; Chen, H. In vitro and in vivo evaluation of liposomes modified with polypeptides and red cell membrane as a novel drug delivery system for myocardium targeting. *Drug Deliv.* **2020**, *27*, 599–606. [CrossRef] [PubMed]
64. Hu, X.; Li, H.; Huang, X.; Zhu, Z.; Zhu, H.; Gao, Y.; Zhu, Z.; Chen, H. Cell membrane-coated gold nanoparticles for apoptosis imaging in living cells based on fluorescent determination. *Microchim. Acta* **2020**, *187*, 175. [CrossRef] [PubMed]
65. Peng, H.; Xu, Z.; Wang, Y.; Feng, N.; Yang, W.; Tang, J. Biomimetic mesoporous silica nanoparticles for enhanced blood circulation and cancer therapy. *ACS Appl. Bio Mater.* **2020**, *3*, 7849–7857. [CrossRef]
66. Cai, D.; Liu, L.; Han, C.; Ma, X.; Qian, J.; Zhou, J.; Zhu, W. Cancer cell membrane-coated mesoporous silica loaded with superparamagnetic ferroferric oxide and paclitaxel for the combination of chemo/magnetocaloric therapy on MDA-MB-231 cells. *Sci. Rep.* **2019**, *9*, 14475. [CrossRef]
67. Meng, Q.-F.; Rao, L.; Zan, M.; Chen, M.; Yu, G.-T.; Wei, X.; Wu, Z.; Sun, Y.; Guo, S.-S.; Zhao, X.-Z.; et al. Macrophage membrane-coated iron oxide nanoparticles for enhanced photothermal tumor therapy. *Nanotechnology* **2018**, *29*, 134004. [CrossRef]
68. Sherwood, J.; Sowell, J.; Beyer, N.; Irvin, J.; Stephen, C.; Antone, A.J.; Bao, Y.; Ciesla, L.M. Cell-membrane coated iron oxide nanoparticles for isolation and specific identification of drug leads from complex matrices. *Nanoscale* **2019**, *11*, 6352–6359. [CrossRef]

69. Liang, X.; Ye, X.; Wang, C.; Xing, C.; Miao, Q.; Xie, Z.; Chen, X.; Zhang, X.; Zhang, H.; Mei, L. Photothermal cancer immunotherapy by erythrocyte membrane-coated black phosphorus formulation. *J. Control. Release* **2019**, *296*, 150–161. [CrossRef] [PubMed]
70. Su, Y.; Wang, T.; Su, Y.; Li, M.; Zhou, J.; Zhang, W.; Wang, W. A neutrophil membrane-functionalized black phosphorus riding inflammatory signal for positive feedback and multimode cancer therapy. *Mater. Horiz.* **2020**, *7*, 574–585. [CrossRef]
71. Shang, Y.; Wang, Q.; Wu, B.; Zhao, Q.; Li, J.; Huang, X.; Chen, W.; Gui, R. Platelet-membrane-camouflaged black phosphorus quantum dots enhance anticancer effect mediated by apoptosis and autophagy. *ACS Appl. Mater. Interfaces* **2019**, *11*, 28254–28266. [CrossRef]
72. Ben-Akiva, E.; Meyer, R.A.; Yu, H.; Smith, J.T.; Pardoll, D.M.; Green, J.J. Biomimetic anisotropic polymeric nanoparticles coated with red blood cell membranes for enhanced circulation and toxin removal. *Sci. Adv.* **2020**, *6*, eaay9035. [CrossRef]
73. Zhang, L.; Xie, X.; Liu, D.; Xu, Z.P.; Liu, R. Efficient co-delivery of neo-epitopes using dispersion-stable layered double hydroxide nanoparticles for enhanced melanoma immunotherapy. *Biomaterials* **2018**, *174*, 54–66. [CrossRef] [PubMed]
74. Wang, Q.; Shen, J.; Mo, E.; Zhang, H.; Wang, J.; Hu, X.; Zhou, J.; Bai, H.; Tang, G. A versatile ultrafine and super-absorptive H^+-modified montmorillonite: Application for metabolic syndrome intervention and gastric mucosal protection. *Biomater. Sci.* **2020**, *8*, 3370–3380. [CrossRef] [PubMed]
75. Zhang, L.-X.; Hu, J.; Jia, Y.-B.; Liu, R.-T.; Cai, T.; Xu, Z.P. Two-dimensional layered double hydroxide nanoadjuvant: Recent progress and future direction. *Nanoscale* **2021**. [CrossRef]
76. Li, M.; Fang, H.; Liu, Q.; Gai, Y.; Yuan, L.; Wang, S.; Li, H.; Hou, Y.; Gao, M.; Lan, X. Red blood cell membrane-coated upconversion nanoparticles for pretargeted multimodality imaging of triple-negative breast cancer. *Biomater. Sci.* **2020**, *8*, 1802–1814. [CrossRef]
77. Xu, L.; Wu, S.; Wang, J. Cancer cell membrane—Coated nanocarriers for homologous target inhibiting the growth of hepatocellular carcinoma. *J. Bioact. Compat. Polym.* **2019**, *34*, 58–71. [CrossRef]
78. Hu, C.-M.J.; Fang, R.H.; Wang, K.-C.; Luk, B.T.; Thamphiwatana, S.; Dehaini, D.; Nguyen, P.; Angsantikul, P.; Wen, C.H.; Kroll, A.V.; et al. Nanoparticle biointerfacing by platelet membrane cloaking. *Nature* **2015**, *526*, 118–121. [CrossRef]
79. Pernow, J.; Mahdi, A.; Yang, J.; Zhou, Z. Red blood cell dysfunction: A new player in cardiovascular disease. *Cardiovasc. Res.* **2019**, *115*, 1596–1605. [CrossRef]
80. Gregg, D.; Goldschmidt-Clermont, P.J. Platelets and cardiovascular disease. *Circulation* **2003**, *108*. [CrossRef]
81. Silvestre-Roig, C.; Braster, Q.; Ortega-Gomez, A.; Soehnlein, O. Neutrophils as regulators of cardiovascular inflammation. *Nat. Rev. Cardiol.* **2020**, *17*, 327–340. [CrossRef]
82. Xia, Q.; Zhang, Y.; Li, Z.; Hou, X.; Feng, N. Red blood cell membrane-camouflaged nanoparticles: A novel drug delivery system for antitumor application. *Acta Pharm. Sin. B* **2019**, *9*, 675–689. [CrossRef]
83. Wang, S.; Duan, Y.; Zhang, Q.; Komarla, A.; Gong, H.; Gao, W.; Zhang, L. Drug targeting via platelet membrane—Coated nanoparticles. *Small Struct.* **2020**, *1*, 2000018. [CrossRef] [PubMed]
84. Thamphiwatana, S.; Angsantikul, P.; Escajadillo, T.; Zhang, Q.; Olson, J.; Luk, B.T.; Zhang, S.; Fang, R.H.; Gao, W.; Nizet, V.; et al. Macrophage-like nanoparticles concurrently absorbing endotoxins and proinflammatory cytokines for sepsis management. *Proc. Natl. Acad. Sci. USA* **2017**, *114*, 11488–11493. [CrossRef] [PubMed]
85. Peng, R.; Ji, H.; Jin, L.; Lin, S.; Huang, Y.; Xu, K.; Yang, Q.; Sun, D.; Wu, W. Macrophage-based therapies for atherosclerosis management. *J. Immunol. Res.* **2020**, *2020*, 1–11. [CrossRef] [PubMed]
86. Chu, D.; Dong, X.; Shi, X.; Zhang, C.; Wang, Z. Neutrophil-based drug delivery systems. *Adv. Mater.* **2018**, *30*, 1706245. [CrossRef] [PubMed]
87. Fang, R.H.; Hu, C.-M.J.; Luk, B.T.; Gao, W.; Copp, J.A.; Tai, Y.; O'Connor, D.E.; Zhang, L. Cancer cell membrane-coated nanoparticles for anticancer vaccination and drug delivery. *Nano Lett.* **2014**, *14*, 2181–2188. [CrossRef]
88. Wang, M.; Xin, Y.; Cao, H.; Li, W.; Hua, Y.; Webster, T.J.; Zhang, C.; Tang, W.; Liu, Z. Recent advances in mesenchymal stem cell membrane-coated nanoparticles for enhanced drug delivery. *Biomater. Sci.* **2021**, *9*, 1088–1103. [CrossRef]
89. Wang, D.; Liu, C.; You, S.; Zhang, K.; Li, M.; Cao, Y.; Wang, C.; Dong, H.; Zhang, X. Bacterial vesicle-cancer cell hybrid membrane-coated nanoparticles for tumor specific immune activation and photothermal therapy. *ACS Appl. Mater. Interfaces* **2020**, *12*, 41138–41147. [CrossRef] [PubMed]
90. Zhang, Y.; Chen, Y.; Lo, C.; Zhuang, J.; Angsantikul, P.; Zhang, Q.; Wei, X.; Zhou, Z.; Obonyo, M.; Fang, R.H.; et al. Inhibition of pathogen adhesion by bacterial outer membrane-coated nanoparticles. *Angew. Chem. Int. Ed.* **2019**, *58*, 11404–11408. [CrossRef]
91. Oldenborg, P.-A.; Zheleznyak, A.; Fang, Y.-F.; Lagenaur, C.F.; Gresham, H.D.; Lindberg, F.P. Role of CD47 as a marker of self on red blood cells. *Science* **2000**, *288*, 2051–2054. [CrossRef] [PubMed]
92. Hu, C.-M.J.; Fang, R.H.; Copp, J.; Luk, B.T.; Zhang, L. A biomimetic nanosponge that absorbs pore-forming toxins. *Nat. Nanotechnol.* **2013**, *8*, 336–340. [CrossRef] [PubMed]
93. Hu, C.-M.J.; Fang, R.H.; Luk, B.T.; Zhang, L. Nanoparticle-detained toxins for safe and effective vaccination. *Nat. Nanotechnol.* **2013**, *8*, 933–938. [CrossRef]
94. Wang, Y.; Zhang, K.; Qin, X.; Li, T.; Qiu, J.; Yin, T.; Huang, J.; McGinty, S.; Pontrelli, G.; Ren, J.; et al. Biomimetic nanotherapies: Red blood cell based core–shell structured nanocomplexes for atherosclerosis management. *Adv. Sci.* **2019**, *6*, 1900172. [CrossRef] [PubMed]
95. Shao, J.; Abdelghani, M.; Shen, G.; Cao, S.; Williams, D.S.; van Hest, J.C.M. Erythrocyte membrane modified janus polymeric motors for thrombus therapy. *ACS Nano* **2018**, *12*, 4877–4885. [CrossRef] [PubMed]

96. Van der Meijden, P.E.J.; Heemskerk, J.W.M. Platelet biology and functions: New concepts and clinical perspectives. *Nat. Rev. Cardiol.* **2019**, *16*, 166–179. [CrossRef]
97. Wang, S.; Wang, R.; Meng, N.; Guo, H.; Wu, S.; Wang, X.; Li, J.; Wang, H.; Jiang, K.; Xie, C.; et al. Platelet membrane-functionalized nanoparticles with improved targeting ability and lower hemorrhagic risk for thrombolysis therapy. *J. Control. Release* **2020**, *328*, 78–86. [CrossRef] [PubMed]
98. Zhao, Y.; Xie, R.; Yodsanit, N.; Ye, M.; Wang, Y.; Wang, B.; Guo, L.-W.; Kent, K.C.; Gong, S. Hydrogen peroxide-responsive platelet membrane-coated nanoparticles for thrombus therapy. *Biomater. Sci.* **2021**. [CrossRef]
99. Ma, Y.; Ma, Y.; Gao, M.; Han, Z.; Jiang, W.; Gu, Y.; Liu, Y. Platelet-mimicking therapeutic system for noninvasive mitigation of the progression of atherosclerotic plaques. *Adv. Sci.* **2021**, 2004128. [CrossRef]
100. Kolaczkowska, E.; Kubes, P. Neutrophil recruitment and function in health and inflammation. *Nat. Rev. Immunol.* **2013**, *13*, 159–175. [CrossRef]
101. Sreeramkumar, V.; Adrover, J.M.; Ballesteros, I.; Cuartero, M.I.; Rossaint, J.; Bilbao, I.; Nácher, M.; Pitaval, C.; Radovanovic, I.; Fukui, Y.; et al. Neutrophils scan for activated platelets to initiate inflammation. *Science* **2014**, *346*, 1234–1238. [CrossRef]
102. Schofield, Z.V.; Woodruff, T.M.; Halai, R.; Wu, M.C.-L.; Cooper, M.A. Neutrophils—A key component of ischemia-reperfusion injury. *Shock* **2013**, *40*, 463–470. [CrossRef]
103. Tang, C.; Wang, C.; Zhang, Y.; Xue, L.; Li, Y.; Ju, C.; Zhang, C. Recognition, intervention, and monitoring of neutrophils in acute ischemic stroke. *Nano Lett.* **2019**, *19*, 4470–4477. [CrossRef] [PubMed]
104. Khoury, M.K.; Yang, H.; Liu, B. Macrophage biology in cardiovascular diseases. *ATVB* **2021**, *41*. [CrossRef] [PubMed]
105. Yap, J.; Cabrera-Fuentes, H.A.; Irei, J.; Hausenloy, D.J.; Boisvert, W.A. Role of macrophages in cardioprotection. *Int. J. Mol. Sci.* **2019**, *20*, 2474. [CrossRef]
106. Lim, S.Y.; Yuzhalin, A.E.; Gordon-Weeks, A.N.; Muschel, R.J. Targeting the CCL2-CCR2 signaling axis in cancer metastasis. *Oncotarget* **2016**, *7*, 28697–28710. [CrossRef] [PubMed]
107. Zhao, H.; Li, L.; Zhang, J.; Zheng, C.; Ding, K.; Xiao, H.; Wang, L.; Zhang, Z. C–C Chemokine Ligand 2 (CCL2) recruits macrophage-membrane-camouflaged hollow bismuth selenide nanoparticles to facilitate photothermal sensitivity and inhibit lung metastasis of breast cancer. *ACS Appl. Mater. Interfaces* **2018**, *10*, 31124–31135. [CrossRef] [PubMed]
108. Gao, C.; Huang, Q.; Liu, C.; Kwong, C.H.T.; Yue, L.; Wan, J.-B.; Lee, S.M.Y.; Wang, R. Treatment of atherosclerosis by macrophage-biomimetic nanoparticles via targeted pharmacotherapy and sequestration of proinflammatory cytokines. *Nat. Commun.* **2020**, *11*, 2622. [CrossRef]
109. Wang, Y.; Zhang, K.; Li, T.; Maruf, A.; Qin, X.; Luo, L.; Zhong, Y.; Qiu, J.; McGinty, S.; Pontrelli, G.; et al. Macrophage membrane functionalized biomimetic nanoparticles for targeted anti-atherosclerosis applications. *Theranostics* **2021**, *11*, 164–180. [CrossRef] [PubMed]
110. Xue, Y.; Zeng, G.; Cheng, J.; Hu, J.; Zhang, M.; Li, Y. Engineered macrophage membrane-enveloped nanomedicine for ameliorating myocardial infarction in a mouse model. *Bioeng. Transl. Med.* **2020**. [CrossRef] [PubMed]
111. Xue, J.; Zhao, Z.; Zhang, L.; Xue, L.; Shen, S.; Wen, Y.; Wei, Z.; Wang, L.; Kong, L.; Sun, H.; et al. Neutrophil-mediated anticancer drug delivery for suppression of postoperative malignant glioma recurrence. *Nat. Nanotechnol.* **2017**, *12*, 692–700. [CrossRef]
112. Zhang, Q.; Dehaini, D.; Zhang, Y.; Zhou, J.; Chen, X.; Zhang, L.; Fang, R.H.; Gao, W.; Zhang, L. Neutrophil membrane-coated nanoparticles inhibit synovial inflammation and alleviate joint damage in inflammatory arthritis. *Nat. Nanotechnol.* **2018**, *13*, 1182–1190. [CrossRef] [PubMed]
113. Dong, X.; Gao, J.; Zhang, C.Y.; Hayworth, C.; Frank, M.; Wang, Z. Neutrophil membrane-derived nanovesicles alleviate inflammation to protect mouse brain injury from ischemic stroke. *ACS Nano* **2019**. [CrossRef]
114. Feng, L.; Dou, C.; Xia, Y.; Li, B.; Zhao, M.; Yu, P.; Zheng, Y.; El-Toni, A.M.; Atta, N.F.; Galal, A.; et al. Neutrophil-like cell-membrane-coated nanozyme therapy for ischemic brain damage and long-term neurological functional recovery. *ACS Nano* **2021**, *15*, 2263–2280. [CrossRef] [PubMed]
115. Yellowley, C. CXCL12/CXCR4 signaling and other recruitment and homing pathways in fracture repair. *BoneKEy Rep.* **2013**, *2*. [CrossRef]
116. Lee, S.-P.; Youn, S.-W.; Cho, H.-J.; Li, L.; Kim, T.-Y.; Yook, H.-S.; Chung, J.-W.; Hur, J.; Yoon, C.-H.; Park, K.-W.; et al. Integrin-linked kinase, a hypoxia-responsive molecule, controls postnatal vasculogenesis by recruitment of endothelial progenitor cells to ischemic tissue. *Circulation* **2006**, *114*, 150–159. [CrossRef] [PubMed]
117. Bose, R.J.C.; Kim, B.J.; Arai, Y.; Han, I.; Moon, J.J.; Paulmurugan, R.; Park, H.; Lee, S.-H. Bioengineered stem cell membrane functionalized nanocarriers for therapeutic targeting of severe hindlimb ischemia. *Biomaterials* **2018**, *185*, 360–370. [CrossRef] [PubMed]
118. Kim, H.Y.; Kim, T.J.; Kang, L.; Kim, Y.-J.; Kang, M.K.; Kim, J.; Ryu, J.H.; Hyeon, T.; Yoon, B.-W.; Ko, S.-B.; et al. Mesenchymal stem cell-derived magnetic extracellular nanovesicles for targeting and treatment of ischemic stroke. *Biomaterials* **2020**, *243*, 119942. [CrossRef]
119. Oroojalian, F.; Beygi, M.; Baradaran, B.; Mokhtarzadeh, A.; Shahbazi, M. Immune cell membrane-coated biomimetic nanoparticles for targeted cancer therapy. *Small* **2021**, *17*, 2006484. [CrossRef]
120. Jin, J.; Bhujwalla, Z.M. Biomimetic nanoparticles camouflaged in cancer cell membranes and their applications in cancer theranostics. *Front. Oncol.* **2020**, *9*, 1560. [CrossRef]
121. Strobel, E. Hemolytic transfusion reactions. *Transfus. Med. Hemother.* **2008**, *35*, 346–353. [CrossRef] [PubMed]

122. Song, Y.; Huang, Z.; Liu, X.; Pang, Z.; Chen, J.; Yang, H.; Zhang, N.; Cao, Z.; Liu, M.; Cao, J.; et al. Platelet membrane-coated nanoparticle-mediated targeting delivery of rapamycin blocks atherosclerotic plaque development and stabilizes plaque in apolipoprotein e-deficient (ApoE−/−) mice. *Nanomed. Nanotechnol. Biol. Med.* **2019**, *15*, 13–24. [CrossRef] [PubMed]
123. Huang, K.; Wen, S.; Wang, W.; Zhou, J.; Huang, J.; Wang, F.; Pang, L.; Wang, Y.; Sun, X. Erythrocyte membrane coated nanoparticle-based control releasing hydrogen sulfide system protects ischemic myocardium. *Nanomedicine* **2021**, *16*, 465–480. [CrossRef] [PubMed]
124. Li, M.; Li, J.; Chen, J.; Liu, Y.; Cheng, X.; Yang, F.; Gu, N. Platelet membrane biomimetic magnetic nanocarriers for targeted delivery and in situ generation of nitric oxide in early ischemic stroke. *ACS Nano* **2020**, *14*, 2024–2035. [CrossRef]
125. Ma, J.; Zhang, S.; Liu, J.; Liu, F.; Du, F.; Li, M.; Chen, A.T.; Bao, Y.; Suh, H.W.; Avery, J.; et al. Targeted drug delivery to stroke via chemotactic recruitment of nanoparticles coated with membrane of engineered neural stem cells. *Small* **2019**, *15*, 1902011. [CrossRef]
126. Dehaini, D.; Wei, X.; Fang, R.H.; Masson, S.; Angsantikul, P.; Luk, B.T.; Zhang, Y.; Ying, M.; Jiang, Y.; Kroll, A.V.; et al. Erythrocyte-platelet hybrid membrane coating for enhanced nanoparticle functionalization. *Adv. Mater.* **2017**, *29*, 1606209. [CrossRef] [PubMed]
127. Han, X.; Shen, S.; Fan, Q.; Chen, G.; Archibong, E.; Dotti, G.; Liu, Z.; Gu, Z.; Wang, C. Red blood cell–derived nanoerythrosome for antigen delivery with enhanced cancer immunotherapy. *Sci. Adv.* **2019**, *5*, eaaw6870. [CrossRef] [PubMed]
128. Zinger, A.; Sushnitha, M.; Naoi, T.; Baudo, G.; De Rosa, E.; Chang, J.; Tasciotti, E.; Taraballi, F. Enhancing inflammation targeting using tunable leukocyte-based biomimetic nanoparticles. *ACS Nano* **2021**, acsnano.0c05792. [CrossRef] [PubMed]
129. Cheng, Q.; Wei, T.; Farbiak, L.; Johnson, L.T.; Dilliard, S.A.; Siegwart, D.J. Selective organ targeting (SORT) nanoparticles for tissue-specific MRNA delivery and CRISPR–Cas gene editing. *Nat. Nanotechnol.* **2020**, *15*, 313–320. [CrossRef]
130. Cheng, B.; Xie, R.; Dong, L.; Chen, X. Metabolic remodeling of cell-surface sialic acids: Principles, applications, and recent advances. *ChemBioChem* **2016**, *17*, 11–27. [CrossRef]
131. Stephan, M.T.; Irvine, D.J. Enhancing cell therapies from the outside in: Cell surface engineering using synthetic nanomaterials. *Nano Today* **2011**, *6*, 309–325. [CrossRef] [PubMed]
132. Yan, H.; Shao, D.; Lao, Y.; Li, M.; Hu, H.; Leong, K.W. Engineering cell membrane-based nanotherapeutics to target inflammation. *Adv. Sci.* **2019**, *6*, 1900605. [CrossRef] [PubMed]
133. Ai, X.; Wang, S.; Duan, Y.; Zhang, Q.; Chen, M.S.; Gao, W.; Zhang, L. Emerging approaches to functionalizing cell membrane-coated nanoparticles. *Biochemistry* **2021**, *60*, 941–955. [CrossRef] [PubMed]

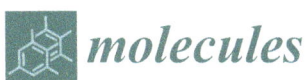

Review

Exploiting a New Approach to Destroy the Barrier of Tumor Microenvironment: Nano-Architecture Delivery Systems

Yanting Sun [1,†], Yuling Li [2,†], Shuo Shi [1,*] and Chunyan Dong [1,*]

1. Department of Oncology, Shanghai East Hospital, Shanghai Key Laboratory of Chemical Assessment and Sustainability, School of Chemical Science and Engineering, Tongji University, Shanghai 200120, China; sunyanting0210@163.com
2. Department of Pharmacy, Shanghai East Hospital, Tongji University School of Medicine, Shanghai 200120, China; yuling19893@163.com
* Correspondence: shishuo@tongji.edu.cn (S.S.); cy_dong@tongji.edu.cn (C.D.)
† These authors contribute equally to this work.

Abstract: Recent findings suggest that tumor microenvironment (TME) plays an important regulatory role in the occurrence, proliferation, and metastasis of tumors. Different from normal tissue, the condition around tumor significantly altered, including immune infiltration, compact extracellular matrix, new vasculatures, abundant enzyme, acidic pH value, and hypoxia. Increasingly, researchers focused on targeting TME to prevent tumor development and metastasis. With the development of nanotechnology and the deep research on the tumor environment, stimulation-responsive intelligent nanostructures designed based on TME have attracted much attention in the anti-tumor drug delivery system. TME-targeted nano therapeutics can regulate the distribution of drugs in the body, specifically increase the concentration of drugs in the tumor site, so as to enhance the efficacy and reduce adverse reactions, can utilize particular conditions of TME to improve the effect of tumor therapy. This paper summarizes the major components and characteristics of TME, discusses the principles and strategies of relevant nano-architectures targeting TME for the treatment and diagnosis systematically.

Keywords: tumor microenvironment; targeted therapy; nanoparticles; nano therapeutics; tumor imaging

1. Introduction

Owing to the complex and continuously evolving tumor microenvironment (TME), cancer becomes one of the most difficult diseases to cure all over the world. The bidirectional interactions between tumor and the TME bring about the progression, therapeutic resistance, and metastasis of cancer [1]. TME composes various supporting cells such as immune cells, fibroblasts, endothelial cells, and extra components like exosomes, cytokines, enzymes, growth factors, and extracellular matrix (ECM), etc. [2,3]. In addition, the tumor microenvironment displays unique pH values, hypoxic condition, high ATP concentration, and abundant tumor microvasculature [4–6]. The communications between tumor cells and the microenvironment result in drug resistance by changing the phenotypes of tumor cells as well [7]. Therefore, treatment targeting the microenvironment has attracted increasing attention.

The rapid development of nanotechnology has provided a good platform for early diagnosis and more effective therapy of tumors [8]. Nanoparticles (NPs) can effectively improve the pharmacokinetic and pharmacodynamics properties of drugs and improve the therapeutic effect due to its special size, shape, and material [9]. Coated with folic acid, hyaluronic acid, and other molecules, nanoparticles can be used as good carriers concentrating drugs at the tumor site much better. Due to the high biocompatibility, good targeting property and low toxicity of organic nanomaterials, related materials have been developed in large quantities. Some organic nanomaterials like liposomes (pegylated liposomal doxorubicin, paclitaxel liposome, vincristine sulfate liposome, etc.) have been used in clinical chemotherapy very well [9]. Inorganic materials are also widely used in the preparation of nanomaterials. Mesoporous silica nanoparticles (MSNs) have great advantages in the fields of adsorption, separation, catalysis, and drug delivery [10]. Magnetic Nanoparticles (MNPs), by means of an external magnetic field, can increase the aggregation of MNPs at the tumor site and reduce the distribution in normal tissues. Furthermore, MNPs have the functions of hyperthermia and imaging, and its super paramagnetism makes it an obvious advantage as MRI (magnetic resonance imaging) contrast agent [11]. Other metal nanoparticles, such as gold nanoparticles (GNPs), can inhibit tumor angiogenesis by themselves and have photothermal effects as well [12]. However, these nanomaterials have shown great success in treating tumors and reducing adverse reactions. The presence of TME still bring limitations for nanomedicines to treat tumors. Aiming for the acidic pH, hypoxia and abundant ATP quantity conditions of TME, NPs response to different stimuli were developed, which could remove the obstacle of low accumulation with enhanced permeation and retention (EPR) effect in the tumor [13]. Nano-architectures established by virus-like particles, polymer, inorganics, micelle, self-assembled proteins, liposomes, polypeptides with suitable volume ratio, and tunable morphologies can achieve the purpose of broad spectrum, low toxicity, and low drug resistance. These NPs can not only reach the tumor site precisely, but also load much more lipophilic drug molecules by its special hollow structure, cut off the interaction between tumor cells and the microenvironment, and inhibit the proliferation of tumor cells more efficiently [14–16].

The role of the TME during nano-targeted tumor treatment strategies has been reviewed somewhere, however, most research just focused on part of the compositions or stimuli categories [17–19]. This review aims to elaborate the components and physiological conditions of TME, summarize the nano-architectures response to physiological barriers or unique constituents, and discuss the prospect of nano therapeutics in TME (Figure 1).

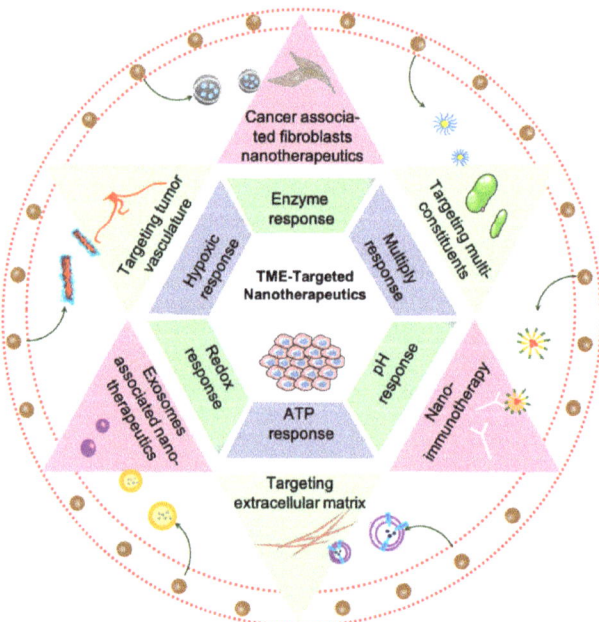

Figure 1. Schematic of nano therapeutics target tumor microenvironment.

2. Special Characteristics of Tumor Microenvironment

2.1. Major Constituents of TME

Immune cells, ECM, cancer associated fibroblasts (CAFs), tumor vessels, exosomes and chemokines are vital constituents of TME, all of which participate in tumor progression and invasion particularly (Figure 2). Here, we will concentrate on the principles of their respective activities.

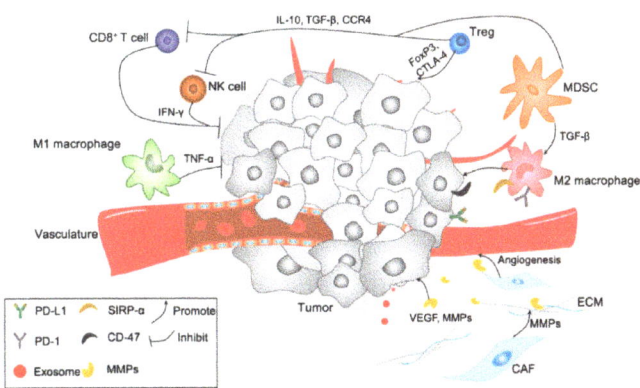

Figure 2. The main components of the tumor microenvironment, including tumor cell, immune cells (such as B cells, T cells, DC cells, NK cells, M1/M2 macrophages), tumor vasculature, ECM, fibroblast, exosomes and cytokines.

2.1.1. Immune Cells and Chemokines

The functions of immune cells and chemokines are controversial in TME. Current research showed that there were a variety of immune cells in the inflammatory microenvironment, including adaptive immune cells as T lymphocytes (T cells) and B lymphocytes (B cells), innate immune defense cells as macrophages, natural killer (NK) cells, dendritic cells (DCs), and myeloid-derived suppressor cells (MDSCs) [20–22]. In the inflammatory microenvironment, the special phenomenon-"immune escape" prevents cancer cells from being recognized by killer cells such as CD8$^+$ T cells and NK cells, making it easier for cancer cells to survive, infiltrate, and metastasize [5,23,24]. Among them, tumor associated macrophages (TAMs), regulatory T cells (Tregs) and MDSCs play vital roles in the tumor immunosuppression environment. Recruitment and differentiation of these immunosuppressive cells depend on the presence of numerous cytokines in the microenvironment [25–27].

Macrophages can be divided into M1 and M2 type according to different phenotypes and functions. M1 macrophages with tumoricidal effects can inhibit tumor growth and secrete pro-inflammatory cytokines like tumor necrosis factor-α (TNF-α), interleukin (IL)-6, and IL-12 [26,28]. M2 macrophages activated by IL-4, IL-10, and IL-13 hold the function of secreting cytokines such as vascular endothelial growth factor (VEGF), epidermal growth factor (EGF), and transforming growth factor-β (TGF-β). All of them participate in promoting repair, suppressing immune response, and angiogenesis [29,30]. M2 macrophages in the tumor microenvironment account for a much higher proportion than M1 macrophages [26]. Programmed cell death 1 (PD-1) expressed on M2 macrophages combining with the programmed cell death ligand 1 (PD-L1) expressed on tumor cells exerted immunosuppressive effect [31]. Meanwhile, tumor cells highly express CD47, which is the ligand of signaling regulatory protein α (SIRPα), an immune checkpoint found on macrophages [32,33]. Binding of CD47-SIRPα axis will suppress phagocytosis effectively. Therefore, effectively improving phagocytosis of macrophages or transforming M2 macrophages into M1 type is the main therapeutic direction in current research.

Tregs, which are abundant in the tumor stroma is a specific subgroup of $CD4^+$ T cells expressing the transcription factor Foxp3, CD25 and cytotoxic T-lymphocyte-associated antigen-4 (CTLA-4) [34–36]. The chemokine ligand (CCL) 22 produced by macrophages and tumor cells can bind to chemokine receptor (CCR) 4 expressed on Tregs, consequently recruiting Treg into TME and leading to tumor growth and poor patients' outcomes with its immunosuppressive function [37]. Tregs create an immunosuppressive environment through the activities of cell surface molecules (Foxp3, CTLA-4, CD25, CD39, CD73, TIGIT), secretion of cytokines (IL-2, IL-10, TGF-β, CCR4) and immune molecules (granzyme, cyclic AMP, and indole-amine-2,3-dioxygenase (IDO)) [36,38–42]. Therefore, blocking the functional molecules expressed on Tregs such as CTLA-4, PD-1, CCR4, TGF-β, Foxp3, or completely eliminating the presence of Tregs can improve the immune escape effect of tumor inflammatory microenvironment.

MDSCs are a group of heterogeneous cells that lack lymphoid markers with multidirectional differentiation potential and immunosuppressive function. This group includes immature DCs, macrophages, granulocytes, and other myeloid cells in the early stage of differentiation [43]. Immune suppression by MDSC involves several complex mechanisms. Due to its suppression of T cells and NK cells in TME, the accumulation of MDSCs is one of the main reasons for tumor immune unresponsiveness [44]. MDSCs can reduce local tryptophan levels due to the activity of IDO to reduce the proliferation of T cells [45]. Peroxynitrite (PNT) produced by MDSCs can alter chemokines and block the entrance of $CD8^+$ T cells. MDSC also induce Tregs and affect function of NK cells by producing immunosuppressive cytokines like IL-10 and TGF-β [46]. Besides the influence of differentiation of TAMs, MDSCs also promote angiogenesis by secreting factors compensating for VEGF [27,47]. Immunotherapy targeting MDSCs provides a new therapeutic strategy for anti-tumor therapy.

2.1.2. Extracellular Matrix

ECM contains proteins, glycoproteins, proteoglycans, polysaccharides, and other components. All of them provide structural support for tissue organization and promote information transmission between cells [48]. In normal tissues, connective proteins and adhesive proteins in ECM keep connection between cells and maintain tissue homeostasis [49]. However, in solid tumors, remodeled ECM affects the migration and invasion of cells, and promotes the occurrence and malignant progression of tumors. Working as information transmitter between ECM and other cells, integrins are highly expressed on tumor cells and vascular endothelial cells, and usually affect the function of some immune cells and fibroblasts. Integrins on the surface of tumor cells regulate cell protrusion and adhesion in the process of tumor migration. Meanwhile, they mediate the function of multiple matrix metalloproteinases (MMPs) like MMP2, MMP9, and MMP14 to remodel ECM [50,51]. ECM remodeling is mainly regulated by MMPs, and proteases such as serine acid/cysteine [52]. In addition, the remodeled dense ECM slows the penetration and diffusion of large molecules to create a high-pressure environment, thereby resulting in therapy limitation [53,54].

2.1.3. Cancer Associated Fibroblasts

CAFs are one of the main components of TME. Unlike resting fibroblasts, CAFs metabolize vigorously and secrete large amounts of proteome, including cytokines, chemokines, and various protease CAF spindles [55,56]. CAFs also provide structural support for tissues and act as a transmitter of information between cells [57]. Due to the expression of serine protease, fibrinogen activator, and MMPs on CAFs, ECM is hydrolyzed and reconstructed. In addition, CAFs can also express a variety of cytokines and proteases, such as stromal cell-derived factor 1 (SDF1), VEGF, MMPs, and monocyte chemotactic protein-1 (MCP-1) to promote tumor growth, metastasis, and angiogenesis [58–60]. In addition, CAFs support cancer progression through changes of metabolism. In tumors, p38 signal of CAFs activates by cancer cells, the fibroblast-derived p38-regulated cytokines mobilize glycogen in cancer cells, which utilizes by cancer cells for glycolysis, promoting cancer invasion and metastasis [61]. In breast cancer, glycolytic CAFs provide extra pyruvate and lactate for augmentation of mitochondrial activity of tumor cells, which confers tumor cells with multiple drug resistance [62]. CAFs also regulate cancer cell metabolism independently of genetic mutations of cancer cell. FAK-depletion in CAFs promoting chemokin production, enhancing malignant cell glycolysis by activating protein kinase A via CCR1/CCR2 axis [63]. Therefore, NPs targeting CAFs can prevent tumor cells growing in numerous ways.

2.1.4. Exosomes

Exosomes are extracellular vesicles typically ~30 to ~200 nm in diameter and containing genetic material, proteins, and lipids [64]. They act as powerful signaling molecules connecting cancer cells and the surrounding components. Exosomes secreted by tumor cells carry miRNAs to regulate vascular endothelial cells. This phenomenon destroys the barrier of endothelial cells, and then allows cancer cells to enter the blood vessels, promoting tumor spread and metastasis [65]. Exosomes secreted by leukemia cells can promote the activation of CAFs. In breast cancer research, exosomes secreted by CAFs promote the invasion and metastasis of cancer by activating the Wnt-pathway [66]. Astrocytes in the brain metastatic microenvironment secrete exosomes loading miRNAs, which specifically downregulate tumor suppressor gene PTEN and lead to metastatic colonization [67]. Cancer exosomes inhibit the cytotoxic of $CD4^+$ T cells, $CD8^+$ T cells, and NK cells [68]. Exosomes also inhibit the differentiation of DCs and MDSCs [69,70]. Exosomes derived from cancer cells definitely have short-and long-term effects on cancer progress. Treatments targeting exosomes might be new directions of tumor therapy.

2.1.5. Tumor Vasculature

The regeneration of vasculatures is a very complicated progress in TME. Vascular endothelial cells regulated by the angiogenic factors can affect the migration and proliferation of tumor. The new vessels formed by adhesion of loosely endothelial cells provide chances for tumor growth and distant metastasis [71]. A variety of cells and growth factors are involved in this process, such as vascular cell adhesion molecule-1 (VCAM-1), $\alpha(v)\beta(3)$ integrin, VEGF, TGF, platelet-derived growth factor (PDGF), and angiogenin. Among them, VCAM-1 and $\alpha(v)\beta(3)$ integrin not only promote the proliferation and differentiation of endothelial cells but also improve vascular permeability [72,73]. PDGF, angiopoietin, and TGF secreted by tumor cells can also affect the action of peripheral cells, vascular maturation, and integrity. In addition, the highly abnormal and dysfunctional system of tumor blood vessels can also lead to impaired ability of immune effector cells to penetrate solid tumors. Therefore, the normalization of tumor blood vessels can enhance tissue perfusion and improve the infiltration of immune effector cells, thus enhancing therapy effects [74,75].

2.2. Physiological Condition of TME for Imaging and Targeting
2.2.1. Hypoxic Condition and Acid Microenvironment

Normal tissue is powered by mitochondrial oxidative decomposition, while cancer cells are mostly powered by glycolysis, a reprogrammed way known as the "Warburg effect" [76]. The majority of tumors are lack of adequate blood supply, and then hypoxic regions appear, where metabolize glucose into lactic acid through anaerobic glycolysis. When a large amount of lactic acid accumulates in the tumor cell, the proton pump transports H+ to the extracellular environment, resulting in an acidic extracellular environment (pH = 5.6–6.8) [77]. During glycolysis, the hypoxia inducible factor (HIF) can regulate glycolysis enzymes (HK1, HK3, TGF-2, et al.) to affect the energy metabolism and proliferation of tumor cells [78,79]. Therefore, utilizing the acid environment of the TME to design a platform acting on HIF-1 could be a new treatment strategy for tumors [80].

2.2.2. Extracellular ATP Content

It is an established notion that extracellular adenosine-5'-triphos-phate (ATP) is one of the major biochemical constituents of TME [81]. Mitochondria are where ATP is produced. It is different between normal cells and cancer cells with mitochondrial metabolism. Although there is little oxygen in cancer cells, in mitochondria, glycolysis is preferential for providing energy, which is called Warburg effect. The reprogramming metabolism in cancer is regulated by central regulators of glycolysis such as HIF-1, Myc, p53, and the PI3K/Akt/mTOR pathways [82]. In tumor tissues, these active pathways promote glycolysis in hypoxia, promoting mitochondria to produce large amounts of ATP. The sharp different concentration of ATP contrast between extracellular (<0.4 mM) and intracellular (1–10 mM) is a characteristic of TME, and the use of ATP can be a practical way for regulating drug release [83,84]. In addition, tumor cells usually metabolize vigorously, and once there is a lack of energy, cell damage happens. The damage of plasma membrane is a recognizable origin of ATP upregulating. Besides the cell injury, the hypoxic-induced stress of TME is also a strong stimulus for ATP release [85]. The ATP concentration in TME is remarkably more than those in normal tissues (10–100 nM) [84]. Based on such a concentration difference, the ATP stimulating response system can be designed to ensure the drugs reach the tumor site more accurately.

2.2.3. Redox Condition

Many organelles, such as cytosol, mitochondrion, and nucleus, contain very high concentrations of glutathione (GSH). In cancer cells, the concentration of GSH is 100–1000 folds of the normal tissue. Due to the existence of thiol groups, GSH can act as electron donors (reducing agents) for developing smart NPs [86].

3. Microenvironment-Targeted Nano-Delivery System as a Promising Strategy

The drug therapy for cancer has been unable to exert its maximum effect due to insufficient orientation, pharmacokinetic obstacles. In order to overcome the shortcomings of traditional drug delivery methods, a new method, a nano-delivery system, is being researched. It can bring drugs accurately to the tumor site and prolong the half-life of the drug in vivo. According to different conditions between TME and normal tissue, NPs are designed to be new solutions for tumor imaging and treatment (Figure 3). All the works mentioned were summarized in Table 1 to reflect the latest development of nano-target strategies applied to TME.

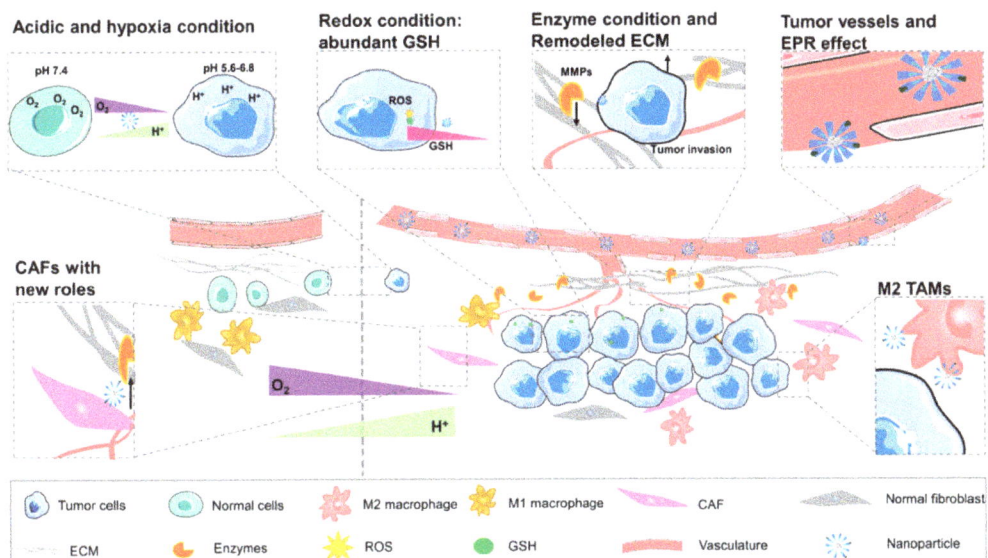

Figure 3. The difference between tumor microenvironment and normal cellular environment (N: normal cellular environment, T: tumor microenvironment). The picture shows new curved blood vessels in TME and EPR effect. Redox condition created by the high content of GSH in tumor cells. Compared with the normal tissue, TME contains a large number of enzymes, anoxic and acidic environments. The percentage of M2 TAM in tumor tissue is larger than that in normal tissue. Special ECM and CAF cells contact with vasculature provides a good condition for angiogenesis and tumor progression.

3.1. Major Composition Mediated Nanoparticles in TME

3.1.1. Nanoparticles Targeting Immune Cells

The immunosuppressive microenvironment is one of the main reasons for the poor antitumor effect in vivo [87]. For M2 macrophages, the most popular methods are reducing M2 macrophages, blocking the immune suppressive function of M2 by blocking PD-1/PD-L1 and the CD47-SIRPα axis [88]. Qian and others designed a fibrin gel capsulate calcium carbonate NPs used in the surgical wound which would polarize M2-like macrophages to a M1-like phenotype. The pre-loaded anti-CD47 antibody in this vector further block the "don't eat me" signal in cancer cells [89]. Shi et al. utilized precision nanoparticle-based reactive oxygen species photogeneration to reprogram M2 macrophages to M1 macrophages, then recruited cytotoxic lymphocyte (CTL) and direct memory T-cells to make the tumoricidal response more effective [90]. Both gold nanoparticles (AuNPs) and silver nanoparticles (AgNPs) can modulate ROS and reactive nitrogen species (RNS) to activate inflammatory signaling pathways, which can re-polarize macrophages to M1-like phenotypes [91]. We built a multifunctional nanoplatform (FA-CuS/DTX@PEI-PpIX-CpG nanocomposites) for synergistic PDT, PTT, loading DTX to enhance immunotherapy of anti-PD-L1, and polarizing myeloid-derived suppressor cells (MDSCs) toward M1 phenotype successfully in breast cancer (Figure 4) [92].

Recently, interaction between the tumor metabolism and immunity has been proved to be a potential therapeutic strategy. A mannosylated lactoferrin nanoparticulate system (Man-LF NPs) is developed. It facilitated dual-targeting biomimetic codelivery of shikonin and JQ1 to target the macrophage marker mannose receptor and LRP-1. JQ1 itself is a PD-L1 checkpoint blockage that can combine with Man-LF NPs and reduce the generation of immune cells such as Tregs [93]. Macrophages in TME have also contributed to tumor diagnosis and localization, Kim et al. made imaging macrophages in tumors possible towards a pharmacokinetically optimized, ^{64}Cu-labeled polyglucose nanoparticle (Macrin) for quantitative positron emission tomography (PET). This technique not only detected the number of macrophages, but also contributed to the effective image of tumor location [94].

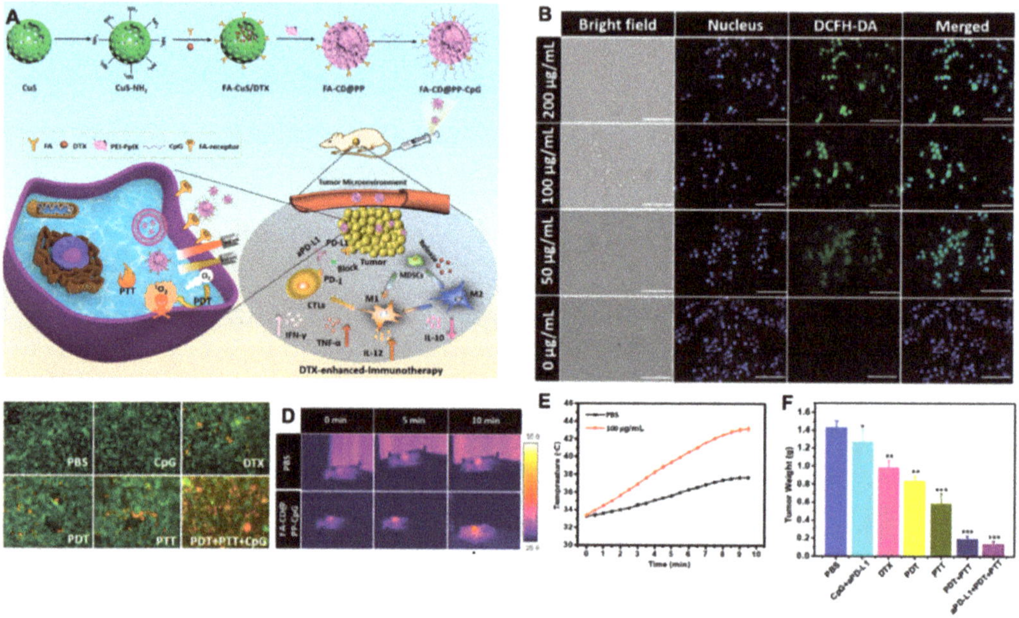

Figure 4. (**A**) Rational design and synthesis, its application in cancer treatment (left), and illustration of FA-CD@PP-CpG for docetaxel-enhanced immunotherapy (right); (**B**) intracellular ROS detection in 4T1 cells incubated with various concentrations of FA-CD@PP-CpG under 650 nm irradiation; (**C**) corresponding fluorescence images of 4T1 cells constrained with calcein AM (live cells, green) and propidium iodide (dead cells, red) after being treated with different conditions. (**D**) The in vivo thermal images of the mice after intravenous injection of PBS and FA-CD@PP-CpG under 808 nm irradiation; (**E**) temperature change curve of tumor sites as a function of irradiation time; (**F**) the weight of tumor tissue in different groups obtained on day 14, adapted with permission from [92].

In general, the expression of receptor tyrosine kinases (RTKs) in cancer cells can activate the STAT3/5 signaling pathway, which promotes the secretion of TH2 cytokines and then promotes the survival of $CD4^+$ $Foxp3^+$ Tregs [95,96]. Thus, the sunitinib-targeting receptor tyrosine kinase drug transferred by nanomaterial has been used to decrease $CD4^+$ $Foxp3^+$ Tregs and MDSCs [97]. Tlyp1 peptide coupled nanoparticles, combined with anti-CTLA4 immuno-checkpoint inhibitors targeting microenvironments, can also enhance imatinib's ability of decrease Tregs by inhibiting the phosphorylation of STAT3 and STAT5 signaling pathways [98]. A CpG self-crosslinked nanoparticles-loaded IR820-conjugated hydrogel with dual self-fluorescence to exert the combined photothermal-immunotherapy was designed in a melanoma model. These NPs improve the immune response of adjuvant through adjusting the quantity of $CD8^+$ T cells, DCs, Tregs, and MDSCs in TME [99].

Stimulator of interferon genes (STING) could enhance tumor immunogenicity, and researchers found, when packing STING into NPs, that its activity to 2'3' cyclic guanosine monophosphate-adenosine monophosphate (cGAMP) enhanced [100]. IDO,TGF-β, IL-10, and IL-35 also have the abilities to modulate the immune microenvironment [101]. IDO is a rate-limiting enzyme of human tryptophan metabolic that can oxidize tryptophan into canine urine. IDO directly inhibits the function of T cells and enhances the immunosuppressant effect of Tregs, thereby mediating the effect of local immune tolerance and promoting the immune escape of tumors [102,103]. IDO is increasingly incorporated into the nano therapeutics system to regulate the outcome of immunotherapy interventions. In melanoma,

Cheng and colleagues built a peptide assembling nanoparticle, which concurrently blockade immune checkpoints and tryptophan metabolism towards on-demand release of a short d-peptide antagonist of programmed cell PD-1 and an inhibitor of IDO [104]. Aimed at TGF-β, Xu et al. silenced TGF-β in microenvironments to solve the problem that the combined vaccine of tumor antigen (Trp 2 peptide) and adjuvant (CpG oligonucleotide) has a poor effect on melanoma [105]. Our team constructed CpG capsuled Cu_9S_5@$mSiO_2$-PpIX@MnO_2 NPs to promote infiltration of CTLs in tumor tissue, and further upregulated interferon gamma (IFN-γ) to promote immune response [106].

Suppressing the function of immune-tolerant cells and promoting the anti-tumor effect of cells have been the key points of tumor immunotherapy. Regulation of immune tolerance in TME combined with nanomaterials can effectively avoid the obstacles caused by microenvironments for drug entry. Therefore, regulating the function of immune cells in microenvironments is one of the key tasks of the nanomaterials system.

3.1.2. Nanoparticles Targeting CAF

CAF is the main source of growth factors, chemokines, ECM proteins, and matrix degrading enzymes in TME. It can produce a variety of growth factors and cytokines to promote the survival and invasion of tumor cells [107]. Kovacs and colleagues found that gold-core silver-shell hybrid nanomaterials could reduce the tumor promotion by attenuating behavior of CAFs [108].

According to the regulation of CAFs of immune cells, Hou et al. developed a nanoemulsion (NE) formulation to deliver fraxinellone (Frax). This NP was around 145 nm length, could be taken by CAFs efficiently, and accumulated in the TME. Combining with a tumor-specific peptide vaccine will enhance tumor-specific T-cell infiltration and activate death receptors on the tumor cell surface (Figure 5) [109]. Recently, NPs targeting CAFs for tumor therapy mainly focused on destroying the tumor tissue to promote drug penetration and reprogramming immune TME. Since CAFs participate in cancer glucose metabolism immediately, NPs targeting CAFs about decreasing glycolysis of cancer cells remain to be developed.

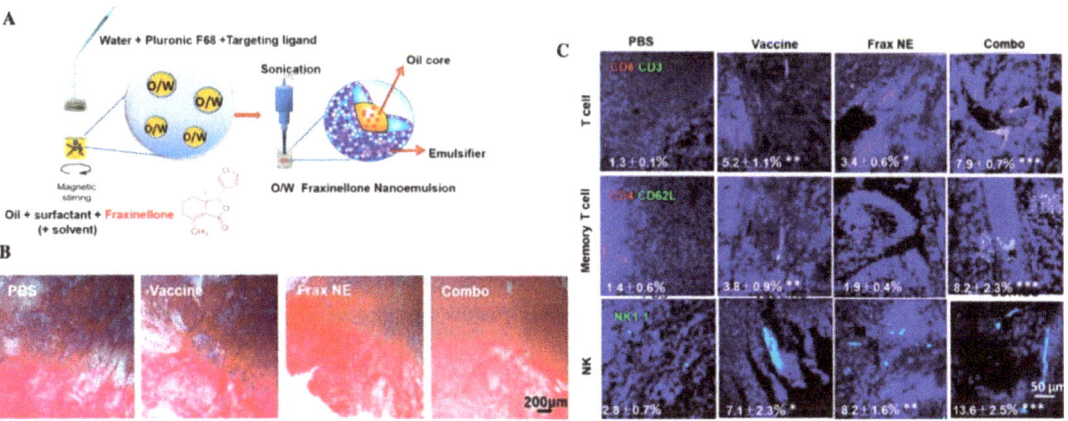

Figure 5. (**A**) Scheme depicting the preparation process of Frax NE; (**B**) Masson's trichrome stain for collagen; (**C**) confocal and flow cytometric analysis of immune cells infiltration in the TME, adapted with permission from [109].

3.1.3. Nanoparticles Targeting ECM

People try to find ways to destruct the structure of ECM. As the most well-known matrix enzyme, MMPs, particularly MMP2 and MMP9, were frequently applied in NPs [110,111]. Many systems that respond to enzymes such as MMPs are also used in drug delivery and imaging. Ji et al. utilized pirfenidone (PFD) loaded MRPL (MRPL-

PFD), a MMP2 responsive peptide-hybrid liposome, to downregulate the components of ECM, thus increasing the penetration of drugs in pancreatic cancer tissue (Figure 6) [112]. Other enzymes acting on the microenvironment can also degrade the structure of ECM. Hyaluronidase (HAase) can break down hyaluronan and then enhance the efficacy of nanoparticle-based PDT. Utilizing HAase and DOX together will also increase cancer mortality [113–115]. Blocking collagen and integrin signaling for anti-fibrotic therapeutic strategy can also be considered in future treatment for ECM to improve drug delivery [116].

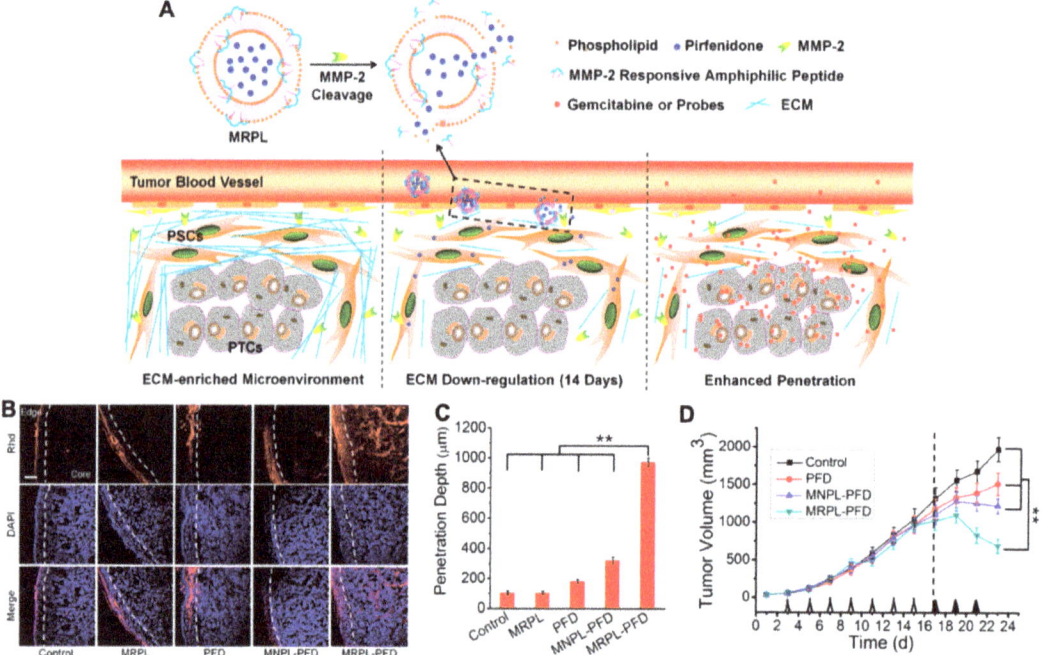

Figure 6. (**A**) Mechanism of MMP-2 Responsive Peptide Hybrid Liposome (MRPL) for downregulation of ECM in pancreatic tumors; (**B**) Rhd penetration and distribution in pancreatic tumor (PSCs/Mia-paca-2 co-implanted) tissues after 2 weeks' treatment of the different PFD formulations; (**C**) quantification of the depth of Rhd penetration in tumors treated by the PFD formulations; (**D**) the growth curves of PSCs and Mia-paca-2 co-implanted pancreatic tumors in mice treated by the different PFD formulations, adapted with permission from [112].

3.1.4. Nanoparticles Targeting Exosomes

As a natural intercellular shuttle of miRNA, exosomes affect a series of physiological and pathological processes in receptor cells or tissues, and are ideal nano carriers for nucleic acid targeted delivery in vivo [117]. The antigen presenting function of dendritic cells was utilized to develop a single membrane vesicle-based vaccine, which would participate in repressing both melanoma (B16) and Lewis lung carcinoma (LLC) tumor growth [118]. Utilizing exosomes to load NPs showed perfect biocompatibility. Xiong and co-workers built NPs together laurate-functionalized Pt (IV) prodrug (Pt(lau)) and human serum albumin (HSA) with lecithin, capsuled by the exosomes, had a good platinum chemotherapy efficiency (Figure 7) [119].

Exosomes shed by cancer cells have also been designed on cancer diagnosis. Liu et al. made exosomes immobilize on magnetic microbeads to produce fluorescent signal. They qualified the exosomes in plasma samples from breast cancer patients for early diagnosis of cancer in vitro [120]. Lewis et al. built an in vitro probe screening of bio-membrane chips, which was composed of the captured exosomes and other extracellular vesicles in the plasma, and tested the express of glypican-1 and CD63 to diagnose pancreatic ductal adenocarcinom in vitro [121].

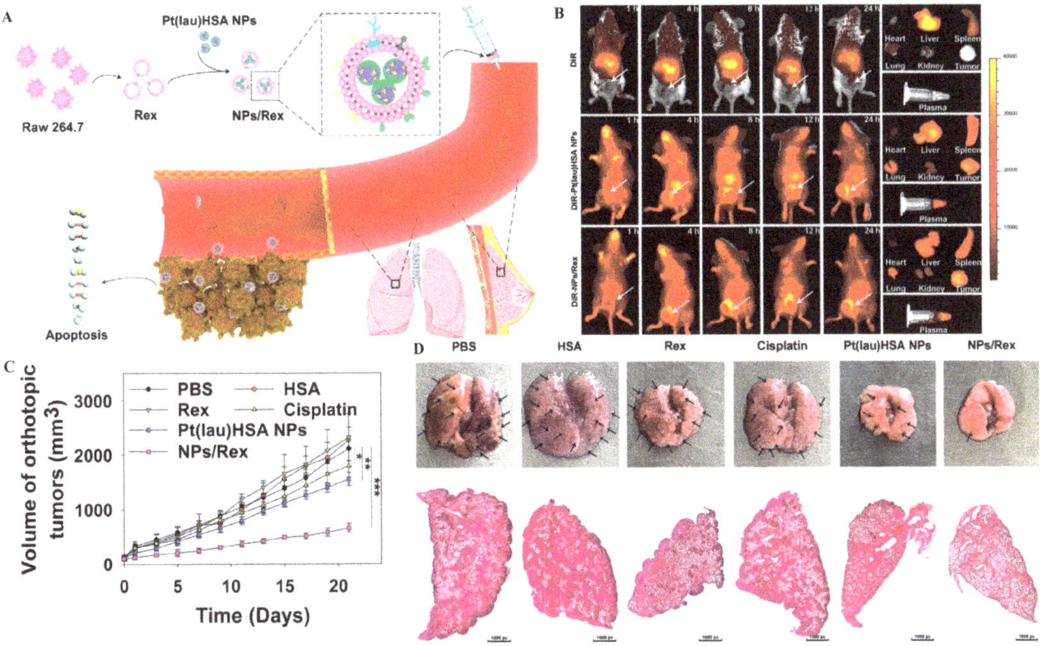

Figure 7. (**A**) Schematic illustration of the Pt(lau)HSA NP-loaded exosome platform (NPs/Rex) for efficient chemotherapy of breast cancer; (**B**) biodistribution of DiR, DiR-Pt(lau)HSA NPs, and DiR-NPs/Rex in 4T1 tumor-bearing BALB/c mice; (**C**) the volume of orthotopic tumors; (**D**) typical lung tissues with visualized metastatic nodules (black arrows) and H&E for metastatic nodules of lungs in each group, adapted with permission from [119].

3.1.5. Nanoparticles Targeting Tumor Vasculature

Using EPR more effectively and enhancing the permeability of vascular have been widely studied in the latest nano therapeutics [122,123]. There are some reports that used NO to improve the EPR effect in pancreatic cancer and other diseases with low vascular permeability [122,124,125]. Other delivery systems like actively targeting VEGF and $\alpha(v)\beta(3)$ integrin were also used widely [126]. Integrins play important roles in cell adhesion and cell signaling, and $\alpha(v)\beta(3)$ integrin is one type of them that can modulate angiogenic endothelial cells. Graf et al. described a NP using cyclic pentapeptide c(RGDfK) to active target $\alpha(v)\beta(3)$ integrin on cancer cells and tumor neovasculature [127].

To improve the diagnosis of tumor, Youbin and co-workers proposed the poly(acrylicacid) (PAA)-modified NaLnF$_4$:40Gd/20Yb/2Er nanorods ((Ln = Y, Yb, Lu, PAA-Ln-NRs) to enhance the shifting of NIR-IIb (a general in vivo fluorescence imaging technology), which successfully imaged the vessels of small tumors (about 4 mm), metastatic tissue (about 3 mm), and even brain vasculatures (Figure 8) [128]. Cecchini et al. reported a nanoMIPs against VEGF coupled with quantum dots (QDs) for tumor imaging in melanoma [129]. In cholangiocarcinoma, $\alpha(v)\beta(3)$ integrin also combined with aggregation induced emission (AIE) for image-guided PDT, and presented a good antitumor response [130].

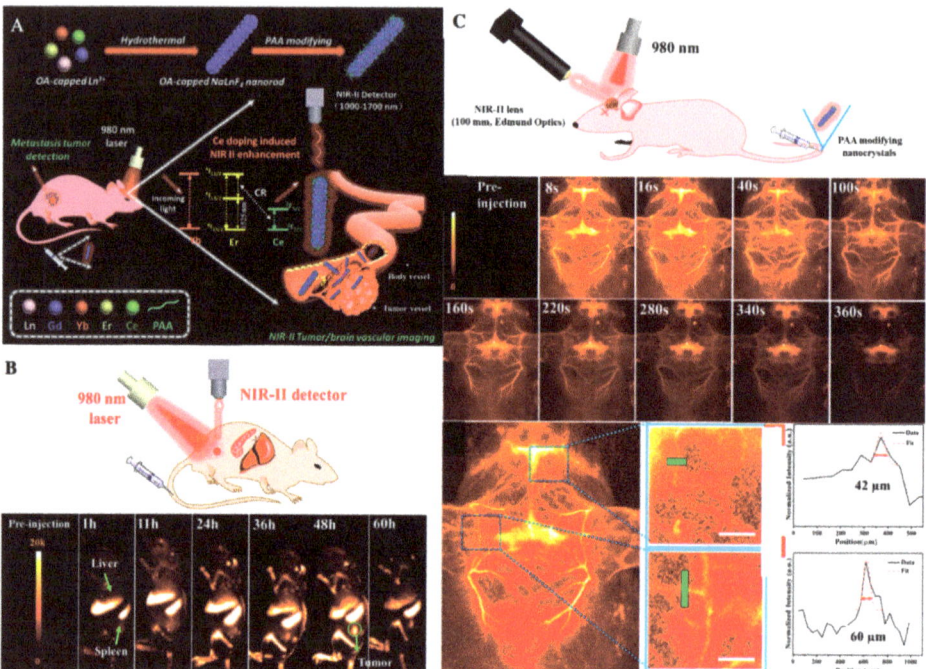

Figure 8. (**A**) Schematic illustration of the enhanced NIR-IIb emission of PAA-Ln-NRs via Ce^{3+} doping for non-invasive tumor metastasis/vascular visualization and brain vessel imaging; (**B**) schematic illustration of in vivo small tumor diagnosis by using PAA-Lu-NRs, and the NIR-IIb bioimaging of tumor-bearing mouse after intravenously injecting PAA-Lu-NRs at different time periods; (**C**) schematic illustration of in vivo noninvasive brain vessel imaging by using the in vivo imaging system, fast brain vascular imaging of a mouse with hair removed and cross-sectional fluorescence intensity profiles along the green lines of the mouse, adapted with permission from [128].

3.1.6. Nanoparticles Targeting Multiconstituents

In addition to targeting single constituents, some NPs can regulate multiple barriers and have also been simultaneously designed for tumor therapies. Targeting tumor cells and immune cells simultaneously can effectively reduce the immune escape phenomenon of TME. Shi et al. designed a versatile calcium ion nanogenerator. The degradation and release of Ca^{2+} by nanoparticles can promote the maturation of DCs by promoting autophagy of DCs, and it can promote tumor cells to produce damage-associated molecular patterns (DAMPs), further maturing DCs and the enhanced infiltration of CTLs at the same time [131]. In addition, researchers have combined exosomes with immunotherapy. Xie's team synthesized responsive exosome nano-bioconjugates. They modified exosomes derived from M1 macrophages with antibodies of CD47 and SIRPα. The broken benzoic-imine bonds are cleaved to release antibodies of SIRPα and CD47 in the acidic TME abolished the "don't eat me" signal between tumor cell and macrophages [132]. The native M1 exosomes reprogram the M2 macrophages to M1 effectively at the same time [132].

3.2. *Physiological Condition Mediated Nanoparticles in TME*

3.2.1. Hypoxic Stimulus

The hypoxic condition in tumor microenvironment is considered to play an important role in malignancy and progression of cancer. Hypoxic areas of tumors also bring obstacles to radiation therapy due to the oxygen free radicals [133]. Utilizing this characteristic, the low oxygen response nano-delivery systems were produced.

The approaches developed thus far can be classified into three categories: countering hypoxia, exploiting hypoxia, and disregarding hypoxia [134]. (i) Directly or indirectly elevating O_2 concentration to counter hypoxia is a promising way to improve the efficiency of tumor therapy, especially for photodynamic therapy (PDT) and radiation therapy (RT). PDT generates reactive oxygen species (ROS) by using light-excited photosensitizer (PS), resulting in cell apoptosis and microvascular damage [125]. Red blood cells (RBCs) carrying hemoglobin molecules are primary oxygen sources in our body. Because the efficacy of PDT is deeply oxygen-dependent, a technique named RBC-facilitated PDT was developed to improve hypoxia conditions in tumors. Wei et al. showed a nanocapsule that encapsulated photosensitizers and tethered the conjugates onto RBC surface. By using biotin-neutravidin-mediated coupling, they conjugated ZnF16Pc (photosensitizer)-loaded ferritins onto each RBC [135]. This new structure, which could overcome low oxygen conditions, showed efficient $^1O_2$ production to overcome low oxygen conditions and enhanced PDT capacity [135]. For RT, an artificial nanoscale RBC will remarkably enhance the treatment efficacy as well. For example, an artificial blood substitute perfluorocarbon (PFC) was encapsulated with biocompatible poly(d,l-lactide-co-glycolide) (PLGA) and then further coated with a red-blood-cell membrane (RBCM), showing efficient loading of oxygen and significantly enhanced treatment efficiency during RT [136]. With increasing production of H_2O_2 in cancer cells, NPs converting endogenous H_2O_2 to toxic ROS and decomposing endogenous H_2O_2 to O_2 were rapidly developed. Noble metal nanoparticles like Mn, Au, Pt, and Ir are well known for their catalytic performances in various fields [137]. MnO_2 is a common material to enhance PDT treatment and imaging. Mn^{2+} could react with H_2O_2 in the tumor, then downregulate the expression of HIF-1 to increase oxygen content and optimize MRI imaging [138,139]. A nanoplatform based on mesoporous polydopamine (MPDA) modified with Pt also produces O_2 by decomposing overexpressed H_2O_2 in the tumor. Meanwhile, the existence of Pt can act as a nano-factory to provide support for PDT (Figure 9) [140]. (ii) Taking advantage of the deficiency of oxygen molecules is a new approach for drug release and PDT. Yin et al. developed a novel amphiphilic block copolymer radiosensitizers. After optimizing the ratios of carboxyl and metronidazole (MN) groups, PEG-b-P(LG-g-MN) micelles could be used to encapsulate doxorubicin (DOX@HMs) efficiently [141]. Hypoxia-responsive structural transformation of MN into hydrophilic aminoimidazole triggers fast DOX release from DOX@HMs, which acted as high-efficiency radiosensitizers and hypoxia-responsive DOX nanocarriers [141]. Some drugs that are selectively toxic to hypoxic cells like Tirapazamine (TPZ) were designed to combine with oxygen-dependent PDT to enhance bioreductive therapy. Shao's group developed a core-shell upconversion nanoparticle@porphyrinic MOFs (UCSs) for combinational therapy against hypoxic tumors [142]. TPZ was encapsulated in nanopores of the MOF shell of the heterostructures (TPZ/UCSs), which enables the near-infrared light-triggered production of cytotoxic reactive oxygen species [142]. Furthermore, with the combination of PD-L1, this nanoplatform recruited specific tumor infiltration of cytotoxic T cells and inhibited the metastasis of the tumor as well. Other methods like eliminating the oxygen in the tumor, inhibiting the growth of tumor vessels, and stopping the nutrient delivery to starve the tumor cells still have many challenges [143,144]. (iii) Using new anticancer modalities to disregard hypoxia conditions becomes another innovative antitumor strategy. PDT with diminished O_2 dependence will effectively overcome its strong oxygen dependence and limitation of treating deep tumors. It has been reported that fractional light delivery may be a superior way to enhance PDT effects due to the reduction of short-term oxygen consumption during PDT [145]. Since the generation of oxygen-irrelevant free radicals is oxygen-independent, and the exploration of UCNP is an inner light source to activate most organic photosensitizers (PSs) to create cytotoxic $^1O_2$, researchers discovered that the Ru complex displayed excellent type I PDT activity [142,146]. Due to its special Fenton reaction, Fe nanoparticles can produce reactive •OH species with endogenous H_2O_2 ($Fe^{2+} + H_2O_2 \rightarrow Fe^{3+} + •OH + OH^-$) and produce cytotoxic effects without external energy through chemotherapeutic therapy (CDT). Yu et al. fabricated a core-shell structured iron-based NPs (Fe_5C_2@Fe_3O_4) to release ferrous ions in acidic environments to disproportionate H_2O_2 into •OH radicals, and its high magnetization is favorable for both magnetic targeting and T2-weighted MRI [147]. In addition, gold nanospheres, graphene oxide, polydopamine (PDA), and other materials have been widely used as PTT reagents and nano carriers to deliver PDT reagents, so as to overcome the therapeutic limitations of PDT [148–150].

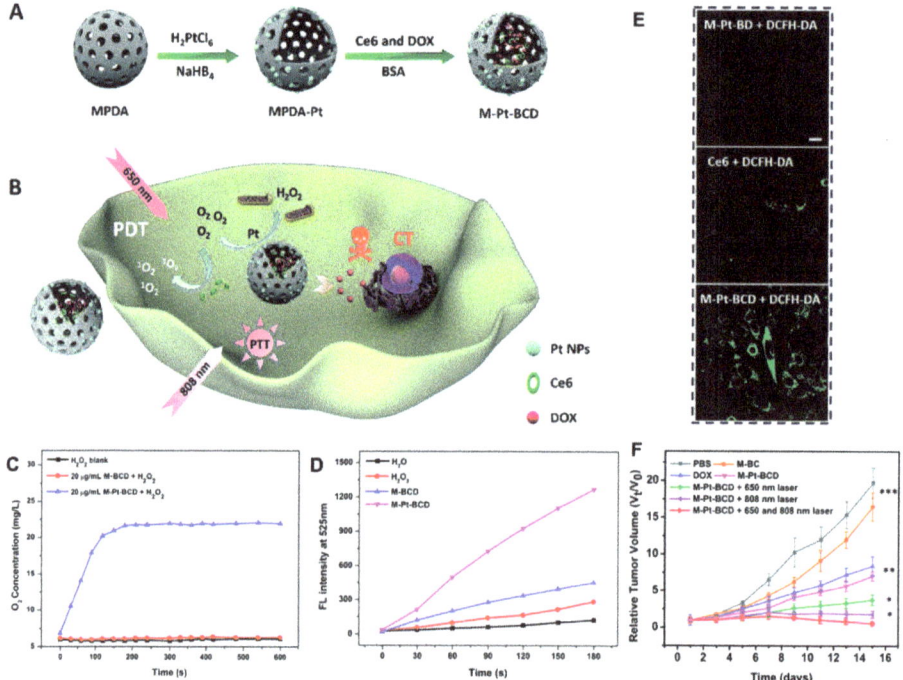

Figure 9. (**A**) Schematic illustration of the synthesis of MPDA-Pt-BSA/ Ce6/DOX (M-Pt-BCD); (**B**) schematic illustration of the application of M-Pt-BCD for enhanced- PDT and synergistic therapy; (**C**) O_2 generation of H_2O_2 blank, M-BCD and M-Pt-BCD; (**D**) $^1O_2$ production efficiency of H_2O, H_2O_2, M-BCD and M-Pt-BCD; (**E**) confocal microscopic images of cellular $^1O_2$ levels detected by DCFH-DA staining upon 650 nm irradiation; (**F**) tumor growth curves, reproduced by permission of The Royal Society of Chemistry [140].

3.2.2. pH Response

pH responsive nano-vectors are one of the typical carriers for TME. Chemical bond response to pH is one of the most widely used strategies in pH responsive nano delivery systems. The most common pH sensitive bonds include hydrazone bond, imine bond, oxime bond, amide bond, benzoic-imine bond, orthoesters, polyacetals, and ketals [151,152]. These chemical bonds break in acidic environments to degrade the carrier, and then increase the uptake of tumor cells or accelerate drug release. When it comes to the design of pH-sensitive materials, besides pH sensitive chemical bonds, other main strategies are conformational change, protonation, and charge reversal with pH change [151]. For example, Chen's team developed a DNA-based stimulus-responsive drug delivery system precisely responding to pH variations in the range of 5.0–7.0. On the face of the gold nanoparticles, one DNA strand was an acti-MUC1 aptamer targeting tumor membrane, the other DNA strand was switchable DNA, which has a linear conformation under neutral or alkaline conditions and self-folds into a triplex under acidic conditions [153].

In cells, nano-switches can react with endosomes and lysosomes and switch to triplex in lysosomes, so as to achieve the goal of accurately drug release (Figure 10) [153]. Nanocarriers involved in protonation/deprotonation are mainly nano liposomes, peptides, and polymers. The phospholipid components in liposomes are usually destabilized under acidic conditions, so as to deliver the contents of liposomes to cells. In mouse cancer models, Guangna et al. combined platelet membrane with the functionalized synthetic liposome; because of its camouflage based on the platelet membrane, this platform enhanced tumor affinity and released DOX in acidic microenvironment more selectively and efficiently [154]. The anionic/cationic polymers with different groups deform various nanocarriers through the change of their hydrophilicity, which lead to drug release [155]. Inorganic salts such as MnO2, CaP, and $CaCO_3$ are widely used for pH response NPs because of their acid solubility [156–158]. Ma et al. designed a pH-sensitive dye linked peptide substrate of MMP-9 with Fe_3O_4 nanoparticles, establishing a Forster resonance energy transfer (FRET) system to detect the invasion and metastasis of tumor by detecting the overexpression of MMP9 [159]. A pH responsive magnetic nanoparticle can combine magnetic hyperthermia with drug delivery dependent on magnetic stimulation, achieving the purpose of targeting TME and tumor treatment at the same time [160].

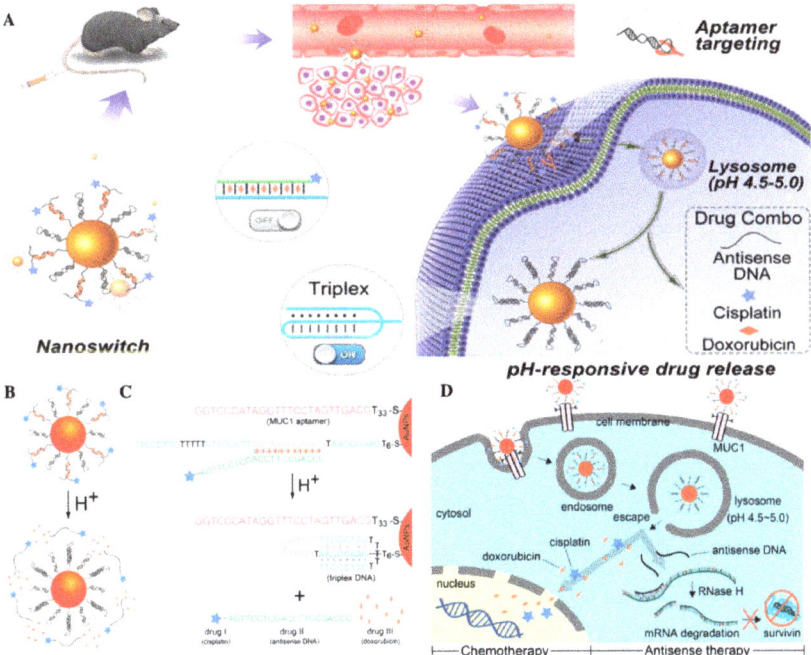

Figure 10. (**A**) Schematic illustration of the DNA-based stimulus-responsive drug delivery system; (**B**) pH-responsive regulation of the nanoswitch and drug release; (**C**) schematic illustration of DNA strands and the multidrug loaded on the surface of AuNPs; (**D**) intracellular pH-responsive multidrug delivery and release, adapted with permission from [153].

3.2.3. ATP Response

Since the concentration of ATP in tumor cells is much higher than extracellular environments and ATP is involved in many biochemical reactions in cells, NPs response to ATP were widely developed. ATP sensitive NPs can release drugs without the help of external forces. Zhenqi et al. developed nano ZIF-90 self-assembled from zinc ions and imidazole-2-carboxaldehyde (2-ICA) to deliver DOX. Because the coordination between ATP and Zn^{2+} is much stronger than that between imidazole and Zn^{2+}, nano ZIF-90 can be decomposed and respond to ATP [161]. Graphene oxide (GO) has been shown to bind single stranded DNA. When the template DNA contains ATP binding domain and reached ATP specific recognition, it could be circularized upon proximity ligation after hybridizing to linker DNA on the surface of GO [162]. Then, rolling circle amplification was initiated from the 3′-end of the template DNA, and the elongated sequence was hybridized with thousands of signal DNA (conjugated with Cy3), so as to amplify the template DNA, generate fluorescent signals, and achieve the purpose of tumor monitoring [162]. Yuan et al. exploited a ATP binding natural protein, GroEL (a bacterial chaperonin) loading DOX, once in the presence of a critical concentration of ATP in tumor site, it releases drugs [163]. In addition to using ATP as a switch for drug release, another way in which ATP participates is to regulate its expression in cells with nanosystems. Xiao's team exploited a multifunctional theranostic platform combing CDT with limotherapy. While enhancing the CDT effect to induce apoptosis of cancer cells, nano Se and Mn^{2+} ions inhibited the production of ATP, which made cancer cells starve and further killed tumor cells, monitoring the treatment of tumors by MRI simultaneously [164].

3.2.4. Reduction Response

In addition to GSH, tumor cells also contain thioprotein, Fe^{2+}, cysteine, and other reductive substances, and the difference of GSH concentration between tumor cells and TME makes a reduction-responsive drug carrier come true [165,166]. GSH/glutathione disulfide (GSSG) is one of the major redox couples in cells, and adding disulfide bonds to drug carriers is one of the most commonly used methods to build GSH responsive drug carriers. There are many forms of GSH-responsive nano-vehicles (like micelles, nanogels, nanoparticles), so as to improve the drug release successfully. For example, in order to solve the problems of drug resistance caused by cancer stem cells (CSC), Rubone (RUB, a miR-34 activator for targeting CSCs) and DTX were utilized to treat taxane resistant prostate patients. A self-assembled DTX/p-RUB micelles showed good stability in vitro and could be accurately delivered to tumor cells though the EPR effect. After the tumor cells endocytosed the micelles, the micelles expanded and disintegrated due to the protonation of diisopropylaminoethanol (DIPAE) and GSH induced disulfide bond cleavage of acid endocytosis vesicles, which led to the rapid release of DTX and RUB. The release of RUB upregulated miR-34a and regulated the expression of chemoresistance related proteins, thus making tumor cells sensitive to DTX, significantly inhibiting the progress of drug resistance [167]. Ling and colleagues constructed a self-assembled NP platform composed of amphiphilic lipid polyethylene glycol (PEG), and it can effectively deliver Pt (IV) precursor drugs through the elimination of GSH [168].

Some metal oxides like MnO_2 also have the potential of GSH response. MnO_2 reacts with GSH in cells to form glutathione disulfide and Mn^{2+}, which leads to the consumption of GSH and enhancement of CDT. In addition to the MRI features of Mn^{2+}, MRI monitored chemo- chemical combination therapy is realized [167].

3.2.5. Enzyme Response

Many enzymes like MMPs regulate the function of cellular components and take part in tumor progression. From this prospect, the presence of these abnormal enzymes gives the chance for researchers to build a sensitive system for drug release. The presence of NO can activate endogenous MMP1 and MMP2, and researchers have developed an MSN loaded with a doxorubicin (DOX) and NO donor to enhance the antitumor effect [169]. In addition, PLGLAG peptide and gelatin are both main target proteins of MMP9 and MMP2, which can be widely used to MMP responsive NPs [170–172].

According to the Warburg effect, the proliferation of tumor cells mainly depends on aerobic glycolysis, so tumor cells are more sensitive to the change of glucose concentration. Glucose oxidase (GOx), an endogenous oxidoreductase, reacts with glucose and O2 in cells then produce gluconic acid and H_2O_2, which can inhibit the proliferation of cancer cells through starvation therapy. In addition, H_2O_2 can be transformed into

•OH free radical to kill cancer cells and enhance the oxidative stress response of cancer cells [173]. Through GOx, starvation therapy can together with chemotherapy, CDT, PDT, or immunotherapy to explore new strategies for cancer treatment. For example, Mengyu et al. constructed a multifunctional cascade bioreactor based on hollow mesoporous Cu2MoS4 (CMS) loaded with GOx for synergetic cancer therapy by CDT/starvation therapy/phototherapy/immunotherapy [174]. First of all, CMS containing multivalent elements ($Cu^{1+}/^{2+}$, $Mo^{4+}/^{6+}$) showed Fenton like activity, which could produce · OH and reduce GSH, thus reducing the antioxidant capacity of tumor. Secondly, in hypoxic TME conditions, hydrogen peroxide like CMS can react with H_2O_2 to generate O_2, activate the effect of GOx, start starvation therapy, and regenerate H_2O_2. Finally, the regenerated H_2O_2 can participate in Fenton like reactions to realize GOx-catalysis-enhanced CDT. At the same time, because of the excellent photothermal conversion efficiency under 1064 nm laser irradiation, CMS killed tumor cells significantly in PDT. More importantly, the PEGylated CMS@GOx-based synergistic therapy combined with anti-CTLA4 can stimulate a robust immune response [174].

3.2.6. Multiply Response

A mesoporous silica-coated gold cube-in-cubes core/shell nanocomposites loading DOX was combined with ArgGlyAsp (RGD) peptide to achieve a platform that can deliver drugs and produce O_2 in situ. This nano platform simultaneously enhanced photodynamic efficacy, achieving heat- and pH-sensitive drug release and location imaging (Figure 11) [175]. Lan et al. decorated an emerging class of highly tunable two-dimensional material: cationic Hf12-Ru nanoscale metal-organic frameworks (Hf12-Ru nMOF), then functionalized with pH-sensitive fluorescein isothiocyanate and targeting mitochondria, utilized the pH and quantities of O_2 in the mitochondria to image living cells [176]. Yi and colleagues developed a redox/ATP switchable theranostic NPs. They conjugated a fluorescent probe (FAM) and a quencher (BHQ-1) to ATP, complexed with a GSH-sensitive cationic polymer. This smart NPs loading fluorescent probes can monitor drug release in vivo [177].

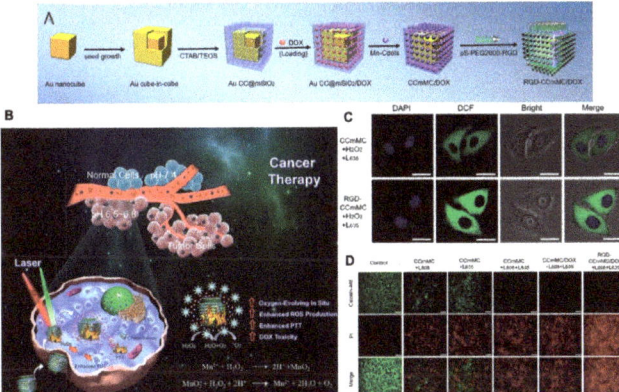

Figure 11. (A) Schematic illustration of the synthesis process for the versatile RGD-CCmMC/DOX nanovehicles; (B) schematic illustration of the therapeutic mechanism of the RGD-CCmMC/DOX nanoplatforms to enhance the overall anticancer efficiency of triple-combination photodynamic/photothermal/chemo-therapy in a solid tumor; (C) CLSM images of 4T1 cells treated with different formulations under laser irradiation. The production of intracellular ROS and O_2 generation were measured by the green fluorescence intensity of DCF; (D) fluorescence microscopy images of 4T1 cells with various treatments using Calcein AM/PI staining, adapted with permission from [175].

Table 1. Nanoparticle approaches for targeting TME in this review.

Target	Loading Drugs	Nanocomposites and Outcomes	Animal Models/Cell Lines	Ref.
1. Physiological condition				
Hypoxia response	-	P-FRT-RBCs to enhance PDT, show efficient $^1O_2$ production	U87MG-bearing subcutaneous models	[135]
	-	PFC@PLGA-RBCM NPs to enhance RT	4T1 tumor-bearing mice model	[136]
	acriflavine	ROS responsive ACF@MnO$_2$ NPs to guide RT and MRI	CT26-bearing mice model	[138]
	DOX	MPDA-Pt-BSA/Ce6/DOX combined PDT and PTT	MDA-MB-231 tumor-bearing mice model	[140]
	DOX	DOX@HMs to enhance chemoradiotherapy	4T1 tumor-bearing mice model	[141]
	TPZ and a-PD-L1	TPZ/UCSs combined with PDT to activate chemotherapy and immunotherapy	CT26-bearing mice model	[142]
	coumarin	coumarin-modified cyclometalated Ru (II) complexes for better PDT effect	HeLa cell-bearing mice model	[146]
	-	PEG/Fe$_5$C$_2$@Fe$_3$O$_4$ NPs with magnetic targeting for produce reactive •OH species and MRI imaging	4T1 tumor-bearing mice model	[147]
pH response	DOX, cisplatin, and asDNA	AuNPs with DNA bands, release three drugs due to nanoswitch changes conformation in acidic condition	MCF-7, Hela, L02 cells/Balb/c nude mice model	[153]
	DOX	pH-sensitive PEOz-liposome-dox NPs for drug delivery	CT26 and 4T1 -bearing mice model	[154]
	-	ANNA/ MMP-9/PEGylated Fe$_3$O$_4$ particle for MR imaging to guide tumor invasion in vivo	BALB/c nude mice bearing human colon cancer	[159]
ATP response	DOX	AP-ZIF-90@DOX, dual responsive to high ATP and low pH condition to release DOX in tumor cells	MDA-MB-231 tumor bearing mouse	[161]
	DOX	DNA/MSN/FA/DOX NPs for drug release and fluorescence imaging	HeLa cells	[162]
	-	MCDION-Se with CDT, inhibit the generation of ATP, thus starving cancer cells	HeLa and HK-2 cells/BALB/C nude mice model	[164]
Reduction response	DTX and RUB	DTX/p-RUB micelles, regulate the expression of chemoresistance	DU145-TXR and PC3-TXR cells/mice model	[167]
	Pt prodrug	self-assembled PEG/Pt (IV) NP through GSH-exhausting effect to delivery safer and more effective	A2780cis tumor-bearing athymic nude mice	[168]
Enzyme response	DOX	MSN loaded with DOX and NO donor (S-nitrosothiol) to create DN@MSN, activate MMP and degrade collagen in the tumor ECM	4T1 tumor-bearing mice model	[169]
	anti-CTLA4	PEGylated Cu$_2$MoS$_4$ (CMS)@GOx, promote CDT, PDT, PTT and starvation therapy	HeLa cell-bearing mice model	[174]
Multiply response	DOX	RGD-CCmMC/DOX nanovehicles achieve heat- and pH-sensitive drug release with precise control to specific tumor site	4T1 tumor-bearing mice model	[175]
	-	Hfl2-Ru nMOF for ratiometric pH and oxygen sensing in mitochondria for monitoring pH and O$_2$ in live cells	CT26 cell line	[154]
	DOX	FAM-ATP/BHQ-1-cDNA@DOX NPs,can monitor drug release in vivo	HeLa, HepG2, or MCF-7 cell line	[177]

Table 1. Cont.

Target	Loading Drugs	Nanocomposites and Outcomes	Animal Models/Cell Lines	Ref.
2. Immune cells				
Macrophages	anti-CD47 antibody	aCD47@CaCO$_3$ nanoparticles encapsulated in fibrin gel to scavenge H$^+$ in the surgical wound, polarize TAM	Female C57BL/6 mice; B16F10 cell line	[89]
	-	MAN-PLGA and MAN-PLGA-N NPs affected by acidic pH, disrupt the endosome/lysosome membrane help rise ROS and M1 macrophages	BALB/C mice; 4T1, B16, RAW264.7 cell lines	[90]
	-	AuNPs and AgNPs modulate the reactive ROS and RNS production, downregulate TNF-α and IL-10	murine fibrosarcoma model	[91]
	DTX	FA-CuS/DTX@PEI-PpIX- CpG nanocomposites cooperated with PDT and PTT, enhance immunotherapy successfully	4T1-tumor-bearing mice model	[92]
	shikonin and JQ1	Man-LF NPs targeting mannose receptor and LRP-1 expressed on cancer cells and TAMs, inducing immune cell death, repressing glucose metabolism and repolarizing TAMs	CT26-tumor-bearing mice model	[93]
	-	^{64}Cu-labeled polyglucose nanoparticle (Macrin) for PET can image the macrophages in tumor, to evaluate TAM-targeted therapy	KP-tumor bearing lungs-C57BL/6 mice,4T1-bearing-BALB/c mice	[94]
		polymeric micelle nano-delivery system (SUNb-PM) to increase cytotoxic		
Tregs and MDSCs	sunitinib	T-cell infiltration and decrease the percentage of MDSCs and Tregs in the TME	C57BL/6 mice bearing B16F10 tumors	[97]
Tregs	imatinib	tLyp1 peptide-modified hybrid NPs, downregulate Tregs suppression and elevate intratumoral CD8$^+$ T cells	C57BL/6 mice bearing B16/BL6 tumors	[98]
	-	CpG NPs/IR820-hydrogel, combined photothermal-immunotherapy by the dual fluorescence imaging method without additional fluorescent labeling	BALB/c mice, B16 cell line	[99]
Other immune molecules	-	NLG919@DEAP-DPPA-1 NPs, concurrent blockade of immune checkpoints and tryptophan metabolism	B16-F10 bearing mice model	[104]
	siRNA	LPH NP delivery TGF-β siRNA, increase tumor infiltrating CD8$^+$ T cells and decrease Tregs	C57BL/6mice, B16F10 melanoma cell	[105]
	-	CSPM@CpG and synergist c PTT/PDT/immunotherapy	4T1-tumor-bearing mice model	[106]
3. CAF				
	fraxinelloneand vaccine	Au@Ag NP, attenuate the tumor cell-promoting behavior of CAFs nanoemulsion deliver fraxinellone and tumor-specific peptide vaccine, enhance anti-fibrosis ability and tumor-specific T-cell infiltration	NIH/3T3, MRC-5 fibroblast cells Famale C57BL/6 mice, Murine BRAF-mutant melanoma cell line BPD6	[108] [109]
4. ECM				
	pirfenidone	MRPL-PFD, downregulate ECM levels and enhance penetration of therapeutic drugs	Mia-paca-2 co-implanted tumor-bearing mice model	[112]

Table 1. Cont.

Target	Loading Drugs	Nanocomposites and Outcomes	Animal Models/Cell Lines	Ref.
5. Exosomes	Pt prodrug	exosome capsule Pt(Iau)-HSA-lecithin NPs develop chemotherapy for breast cancer	4T1 tumor bearing lung metastasis mice model	[119]
	-	AC electrokinetic direct immunoassay procedure permits specific identification and quantification of target biomarkers within as little as 30 min total time	Blood samples from patients	[120]
	-	magnetic beads conjugated with CD63 antibody for early diagnosis of cancer exosome	MDA-MB-231 cell line	[121]
6. Vasculature	cisplatin prodrug	cyclic pentapeptide and Pt (IV) loaded PLGA- PEG NPs targeting α(v)β(3) integrin were more efficacious and better tolerated	Female nude mice, DU145, MCF-7 cell line	[127]
	-	poly (acrylic acid) (PAA)-modified NaLnF4:40Gd/20Yb/2Er nanorods, for in vivo optical-guided tumor vessel/metastasis and noninvasive brain vascular imaging	LLC tumor bearing mice model	[128]
	-	anti-hVEGF molecularly imprinted polymer nanoparticles coupled with quantum dots for cancer imaging	WM-266 hVEGF(+) and A-375 hVEGF(−) model	[129]
	-	aggregation-induced emission (AIE) photosensitizer to fabricate integrin α(v)β(3) for image-guided and PDT	Nude mice, QBC939, L-O2, and HK-2 cells	[130]
7. Multiconstituents	-	Ca^{2+} in NPs can promote the maturation of DCs and release DAMPs from tumor cell to enhance infiltration of CTLs		[131]
	anti-CD47 and anti-SIRPα	exosomes NPs from M1 macrophages stopped SIRPα—CD47 axis in the acidic TME abolished the "don't eat me" signal between tumor cell and macrophages and reprogram the M2 macrophages to M1 type	4T1 tumor-bearing BALB/c mice	[132]

4. Conclusions and Outlook

Traditional cancer diagnosis, chemotherapy, radiotherapy, surgery, and other treatments have kept the high mortality rate of cancer patients, and this led us to develop new strategies with more accurate diagnoses and more effective treatments. Using NPs to treat cancers is an emerging approach. In addition to targeting tumors themselves, utilizing TME and physicochemical properties to treat and orientate tumors have been a great inspiration and challenge for the development of nanoparticles. More evidence is needed for the clinical application of NPs, and here we summarize current results and several challenges of NPs.

The special conditions of the tumor microenvironment give us superior delivery conditions. The immunosuppressed environment of tumor causes "immune escape" and serves as a good direction for the treatment of tumors. The extracellular matrix, enzymes, and inflammatory factors also provide promising therapeutic targets. The physiological features such as hypoxia, acidic microenvironment, and abundant angiogenesis also give NPs good access conditions to reach tumor site and release drugs.

How to use the particular microenvironment of tumor to design delivered nanoparticles is a big hurdle. A question that remains to be solved is how to deliver drugs to tumor tissues more efficiently and specifically. PEG and zwitterionic materials can effectively reduce the blood clearance rate. In order to improve the biocompatibility, it is also a breakthrough for people to use the biological membranes to cover the material. According to the EPR effect and the abundance of blood vessels in tumors, drugs will be delivered to tumor tissue precisely, hence improving therapeutic efficiency for tumors. However, there is a huge difference between the internal environment of human beings and that of animal models, and how to reduce the side effects of materials and systems is what we need to work on. Clinical trials on nanoparticles are yet to be developed, and we should make more efforts to develop safe and efficient therapy strategies.

Author Contributions: Conceptualization, methodology, software, writing-original draft preparation, editing, Y.S. and Y.L.; project administration, and review, S.S. and C.D. All authors have read and agreed to the published version of the manuscript.

Funding: This work was supported by the Science and Technology Commission of Shanghai Municipality (Grant No. 14DZ2261100, 15DZ1940106), the Joint Project of Health and Family Planning Committee of Pudong New Area (Grant No. PW2017D-10) and the National Natural Science Foundation of China (Grant Nos. 81860547, 81573008, 21671150, 21877084, 81171646, 31170776, and 21472139).

Institutional Review Board Statement: Not applicable.

Informed Consent Statement: Not applicable.

Data Availability Statement: Not applicable.

Conflicts of Interest: There are no conflict to declare.

Abbreviations

Abbreviation	Full terms
TME	Tumor microenvironment
ECM	Extracellular matrix
NPs	Nanoparticles
EPR	Enhanced permeation and retention
MSNs	Mesoporous silica nanoparticles
MNPs	Magnetic nanoparticles
GNPs	Gold nanoparticles
CAFs	Cancer associated fibroblasts
T cell	T lymphocyte
B cell	B lymphocyte
ROS	Reactive oxygen species

NK	Natural killer
DCs	Dendritic cells
SIRPα	Signaling regulatory protein α
Tregs	Regulatory T cells
TAMs	Tumor associated macrophages
TNF-α	Tumor necrosis factor-α-T
IL	Interleukin
CTLA-4	Cytotoxic T-lymphocyte-associated antigen-4
CCL	Chemokine ligand
CCR	Chemokine recepter
MDSCs	Myeloid-derived suppressor cells
VEGF	Vascular endothelial growth factor
EGF	Epidermal growth factor
TGF-β	Transforming growth factor-β
MMP	Matrix metalloproteinase
SDF1	Stromal cell- derived factor 1
MCP-1	Monocyte chemotactic protein-1
VCAM-1	Vascular cell adhesion molecule-1
PDGF	Platelet-derived growth factor
DAMPs	produce damage-associated molecular patterns
HIF	Hypoxia inducible factor
ATP	Adenosine-5′-triphos-phate
GSH	Glutathione
MPDA	Mesoporous polydopamine
FRET	Forster resonance energy transfer
ssDNA	Single-stranded DNA
GSSG	GSH/glutathione disulfide
CSC	Cancer stem cells
PEG	polyethylene glycol
DOX	Doxorubicin
CTL	Cytotoxic lymphocyte
AuNPs	Gold nanoparticles
AgNPs	Silver nanoparticles
RNS	Reactive nitrogen species
PTT	Photothermal therapy
PDT	Photodynamic therapy
DTX	Docetaxel
ROS	Reactive oxygen species
Man-LF NPs	Mannosylated lactoferrin nanoparticulate system
cGAMP	Cyclic guanosine monophosphate-adenosine monophosphate
STING	Stimulator of interferon genes
PD-1	Programmed cell death 1
PD-L1	Programmed cell death ligand 1
IDO	Indole-amine-2,3-dioxygenase
NE	Nanoemulsion
PFD	Pirfenidone
LLC	Lewis lung carcinoma
HSA	Human serum albumin
QDs	Quantum dots
ACF	Acriflavine

References

1. Cheng, H.S.; Lee, J.X.T.; Wahli, W.; Tan, N.S. Exploiting vulnerabilities of cancer by targeting nuclear receptors of stromal cells in tumor microenvironment. *Mol. Cancer* **2019**, *18*, 51. [CrossRef]
2. Lord, E.M.; Penney, D.P.; Sutherland, R.M.; Cooper, R.A., Jr. Morphological and functional characteristics of cells infiltrating and destroying tumor multicellular spheroids in vivo. *Virchows Arch. B Cell Pathol. Incl. Mol. Pathol.* **1979**, *31*, 103–116. [CrossRef]
3. Zhu, L.; Wang, T.; Perche, F.; Taigind, A.; Torchilin, V.P. Enhanced anticancer activity of nanopreparation containing an MMP2-sensitive PEG-drug conjugate and cell-penetrating moiety. *Proc. Natl. Acad. Sci. USA* **2013**, *110*, 17047–17052. [CrossRef]

4. Fane, M.; Weeraratna, A.T. How the ageing microenvironment influences tumour progression. *Nat. Rev. Cancer* **2020**, *20*, 89–106. [CrossRef]
5. Binnewies, M.; Roberts, E.W.; Kersten, K.; Chan, V.; Fearon, D.F.; Merad, M.; Coussens, L.M.; Gabrilovich, D.I.; Ostrand-Rosenberg, S.; Hedrick, C.C.; et al. Understanding the tumor immune microenvironment (TIME) for effective therapy. *Nat. Med.* **2018**, *24*, 541–550. [CrossRef] [PubMed]
6. Quail, D.F.; Joyce, J.A. The Microenvironmental Landscape of Brain Tumors. *Cancer Cell* **2017**, *31*, 326–341. [CrossRef] [PubMed]
7. Qu, Y.; Dou, B.; Tan, H.; Feng, Y.; Wang, N.; Wang, D. Tumor microenvironment-driven non-cell-autonomous resistance to antineoplastic treatment. *Mol. Cancer* **2019**, *18*, 69. [CrossRef] [PubMed]
8. Musetti, S.; Huang, L. Nanoparticle-Mediated Remodeling of the Tumor Microenvironment to Enhance Immunotherapy. *ACS Nano* **2018**, *12*, 11740–11755. [CrossRef] [PubMed]
9. Gabizon, A.A.; Patil, Y.; La-Beck, N.M. New insights and evolving role of pegylated liposomal doxorubicin in cancer therapy. *Drug. Resist. Update* **2016**, *29*. [CrossRef]
10. Wang, Y.; Zhao, Q.; Han, N.; Bai, L.; Li, J.; Liu, J.; Che, E.; Hu, L.; Zhang, Q.; Jiang, T.; et al. Mesoporous silica nanoparticles in drug delivery and biomedical applications. *Nanomedicine* **2015**, *11*, 313–327. [CrossRef]
11. Pastucha, M.; Farka, Z.; Lacina, K.; Mikušová, Z.; Skládal, P. Magnetic nanoparticles for smart electrochemical immunoassays: A review on recent developments. *Mikrochim. Acta* **2019**, *186*, 312. [CrossRef]
12. Singh, P.; Pandit, S.; Mokkapati, V.R.S.S.; Garg, A.; Ravikumar, V.; Mijakovic, I. Gold Nanoparticles in Diagnostics and Therapeutics for Human Cancer. *Int. J. Mol. Sci.* **2018**, *19*, 1979. [CrossRef]
13. Maeda, H.; Nakamura, H.; Fang, J. The EPR effect for macromolecular drug delivery to solid tumors: Improvement of tumor uptake, lowering of systemic toxicity, and distinct tumor imaging in vivo. *Adv. Drug Deliv. Rev.* **2013**, *65*, 71–79. [CrossRef]
14. Keren, L.; Bosse, M.; Marquez, D.; Angoshtari, R.; Jain, S.; Varma, S.; Yang, S.-R.; Kurian, A.; Van Valen, D.; West, R.; et al. A Structured Tumor-Immune Microenvironment in Triple Negative Breast Cancer Revealed by Multiplexed Ion Beam Imaging. *Cell* **2018**, *174*, 1373–1387.e1319. [CrossRef] [PubMed]
15. Meurette, O.; Mehlen, P. Notch Signaling in the Tumor Microenvironment. *Cancer Cell* **2018**, *34*, 536–548. [CrossRef] [PubMed]
16. Cong, V.T.; Gaus, K.; Tilley, R.D.; Gooding, J.J. Rod-shaped mesoporous silica nanoparticles for nanomedicine: Recent progress and perspectives. *Expert Opin. Drug Deliv.* **2018**, *15*, 881–892. [CrossRef] [PubMed]
17. El-Sawy, H.S.; Al-Abd, A.M.; Ahmed, T.A.; El-Say, K.M.; Torchilin, V.P. Stimuli-Responsive Nano-Architecture Drug-Delivery Systems to Solid Tumor Micromilieu: Past, Present, and Future Perspectives. *ACS Nano* **2018**, *12*, 10636–10664. [CrossRef]
18. Shi, Y.; Lammers, T. Combining Nanomedicine and Immunotherapy. *Acc. Chem. Res.* **2019**, *52*, 1543–1554. [CrossRef]
19. Peng, J.; Yang, Q.; Shi, K.; Xiao, Y.; Wei, X.; Qian, Z. Intratumoral fate of functional nanoparticles in response to microenvironment factor: Implications on cancer diagnosis and therapy. *Adv. Drug Deliv. Rev.* **2019**, *143*, 37–67. [CrossRef] [PubMed]
20. Jiménez-Sánchez, A.; Memon, D.; Pourpe, S.; Veeraraghavan, H.; Li, Y.; Vargas, H.A.; Gill, M.B.; Park, K.J.; Zivanovic, O.; Konner, J.; et al. Heterogeneous Tumor-Immune Microenvironments among Differentially Growing Metastases in an Ovarian Cancer Patient. *Cell* **2017**, *170*, 927–938.e920. [CrossRef]
21. Hinshaw, D.C.; Shevde, L.A. The Tumor Microenvironment Innately Modulates Cancer Progression. *Cancer Res.* **2019**, *79*, 4557–4566. [CrossRef] [PubMed]
22. Zhao, J.; Guo, C.; Xiong, F.; Yu, J.; Ge, J.; Wang, H.; Liao, Q.; Zhou, Y.; Gong, Q.; Xiang, B.; et al. Single cell RNA-seq reveals the landscape of tumor and infiltrating immune cells in nasopharyngeal carcinoma. *Cancer Lett.* **2020**, *477*, 131–143. [CrossRef] [PubMed]
23. Thommen, D.S.; Schumacher, T.N. T Cell Dysfunction in Cancer. *Cancer Cell* **2018**, *33*, 547–562. [CrossRef]
24. Zhang, Y.; Kurupati, R.; Liu, L.; Zhou, X.Y.; Zhang, G.; Hudaihed, A.; Filisio, F.; Giles-Davis, W.; Xu, X.; Karakousis, G.C.; et al. Enhancing CD8 T Cell Fatty Acid Catabolism within a Metabolically Challenging Tumor Microenvironment Increases the Efficacy of Melanoma Immunotherapy. *Cancer Cell* **2017**, *32*, 377–391.e379. [CrossRef]
25. Griffith, J.W.; Sokol, C.L.; Luster, A.D. Chemokines and chemokine receptors: Positioning cells for host defense and immunity. *Annu Rev. Immunol.* **2014**, *32*, 659–702. [CrossRef] [PubMed]
26. Vitale, I.; Manic, G.; Coussens, L.M.; Kroemer, G.; Galluzzi, L. Macrophages and Metabolism in the Tumor Microenvironment. *Cell Metab.* **2019**, *30*, 36–50. [CrossRef] [PubMed]
27. Baert, T.; Vankerckhoven, A.; Riva, M.; Van Hoylandt, A.; Thirion, G.; Holger, G.; Mathivet, T.; Vergote, I.; Coosemans, A. Myeloid Derived Suppressor Cells: Key Drivers of Immunosuppression in Ovarian Cancer. *Front. Immunol.* **2019**, *10*, 1273. [CrossRef]
28. Shabani, M.; Sadeghi, A.; Hosseini, H.; Teimouri, M.; Babaei Khorzoughi, R.; Pasalar, P.; Meshkani, R. Resveratrol alleviates obesity-induced skeletal muscle inflammation via decreasing M1 macrophage polarization and increasing the regulatory T cell population. *Sci. Rep.* **2020**, *10*, 3791. [CrossRef]
29. Mathivet, T.; Bouleti, C.; Van Woensel, M.; Stanchi, F.; Verschuere, T.; Phng, L.-K.; Dejaegher, J.; Balcer, M.; Matsumoto, K.; Georgieva, P.B.; et al. Dynamic stroma reorganization drives blood vessel dysmorphia during glioma growth. *EMBO Mol. Med.* **2017**, *9*, 1629–1645. [CrossRef]
30. Nawaz, A.; Aminuddin, A.; Kado, T.; Takikawa, A.; Yamamoto, S.; Tsuneyama, K.; Igarashi, Y.; Ikutani, M.; Nishida, Y.; Nagai, Y.; et al. CD206 M2-like macrophages regulate systemic glucose metabolism by inhibiting proliferation of adipocyte progenitors. *Nat. Commun.* **2017**, *8*, 286. [CrossRef]

31. Gordon, S.R.; Maute, R.L.; Dulken, B.W.; Hutter, G.; George, B.M.; McCracken, M.N.; Gupta, R.; Tsai, J.M.; Sinha, R.; Corey, D.; et al. PD-1 expression by tumour-associated macrophages inhibits phagocytosis and tumour immunity. *Nature* **2017**, *545*, 495–499. [CrossRef]
32. Logtenberg, M.E.W.; Jansen, J.H.M.; Raaben, M.; Toebes, M.; Franke, K.; Brandsma, A.M.; Matlung, H.L.; Fauster, A.; Gomez-Eerland, R.; Bakker, N.A.M.; et al. Glutaminyl cyclase is an enzymatic modifier of the CD47- SIRPα axis and a target for cancer immunotherapy. *Nat. Med.* **2019**, *25*, 612–619. [CrossRef] [PubMed]
33. Veillette, A.; Tang, Z. Signaling Regulatory Protein (SIRP)α-CD47 Blockade Joins the Ranks of Immune Checkpoint Inhibition. *J. Clin. Oncol.* **2019**, *37*, 1012–1014. [CrossRef] [PubMed]
34. Arce Vargas, F.; Furness, A.J.S.; Solomon, I.; Joshi, K.; Mekkaoui, L.; Lesko, M.H.; Miranda Rota, E.; Dahan, R.; Georgiou, A.; Sledzinska, A.; et al. Fc-Optimized Anti-CD25 Depletes Tumor-Infiltrating Regulatory T Cells and Synergizes with PD-1 Blockade to Eradicate Established Tumors. *Immunity* **2017**, *46*, 577–586. [CrossRef]
35. Matoba, T.; Imai, M.; Ohkura, N.; Kawakita, D.; Ijichi, K.; Toyama, T.; Morita, A.; Murakami, S.; Sakaguchi, S.; Yamazaki, S. Regulatory T cells expressing abundant CTLA-4 on the cell surface with a proliferative gene profile are key features of human head and neck cancer. *Int. J. Cancer* **2019**, *144*, 2811–2822. [CrossRef]
36. Lu, L.; Barbi, J.; Pan, F. The regulation of immune tolerance by FOXP3. *Nat. Rev. Immunol.* **2017**, *17*, 703–717. [CrossRef]
37. Pierini, A.; Nishikii, H.; Baker, J.; Kimura, T.; Kwon, H.-S.; Pan, Y.; Chen, Y.; Alvarez, M.; Strober, W.; Velardi, A.; et al. Foxp3 regulatory T cells maintain the bone marrow microenvironment for B cell lymphopoiesis. *Nat. Commun.* **2017**, *8*, 15068. [CrossRef]
38. Sakaguchi, S.; Mikami, N.; Wing, J.B.; Tanaka, A.; Ichiyama, K.; Ohkura, N. Regulatory T Cells and Human Disease. *Annu Rev. Immunol.* **2020**, 541–566. [CrossRef] [PubMed]
39. Mariathasan, S.; Turley, S.J.; Nickles, D.; Castiglioni, A.; Yuen, K.; Wang, Y.; Kadel, E.E.; Koeppen, H.; Astarita, J.L.; Cubas, R.; et al. TGFβ attenuates tumour response to PD-L1 blockade by contributing to exclusion of T cells. *Nature* **2018**, *554*, 544–548. [CrossRef] [PubMed]
40. Zhao, H.; Liao, X.; Kang, Y. Tregs: Where We Are and What Comes Next? *Front. Immunol.* **2017**, *8*, 1578. [CrossRef]
41. Kryczek, I.; Wang, L.; Wu, K.; Li, W.; Zhao, E.; Cui, T.; Wei, S.; Liu, Y.; Wang, Y.; Vatan, L.; et al. Inflammatory regulatory T cells in the microenvironments of ulcerative colitis and colon carcinoma. *Oncoimmunology* **2016**, *5*, e1105430. [CrossRef]
42. Altorki, N.K.; Markowitz, G.J.; Gao, D.; Port, J.L.; Saxena, A.; Stiles, B.; McGraw, T.; Mittal, V. The lung microenvironment: An important regulator of tumour growth and metastasis. *Nat. Rev. Cancer* **2019**, *19*, 9–31. [CrossRef] [PubMed]
43. Riera-Domingo, C.; Audigé, A.; Granja, S.; Cheng, W.-C.; Ho, P.-C.; Baltazar, F.; Stockmann, C.; Mazzone, M. Immunity, Hypoxia, and Metabolism-the Ménage à Trois of Cancer: Implications for Immunotherapy. *Physiol. Rev.* **2020**, *100*, 1–102. [CrossRef] [PubMed]
44. Valanparambil, R.M.; Tam, M.; Gros, P.-P.; Auger, J.-P.; Segura, M.; Gros, P.; Jardim, A.; Geary, T.G.; Ozato, K.; Stevenson, M.M. IRF-8 regulates expansion of myeloid-derived suppressor cells and Foxp3+ regulatory T cells and modulates Th2 immune responses to gastrointestinal nematode infection. *PLoS Pathog.* **2017**, *13*, e1006647. [CrossRef] [PubMed]
45. Yu, J.; Du, W.; Yan, F.; Wang, Y.; Li, H.; Cao, S.; Yu, W.; Shen, C.; Liu, J.; Ren, X. Myeloid-derived suppressor cells suppress antitumor immune responses through IDO expression and correlate with lymph node metastasis in patients with breast cancer. *J. Immunol.* **2013**, *190*, 3783–3797. [CrossRef] [PubMed]
46. Kumar, V.; Patel, S.; Tcyganov, E.; Gabrilovich, D.I. The Nature of Myeloid-Derived Suppressor Cells in the Tumor Microenvironment. *Trends Immunol.* **2016**, *37*, 208–220. [CrossRef]
47. Su, X.; Fan, Y.; Yang, L.; Huang, J.; Qiao, F.; Fang, Y.; Wang, J. Dexmedetomidine expands monocytic myeloid-derived suppressor cells and promotes tumour metastasis after lung cancer surgery. *J. Transl. Med.* **2018**, *16*, 347. [CrossRef]
48. Niklason, L.E. Understanding the Extracellular Matrix to Enhance Stem Cell-Based Tissue Regeneration. *Cell Stem Cell* **2018**, *22*, 302–305. [CrossRef]
49. Kalluri, R. Basement membranes: Structure, assembly and role in tumour angiogenesis. *Nat. Rev. Cancer* **2003**, *3*, 422–433. [CrossRef]
50. Chen, H.; Qu, J.; Huang, X.; Kurundkar, A.; Zhu, L.; Yang, N.; Venado, A.; Ding, Q.; Liu, G.; Antony, V.B.; et al. Mechanosensing by the α6-integrin confers an invasive fibroblast phenotype and mediates lung fibrosis. *Nat. Commun.* **2016**, *7*, 12504. [CrossRef]
51. Yosef, G.; Arkadash, V.; Papo, N. Targeting the MMP-14/MMP-2/integrin αβ axis with multispecific N-TIMP2-based antagonists for cancer therapy. *J. Biol. Chem.* **2018**, *293*, 13310–13326. [CrossRef] [PubMed]
52. Castro-Castro, A.; Marchesin, V.; Monteiro, P.; Lodillinsky, C.; Rossé, C.; Chavrier, P. Cellular and Molecular Mechanisms of MT1-MMP-Dependent Cancer Cell Invasion. *Annu Rev. Cell Dev. Biol.* **2016**, *32*, 555–576. [CrossRef] [PubMed]
53. Huels, D.J.; Medema, J.P. Think About the Environment: Cellular Reprogramming by the Extracellular Matrix. *Cell Stem Cell* **2018**, *22*, 7–9. [CrossRef] [PubMed]
54. Hawk, M.A.; Gorsuch, C.L.; Fagan, P.; Lee, C.; Kim, S.E.; Hamann, J.C.; Mason, J.A.; Weigel, K.J.; Tsegaye, M.A.; Shen, L.; et al. RIPK1-mediated induction of mitophagy compromises the viability of extracellular-matrix-detached cells. *Nat. Cell Biol.* **2018**, *20*, 272–284. [CrossRef] [PubMed]
55. Cadamuro, M.; Brivio, S.; Mertens, J.; Vismara, M.; Moncsek, A.; Milani, C.; Fingas, C.; Cristina Malerba, M.; Nardo, G.; Dall'Olmo, L.; et al. Platelet-derived growth factor-D enables liver myofibroblasts to promote tumor lymphangiogenesis in cholangiocarcinoma. *J. Hepatol.* **2019**, *70*, 700–709. [CrossRef] [PubMed]

56. Roswall, P.; Bocci, M.; Bartoschek, M.; Li, H.; Kristiansen, G.; Jansson, S.; Lehn, S.; Sjölund, J.; Reid, S.; Larsson, C.; et al. Microenvironmental control of breast cancer subtype elicited through paracrine platelet-derived growth factor-CC signaling. *Nat. Med.* **2018**, *24*, 463–473. [CrossRef]
57. Kumar, V.; Donthireddy, L.; Marvel, D.; Condamine, T.; Wang, F.; Lavilla-Alonso, S.; Hashimoto, A.; Vonteddu, P.; Behera, R.; Goins, M.A.; et al. Cancer-Associated Fibroblasts Neutralize the Anti-tumor Effect of CSF1 Receptor Blockade by Inducing PMN-MDSC Infiltration of Tumors. *Cancer Cell* **2017**, *32*, 654–668.e655. [CrossRef]
58. Zhang, J.; Chen, L.; Xiao, M.; Wang, C.; Qin, Z. FSP1+ fibroblasts promote skin carcinogenesis by maintaining MCP-1-mediated macrophage infiltration and chronic inflammation. *Am. J. Pathol.* **2011**, *178*, 382–390. [CrossRef]
59. Moore-Smith, L.D.; Isayeva, T.; Lee, J.H.; Frost, A.; Ponnazhagan, S. Silencing of TGF-β1 in tumor cells impacts MMP-9 in tumor microenvironment. *Sci. Rep.* **2017**, *7*, 8678. [CrossRef]
60. Yang, J.; Lu, Y.; Lin, Y.-Y.; Zheng, Z.-Y.; Fang, J.-H.; He, S.; Zhuang, S.-M. Vascular mimicry formation is promoted by paracrine TGF-β and SDF1 of cancer-associated fibroblasts and inhibited by miR-101 in hepatocellular carcinoma. *Cancer Lett.* **2016**, *383*, 18–27. [CrossRef]
61. Curtis, M.; Kenny, H.A.; Ashcroft, B.; Mukherjee, A.; Johnson, A.; Zhang, Y.; Helou, Y.; Batlle, R.; Liu, X.; Gutierrez, N.; et al. Fibroblasts Mobilize Tumor Cell Glycogen to Promote Proliferation and Metastasis. *Cell Metab.* **2019**, *29*. [CrossRef] [PubMed]
62. Yu, T.; Yang, G.; Hou, Y.; Tang, X.; Wu, C.; Wu, X.A.; Guo, L.; Zhu, Q.; Luo, H.; Du, Y.E.; et al. Cytoplasmic GPER translocation in cancer-associated fibroblasts mediates cAMP/PKA/CREB/glycolytic axis to confer tumor cells with multidrug resistance. *Oncogene* **2017**, *36*, 2131–2145. [CrossRef] [PubMed]
63. Demircioglu, F.; Wang, J.; Candido, J.; Costa, A.S.H.; Casado, P.; de Luxan Delgado, B.; Reynolds, L.E.; Gomez-Escudero, J.; Newport, E.; Rajeeve, V.; et al. Cancer associated fibroblast FAK regulates malignant cell metabolism. *Nat. Commun.* **2020**, *11*, 1290. [CrossRef] [PubMed]
64. Pegtel, D.M.; Gould, S.J. Exosomes. *Annu. Rev. Biochem.* **2019**, *88*, 487–514. [CrossRef]
65. Zhou, W.; Fong, M.Y.; Min, Y.; Somlo, G.; Liu, L.; Palomares, M.R.; Yu, Y.; Chow, A.; O'Connor, S.T.F.; Chin, A.R.; et al. Cancer-secreted miR-105 destroys vascular endothelial barriers to promote metastasis. *Cancer Cell* **2014**, *25*, 501–515. [CrossRef]
66. Luga, V.; Zhang, L.; Viloria-Petit, A.M.; Ogunjimi, A.A.; Inanlou, M.R.; Chiu, E.; Buchanan, M.; Hosein, A.N.; Basik, M.; Wrana, J.L. Exosomes mediate stromal mobilization of autocrine Wnt-PCP signaling in breast cancer cell migration. *Cell* **2012**, *151*, 1542–1556. [CrossRef] [PubMed]
67. Zhang, L.; Zhang, S.; Yao, J.; Lowery, F.J.; Zhang, Q.; Huang, W.-C.; Li, P.; Li, M.; Wang, X.; Zhang, C.; et al. Microenvironment-induced PTEN loss by exosomal microRNA primes brain metastasis outgrowth. *Nature* **2015**, *527*, 100–104. [CrossRef] [PubMed]
68. Théry, C.; Ostrowski, M.; Segura, E. Membrane vesicles as conveyors of immune responses. *Nat. Rev. Immunol.* **2009**, *9*, 581–593. [CrossRef]
69. Guo, X.; Qiu, W.; Wang, J.; Liu, Q.; Qian, M.; Wang, S.; Zhang, Z.; Gao, X.; Chen, Z.; Guo, Q.; et al. Glioma exosomes mediate the expansion and function of myeloid-derived suppressor cells through microRNA-29a/Hbp1 and microRNA-92a/Prkar1a pathways. *Int. J. Cancer* **2019**, *144*, 3111–3126. [CrossRef]
70. Guo, X.; Qiu, W.; Liu, Q.; Qian, M.; Wang, S.; Zhang, Z.; Gao, X.; Chen, Z.; Xue, H.; Li, G. Immunosuppressive effects of hypoxia-induced glioma exosomes through myeloid-derived suppressor cells via the miR-10a/Rora and miR-21/Pten Pathways. *Oncogene* **2018**, *37*, 4239–4259. [CrossRef]
71. Matsumoto, Y.; Nichols, J.W.; Toh, K.; Nomoto, T.; Cabral, H.; Miura, Y.; Christie, R.J.; Yamada, N.; Ogura, T.; Kano, M.R.; et al. Vascular bursts enhance permeability of tumour blood vessels and improve nanoparticle delivery. *Nat. Nanotechnol.* **2016**, *11*, 533–538. [CrossRef]
72. Chen, Z.; Zhu, S.; Hong, J.; Soutto, M.; Peng, D.; Belkhiri, A.; Xu, Z.; El-Rifai, W. Gastric tumour-derived ANGPT2 regulation by DARPP-32 promotes angiogenesis. *Gut* **2016**, *65*, 925–934. [CrossRef] [PubMed]
73. Patel, N.; Duffy, B.A.; Badar, A.; Lythgoe, M.F.; Årstad, E. Bimodal Imaging of Inflammation with SPECT/CT and MRI Using Iodine-125 Labeled VCAM-1 Targeting Microparticle Conjugates. *Bioconjug. Chem.* **2015**, *26*, 1542–1549. [CrossRef] [PubMed]
74. Huang, Y.; Kim, B.Y.S.; Chan, C.K.; Hahn, S.M.; Weissman, I.L.; Jiang, W. Improving immune-vascular crosstalk for cancer immunotherapy. *Nat. Rev. Immunol.* **2018**, *18*, 195–203. [CrossRef] [PubMed]
75. Maman, S.; Witz, I.P. A history of exploring cancer in context. *Nat. Rev. Cancer* **2018**, *18*, 359–376. [CrossRef] [PubMed]
76. Li, L.; Liang, Y.; Kang, L.; Liu, Y.; Gao, S.; Chen, S.; Li, Y.; You, W.; Dong, Q.; Hong, T.; et al. Transcriptional Regulation of the Warburg Effect in Cancer by SIX1. *Cancer Cell* **2018**, *33*, 368–385. [CrossRef]
77. Lin, B.; Chen, H.; Liang, D.; Lin, W.; Qi, X.; Liu, H.; Deng, X. Acidic pH and High-H0 Dual Tumor Microenvironment-Responsive Nanocatalytic Graphene Oxide for Cancer Selective Therapy and Recognition. *ACS Appl. Mater. Interfaces* **2019**, *11*, 11157–11166. [CrossRef] [PubMed]
78. Keith, B.; Johnson, R.S.; Simon, M.C. HIF1α and HIF2α: Sibling rivalry in hypoxic tumour growth and progression. *Nat. Rev. Cancer* **2011**, *12*, 9–22. [CrossRef]
79. Massari, F.; Ciccarese, C.; Santoni, M.; Iacovelli, R.; Mazzucchelli, R.; Piva, F.; Scarpelli, M.; Berardi, R.; Tortora, G.; Lopez-Beltran, A.; et al. Metabolic phenotype of bladder cancer. *Cancer Treat. Rev.* **2016**, *45*, 46–57. [CrossRef]
80. Chen, F.; Chen, J.; Yang, L.; Liu, J.; Zhang, X.; Zhang, Y.; Tu, Q.; Yin, D.; Lin, D.; Wong, P.-P.; et al. Extracellular vesicle-packaged HIF-1α-stabilizing lncRNA from tumour-associated macrophages regulates aerobic glycolysis of breast cancer cells. *Nat. Cell Biol.* **2019**, *21*, 498–510. [CrossRef]

81. Kepp, O.; Loos, F.; Liu, P.; Kroemer, G. Extracellular nucleosides and nucleotides as immunomodulators. *Immunol. Rev.* **2017**, *280*, 83–92. [CrossRef] [PubMed]
82. Abdel-Wahab, A.F.; Mahmoud, W.; Al-Harizy, R.M. Targeting glucose metabolism to suppress cancer progression: Prospective of anti-glycolytic cancer therapy. *Pharmacol. Res.* **2019**, *150*, 104511. [CrossRef]
83. Mo, R.; Jiang, T.; DiSanto, R.; Tai, W.; Gu, Z. ATP-triggered anticancer drug delivery. *Nat. Commun.* **2014**, *5*, 3364. [CrossRef] [PubMed]
84. Sameiyan, E.; Bagheri, E.; Dehghani, S.; Ramezani, M.; Alibolandi, M.; Abnous, K.; Taghdisi, S.M. Aptamer-based ATP-responsive delivery systems for cancer diagnosis and treatment. *Acta Biomater.* **2021**, *123*, 110–122. [CrossRef] [PubMed]
85. Hatfield, S.M.; Kjaergaard, J.; Lukashev, D.; Schreiber, T.H.; Belikoff, B.; Abbott, R.; Sethumadhavan, S.; Philbrook, P.; Ko, K.; Cannici, R.; et al. Immunological mechanisms of the antitumor effects of supplemental oxygenation. *Sci. Transl. Med.* **2015**, *7*, 277ra230. [CrossRef]
86. Ogiwara, H.; Takahashi, K.; Sasaki, M.; Kuroda, T.; Yoshida, H.; Watanabe, R.; Maruyama, A.; Makinoshima, H.; Chiwaki, F.; Sasaki, H.; et al. Targeting the Vulnerability of Glutathione Metabolism in ARID1A-Deficient Cancers. *Cancer Cell* **2019**, *35*, 9–22. [CrossRef]
87. Yang, J.; Wang, C.; Shi, S.; Dong, C. Nanotechnologies for enhancing cancer immunotherapy. *Nano Res.* **2020**, 1–22. [CrossRef]
88. Peranzoni, E.; Lemoine, J.; Vimeux, L.; Feuillet, V.; Barrin, S.; Kantari-Mimoun, C.; Bercovici, N.; Guérin, M.; Biton, J.; Ouakrim, H.; et al. Macrophages impede CD8 T cells from reaching tumor cells and limit the efficacy of anti-PD-1 treatment. *Proc. Natl. Acad. Sci. USA* **2018**, *115*, E4041–E4050. [CrossRef] [PubMed]
89. Chen, Q.; Wang, C.; Zhang, X.; Chen, G.; Hu, Q.; Li, H.; Wang, J.; Wen, D.; Zhang, Y.; Lu, Y.; et al. In situ sprayed bioresponsive immunotherapeutic gel for post-surgical cancer treatment. *Nat. Nanotechnol.* **2019**, *14*, 89–97. [CrossRef]
90. Shi, C.; Liu, T.; Guo, Z.; Zhuang, R.; Zhang, X.; Chen, X. Reprogramming Tumor-Associated Macrophages by Nanoparticle-Based Reactive Oxygen Species Photogeneration. *Nano Lett.* **2018**, *18*, 7330–7342. [CrossRef]
91. Pal, R.; Chakraborty, B.; Nath, A.; Singh, L.M.; Ali, M.; Rahman, D.S.; Ghosh, S.K.; Basu, A.; Bhattacharya, S.; Baral, R.; et al. Noble metal nanoparticle-induced oxidative stress modulates tumor associated macrophages (TAMs) from an M2 to M1 phenotype: An in vitro approach. *Int. Immunopharmacol.* **2016**, *38*, 332–341. [CrossRef]
92. Chen, L.; Zhou, L.; Wang, C.; Han, Y.; Lu, Y.; Liu, J.; Hu, X.; Yao, T.; Lin, Y.; Liang, S.; et al. Tumor-Targeted Drug and CpG Delivery System for Phototherapy and Docetaxel-Enhanced Immunotherapy with Polarization toward M1-Type Macrophages on Triple Negative Breast Cancers. *Adv. Mater.* **2019**, *31*, e1904997. [CrossRef] [PubMed]
93. Wang, H.; Tang, Y.; Fang, Y.; Zhang, M.; Wang, H.; He, Z.; Wang, B.; Xu, Q.; Huang, Y. Reprogramming Tumor Immune Microenvironment (TIME) and Metabolism via Biomimetic Targeting Codelivery of Shikonin/JQ1. *Nano Lett.* **2019**, *19*, 2935–2944. [CrossRef]
94. Kim, H.-Y.; Li, R.; Ng, T.S.C.; Courties, G.; Rodell, C.B.; Prytyskach, M.; Kohler, R.H.; Pittet, M.J.; Nahrendorf, M.; Weissleder, R.; et al. Quantitative Imaging of Tumor-Associated Macrophages and Their Response to Therapy Using Cu-Labeled Macrin. *ACS Nano* **2018**, *12*, 12015–12029. [CrossRef] [PubMed]
95. Johnson, D.E.; O'Keefe, R.A.; Grandis, J.R. Targeting the IL-6/JAK/STAT3 signalling axis in cancer. *Nat. Rev. Clin. Oncol.* **2018**, *15*, 234–248. [CrossRef] [PubMed]
96. Yu, H.; Lee, H.; Herrmann, A.; Buettner, R.; Jove, R. Revisiting STAT3 signalling in cancer: New and unexpected biological functions. *Nat. Rev. Cancer* **2014**, *14*, 736–746. [CrossRef] [PubMed]
97. Huo, M.; Zhao, Y.; Satterlee, A.B.; Wang, Y.; Xu, Y.; Huang, L. Tumor-targeted delivery of sunitinib base enhances vaccine therapy for advanced melanoma by remodeling the tumor microenvironment. *J. Control. Release* **2017**, *245*, 81–94. [CrossRef]
98. Ou, W.; Thapa, R.K.; Jiang, L.; Soe, Z.C.; Gautam, M.; Chang, J.-H.; Jeong, J.-H.; Ku, S.K.; Choi, H.-G.; Yong, C.S.; et al. Regulatory T cell-targeted hybrid nanoparticles combined with immuno-checkpoint blockage for cancer immunotherapy. *J. Control. Release* **2018**, *281*, 84–96. [CrossRef]
99. Dong, X.; Liang, J.; Yang, A.; Qian, Z.; Kong, D.; Lv, F. Fluorescence imaging guided CpG nanoparticles-loaded IR820-hydrogel for synergistic photothermal immunotherapy. *Biomaterials* **2019**, *209*, 111–125. [CrossRef]
100. Shae, D.; Becker, K.W.; Christov, P.; Yun, D.S.; Lytton-Jean, A.K.R.; Sevimli, S.; Ascano, M.; Kelley, M.; Johnson, D.B.; Balko, J.M.; et al. Endosomolytic polymersomes increase the activity of cyclic dinucleotide STING agonists to enhance cancer immunotherapy. *Nat. Nanotechnol.* **2019**, *14*, 269–278. [CrossRef]
101. Prendergast, G.C.; Malachowski, W.P.; DuHadaway, J.B.; Muller, A.J. Discovery of IDO1 Inhibitors: From Bench to Bedside. *Cancer Res.* **2017**, *77*, 6795–6811. [CrossRef]
102. Medzhitov, R.; Shevach, E.M.; Trinchieri, G.; Mellor, A.L.; Munn, D.H.; Gordon, S.; Libby, P.; Hansson, G.K.; Shortman, K.; Dong, C.; et al. Highlights of 10 years of immunology in Nature Reviews Immunology. *Nat. Rev. Immunol.* **2011**, *11*, 693–702. [CrossRef]
103. Smith, C.; Chang, M.Y.; Parker, K.H.; Beury, D.W.; DuHadaway, J.B.; Flick, H.E.; Boulden, J.; Sutanto-Ward, E.; Soler, A.P.; Laury-Kleintop, L.D.; et al. IDO is a nodal pathogenic driver of lung cancer and metastasis development. *Cancer Discov.* **2012**, *2*, 722–735. [CrossRef]
104. Cheng, K.; Ding, Y.; Zhao, Y.; Ye, S.; Zhao, X.; Zhang, Y.; Ji, T.; Wu, H.; Wang, B.; Anderson, G.J.; et al. Sequentially Responsive Therapeutic Peptide Assembling Nanoparticles for Dual-Targeted Cancer Immunotherapy. *Nano Lett.* **2018**, *18*, 3250–3258. [CrossRef]

105. Xu, Z.; Wang, Y.; Zhang, L.; Huang, L. Nanoparticle-delivered transforming growth factor-β siRNA enhances vaccination against advanced melanoma by modifying tumor microenvironment. *ACS Nano* **2014**, *8*, 3636–3645. [CrossRef]
106. Zhou, L.; Chen, L.; Hu, X.; Lu, Y.; Liu, W.; Sun, Y.; Yao, T.; Dong, C.; Shi, S. A CuS nanoparticle-based CpG delivery system for synergistic photothermal-, photodynamic- and immunotherapy. *Commun. Biol.* **2020**, *3*, 343. [CrossRef] [PubMed]
107. Kalluri, R. The biology and function of fibroblasts in cancer. *Nat. Rev. Cancer* **2016**, *16*, 582–598. [CrossRef] [PubMed]
108. Kovács, D.; Igaz, N.; Marton, A.; Rónavári, A.; Bélteky, P.; Bodai, L.; Spengler, G.; Tiszlavicz, L.; Rázga, Z.; Hegyi, P.; et al. Core-shell nanoparticles suppress metastasis and modify the tumour-supportive activity of cancer-associated fibroblasts. *J. Nanobiotechnol.* **2020**, *18*, 18. [CrossRef] [PubMed]
109. Hou, L.; Liu, Q.; Shen, L.; Liu, Y.; Zhang, X.; Chen, F.; Huang, L. Nano-delivery of fraxinellone remodels tumor microenvironment and facilitates therapeutic vaccination in desmoplastic melanoma. *Theranostics* **2018**, *8*, 3781–3796. [CrossRef]
110. Yu, Z.; Zhou, L.; Zhang, T.; Shen, R.; Li, C.; Fang, X.; Griffiths, G.; Liu, J. Sensitive Detection of MMP9 Enzymatic Activities in Single Cell-Encapsulated Microdroplets as an Assay of Cancer Cell Invasiveness. *ACS Sens.* **2017**, *2*, 626–634. [CrossRef]
111. Van Rijt, S.H.; Bölükbas, D.A.; Argyo, C.; Datz, S.; Lindner, M.; Eickelberg, O.; Königshoff, M.; Bein, T.; Meiners, S. Protease-mediated release of chemotherapeutics from mesoporous silica nanoparticles to ex vivo human and mouse lung tumors. *ACS Nano* **2015**, *9*, 2377–2389. [CrossRef]
112. Ji, T.; Lang, J.; Wang, J.; Cai, R.; Zhang, Y.; Qi, F.; Zhang, L.; Zhao, X.; Wu, W.; Hao, J.; et al. Designing Liposomes to Suppress Extracellular Matrix Expression to Enhance Drug Penetration and Pancreatic Tumor Therapy. *ACS Nano* **2017**, *11*, 8668–8678. [CrossRef]
113. Gong, H.; Chao, Y.; Xiang, J.; Han, X.; Song, G.; Feng, L.; Liu, J.; Yang, G.; Chen, Q.; Liu, Z. Hyaluronidase To Enhance Nanoparticle-Based Photodynamic Tumor Therapy. *Nano Lett.* **2016**, *16*, 2512–2521. [CrossRef] [PubMed]
114. Zhou, H.; Fan, Z.; Deng, J.; Lemons, P.K.; Arhontoulis, D.C.; Bowne, W.B.; Cheng, H. Hyaluronidase Embedded in Nanocarrier PEG Shell for Enhanced Tumor Penetration and Highly Efficient Antitumor Efficacy. *Nano Lett.* **2016**, *16*, 3268–3277. [CrossRef] [PubMed]
115. Guan, X.; Chen, J.; Hu, Y.; Lin, L.; Sun, P.; Tian, H.; Chen, X. Highly enhanced cancer immunotherapy by combining nanovaccine with hyaluronidase. *Biomaterials* **2018**, *171*, 198–206. [CrossRef] [PubMed]
116. An, B.; Lin, Y.-S.; Brodsky, B. Collagen interactions: Drug design and delivery. *Adv. Drug Deliv. Rev.* **2016**, *97*, 69–84. [CrossRef] [PubMed]
117. Van den Boorn, J.G.; Dassler, J.; Coch, C.; Schlee, M.; Hartmann, G. Exosomes as nucleic acid nanocarriers. *Adv. Drug Deliv. Rev.* **2013**, *65*, 331–335. [CrossRef] [PubMed]
118. Tian, X.; Zhu, M.; Tian, Y.; Ramm, G.A.; Zhao, Y.; Nie, G. A membrane vesicle-based dual vaccine against melanoma and Lewis lung carcinoma. *Biomaterials* **2012**, *33*, 6147–6154. [CrossRef]
119. Xiong, F.; Ling, X.; Chen, X.; Chen, J.; Tan, J.; Cao, W.; Ge, L.; Ma, M.; Wu, J. Pursuing Specific Chemotherapy of Orthotopic Breast Cancer with Lung Metastasis from Docking Nanoparticles Driven by Bioinspired Exosomes. *Nano Lett.* **2019**, *19*, 3256–3266. [CrossRef]
120. Liu, C.; Xu, X.; Li, B.; Situ, B.; Pan, W.; Hu, Y.; An, T.; Yao, S.; Zheng, L. Single-Exosome-Counting Immunoassays for Cancer Diagnostics. *Nano Lett.* **2018**, *18*, 4226–4232. [CrossRef]
121. Lewis, J.M.; Vyas, A.D.; Qiu, Y.; Messer, K.S.; White, R.; Heller, M.J. Integrated Analysis of Exosomal Protein Biomarkers on Alternating Current Electrokinetic Chips Enables Rapid Detection of Pancreatic Cancer in Patient Blood. *ACS Nano* **2018**, *12*, 3311–3320. [CrossRef]
122. Goos, J.A.C.M.; Cho, A.; Carter, L.M.; Dilling, T.R.; Davydova, M.; Mandleywala, K.; Puttick, S.; Gupta, A.; Price, W.S.; Quinn, J.F.; et al. Delivery of polymeric nanostars for molecular imaging and endoradiotherapy through the enhanced permeability and retention (EPR) effect. *Theranostics* **2020**, *10*, 567–584. [CrossRef]
123. Tee, J.K.; Yip, L.X.; Tan, E.S.; Santitewagun, S.; Prasath, A.; Ke, P.C.; Ho, H.K.; Leong, D.T. Nanoparticles' interactions with vasculature in diseases. *Chem. Soc. Rev.* **2019**, *48*, 5381–5407. [CrossRef]
124. Kinoshita, R.; Ishima, Y.; Chuang, V.T.G.; Nakamura, H.; Fang, J.; Watanabe, H.; Shimizu, T.; Okuhira, K.; Ishida, T.; Maeda, H.; et al. Improved anticancer effects of albumin-bound paclitaxel nanoparticle via augmentation of EPR effect and albumin-protein interactions using S-nitrosated human serum albumin dimer. *Biomaterials* **2017**, *140*, 162–169. [CrossRef] [PubMed]
125. Kwon, S.; Ko, H.; You, D.G.; Kataoka, K.; Park, J.H. Nanomedicines for Reactive Oxygen Species Mediated Approach: An Emerging Paradigm for Cancer Treatment. *Acc. Chem. Res.* **2019**, *52*, 1771–1782. [CrossRef] [PubMed]
126. Goel, S.; Chen, F.; Hong, H.; Valdovinos, H.F.; Hernandez, R.; Shi, S.; Barnhart, T.E.; Cai, W. VEGF$_{121}$-conjugated mesoporous silica nanoparticle: A tumor targeted drug delivery system. *ACS Appl. Mater. Interfaces* **2014**, *6*, 21677–21685. [CrossRef] [PubMed]
127. Graf, N.; Bielenberg, D.R.; Kolishetti, N.; Muus, C.; Banyard, J.; Farokhzad, O.C.; Lippard, S.J. α(V)β(3) integrin-targeted PLGA-PEG nanoparticles for enhanced anti-tumor efficacy of a Pt(IV) prodrug. *ACS Nano* **2012**, *6*, 4530–4539. [CrossRef]
128. Li, Y.; Zeng, S.; Hao, J. Non-Invasive Optical Guided Tumor Metastasis/Vessel Imaging by Using Lanthanide Nanoprobe with Enhanced Down-Shifting Emission beyond 1500 nm. *ACS Nano* **2019**, *13*, 248–259. [CrossRef] [PubMed]
129. Cecchini, A.; Raffa, V.; Canfarotta, F.; Signore, G.; Piletsky, S.; MacDonald, M.P.; Cuschieri, A. In Vivo Recognition of Human Vascular Endothelial Growth Factor by Molecularly Imprinted Polymers. *Nano Lett.* **2017**, *17*, 2307–2312. [CrossRef]

130. Li, M.; Gao, Y.; Yuan, Y.; Wu, Y.; Song, Z.; Tang, B.Z.; Liu, B.; Zheng, Q.C. One-Step Formulation of Targeted Aggregation-Induced Emission Dots for Image-Guided Photodynamic Therapy of Cholangiocarcinoma. *ACS Nano* **2017**, *11*, 3922–3932. [CrossRef] [PubMed]
131. An, J.; Zhang, K.; Wang, B.; Wu, S.; Wang, Y.; Zhang, H.; Zhang, Z.; Liu, J.; Shi, J. Nanoenabled Disruption of Multiple Barriers in Antigen Cross-Presentation of Dendritic Cells Calcium Interference for Enhanced Chemo-Immunotherapy. *ACS Nano* **2020**, *14*, 7639–7650. [CrossRef]
132. Nie, W.; Wu, G.; Zhang, J.; Huang, L.-L.; Ding, J.; Jiang, A.; Zhang, Y.; Liu, Y.; Li, J.; Pu, K.; et al. Responsive Exosome Nano-bioconjugates for Synergistic Cancer Therapy. *Angew. Chem. Int. Ed. Engl.* **2020**, *59*, 2018–2022. [CrossRef] [PubMed]
133. Rey, S.; Schito, L.; Koritzinsky, M.; Wouters, B.G. Molecular targeting of hypoxia in radiotherapy. *Adv. Drug. Deliv. Rev.* **2017**, *109*, 45–62. [CrossRef] [PubMed]
134. Liu, Y.; Jiang, Y.; Zhang, M.; Tang, Z.; He, M.; Bu, W. Modulating Hypoxia via Nanomaterials Chemistry for Efficient Treatment of Solid Tumors. *Acc. Chem. Res.* **2018**, *51*, 2502–2511. [CrossRef]
135. Tang, W.; Zhen, Z.; Wang, M.; Wang, H.; Chuang, Y.-J.; Zhang, W.; Wang, G.D.; Todd, T.; Cowger, T.; Chen, H.; et al. Red Blood Cell-Facilitated Photodynamic Therapy for Cancer Treatment. *Adv. Funct. Mater.* **2016**, *26*, 1757–1768. [CrossRef] [PubMed]
136. Gao, M.; Liang, C.; Song, X.; Chen, Q.; Jin, Q.; Wang, C.; Liu, Z. Erythrocyte-Membrane-Enveloped Perfluorocarbon as Nanoscale Artificial Red Blood Cells to Relieve Tumor Hypoxia and Enhance Cancer Radiotherapy. *Adv. Mater.* **2017**, *29*, 10. [CrossRef]
137. Dong, Z.; Yang, Z.; Hao, Y.; Feng, L. Fabrication of HO-driven nanoreactors for innovative cancer treatments. *Nanoscale* **2019**, *11*, 16164–16186. [CrossRef]
138. Meng, L.; Cheng, Y.; Tong, X.; Gan, S.; Ding, Y.; Zhang, Y.; Wang, C.; Xu, L.; Zhu, Y.; Wu, J.; et al. Tumor Oxygenation and Hypoxia Inducible Factor-1 Functional Inhibition via a Reactive Oxygen Species Responsive Nanoplatform for Enhancing Radiation Therapy and Abscopal Effects. *ACS Nano* **2018**, *12*, 8308–8322. [CrossRef]
139. Hu, X.; Xu, Z.; Hu, J.; Dong, C.; Lu, Y.; Wu, X.; Wumaier, M.; Yao, T.; Shi, S. A redox-activated theranostic nanoplatform: Toward glutathione-response imaging guided enhanced-photodynamic therapy. *Inorg. Chem. Front.* **2019**, *6*, 2865–2872. [CrossRef]
140. Hu, X.; Lu, Y.; Shi, X.; Yao, T.; Dong, C.; Shi, S. Integrating in situ formation of nanozymes with mesoporous polydopamine for combined chemo, photothermal and hypoxia-overcoming photodynamic therapy. *Chem. Commun.* **2019**, *55*, 14785–14788. [CrossRef] [PubMed]
141. Yin, W.; Qiang, M.; Ke, W.; Han, Y.; Mukerabigwi, J.F.; Ge, Z. Hypoxia-responsive block copolymer radiosensitizers as anticancer drug nanocarriers for enhanced chemoradiotherapy of bulky solid tumors. *Biomaterials* **2018**, *181*, 360–371. [CrossRef]
142. Shao, Y.; Liu, B.; Di, Z.; Zhang, G.; Sun, L.-D.; Li, L.; Yan, C.-H. Engineering of Upconverted Metal–Organic Frameworks for Near-Infrared Light-Triggered Combinational Photodynamic/Chemo-/Immunotherapy against Hypoxic Tumors. *J. Am. Chem. Soc.* **2020**, *142*, 3939–3946. [CrossRef] [PubMed]
143. Li, S.Y.; Cheng, H.; Xie, B.R.; Qiu, W.X.; Zeng, J.Y.; Li, C.X.; Wan, S.S.; Zhang, L.; Liu, W.L.; Zhang, X.Z. Cancer Cell Membrane Camouflaged Cascade Bioreactor for Cancer Targeted Starvation and Photodynamic Therapy. *ACS Nano* **2017**, *11*, 7006–7018. [CrossRef]
144. Yu, Z.; Zhou, P.; Pan, W.; Li, N.; Tang, B. A biomimetic nanoreactor for synergistic chemiexcited photodynamic therapy and starvation therapy against tumor metastasis. *Nat. Commun.* **2018**, *9*, 5044. [CrossRef]
145. de Souza, A.L.R.; Marra, K.; Gunn, J.; Samkoe, K.S.; Kanick, S.C.; Davis, S.C.; Chapman, M.S.; Maytin, E.V.; Hasan, T.; Pogue, B.W. Comparing desferrioxamine and light fractionation enhancement of ALA-PpIX photodynamic therapy in skin cancer. *Br. J. Cancer* **2016**, *115*, 805–813. [CrossRef] [PubMed]
146. Lv, Z.; Wei, H.; Li, Q.; Su, X.; Liu, S.; Zhang, K.Y.; Lv, W.; Zhao, Q.; Li, X.; Huang, W. Achieving efficient photodynamic therapy under both normoxia and hypoxia using cyclometalated Ru(ii) photosensitizer through type I photochemical process. *Chem. Sci.* **2018**, *9*, 502–512. [CrossRef]
147. Yu, J.; Zhao, F.; Gao, W.; Yang, X.; Ju, Y.; Zhao, L.; Guo, W.; Xie, J.; Liang, X.-J.; Tao, X.; et al. Magnetic Reactive Oxygen Species Nanoreactor for Switchable Magnetic Resonance Imaging Guided Cancer Therapy Based on pH-Sensitive FeC@FeO Nanoparticles. *ACS Nano* **2019**, *13*, 10002–10014. [CrossRef]
148. Gu, Z.; Zhu, S.; Yan, L.; Zhao, F.; Zhao, Y. Graphene-Based Smart Platforms for Combined Cancer Therapy. *Adv. Mater.* **2019**, *31*, e1800662. [CrossRef]
149. Poinard, B.; Neo, S.Z.Y.; Yeo, E.L.L.; Heng, H.P.S.; Neoh, K.G.; Kah, J.C.Y. Polydopamine Nanoparticles Enhance Drug Release for Combined Photodynamic and Photothermal Therapy. *ACS Appl. Mater. Interfaces* **2018**, *10*, 21125–21136. [CrossRef] [PubMed]
150. Li, W.; Yang, J.; Luo, L.; Jiang, M.; Qin, B.; Yin, H.; Zhu, C.; Yuan, X.; Zhang, J.; Luo, Z.; et al. Targeting photodynamic and photothermal therapy to the endoplasmic reticulum enhances immunogenic cancer cell death. *Nat. Commun.* **2019**, *10*, 3349. [CrossRef]
151. Kanamala, M.; Wilson, W.R.; Yang, M.; Palmer, B.D.; Wu, Z. Mechanisms and biomaterials in pH-responsive tumour targeted drug delivery: A review. *Biomaterials* **2016**, *85*, 152–167. [CrossRef]
152. Nie, W.; Wei, W.; Zuo, L.; Lv, C.; Zhang, F.; Lu, G.-H.; Li, F.; Wu, G.; Huang, L.L.; Xi, X.; et al. Magnetic Nanoclusters Armed with Responsive PD-1 Antibody Synergistically Improved Adoptive T-Cell Therapy for Solid Tumors. *ACS Nano* **2019**, *13*, 1469–1478. [CrossRef]
153. Chen, X.; Chen, T.; Ren, L.; Chen, G.; Gao, X.; Li, G.; Zhu, X. Triplex DNA Nanoswitch for pH-Sensitive Release of Multiple Cancer Drugs. *ACS Nano* **2019**, *13*, 7333–7344. [CrossRef] [PubMed]

154. Liu, G.; Zhao, X.; Zhang, Y.; Xu, J.; Xu, J.; Li, Y.; Min, H.; Shi, J.; Zhao, Y.; Wei, J.; et al. Engineering Biomimetic Platesomes for pH-Responsive Drug Delivery and Enhanced Antitumor Activity. *Adv. Mater.* **2019**, *31*, e1900795. [CrossRef] [PubMed]
155. Ding, D.; Wang, J.; Zhu, Z.; Li, R.; Wu, W.; Liu, B.; Jiang, X. Tumor accumulation, penetration, and antitumor response of cisplatin-loaded gelatin/poly(acrylic acid) nanoparticles. *ACS Appl. Mater. Interfaces* **2012**, *4*, 1838–1846. [CrossRef] [PubMed]
156. Dong, Z.; Feng, L.; Hao, Y.; Chen, M.; Gao, M.; Chao, Y.; Zhao, H.; Zhu, W.; Liu, J.; Liang, C.; et al. Synthesis of Hollow Biomineralized CaCO-Polydopamine Nanoparticles for Multimodal Imaging-Guided Cancer Photodynamic Therapy with Reduced Skin Photosensitivity. *J. Am. Chem. Soc.* **2018**, *140*, 2165–2178. [CrossRef]
157. Wei, R.; Gong, X.; Lin, H.; Zhang, K.; Li, A.; Liu, K.; Shan, H.; Chen, X.; Gao, J. Versatile Octapod-Shaped Hollow Porous Manganese(II) Oxide Nanoplatform for Real-Time Visualization of Cargo Delivery. *Nano Lett.* **2019**, *19*, 5394–5402. [CrossRef] [PubMed]
158. Das, D.K.; Bulow, U.; Diehl, W.E.; Durham, N.D.; Senjobe, F.; Chandran, K.; Luban, J.; Munro, J.B. Conformational changes in the Ebola virus membrane fusion machine induced by pH, Ca2+, and receptor binding. *PLoS Biol.* **2020**, *18*, e3000626. [CrossRef]
159. Ma, T.; Hou, Y.; Zeng, J.; Liu, C.; Zhang, P.; Jing, L.; Shangguan, D.; Gao, M. Dual-Ratiometric Target-Triggered Fluorescent Probe for Simultaneous Quantitative Visualization of Tumor Microenvironment Protease Activity and pH in Vivo. *J. Am. Chem. Soc.* **2018**, *140*, 211–218. [CrossRef] [PubMed]
160. Mai, B.T.; Fernandes, S.; Balakrishnan, P.B.; Pellegrino, T. Nanosystems Based on Magnetic Nanoparticles and Thermo- or pH-Responsive Polymers: An Update and Future Perspectives. *Acc. Chem. Res.* **2018**, *51*, 999–1013. [CrossRef]
161. Jiang, Z.; Wang, Y.; Sun, L.; Yuan, B.; Tian, Y.; Xiang, L.; Li, Y.; Li, Y.; Li, J.; Wu, A. Dual ATP and pH responsive ZIF-90 nanosystem with favorable biocompatibility and facile post-modification improves therapeutic outcomes of triple negative breast cancer in vivo. *Biomaterials* **2019**, *197*, 41–50. [CrossRef]
162. Wang, Y.; Shang, X.; Liu, J.; Guo, Y. ATP mediated rolling circle amplification and opening DNA-gate for drug delivery to cell. *Talanta* **2018**, *176*, 652–658. [CrossRef] [PubMed]
163. Yuan, Y.; Du, C.; Sun, C.; Zhu, J.; Wu, S.; Zhang, Y.; Ji, T.; Lei, J.; Yang, Y.; Gao, N.; et al. Chaperonin-GroEL as a Smart Hydrophobic Drug Delivery and Tumor Targeting Molecular Machine for Tumor Therapy. *Nano Lett.* **2018**, *18*, 921–928. [CrossRef] [PubMed]
164. Xiao, J.; Zhang, G.; Xu, R.; Chen, H.; Wang, H.; Tian, G.; Wang, B.; Yang, C.; Bai, G.; Zhang, Z.; et al. A pH-responsive platform combining chemodynamic therapy with limotherapy for simultaneous bioimaging and synergistic cancer therapy. *Biomaterials* **2019**, *216*, 119254. [CrossRef] [PubMed]
165. Su, L.; Li, R.; Khan, S.; Clanton, R.; Zhang, F.; Lin, Y.-N.; Song, Y.; Wang, H.; Fan, J.; Hernandez, S.; et al. Chemical Design of Both a Glutathione-Sensitive Dimeric Drug Guest and a Glucose-Derived Nanocarrier Host to Achieve Enhanced Osteosarcoma Lung Metastatic Anticancer Selectivity. *J. Am. Chem. Soc.* **2018**, *140*, 1438–1446. [CrossRef]
166. Hu, Y.; Lv, T.; Ma, Y.; Xu, J.; Zhang, Y.; Hou, Y.; Huang, Z.; Ding, Y. Nanoscale Coordination Polymers for Synergistic NO and Chemodynamic Therapy of Liver Cancer. *Nano Lett.* **2019**, *19*, 2731–2738. [CrossRef] [PubMed]
167. Lin, F.; Wen, D.; Wang, X.; Mahato, R.I. Dual responsive micelles capable of modulating miRNA-34a to combat taxane resistance in prostate cancer. *Biomaterials* **2019**, *192*, 95–108. [CrossRef] [PubMed]
168. Ling, X.; Tu, J.; Wang, J.; Shajii, A.; Kong, N.; Feng, C.; Zhang, Y.; Yu, M.; Xie, T.; Bharwani, Z.; et al. Glutathione-Responsive Prodrug Nanoparticles for Effective Drug Delivery and Cancer Therapy. *ACS Nano* **2019**, *13*, 357–370. [CrossRef]
169. Dong, X.; Liu, H.-J.; Feng, H.-Y.; Yang, S.-C.; Liu, X.-L.; Lai, X.; Lu, Q.; Lovell, J.F.; Chen, H.-Z.; Fang, C. Enhanced Drug Delivery by Nanoscale Integration of a Nitric Oxide Donor to Induce Tumor Collagen Depletion. *Nano Lett.* **2019**, *19*, 997–1008. [CrossRef]
170. Liu, J.; Chen, Z.; Wang, J.; Li, R.; Li, T.; Chang, M.; Yan, F.; Wang, Y. Encapsulation of Curcumin Nanoparticles with MMP9-Responsive and Thermos-Sensitive Hydrogel Improves Diabetic Wound Healing. *ACS Appl. Mater. Interfaces* **2018**, *10*, 16315–16326. [CrossRef]
171. Huang, A.; Honda, Y.; Li, P.; Tanaka, T.; Baba, S. Integration of Epigallocatechin Gallate in Gelatin Sponges Attenuates Matrix Metalloproteinase-Dependent Degradation and Increases Bone Formation. *Int. J. Mol. Sci.* **2019**, *20*, 6042. [CrossRef]
172. Qin, S.-Y.; Feng, J.; Rong, L.; Jia, H.-Z.; Chen, S.; Liu, X.-J.; Luo, G.-F.; Zhuo, R.-X.; Zhang, X.-Z. Theranostic GO-based nanohybrid for tumor induced imaging and potential combinational tumor therapy. *Small* **2014**, *10*, 599–608. [CrossRef] [PubMed]
173. Wang, M.; Wang, D.; Chen, Q.; Li, C.; Li, Z.; Lin, J. Recent Advances in Glucose-Oxidase-Based Nanocomposites for Tumor Therapy. *Small* **2019**, *15*, e1903895. [CrossRef]
174. Chang, M.; Wang, M.; Wang, M.; Shu, M.; Ding, B.; Li, C.; Pang, M.; Cui, S.; Hou, Z.; Lin, J. A Multifunctional Cascade Bioreactor Based on Hollow-Structured Cu MoS for Synergetic Cancer Chemo-Dynamic Therapy/Starvation Therapy/Phototherapy/Immunotherapy with Remarkably Enhanced Efficacy. *Adv. Mater.* **2019**, *31*, e1905271. [CrossRef]
175. Zhang, X.; Xi, Z.; Machuki, J.O.a.; Luo, J.; Yang, D.; Li, J.; Cai, W.; Yang, Y.; Zhang, L.; Tian, J.; et al. Gold Cube-in-Cube Based Oxygen Nanogenerator: A Theranostic Nanoplatform for Modulating Tumor Microenvironment for Precise Chemo-Phototherapy and Multimodal Imaging. *ACS Nano* **2019**, *13*, 5306–5325. [CrossRef] [PubMed]
176. Lan, G.; Ni, K.; You, E.; Wang, M.; Culbert, A.; Jiang, X.; Lin, W. Multifunctional Nanoscale Metal-Organic Layers for Ratiometric pH and Oxygen Sensing. *J. Am. Chem. Soc.* **2019**, *141*, 18964–18969. [CrossRef] [PubMed]
177. Lin, Y.; Yang, Y.; Yan, J.; Chen, J.; Cao, J.; Pu, Y.; Li, L.; He, B. Redox/ATP switchable theranostic nanoparticles for real-time fluorescence monitoring of doxorubicin delivery. *J. Mater. Chem. B* **2018**, *6*, 2089–2103. [CrossRef]

MDPI
St. Alban-Anlage 66
4052 Basel
Switzerland
Tel. +41 61 683 77 34
Fax +41 61 302 89 18
www.mdpi.com

Molecules Editorial Office
E-mail: molecules@mdpi.com
www.mdpi.com/journal/molecules

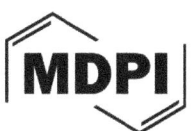

www.ingramcontent.com/pod-product-compliance
Lightning Source LLC
LaVergne TN
LVHW070452100526
838202LV00014B/1712